TEXTBOOK OF
OPERATIVE DENTISTRY

SECOND EDITION

Lloyd Baum, D.M.D., M.S.

Loma Linda University
School of Dentistry
Loma Linda, California

Ralph W. Phillips, M.S., D.Sc.

Associate Dean for Research and
Research Professor of Dental Materials
Indiana University School of Dentistry
Indianapolis, Indiana

Melvin R. Lund, D.M.D., M.S.

Professor and Chairman
Operative Dentistry
Indiana University School of Dentistry
Indianapolis, Indiana

W. B. Saunders Company

PHILADELPHIA □ LONDON □ TORONTO
MEXICO CITY □ RIO DE JANEIRO □ SYDNEY □ TOKYO

W. B. SAUNDERS COMPANY
Harcourt Brace Jovanovich, Inc.

The Curtis Center
Independence Square West
Philadelphia, PA 19106

Library of Congress Cataloging in Publication Data

Baum, Lloyd.

Textbook of operative dentistry.

Includes index.

1. Dentistry, Operative.   I. Phillips, Ralph W.
II. Lund, Melvin R., 1922–   .III. Title. [DNLM:
1. Dentistry, Operative. WU 300 B347t]

RK501.B34   617.6′059   84–20216

ISBN 0–7216–1432–9

Listed here is the latest translated edition of this book together with the language of the translation and the publisher.

Spanish (2nd Edition)—Nueva Editorial Interamericana, Mexico City, Mexico

Textbook of Operative Dentistry   ISBN 0–7216–1432–9

Last digit is the print number: 9   8   7   6   5   4

PREFACE

Traditionally the discipline of operative dentistry has measured its changes or progress in very small increments. In many ways that is still true as there are natural limitations imposed by the environment of the human dentition as we proceed to correct defects in enamel, dentin, and cementum.

The accumulated data and clinical experience of many years bring us to the present state of the art in operative dentistry. This is reflected in a continual barrage of accumulating information regarding the equipment, materials, and technology for restorative dentistry.

It was indicated in the first edition that G. V. Black was deserving of credit for providing a secure beginning of our discipline. His influence is deservedly felt in teaching programs of the present time because of his example in research and academics.

Following him have been many and varied voices and role models, all of which have been important to operative dentistry. It would be fitting to identify these contributors but also impractical as many deserving names would be omitted. These contributors have provided continuity and enrichment to the capabilities and techniques that are essential for success in treatment. The efforts of these highly motivated individuals have provided constructive changes; some are quite subtle and many are obvious. The results of all this activity are most readily apparent during recent years. It has been the good fortune of the authors to personally observe and to participate in these interesting developments.

It is of value to consider these dedicated contributors and the results of their labor for a sense of background and history. It is important for those in the current generation to have an awareness of the accumulated influence that prevails because of the dedication of these pioneers. If our heritage were more fully understood, it could help in the utilization and interpretation of the treatment options that are available.

It is commendable that much of our profession wishes to be in harmony with the times, and this book is dedicated to being helpful in staying abreast of the current state of the art. However, it is well to also consider conservative attitudes as well as conservative preparations. There are many materials and techniques that are effectively promoted as being new. Certainly this is an important consideration but it is also pertinent to evaluate and compare these options with those that preceded. Therefore, this edition maintains features that have a proven track record and that should not be discarded solely because of age. Only when the new concept has a sound foundation based on clinical experience is it included.

When the first edition of this text was published it was apparent that fine tuning would be of value. This has now been accomplished throughout this revision, which continues to emphasize the importance of knowledge of preventive measures and the need to be careful when operating in terms of the patient and the biologic considerations of the tissue being treated. It also reaffirms the importance of isolating the teeth during treatment and the proper use of instrumentation, both rotary and hand.

Beyond this there are some major revisions that are timely. For example, the effort to stay abreast of composite resins now reflects current techniques, including visible light application. The new perspective includes a classification of resin systems such as microfilled, hybrid, and so on, which helps provide an easily understood way of looking at these materials to determine selection and usage. Ancillary phases are the treatment of the eroded area, efficacy of acid etching, and causes for success and failure.

The chapters on amalgam have been reworked to better explain the various types of high copper alloys. They also discuss the delicate and controversial matter of mercury toxicity.

Several new cementing agents have been introduced, and particular emphasis is placed upon the glass ionomer system. Its unique characteristics and usage are explained in detail.

Patients are bringing to the dental office increased concerns regarding dental cosmetics. As a result the practitioner needs to provide answers to these concerns, and reference to this issue occurs frequently throughout the text.

As stated in the first edition, this book is not intended to function as a laboratory manual or to provide in-depth explanation of the many techniques available to operative dentistry but it does focus on a pragmatic approach to treatment. It does not carry bibliographic references to pertinent literature and research findings, which contrasts it with a conventionally referenced text. However, all material presented is consistent with modern research findings.

In summary, the nature of operative dentistry has changed greatly in the past few years and those changes have occurred through an altered pattern of dental disease and through new materials and methodology. This text recognizes these changes and affords a scientific and practical treatment of the subject.

It is hoped that this text will be helpful to the teachers of operative dentistry as they use it to augment their individual courses.

ACKNOWLEDGEMENTS

We are indeed grateful to so many of our colleagues for the direct assistance they have provided as we have prepared this second edition. It is of interest to note that all of us hold a common bond of membership in the Academy of Operative Dentistry. Also, we appreciate the many fine and constructive comments we received from teaching colleagues following the first edition, most of which have now been incorporated in the new edition. The numerous illustrations that have been provided by these friends are duly recognized in the text.

The artwork is a vital segment of this text and we again appreciate the artistic efforts of Dr. Michael Cochran from the Operative Department at Indiana University. In like manner the Dental Illustrations Department at Loma Linda University School of Dentistry, including Ellis Jones, Elwyn Spaulding, and Robert Knabenbauer, has provided effective support. Also helpful in providing photographs were Richard Scott, Michael Halloran, and Alana Fears of the Dental Illustrations Department at Indiana University School of Dentistry.

Likewise, the support of our respective dental school administrations is very important to the success of such a project and is gratefully acknowledged.

We gave been fortunate to have worked with many talented and dedicated colleagues in the teaching of operative dentistry. They willingly provided valuable advice and support; a listing of their names is inadequate but is the best we can do. Currently the operative faculty at Indiana includes William Brackett, Timothy Carlson, Michael Cochran, Ronald Harris, Norris Richmond, and Drexel Boyd. The graduate students of operative dentistry at Indiana continued to make helpful contributions.

We appreciate the fine secretarial help in the typing of the manuscript by Cindy Corbin and Sondra Harvey at Indiana and Kalene Sims at Loma Linda.

The W. B. Saunders Company once again provided their traditional care and concern for excellence in the final product. In this regard we express appreciation to Laura Tarves for arranging the composition of the book and to Karen O'Keefe for its design. We are indebted to Julie Lawley and Betty Gittens for their efforts in production and to Robert Reinhardt, who as Dental Editor followed the progress of the text and offered helpful advice.

CONTENTS

1

PREVENTION OF DENTAL DISEASE

Maintenance of the body in a state of health is a goal to be sought by any practitioner of the healing arts, and the dentist is no exception. It is a careful and wise dentist who protects the oral health of his patients rather than serving only as a repairman for damaged teeth.

He, the dentist, occupies a rather unique position as a therapist because of the nature of the biologic substances with which he works. Unlike his medical colleagues, he deals primarily with tissue that is hard and has no ability to repair itself. Moreover, therapy consists largely of applying a potion, prescribing a drug, or utilizing medications, whereas the dentist's aids are drills, instruments, and filling materials. Surgical procedures performed upon soft tissues depend on normal healing processes, but the dentist has little expectation that a tooth will regrow its missing part following decay removal. Any effective therapeutic measure the dentist initiates must replace the missing part in metal, plastic, or ceramic material. In contrast to the orthopedic surgeon, who also deals with hard bony substances, the dentist cannot cover up the teeth he treats with soft tissues and skin to protect them from a hostile environment.

In performing his health service, the operative dentist (1) prevents or arrests the disease process and (2) restores the missing part. Frequently both objectives are met by the placement of a simple filling (restoration). Often, however, the disease process can be arrested *without* restoring the tooth. In analyzing the dental problem one must differentiate between these two objectives! It is perhaps in relation to the former, the control of disease-causing factors, that the preventive aspects of dental care take on their greatest significance. It does no good to place fine restorations in an environment that will destroy them in a short period of time. Only by simultaneous acts of prevention and restoration can a true health service be rendered.

Control Measures

Dental diseases, like other diseases of the body, are congenital, degenerative, or infectious in nature. Although congenital and degenerative factors require some concern, major attention along preventive lines must be given to infectious processes and action from microbial agents.

By definition, an infectious disease is the invasion of the body by pathogenic organisms. Although not an invasion of the body in the classic

1

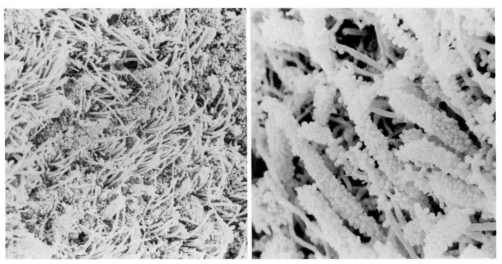

Figure 1–1. Scanning electron microscopic pictures of dental plaque. (Courtesy of Dr. Sheila Jones. Apex 5:93–98, 1971)

sense, a quasi-infectious process takes place when colonies of organisms attach themselves to the teeth (Fig. 1–1). As they grow, these organisms subject the tooth to decalcifying actions, with subsequent destruction and cavitation. Microbial growths on the teeth are known as "plaque." Although it can be removed and tooth surfaces cleansed, plaque will soon reform with new growth, and the destructive process will continue.

It is not the intention of this chapter to discuss the etiology of dental caries or theories of plaque formation. This will be left to other disciplines, where the matter is dealt with in greater detail.

Infectious processes and the relative success achieved in preventing them are dependent upon the pathogenic power of the organism against the resistance of the host (patient). With regard to the host's resistance, one should keep in mind that the tooth is a viable living structure, not a hard piece of inert material. It is a composite structure, consisting of mineral salts blended with organic material. Moreover, in a healthy systemic state small amounts of fluid pass from the pulps of the teeth outward through the dentin, gradually seeping through the enamel into the saliva. Thus the tooth must be looked upon, and treated, as a dynamic substance, not a static, inert material.

Caries Prevention

It should be borne in mind that normal healthy enamel and dentin are largely dependent upon good nutrition during the long formative years of early childhood when the tooth is being developed. Therefore, nutrition as a means of developing host resistance is especially important during the formative years, but it should also be considered in the overall healthy maintenance of the oral tissues throughout life.

Eating proper foods for proper health is only a small part of the role the patient must play in maintaining good teeth and a healthy mouth. His cooperation and assistance are very important in reducing the effect of the microorganisms in the mouth that contribute toward caries. A combined effort on the part of the patient and the dentist can arrest, delay, and eliminate and eliminate many of the carious processes that result in destruction of hard tooth substance. Briefly, the roles of the two might be summarized as follows:

PATIENT

1. Elimination of foods that serve as nutrients for the microorganisms, particularly foods ingested between normal meals.
2. Removal of microbial organisms from the teeth (removal of plaque by brushing, flossing, and so on)
3. Stimulation of circulation of gingival tissues.
4. Use of fluoride-containing dentifrice to make the enamel surface more resistant to caries.
5. Maintenance of good health with the aid of proper nutrition, and so on.

DENTIST

1. Periodic cleansing of the teeth.
2. Application of fluoride to the teeth when indicated.
3. Use of sealants on caries-susceptible areas, especially in pits and fissures, when indicated.
4. Educating, motivating, and assisting the patient in his role of maintenance and care.
5. Repairing early lesions before substantial destruction has occurred.

Dental Examination and Preliminary Treatment

Levels of carious activity are greatest in the early years following tooth eruption and tend to decline with adulthood. The use of fluorides is very important during these years.

It is apparent from the preceding lists that the dentist's role is not as time-consuming as the patient's and that an effective "caries prevention" program is not possible without the patient's cooperation. The wise dentist, therefore, will study his patient to determine whether an active disease process is in progress. Examples of patients with rampant caries are shown in Figures 1–2 and 1–3.

Despite the apparent complexity of dental care, the dentist can usually render an effective patient service if he uses common sense and judgment in

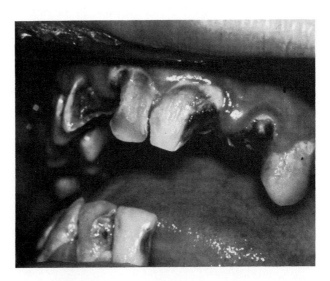

Figure 1–2. Decalcification of gingival enamel. Rapidly advancing caries in a mouth with poor oral hygiene. (Courtesy of Dr. David Krutchkoff)

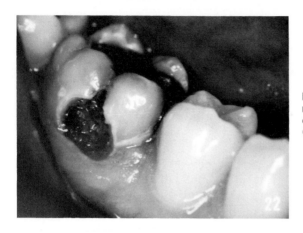

Figure 1–3. Deep carious lesion that has destroyed much of the dentin and enamel on the facial surface of this lower right first molar. (Courtesy of Dr. Eugene Givens)

the application of knowledge already at his disposal. He can determine if the carious process is progressing at a rapid rate by the following observations:

A. *Examination of the Patient with Rampant Caries*

1. The dentin within a cavity will be soft to probing—the result of rapid dissolution and removal of the mineral salts.
2. Enamel surfaces may be covered with diffuse patches of white chalky enamel, showing an attack over a broad front (Fig. 1–4).
3. Dentin within the cavity will be only slightly discolored. Because its surface is being lost at such a rapid rate, it has little opportunity to be stained by coffee, berry juices, and other foods (Fig. 1–5).
4. Teeth in the mouth only a short time (bicuspids of a young teenager) will show evidence of carious lesions.

B. *Examination of the Patient with Slow Caries Activity*

1. The cavities will be dark brown or black in color (see Fig. 1–5). Repeatedly subjected to food stains (e.g., coffee, berries), the dentin absorbs the stains, and its darkness becomes proportional to the long months of exposure. Carious dentin therefore is not identified by its color; it is identified by its texture.
2. The dentin is more dense to probing with a sharp pointed instrument. This is a result of the slow rate of decalcification, as contrasted with rapid decalcification in the acute stage.
3. Fragile crusts of enamel overlying the cavity are more likely to be broken off, whereas intact enamel is more evident in the rapidly developing lesion. Prolonged wear and chewing forces tend to break off the enamel edges, as seen in Figures 1–6 and 1–7.
4. Soft chalky patches of whitish enamel are virtually missing in the older lesion, owing to staining and remineralization of the decalcified areas.

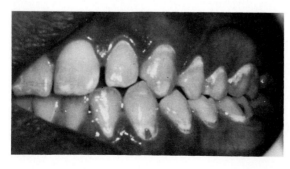

Figure 1–4. Decalcification of gingival enamel. Calcium salts have leached out of the enamel because of the carious activity. Note penetration into dentin of the lower cuspid. (Courtesy of Dr. Ellen Eisenberg)

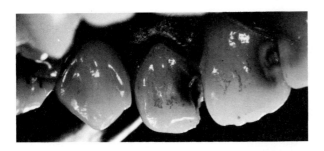

Figure 1–5. Lingual view of two carious lesions. The lesion of the lateral incisor shows more discoloration than the central because it has progressed at a slower rate. The lesion on the central forms a cul-de-sac, which naturally retains debris and microbe activity, whereas the corner on the lateral incisor is missing, allowing a degree of free cleansing. (Courtesy of Dr. Eugene Givens)

C. Initial Treatment of the Caries-Susceptible Patient. Most patients fall within these two extremes, tending to have either rapid or retarded caries activity. Depending upon relative activity of the carious process, one or more of the following treatments should be considered:

1. The soft, diseased dentin should be excavated from the lesions to remove as many microbial agents as possible along with their by-products and other debris.
2. Open cavities within the diseased teeth should be filled with cement dressings to keep out saliva, bacteria, and food particles (such a lesion might be compared to a wound that is cleansed, disinfected, and bandaged; see Chapter 8).
3. Overall microbial activity within the mouth should be reduced by:
   a. modifying the dietary regimen to reduce nutritional components for the microbial colonies (elimination of food and drink rich in carbohydrates and between-meal snacks).
   b. frequent cleansing by brushing and flossing to remove the plaque and microbial colonies from the tooth surfaces.
4. Fluorides should be employed to increase the resistance of enamel to dissolution. This can be accomplished by the application of fluoride in the office, by the home use of aqueous solutions and dentifrices, and by the possible incorporation of fluoride into the drinking water.

Within a few weeks these procedures should provide obvious evidence of caries arrest and control. Nevertheless, the patient should be kept under observation for a period of several months to assure that the disease has been brought under control. As soon as it has been determined that the acute stage of the disease has passed, permanent restorations (e.g., amalgam, gold, composites) can be placed within the teeth without fear of caries recurring adjacent to them.

Although some rapidly advancing and deep lesions need to be treated with a temporary sedative cement, most cavities can be restored at the convenience of the dentist on an appointment basis, and it can be anticipated that the disease will not progress unduly fast.

Figure 1–6. Mouth of a 13 year old boy. Although all the enamel is missing, the underlying black dentin is hard, firm, and insensitive to probing. (Courtesy of Dr. Douglas Foerth)

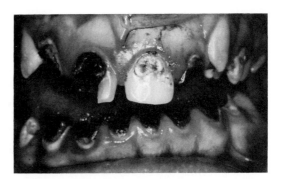

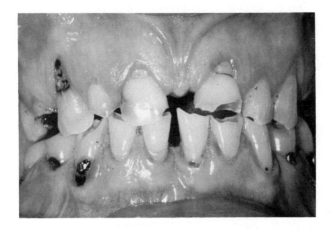

Figure 1–7. Hard tissue pathology of this adult patient is the major area of concern. Restoring the worn anteriors to function and acceptable esthetics is a real challenge. (Courtesy of Captain Richard B. McCoy, U.S.N.)

"Cavities" are not always the result of the carious process. The dentist, in his efforts to protect the patient and prevent additional damage, may discover that a patient's eroded lesions are the result of some obscure cause, such as regurgitated acids from the stomach. Likewise, dissolution of enamel and dentin can occur as a result of dietary habits that permit citrus fruits to have prolonged surface contact with teeth or as a result of abrasive action from incorrect tooth brushing habits.

Dental deterioration may also follow a debilitating disease or a severe emotional disturbance that has had a systemic effect upon the body in general and upon the teeth in particular. Pregnancy in some women often appears to be associated with rampant carious activity. Hormonal changes and other systemic factors combine to modify the oral environment and to lower the ability of the tooth to resist carious activity. When normal systemic activity is restored, the natural tooth defenses become effective again, and the accelerated carious activity is reduced.

The clinician will observe that a time lag of perhaps 6 to 12 months is noted between the onset of systemic change and subsequent manifestations in the teeth. For example, a middle-aged person undergoing a period of extreme

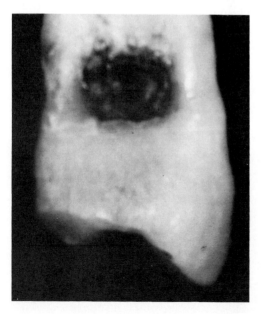

Figure 1–8. Despite the presence of root caries, this premolar was lost because of periodontal disease.

emotional stress in January, during which his health suffers, may not manifest unusual carious activity until October or November of that same year. Similarly, when the period of emotional stress ends and physical health is again restored, several months will pass before the rampant carious activity subsides. During this period of time the treatment should be palliative and involve only the use of temporary restorative materials.

Destructive habit patterns, if present, should be identified and terminated. Although many and varied, the most common habit is the frequent bathing of the teeth with saliva containing nutrient sugar solutions, which serve as food for the microbial colonies. Sucking mints or Life Savers and prolonged sipping of soft drinks or sweetened coffee are but a few of the ways in which nutrients can be supplied to the plaque. Often a smoker endeavoring to "break the habit" resorts to a diversionary habit such as gum chewing or "Coke" sipping, which supplies nutrients to the pathogenic organisms (Fig. 1–8). Improper tooth brushing and flossing habits will severely abrade the teeth, whereas sucking on lemons produces a dissolution of the enamel by the citric acid. Bruxism (clenching or gnashing the teeth) can also be a destructive habit.

Tooth destruction may occur with or without the influence of infectious microbial activity. Occasionally, clinical insight and knowledge from other disciplines is necessary for even the most experienced diagnostician to determine the causes of tooth destruction in some stubborn cases.

A logical question comes to mind, "Is not a tooth with a rapidly developing cavity more painful than a tooth with a slowly developing one?" The answer is "No." Rate of dissolution bears no relationship to pain. A rapidly developing cavity is no more painful than a slowly developing one; indeed, most carious lesions develop asymptomatically, with the development of little or no pain.

Identification of problem areas requiring patient cooperation is only a small part of the problem. Of far greater importance are the human factors that require the patient to exercise self-discipline, to be diligent in plaque removal, and to be careful with his diet. Forgetting to cleanse the mouth after eating is a major problem, as a majority of patients tend to be apathetic or negligent. The dentist must be aware of motivating influences and, insofar as possible, stimulate the patient to be thorough and consistent in the two most important areas, namely, food intake and plaque removal.

Chewable disclosing tablets are also helpful in identifying areas of plaque that have not yet been removed. These tablets stain the plaque a deep red color and provide the patient with a stimulus toward more fastidious brushing habits (Fig. 1–9). Inspection for plaque is recommended before each appointment. If the patient has not been diligent in his efforts to remove plaque, it must be called to his attention and new efforts made to correct this problem.

It is not within the scope of this chapter to describe the training regimen

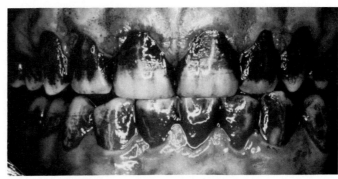

Figure 1–9. Plaque stained with disclosing tablets.

that should be followed or the instructional procedures to be given for flossing and brushing, use of toothpicks, bridge cleaners, and so on.

Pit and Fissure Sealants as a Preventive Measure

In communities where fluoridation is present, reduction in caries may be expected. Because fluoride is effective on smooth surface caries only, the incidence of occlusal caries remains unchanged. Epidemiologic studies show that most molars present in the mouth at 18 years of age will have decay or a restoration on their occlusal surfaces. Pit and fissure sealants are used under the premise that as long as the orifice of a deep fissure remains covered, the carious process is inhibited. The use of sealants is one way to prevent this from occurring and has been recommended at least for the occlusal surfaces of children and adolescents.

Preparation of the teeth for a sealant requires complete isolation of the teeth to be treated, e.g., a rubber dam (see Chapter 9). This is best accomplished with 3% hydrogen peroxide and a pointed-bristle brush on a low-speed rotary handpiece to remove the stain, pellicle, accessible microorganisms, and other debris from the occlusal surface. After proper rinsing and drying, acid etching is employed, as will be discussed in Chapter 10, to prepare the surface to receive the sealant. The surface should be re-rinsed and re-dried. The sealant is applied carefully to minimize the entrapment of bubbles and to insure that no sealant flows into interproximal areas. It is good practice after sealant placement to check the occlusion to determine if an excess of sealant is present that needs to be reduced. When the procedure is completed, there should be a hard resin surface in the grooves.

A major concern with sealants is their ability to remain attached to the enamel and to keep the orifices blocked from entry by microorganisms. If sealants become dislodged, it usually occurs several months after placement and is probably caused by moisture contamination after conditioning the surface. Sealants can be replaced in whole or in part at the discretion of the operator, because new sealant will bond to the old if it has been cleansed properly.

Colored sealants have been recommended for use over transparent types because they can be readily seen by the patients and their parents. Moreover, their presence can readily be identified by the dentist at a recall and examination appointment.

Enamoplasty as a Preventive Measure

As previously mentioned, pit and fissure sealants are one way to prevent microorganisms from entering the fissures and nutrients from becoming available to supply the needs of remaining entrapped bacteria. Instead of covering the fissures with a sealant, enamoplasty results in their removal by grinding them away.

This method has been successfully used and promoted by Dr. Miles Markley for 50 years. Conceptually, the object is to polish out the grooves so they no longer can serve as clefts to harbor organic remnants and microorganisms, which cause carious activity.

Organic remnants that prevent coalescence of the enamel lobes penetrate into the enamel for varying depths, some only a short distance yet others so

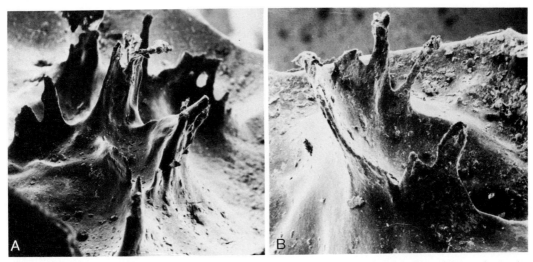

Figure 1–10. Photomicrographs of vinyl resin impressions of the intracoronal morphology of two molar teeth. They show pits arising deep within the crown from the base of the fissures (20 ×). (From Galil, K. A. and Gwinnett, A. J., Three-dimensional replicas of pits and fissures in human teeth. A scanning electron microscope study. Arch. Oral Biol., 20:493–495, 1975)

deep that they virtually penetrate the dento-enamel junction (Fig. 1–10; see also Fig. 2–12). The objective is to polish out the shallow fissures and place small individual restorations in those that are so deep they cannot be polished away (Fig. 1–11). Actually, the grinding and polishing can be carried three quarters of the way through the enamel without any risk to its integrity. The advantage of this method is that the treatment is permanent and needs no examination at a later date for loss of sealant integrity.

The technique for enamoplasty is to use a 330 or 331 pear-shaped bur in the high-speed handpiece. Keeping the bur moving and using tactile sense, the surface is "dished out" as enamel bordering the crevice is removed. Organic remnants can be detected by visual and tactile means. A brown color of the groove is a helpful indicator but does not necessarily indicate a significant cleft in the enamel. Probing with a finely pointed, stiff instrument (Fig. 1–12) is the best method to identify fissure depth (x-rays are of no value).

Figure 1–11. Two alternate preventive methods for treating a developmental fissure along the central groove of an upper molar. Fissure extends approximately 2/3 the distance through the enamel. Lower left: treated by a sealant. Lower right: treated by enamoplasty.

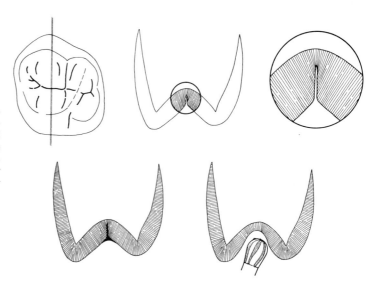

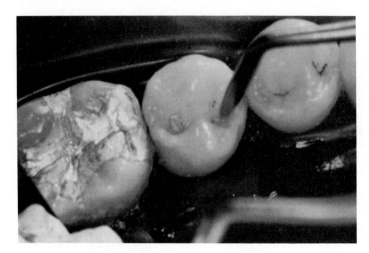

Figure 1–12. Mandibular 2nd premolar treated by enamoplasty. Exploratory enamoplasty with a No. 331 bur reveals only a shallow mesial pit. Rough edges were removed and the area received no other treatment. The distal pit, however, did extend deep into the enamel sufficiently so as to justify making a small cavity preparation, which was restored with amalgam. The sharp, stiff probe ascertains the depth of the pit or fissure much better than an explorer. (Instrument is No. 157–158 manufactured by Suter Dental Mfg. Co., 62 Cedar St., Chico, California 95926)

When the depth of the cleft has been reached, no more reduction is required. If the depth of the cleft continues in a localized spot, approaching the dento-enamel junction, or if perchance actual carious involvement in the dentin has been discovered, a very small pit or groove type cavity is prepared, which in turn is filled and polished.

Molars are particularly indicated for this type of preventive therapy. Most operators agree that a tooth with a proximal lesion, properly prepared, does not require an occlusal extension for anchorage because adequate retention can be obtained within the proximal box. Habitually, however, most proximal lesions are prepared with occlusal extensions because of the presence of developmental occlusal grooves. If these grooves have been "explored" and eliminated, they can be ignored and a slot type of restoration (see Fig. 8–6) placed without fear of occlusal groove caries at a later date. Many operators perform such an exploratory occlusal enamoplasty before preparing a Class II cavity and discover that an occlusal extension is not always necessary. When an occlusal groove, especially a wide groove, is cut across the occlusal surface, the tooth is weakened and may be subject to fracture several years later. This additional effort is considered a small price to pay to avoid unnecessary mutilation of a tooth.

Operative Procedures

Lest one blame only the patient for prevalence of tooth decay and its recurrence around existing restorations, the operative dentist should also direct his attention to restorative procedures per se, which play a very important role in this regard. Far too often, the dentist uses poor judgment in evaluating the defect and in designing its restoration. Designs should be made that obviously take into account the size and shape of the lesion. In addition, however, consideration should be given to congenital defects of the crown, the texture of the enamel at the edges of the lesions, the age of the patient and a prognosis of the patient's ability to care for his mouth, as well as chewing and wear patterns of the tooth in queston.

Many years ago, before the advent of the dental engine, soft carious dentin was removed by a dental instrument, the excavator, which scooped out the soft material of the lesion. Without the aid of local anesthetics, dentists were not expected to cut into sound dentin to anchor a restoration or to terminate the edges of a cavity in sound enamel. It was to be expected that such restorations could be dislodged by chewing forces or subjected to subsequent caries around their edges. It was not until about 1875 that Dr. G. V. Black proposed a rational regimen for "extension for prevention" principles, which made restorations more permanent because they were engineered and designed scientfically. The advent of belt-driven rotary handpieces and electric engines to power them made this new science a practicable modality. In brief, these principles are based on the rule that potentially carious areas should be included within the cavity design, without sacrificing mechanical anchorage for the restoration. Although designs of cavity preparation have changed somewhat in recent years, no significant deviation from these scientific principles has occurred.

The late Dr. Howard R. Raper, who introduced the bite-wing x-ray to the dental profession in 1925, concisely described the role a dentist plays in the prevention of dental disease.*

In the battle for the control of caries there is no substitute, as yet, for the service dentists have to offer. Fractional prevention is certainly not a satisfactory substitute. What does the patient gain if, in a certain tooth otherwise destined to have three cavities, there develop only two? It takes only one cavity to destroy a tooth—unless a dentist comes to the rescue and arrests or cures the disease by filling the tooth.

Take my own personal case for example. Why do I, at the age of 70 odd, still have 26 of my own natural teeth? [Dr. Raper at 88 years still had 26 of his natural teeth.] Is it because I have used any particular brand of medicated toothpaste? No, I have used all kinds of toothpastes and powders, no one kind to the exclusion of others.

Is it because I have always brushed my teeth immediately after eating? No, I have not found it possible to follow this recommended routine.

Is it because I have always consumed a perfectly balanced diet? No, my diet throughout my life has not been one of which dieticians would wholly approve. It has not been either especially good or especially bad.

Is it because I have resisted the impulse to eat sweets? No, I cannot recall ever refusing a piece of candy and demanding a carrot stick.

Is it because I have employed some especially effective brushing technic or a toothbrush guaranteed to "reach the inaccessible areas?" No, my brushing technic has been fair, but nothing to brag about; and I have used all kinds of tooth-brushes—including some with bristles so stiff I had to learn to discriminate against them.

Is it because I drank fluoridated water? No, I have not always had that advantage.

Ah then, you say, it must be because I was blessed with very good teeth by nature. Again the answer is no. It is true that, until recently, I have enjoyed a rather high degree of immunity to periodontal disease; but, looking at the other side of the coin, my susceptibility to caries has been somewhat higher than average.

So I repeat the question: Why do I at my ripe old age still have 26 functionally good teeth? The answer is so simple. It is because, and only because, dentists have saved them for me, by filling the cavities and scaling away the calculus. Had I been denied this service, I would today have no teeth.

With the advent of high-speed handpieces, tungsten carbide burs, and diamond abrading stones, reduction of hard healthy enamel is readily achieved. It is possible, therefore, to overcut when it is not necessary, thereby weakening structural components of the tooth itself (Fig. 1–13). A tooth missing its structural foundation or framework is weakened and likely to fracture (or the restoration is likely to be dislodged) when placed into functional usage. Care must be exercised, therefore, to use judgment in cavity design, lest the restoration actually weaken the tooth and make it more subject

*Paul Barton, *The Prevention of Toothache: One Man [Raper] and His Campaign.* Bulletin, Indiana University, School of Dentistry, 50th Anniversary Edition, Spring Issue. 1975.

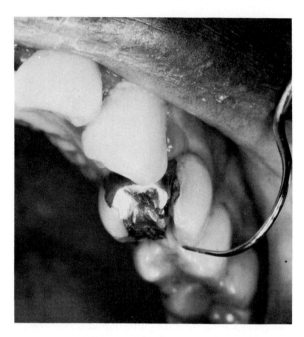

Figure 1–13. Fractured premolar due to weakening of the tooth by an overly deep inlay preparation. The fracture exposed the buccal part of the pulp, and endodontic therapy was required. The fracture extended up the root about 4 mm and required some gingival contouring to obtain an impression for the final crown. Proper tooth preparation could have prevented much discomfort, cost, and effort.

to fracture. Likewise, the cavity must be extended into sound non-susceptible areas where recurrence of the lesion will not take place around the edges. Neither tooth fracture nor dislocation of a restoration is desirable and neither is likely if the operative dentist is exercising true "preventive" concepts as he biomechanically anchors the restorations to the teeth.

Three additional entities within the control of the operative dentist require "preventive" care: the pulp, the gingivae, and the manner in which teeth fit together during closure. If injudicious means are employed in instrumenting the tooth (i.e., dull instruments, heat generation and dehydration, or inadequately insulated fillings), pulps can be insulted or injured, with problems developing at a later date. Improperly contoured restorations may allow fibrous food to lodge between teeth or gouge sensitive gingival tissues.

As he plans his operative procedures, the dentist's attention should be drawn to disharmonies in jaw closure and occlusion of teeth. Improper matching of cusps, ridges, and slopes of the teeth can create occlusal problems—problems that did not occur before the patient had the misfortune to visit the dentist. For example, let us assume that a restoration was placed that was too long, so that the patient could not quite bring his teeth together on closure. Although the restoration would be "high in occlusion," it probably was unrecognized as such by the dentist. A thickness of 15 to 20 micrometers (less than a thousandth of an inch) can usually be detected proprioceptively by a patient. To accommodate himself to the high restoration and assure a comfortable closure pattern, the patient might shift his jaw to one side or the other. Over a period of weeks, months, and years, this abnormal closure pattern, with glancing blows delivered to the teeth, could cause them to migrate to different, inharmoniuous positions. More insidious, with possibly more severe damage, is injury inflicted upon the temporomandibular joint. Many patients have had crippled temporomandibular joints for years, owing to injuries that could be traced back to improperly placed restorations.

It is sad but true that the operative dentist is sometimes guilty of solving one dental problem for a patient only to create new ones for him.

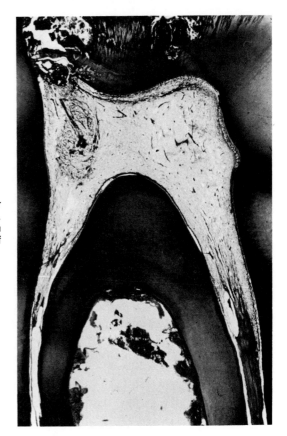

Figure 1–14. Carious pulp exposure of a mandibular molar that could have been prevented by early attention. As is usually the case, the mesial pulp horn, rather than the distal, was penetrated by the lesion. (Courtesy of Dr. David Krutchkoff)

Summary. Prevention consists of plaque control and restricted frequency of refined carbohydrate intake. Self discipline and positive daily habit patterns by the patient are required if these are to be effective. The dentist, on the other hand, can prevent dental problems by early treatment of carious lesions (Fig. 1–14) and optimum fluoride treatment. For children and adolescents, fissure sealants can also be effective as part of a prevention program.

2

CLASSIFICATION OF CAVITIES AND RESTORATIONS

Only in recent years has an edentulous person (one without any teeth) been considered a cripple. Missing teeth have been more or less taken for granted because a large portion of the population was afflicted with tooth loss. In civilized cultures in modern times efforts have been made to retain teeth through operative dentistry and endodontia or to replace them with a prosthodontic appliance. Despite this trend, however, many cultures in the world today, particularly in underdeveloped countries, consider the repair of a tooth a luxury rather than a necessity.

The teeth and the mouth occupy a very important role in the personality of the individual. One needs only to observe the television commercials to appreciate the interest in the teeth and the buying power of the public who are interested in a toothpaste that will "make teeth whiter" or "increase sex appeal."

For similar evidence one needs only to wander among students in an average middle-class high school and count the number of children wearing orthodontic appliances. From the point of view of the parents these orthodontic appliances are placed to improve the child's cosmetic appearance. A missing or broken incisor in the mouth of a teenager or any other major blemish in the appearance of the teeth can create an extreme psychological handicap for

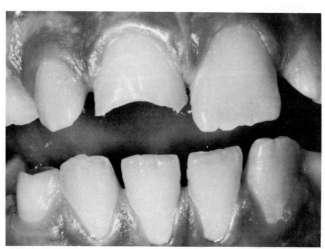

Figure 2–1. Fractured incisor before treatment.

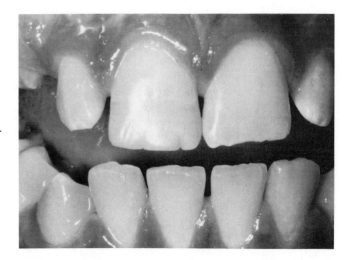

Figure 2–2. Fractured incisor before treatment. (Courtesy of Dr. James Dunn).

the owner as he endeavors to establish his identity among his peers. For this reason the teeth and their appearance can definitely alter the mental health of the individual.

The dentist in his complex role as physician of the mouth, artisan, and mechanic also functions in the role of a psychotherapist. Every dentist has had the experience of treating a withdrawn child for a dental malady, and after correcting an ugly condition has seen the personality of the girl or boy blossom into self-confidence and happiness (Figs. 2–1 and 2–2).

Types of Lesions Involved in Tooth Destruction

Operative dentistry as a discipline does not concern itself with the diseases that occur from missing teeth or the methods by which they are replaced. Operative dentistry relates itself only to the individual tooth, primarily to its treatment and restoration. As a matter of fact, almost all of operative dentistry is related to treatment or control of hard tissue lesions of enamel and dentin, and almost all of the treatment for these lesions is the replacement of missing tooth structure.

Dental Caries. Dental caries is a breakdown or softening of the dentin and enamel. This destructive process progresses more rapidly in dentin than in enamel to create an undermining effect, hence the term "cavity." A layman envisions a tooth as "having a cavity" or "not having a cavity." Such is not actually the case. Disease of hard tooth substance is a relative thing. A lesion or defect in the tooth does not become a "cavity" until its progress has reached the point where surgical intervention is required, usually after the enamel has been penetrated and dentin is involved. Many carious blemishes that have not penetrated the enamel are left untreated, particularly if the process has been aborted.* When the carious process has progressed to the point where penetration of the enamel occurs and the dentin becomes involved, an operative procedure is indicated (Fig. 2–3).

Wear and Abrasion. Abrasive agents can cause destruction in various locations. Wear on the ends of teeth results from their rubbing against each

*Fluoride solutions are often applied as a treatment to remineralize enamel.

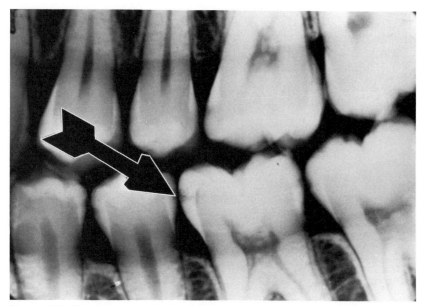

Figure 2–3. Bite-wing x-ray of incipient (early) carious lesions of the posterior teeth. The mesial enamel of the mandibular first molar has been penetrated. (Courtesy of Dr. Wallace W. Johnson)

Figure 2–4. Abrasion of mandibular incisor teeth.

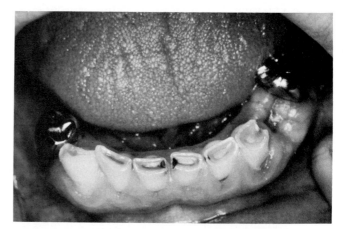

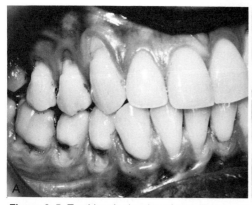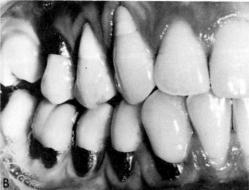

Figure 2–5. Toothbrush abrasion of mandibular and maxillary cervical areas. A, Abrasion was more severe on the left side than the right, an indication of an abnormal pattern of brushing. B, Completed restorations for the right side. Direct gold was used for mandibular restorations. For the sake of esthetics premolar and canine were restored with composite resin. (Courtesy of Dr. David A. Newitter)

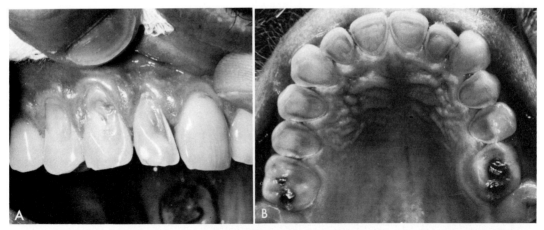

Figure 2–6. Erosion. *A*, Although erosion is very similar to abrasion, close scrutiny can often detect the difference between erosion and abrasion. (Courtesy of Dr. Ellen Eisenberg). *B*, Destruction of the teeth of this 29-year-old patient was caused by gastric acid regurgitaton.

other or from chewing "gritty" food (Fig. 2–4). A classic example is found in the American Indian or Eskimo whose teeth were badly abraded from dietary and cooking habits. Their cooking was done in earthenware bowls into which hot stones were placed to warm and heat the food. Fragments of rocks and sand became mixed with the food and had an abrasive action on the teeth during mastication. Abrasion from incorrect tooth brushing habits is also to be seen as notches on the facial sides of root surfaces (Fig. 2–5).

Bruxism is a common cause of pathologic wear in modern society. Occlusal abnormalities, coupled with nervous tensions, cause a patient to gnash his teeth together. Over a period of several years the occlusal enamel wears away, exposing the softer dentin underneath.

Erosion. Closely related to occlusal wear, but occurring on facial surfaces of the teeth, are gingival lesions. Toothbrush abrasion is manifested as notches in the tooth at the junction of the root and crown. Chemical dissolution is also a frequent cause of tooth breakdown in this region. Like toothbrush abrasion at the gingival, erosion is also manifested as notches in the teeth, but they are of a somewhat different configuration. The exact etiology of much of this erosion is unknown (Figs. 2–5 and 2–6).

Fracture. Injuries of various sorts result in broken teeth (Fig. 2–7). A fracture from an external blow is frequently the cause; however, a molar or a bicuspid may split from only masticatory forces when the individual inadvertently closes down on a hard bony object. Very often these fractures of posterior teeth occur because of previously placed amalgam fillings that leave the remaining tooth structure in a weakened condition. Large pieces of enamel

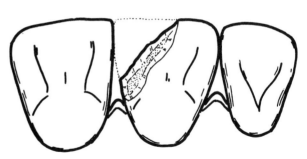

Figure 2–7. Fractured incisor. When an incisal corner is lost by trauma, the usual line of cleavage is as shown.

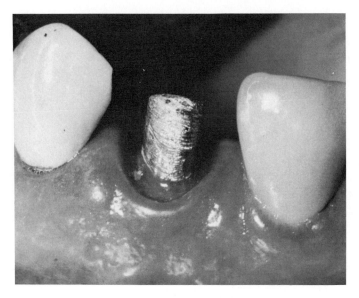

Figure 2–8. Reinforcement of pulpless tooth with a cast gold post and core. The post extends into the canal; the core provides a foundation for a crown. (Courtesy of Dr. Leif Bakland)

Figure 2–9. Two central incisors reinforced with cast gold dowels. After the dowels have been cemented and cut off, two metal-ceramic crowns will be made. Although not always necessary, the insertion of these dowels serves to prevent possible fracture at a later date.

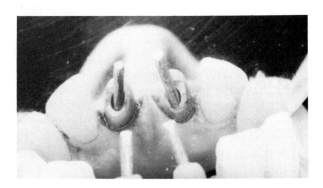

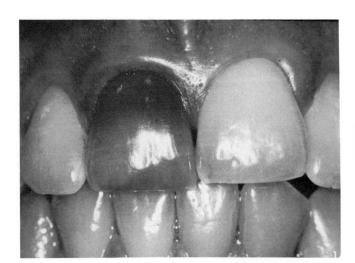

Figure 2–10. Internal staining following pulp death (see Fig. 5–14). (Courtesy of Dr. Leif Bakland)

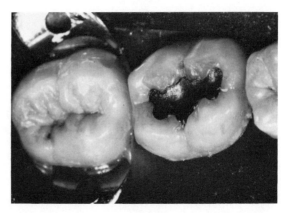

Figure 2–11. Molar with a potential pit and fissure cavity. Diagnosis can be made only after probing with an explorer.

are frequently involved, enough so that some type of crown is required to replace the lost part.

The Endodontically Treated Tooth. Reportedly, endodontically treated teeth contain 9% less fluid than intact teeth in the same mouth. This could explain why vital teeth seem to be more resilient, whereas nonvital teeth are inclined to be more brittle and subject to fracture. Consequently, the roots of nonvital teeth often require reinforcement to prevent fracture (Figs. 2–8 and 2–9) (see Chapter 19).

A tooth with a nonvital pulp is frequently the victim of discoloration. When the enamel of the labial surface is intact but discolored (Fig. 2–10) the tooth may be bleached to restore proper color. When this is not possible, the offending discolored enamel may be ground away and replaced by bonding or in extreme cases by a crown.

ANATOMIC CLASSIFICATION OF CAVITIES

Missing parts of tooth structure can be classified in various ways. One method of classification can be related to the anatomic structure of the tooth

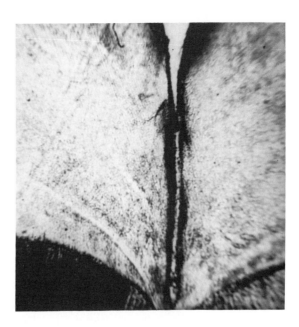

Figure 2–12. Cross-sectional view through a defective developmental fissure. Penetration of this groove closely approached the dento-enamel junction. (Courtesy of Dr. E. E. Kelln)

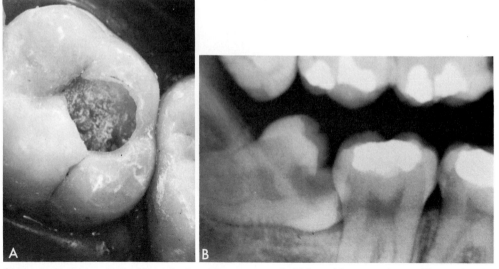

Figure 2–13. Carious lesions through pit and fissure entry. *A*, Oblique ridge area of a maxillary molar. *B*, Impacted mandibular third molar. Except for relatively deep lesions, radiographic examination is not helpful as a diagnostic tool for these lesions.

itself. This method, by and large, is restricted to teeth afflicted by the carious process.

Pit and Fissure Cavity. Where the union of lobes of enamel in the calcification process entraps the organic elements of the enamel-forming organ (Figs. 2–11 and 2–12), a natural pit or thin fin of organic substance separates the lobes. When this organic material is dissolved by enzymatic and bacterial action, a natural passageway into the recesses of the enamel is created. Wherever the depth of penetration is dangerously close to the dentin this natural fissure becomes a miniature culture tube for bacteria. Dissolution of the remaining enamel soon provides a passage into the dentin (Fig. 2–13). Common sites for pit and fissure cavities are shown in Figures 2–14 and 2–15.

Lower incisors and cuspids are seldom afflicted by pit and fissure cavities;

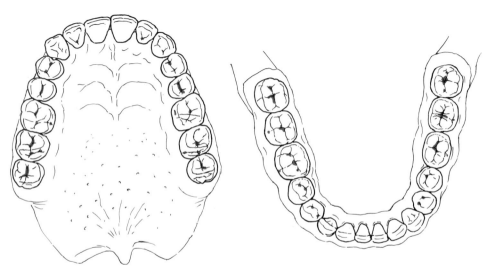

Figure 2–14. Locations where pit and fissure cavities are most likely to be found.

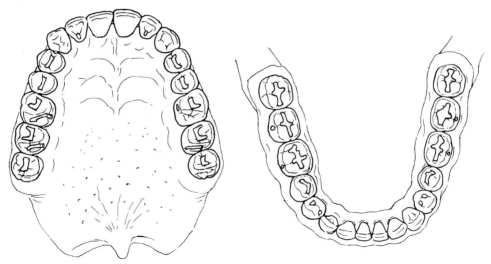

Figure 2–15. Designs of cavities that are located in areas most likely to be congenitally defective.

however, pit and fissure cavities are "where you find them." Aside from the use of sealants, restorative treatment is forthright and direct: namely, the surgical removal of the defective portion and restoration with the proper material.

Smooth Surface Cavity. In contrast to the pit and fissure cavity, the smooth surface cavity is one in which the attacking agent destroys and penetrates the entire thickness of the enamel rather than taking advantage of the preformed penetration provided it by the developmental process. Smooth surface cavities occur on the axial rather than occlusal surface of the crown. Sites of likely occurrence are the buccal and labial surfaces of the teeth, as well as the interproximal regions just below the contact point (Figs. 2–16 to 2–19; see also Fig. 2–3).

Speed of penetration of these cavities through the hard enamel is relatively slow, as compared with that through the softer dentin. Initial evidence of this process is manifested by a whitish area of decalcification on the enamel (see Fig. 1–4). Scraping this surface reveals that the enamel is soft on its outer surface but becomes harder underneath. A smooth surface carious lesion becomes a "cavity," and restoration is indicated only after the carious process has penetrated through the enamel.

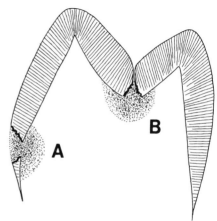

Figure 2–16. Caries penetration through the enamel and into the dentin *(A)* in a smooth surface lesion and *(B)* in an occlusal lesion.

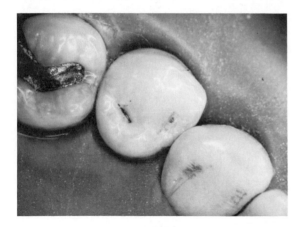

Figure 2–17. Smooth surface cavity on the distal side of lower left first premolar.

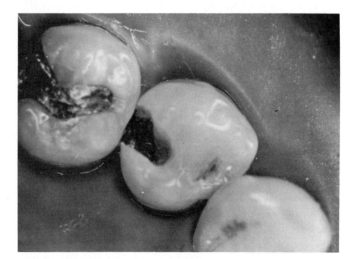

Figure 2–18. Carious dentin exposed by removal of occlusal enamel.

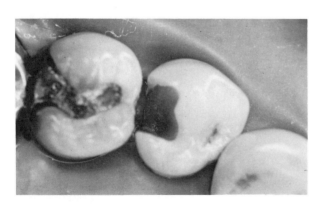

Figure 2–19. Carious dentin removed with excavator, revealing a relatively large cavity (no pulp exposure). (Courtesy of Dr. David A. Newitter)

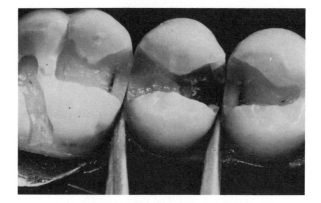

Figure 2–20. Access to proximal lesions is invariably through the marginal ridge. (Courtesy of Dr. Loren Hickey)

Black's Classification

Another method for the classification of lesions is that designed by Dr. G. V. Black about 100 years ago, and it is one that is still widely used today. His classification utilizes the specific location of the common lesions on the teeth as they usually occur. It is as follows:

Class I. Class I lesions occur in pits and fissures of all teeth, but this class is essentially intended for bicuspids and molars. Figures 2–14 and 2–15 illustrate common sites on the teeth where this lesion might occur.

Class II. A cavity occurring on the proximal surface of a *posterior* tooth belongs to a Class II category. A smooth surface cavity or mesial and/or distal

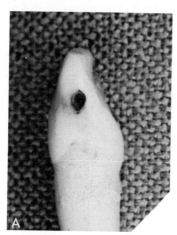

Figure 2–21. Class III lesion. *A,* Small cavity restricted to the proximal surface. *B,* Insofar as possible, access to the lesion is from the lingual. *C,* Extensive lesion, which reaches beyond the proximo-labial line angles of the crown and involves the labial surface.

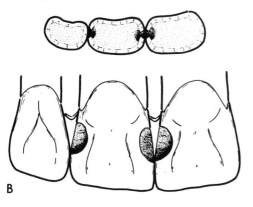

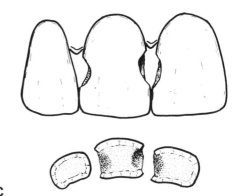

B   C

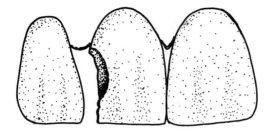

Figure 2–22. One of two types of Class IV cavities. The size of the cavity per se was responsible for loss of this incisal corner.

lesion will usually be below the contact point, where cleanliness is difficult to achieve. By Dr. Black's definition, a Class II lesion can involve both mesial and distal surfaces or only one proximal surface of a tooth and is referred to as an MO, a DO, or an MOD (mesio-occlusal, disto-occlusal, or a mesio-occlusal-distal) cavity.

Because access for repair is from the occlusal (Fig. 2–20), both the side and top of the tooth are restored with a single filling. (See Chapter 11.) By definition, however, the cavity is a proximal lesion and does not necessarily include the occlusal surface. (See Fig. 11–33.)

Class III. As the Class II pertains to posterior teeth, the Class III lesions afflict the *anterior* teeth. By Dr. Black's definition, a Class III cavity may occur on the mesial or distal surface of any incisor or cuspid (Fig. 2–21). Like the Class II, the lesion occurs beneath the contact point, but unlike the molar lesion with its elliptical shape, the Class III is small and quite circular.

Class IV. This cavity is actually an outgrowth of a Class III lesion. Extensive decay or heavy abrasion can weaken an incisal corner and cause it to fracture (Figs. 2–22, 2–23, and 2–24). A Class IV, therefore, as defined by Dr. Black, is a lesion on the proximal surface of an anterior tooth, from which the incisal angle is also missing.

Class V. As indicated earlier, gingival cavities are smooth surface cavities. Regardless of the etiology—caries, abrasion, or erosion— this type of lesion, according to Black's classification, is known as a Class V cavity. By his

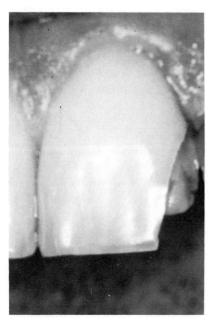

Figure 2–23. A class IV lesion with a defective restoration. The original cause was a large uncontrolled carious lesion that undermined the distoincisal corner of the central incisor.

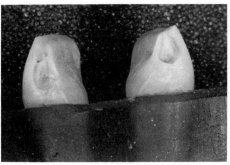

Figure 2–24. Class IV lesions caused primarily by abrasion. The existing proximal cavities were relatively small until shortened by wear; all of the incisal enamel was lost. The resulting lesions now include the incisal corners, thereby becoming class IV cavities.

definition, a Class V cavity could occur on either the facial or the lingual surfaces; however, the predominant occurrence of these lesions is adjacent to the lips and cheeks rather than the tongue (see Fig. 2–5). Class V cavities can involve cementum as well as enamel.

Class VI.* This cavity is found on the tips of cusps or along the biting edges of incisors. Incomplete union at cusp tips or incisal edges infrequently results in a caries-susceptible site.

Auxiliary Classification

In the days of Dr. Black when dentistry was developing into a science, cutting instruments, casting methods, and other technical procedures had not achieved their present-day degrees of sophistication. It is quite understandable then that his classification was not complete and that additional categories are necessary. Other than caries, the following hard tissue pathology of tooth substance requires the attention of the operative dentist:

The Fractured Anterior. By definition, this type of lesion would be a Class IV cavity because it involves the corner of an incisor (see Fig. 2–7). These should be classified separately, however, because the Class IV is the result of cavitation and loss of support for the corner of the tooth; the fractured incisor is the result of trauma (e.g., swimming pool accident or baseball

---

*The Class VI cavity was not actually identified by Dr. Black, but in certain geographic areas it was added to, and became part of, his classification system.

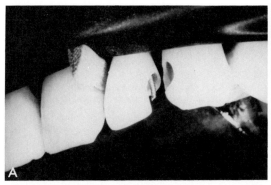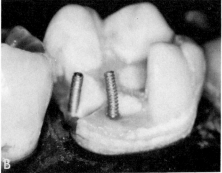

Figure 2–25. Restorations requiring auxiliary anchorage. *A,* Adjacent lesions—class III on central and class IV on lateral. (The threaded pin provides additional support.) *B,* Large amalgam restoration includes restoration of a missing cusp.

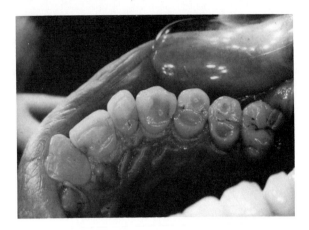

Figure 2–26. Pathologic erosion (or abrasion) of the lingual surface of the canine and cusps of the first premolar.

injury). Moreover, the modality for restoration and repair is quite different for the two. It is also interesting to note that the Class IV lesion is likely to be observed at any age; the fractured incisor is incidental in children and teenagers.

For the fractured incisor, restoration involves bandaging the exposed dentin and restoring the corner in a cosmetic manner. If by chance the fracture passes through the pulp horn, endodontic treatment is usually needed prior to restoring the corner. For restorative procedures for the repair of the fractured incisor, the reader is referred to Chapter 10.

The Cusp Restoration. Large lesions in fractured posterior teeth require major structural replacement. Anchor pegs in the form of miniature threaded retentive pins are used to enhance anchorage for this purpose (Fig. 2–25).

The Abraded Tooth. As people retain their teeth longer and means of restoring them improve, it is expected that teeth worn on the incisal edge and occlusing surfaces must be rebuilt to proper contour. To a certain extent, wear in every mouth is normal, but it reaches pathologic proportions when a considerable amount of dentin is exposed. Such teeth can be rebuilt best with gold castings (Figs. 2–26, 2–27, and 2–28).

The Core for the Vital Tooth (Pin "Build-up"). When a large portion of the enamel and dentin is missing, yet the pulp is healthy and vital, a crown is usually chosen as the proper restorative modality. The problem confronting the operative dentist is one of anchoring and building some "artificial dentin"

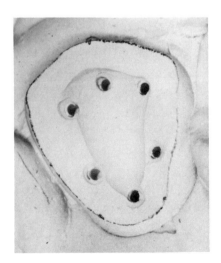

Figure 2–27. Eroded surface of a cuspid with pinholes prepared to receive a casting, which will serve as synthetic enamel over the surface.

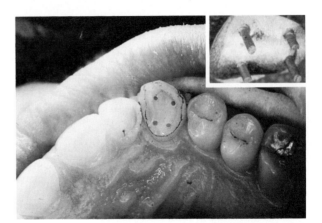

Figure 2–28. Pin-retained gold casting to restore abraded lingual surface.

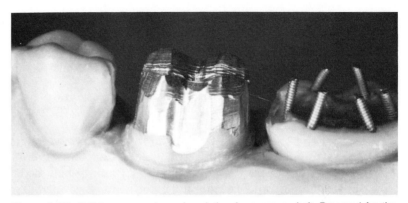

Figure 2–29. Building an amalgam foundation for a crown. *Left*, Prepared for the crown. *Right*, Pins anchored in the root ready to receive the build-up material. (From Baum, L.: Operative Dentistry for the General Practitioner, 1974. Courtesy of Charles C Thomas, Publisher, Springfield, Illinois.)

Figure 2–30. Explorers (probes) commonly used in diagnostic and operative procedures. Available as single-end or double-end instruments, they represent some of the more popular styles. No. 6, Right angle; No. 17, Back action; No. 23, Shepherd's crook; and No. 2, Cow-horn DE with curved ends.

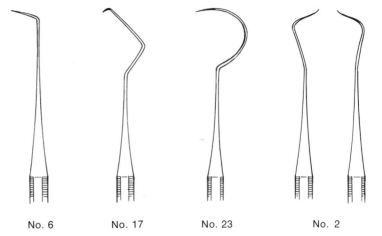

No. 6   No. 17   No. 23   No. 2

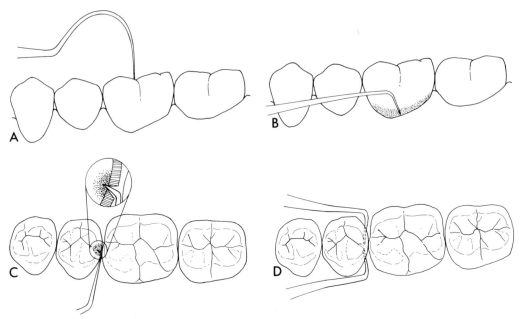

Figure 2–31. Clinical applications of explorers. *A*, No. 23, probing an occlusal groove. *B*, No. 6, probing a gingival lesion. *C*, No. 17, a distal lesion with access from the lingual embrasure. *D*, No. 2, cow-horn probing the cemento-enamel junction on the distal surface of a premolar.

to the root as a foundation upon which a crown can be fabricated. This is usually done in a manner similar to the cusp restoration, namely the anchorage of amalgam or resin to the dentin of the root by the use of miniature threaded stainless steel pins (Fig. 2–29). (See Chapters 11 and 13).

The Coping for the Non-Vital Tooth. When the crown is missing or badly mutilated and the tooth is non-vital, the operative dentist must devise a different method for restoring the defective or missing tooth structure.

Successful anchorage of such a foundation often requires the use of a metal post or dowel extending down into the root canal to provide this foundation. This foundation is usually in the form of a post and core fashioned from a gold casting or a pre-fabricated system (see Figs. 2–8 and 2–9). (See Chapter 19.) Afterward a crown is fabricated for the tooth.

Root Caries. This is a nondescript lesion afflicting root surfaces. It is a softening destructive process that seldom produces cavitation and is frequently found in older patients or those suffering from a debilitating disease. Treatment for these patients does not always involve restoration of the missing part; often the treatment is application of fluorides after caries removal. Insofar as possible the surface is polished so the patient can keep the area clean and free from plaque.

Figure 2–30 shows a number of explorers commonly used in diagnostic and operative procedures. Figure 2–31 demonstrates their clinical applications.

Summary. In summary, it can be said that the operative dentist, in providing a health service to his patient, performs a rather obvious role, which can be achieved only when the restoration is:

1. Hygienic and harmless to the pulp and the surrounding gingival tissues.

2. Strongly and rigidly anchored to the supporting tooth structure to withstand the tremendous forces of mastication brought to bear upon it.

3. Inserted with accuracy and proficiency so that the restoration will be permanent and not likely to succumb to caries or deterioration.

3

INSTRUMENTS AND AGENTS FOR SHAPING TOOTH SUBSTANCE AND FASHIONING METALS

Enamel is the hardest substance found in biological systems. Until the last two decades, the operative dentist had a rather difficult time cutting and shaping enamel because he had no tool suitable to the task. He was forced to penetrate the enamel through natural grooves, undermine it through the softer dentin, and split it along its natural grain structure (enamel rods). Fortunately, the routes of access afforded by carious lesions permitted the entry of an instrument or bur so the enamel could be fractured. With the advent of high-speed cutters and abrading tools (tungsten carbide burs and diamond stones), this no longer poses a problem because enamel can now be cut and shaped at will by the operator.

In the dental office, needs arise for instruments to cut and shape many materials other than enamel. Porcelain, resins, and metals of various types are constantly being fitted, shaped, or polished, both inside the mouth and in the laboratory. Operative dentistry as an art employs the appropriate type of tool with the proper kind of abrasive and cutting or polishing agent to accomplish a given task. Although miniaturized power tools perform most of these tasks, simple hand-held chisels, excavators, and carvers are desirable for certain procedures, e.g., the removal of carious dentin from a deep lesion.

Any craftsman known for his quality of workmanship will not resort to slipshod methods even if certain tools would make it possible to work more rapidly. The skillful and conscientious dentist is no different; the budding dental student should strive to develop the habit of selecting the *right* tool for the *right* purpose.

Table 3–1. KNOOP HARDNESS OF SOME METALS AND ALLOYS
ENCOUNTERED IN DENTISTRY

Gold, annealed	24
Silver, annealed	30
Copper, annealed	65
Nickel, cast	130
Stainless steel, cold worked	300
Steel bur	800
Tooth enamel	300–400
Dentin	60–80
Denture resin	20
Zinc phosphate cement	60
Amalgam	120
Porcelain	800

The development of newer tools does not eliminate the need for older conventional instruments if the operation is to be completed with delicacy and clarity. Because they cut more rapidly, many dentists rely too much upon the use of the high-speed rotating instruments. As a result of this, there frequently occurs needless removal of healthy tooth substance, often resulting in overcut cavities.

Hardness of Materials

In comparison to other materials, enamel is approximately three times as hard as dentin and cementum. Tables 3–1 and 3–2 provide comparative hardness values of common materials, tooth structures, abrasives, and cutting agents.

A desirable characteristic of any abrasive or cutting tool is that it should be harder than the substance to be abraded or cut. If the abrasive cannot indent the surface of the material, then it cannot cut it. In such a case, the abrasive dulls or wears away. Other factors are also involved in abrasive action, such as the body strength of the abrasive and the ductility of the substance being cut. However, hardness is a valuable index of the comparative ability of one material to abrade another. As can be seen in Table 3–1, the soft dentin of a tooth can be more readily cut than can enamel. In fact, being so soft and ductile, dentin may often tend to clog a diamond stone or the flutes of a drill and must be removed in order to retain the instrument's cutting efficiency. Cutting edges can be kept clean of debris by flushing with water or by maintaining an air spray in a dry field. This aspect of cutting will be dealt with at greater length in Chapter 4.

It is not within the scope of this book to describe various brands and designs of available cutting tools, handpieces, and so on. Technical data can be procured from individual manufacturers. The illustrations of a brand or design do not imply that it is necessarily the best one available. For a variety of reasons, individual schools and teachers have their own preferences that may or may not agree with those in this chapter or in other chapters to follow. For this reason, the emphasis will be upon the principles involved in the procedure rather than the particular equipment or instruments employed.

Classification of Rotating Instruments

Rotating instruments can be classified in various ways. One simple classification pertains to the tool itself rather than to the job it is to perform.

Dental Burs. The dental bur has a series of metal cutting blades. Designs vary from that of a twist drill to a multiblade* fissured router. These instruments rotate in a specific direction (counterclockwise) to coincide with the way the blades are formed (Fig. 3–1).

---

*Until recently burs had 6 blades; now designs can include 12 or even 40 blades.

Table 3–2. KNOOP HARDNESS OF ABRASIVE AND CUTTING AGENTS

Silica	800
Garnet	1360
Emery (corundum)	2000
Silicon carbide	2480
Diamond	7000

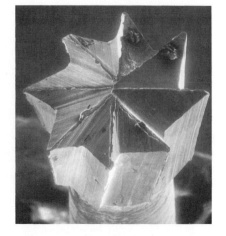

Figure 3–1. End view of a dental bur (inverted cone shape). The bur must rotate counterclockwise in order to cut effectively. (When viewed from the shank, the proper rotation is clockwise.)

Abrading Tools. A second form of rotating instrument is the abrading tool. Unlike the bur, drill, or router, an abrading tool can rotate in either direction. Bonded to its surface or impregnated within it are bits of hard substance (e.g., diamond, garnet, or sand). The hard filler particles vary in size according to use, whether it be for reducing hard enamel or for polishing a soft plastic (Fig. 3–2). Rubber abrasive wheels, diamond and carborundum stones, and sandpaper disks are classic examples of this kind of instrument. As might be expected, bonded abrasives can be either hard and unyielding or soft and flexible.

Polishing Agents. A third category, although not used as often as the others, is a non-bonded abrasive or polishing agent. In the form of a slurry, such as pumice or a polishing compound, these are carried to the working area with a polishing brush, an impregnated cloth wheel, or a rubber cup (Fig. 3–3).

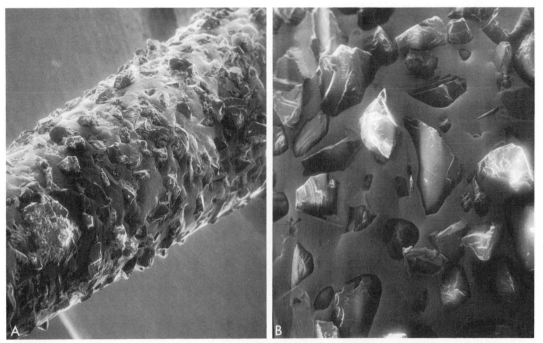

Figure 3–2. Diamond stone. Particles of commercial diamonds are selected by screen sizes and bonding substance. *A*, 80 ×; *B*, 200 ×.

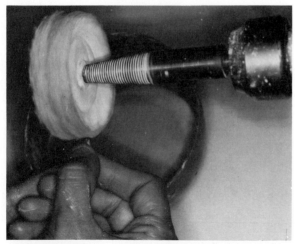

A

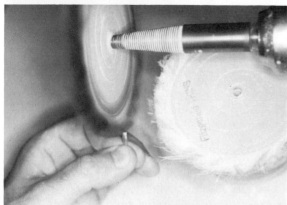

B

Figure 3–3. *A,* Polishing wheel impregnated with pumice slurry. *B,* Cloth buffing wheel specially designed for polishing onlays and small dental castings. The ultimate in polishing efficiency is obtained from a narrow but large diameter cloth wheel mounted on a laboratory lathe.

Classification According to Speed Range

Another method by which classification of rotary instruments can be made is through speed range. Although all instruments may be operated at variable speeds, two basic speed ranges are used: a high-speed range (100,000

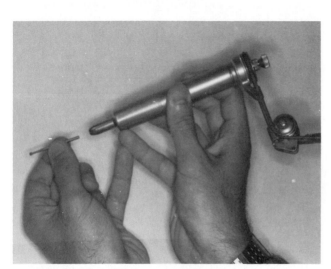

Figure 3–4. Standard Doriot straight handpiece.

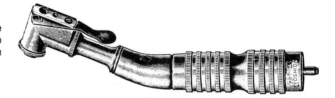

Figure 3–5. Contra-angle handpiece. The gear unit contained in the head generates too much frictional heat for operation at high speeds.

to 300,000 rpm) and a slow-speed range (500 to 15,000 rpm). Until the last two decades only slow-speed cutting or grinding was possible; however, with the advent of the air rotor handpiece,* a new method in tooth reduction and metal cutting became possible. Attendant to this change was a reduction in shaft size of the instrument from 3/32″ diameter to 1/16″ diameter. High-speed cutting requires carbide burs; for slow-speed, either steel or carbide is acceptable. Much less force is applied by the operator in high-speed cutting than in slow-speed cutting. In many respects this is advantageous; however, a loss of tactile sense is a distinct disadvantage with high-speed cutting.

It might be well at this point to classify the handpieces that hold the burs and drills. The slow-speed Doriot straight handpiece (SHP) (Fig. 3–4) may be powered by a belt and pulley system, by an air turbine, or by a direct drive electric motor. It is used when access and direct visibility are good. Burs used in this handpiece have the shank diameter of 3/32″ and operate in the slow-speed range (5,000 to 10,000 rpm). They are engaged in the handpiece by a collet chuck.

Also operating in this speed range is the contra-angle handpiece† (CA or RA) (Fig. 3–5). Burs are engaged by a latch and slot and are used for cutting posterior teeth when the mouth mirror is required for vision. Latch-type burs of 3/32″ diameter* are used in this handpiece and are about 22 mm long. Inaccessible areas can be reached better with a miniature head handpiece and short burs (Fig. 3–6).‡

High-speed handpieces powered by air turbines accept instruments with 1/16″ diameter shanks and are engaged by a collet chuck with a friction grip (FG).

---

*The water turbine handpiece preceded the air turbine, but it is rarely used today.

†Some slow-speed angle handpieces are made to fit burs and stones with a 1/16″ diameter and are engaged by a collet chuck.

‡Burs 28 mm long are available for operating inside root canals, and short neck burs 18 mm long are available for the miniature slow-speed angle handpiece from Brasseler Inc.

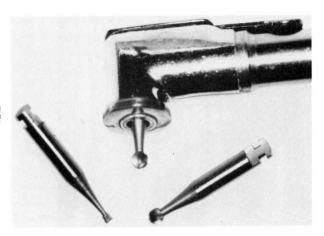

Figure 3–6. Miniature head handpiece with short burs. These can be used in areas of restricted access.

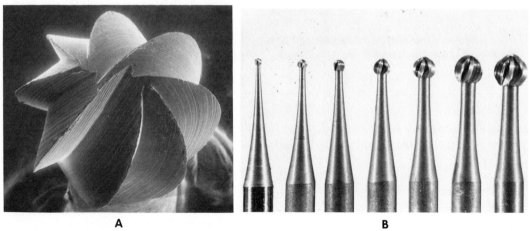

A

B

Figure 3–7. Round burs. *A,* Note the blades, which enable the bur to cut with its end. *B,* Round burs range in size from No. ½, 1, 2, 4, 6, 8, 10 (left to right).

Dental Burs, Stones, Abrasives, and Polishing Agents

Burs

As viewed from the cutting end, the blades of the bur (Fig. 3–1) are formed to cut in a counterclockwise direction. Common designs of these router-type burs are listed below.*

Round Burs (Fig. 3–7). Unique among most burs, this bur is machined so that it will cut on its end as well as on its sides. In its carbide form it cuts enamel with ease and is frequently used expressly to penetrate enamel. In its steel form and at slow speed, it can be used to trim away metal from the inside of a gold casting. In its larger sizes (e.g., No. 6 size) it is used to remove carious dentin.

---

*Numbers for bur identification are arbitrarily established by the manufacturer. Little relevance is seen in numbers between the various designs; however, within a given series, smaller numbers represent small burs; larger numbers, large burs.

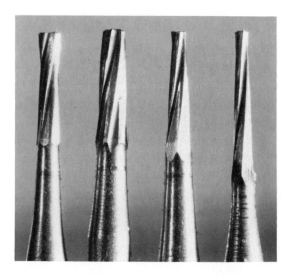

Figure 3–8. Popular sizes of fissure burs (tungsten carbide). Left to right: straight fissure bur No. 57; tapered fissure burs Nos. 171, 170, and 169L ("L" usually means "long").

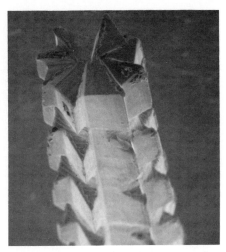

Figure 3–9. Steel cross-cut fissure burs. Steel blades are more fragile and thin than carbide blades, yet their thin cutting edges enable them to shave away dentin better than their carbide counterpart. This is a No. 701 bur. From small to large size, the numbers range from 699, 700, 701, 702.

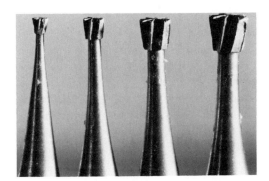

Figure 3–10. Inverted cone burs. Left to right: Nos. 33½, 35, 37, and 39.

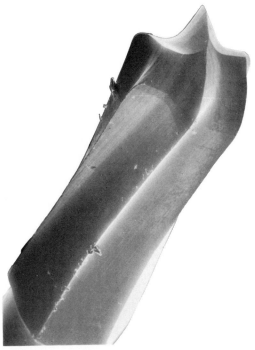

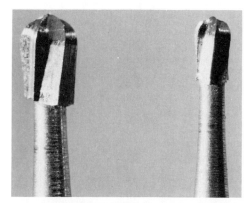

Figure 3–11. Carbide burs (fissure type) with rounded corners. Standard carbide burs have 6 or 8 blades. Pear-shaped burs are numbered (small to large) 329, 330, 331, and 332.

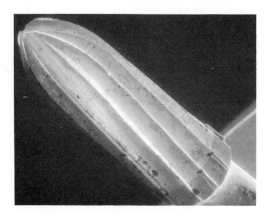

Figure 3–12. Twelve-blade carbide bur. Near the bur shank, notice the union between the tungsten carbide cutting blades and the steel body of the bur where the two dissimilar metals were joined together.

Fissure Burs; Plain Fissure (Fig. 3–8). With either parallel or tapered sides these burs cut enamel and dentin well at high speeds and have the advantage of leaving a smoothly cut surface. Some question their longevity, however.

Fissure Burs; Cross-cut Fissure (Fig. 3–9). These burs are primarily effective for cutting dentin at slow speeds, although in their carbide form at a high speed they effectively reduce enamel and dentin. To prevent fracture the blades are more blunt and the cross grooves less deep than with a steel bur.

Inverted Cone Burs (Fig. 3–10). These burs are most effective for producing undercuts in the preparation. As with other steel burs, they are primarily intended for cutting dentin. Carbide burs are also acceptable but do not cut with the precision of steel burs.

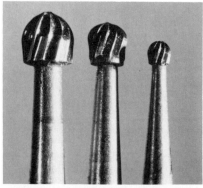
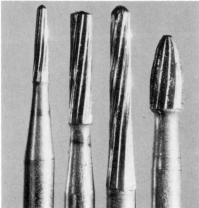

Figure 3–13. Twelve-bladed burs (Midwest gold shank) for cutting metal or beveling enamel margins. They do not cut as rapidly as standard burs, thereby permitting the operator to develop a tactile sense when using them. *Top,* left to right: Nos. 7008, 7006, 7002. *Bottom,* left to right: Nos. 7801, 7583, 7664, 7406. (The No. 7406 is excellent for placing a bevelled margin on a crown preparation.)

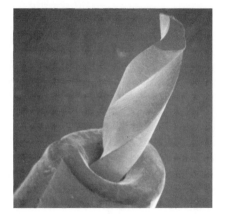

Figure 3–14. Twist drill. A bur cuts on all its sides; a drill cuts only on its end. (See Chapter 13.)

Elliptical Burs (Fig. 3–11). Elliptical or elongated round burs have become popular as a result of a trend toward conservative cavity design. These burs are characterized by round corners and sides with a reverse taper. The pear-shaped bur in its smallest size (No. 329) was introduced to the profession by Dr. Miles Markley and is a classic bur in this family of cutting instruments. It produces a conservative cavity preparation, with rounded internal corners and a minimum removal of tooth structure.

Twelve-Blade Carbide Burs (Fig. 3–12). Available in a variety of shapes and sizes, these burs are intended for beveling and smoothing enamel edges. Operating at high speeds, they are also effective in smoothing the surface of composite resin and for relieving occlusal interferences from gold castings. Because of the increase in cutting surface (more blades) a tactile sense is present when using them.

Finishing Burs (Fig. 3–13). Used for smoothing and polishing amalgam surfaces, these burs are also good for finishing direct gold and casting golds. They do not cut rapidly but provide, at high speed, good tactile sense while being used.

Specialty Cutters (Fig. 3–14). In a miscellaneous category are a variety of rotating instruments for special purposes. There is the twist drill for preparing channels (pinholes) in dentin and Peso reamers and Gates Glidden drills for instrumenting root canals.

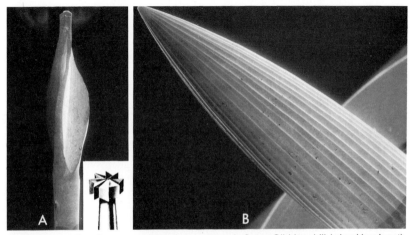

Figure 3–15. Miscellaneous cutting instruments. *A,* Gates Glidden drill (wheel bur inset). *B,* 40-blade bur (carbide).

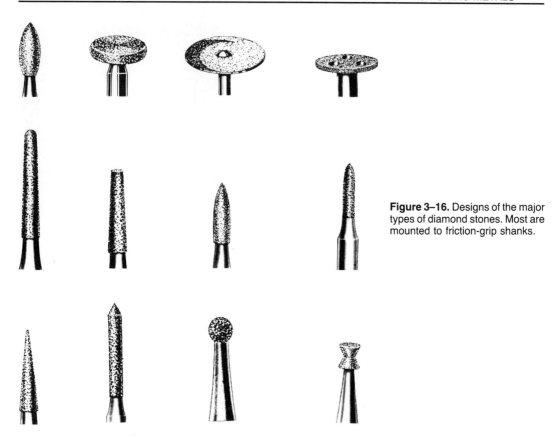

Figure 3–16. Designs of the major types of diamond stones. Most are mounted to friction-grip shanks.

Burs usually bear similar numbers from one manufacturer to another. Infrequently used instruments (e.g., wheel burs, root facers, bi-bevel drills, and lentulo spirals) are best identified by their names (Fig. 3–15).

Diamond Stones*

In various sizes and shapes these abrasive instruments are available in either coarse or fine grits and for either high- or slow-speed (usually high-speed) handpieces. Generally they should not be used to cut metals or unfilled acrylic resin; their use should be limited to the reduction of tooth substance,

---

*Although only a few commonly used designs are shown, scores of shapes and sizes are available from most manufacturers.

Table 3–3. ENGLISH VS. METRIC SYSTEM

Bur Shanks (Diameter)
Slow Speed 3/32″–.094 in.–2.4 mm
High Speed (Friction Grip)1/16″–.0625 in.–1.6 mm

Diameters for Twist Drills
.0315 in.–.80 mm
.0295 in.–.75 mm
.0236 in.–.60 mm
.0197 in.–.50 mm
.0157 in.–.40 mm
.0138 in.–.35 mm

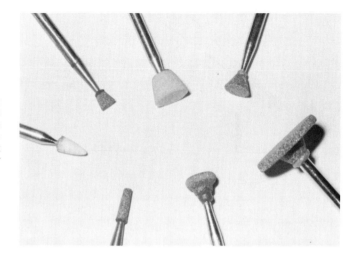

Figure 3–17. Mounted stones. Although a large variety is available, four shapes (and sizes) are usually adequate: large wheel, large inverted cone, small inverted cone, and small taper. Most stones used in the mouth are green or white.

baked porcelain, and composite resin. Some of the common styles are shown in Figure 3–16. Conversion tables for sizes of shank and drill diameters are listed in Table 3–3.

Mounted Stones

Mounted rigidly to a shaft, abrasive stones are available for SHP, RA, and FG usage and are illustrated in Figure 3–17. Mounted stones are generally used to cut and shape metal and are available in various textures depending upon their intended use. For example, a stone used to grind chromium-cobalt alloy in the laboratory would be too harsh to use in an oral environment. The green mounted stone has the proper texture for grinding gold castings in the laboratory or amalgam in the mouth. The abrasive most commonly used is either silicon carbide (SiC) or aluminum oxide (Al_2O_3), The Norton Company's trade name for their synthetic Al_2O_3 is Alundum. The trade name most commonly mentioned for SiC is Carborundum, which is also the company name. Silicon carbide is usually green or black, while Al_2O_3 stones can be white. The color of alumina ranges from white to almost black. The bonding agents in the high-grade stones are vitreous or ceramic. A silicate bonding agent is less common now. The same abrasives chemically are also used in

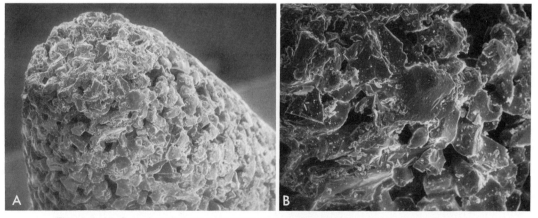

Figure 3–18. Scanning electron microscopy of a mounted green stone. A, 80 ×. B, 200 ×.

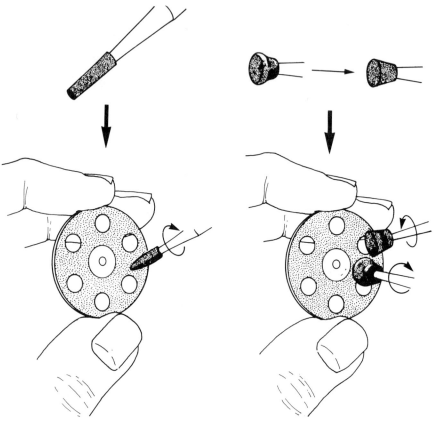

Figure 3–19. Mounted stones can have their shapes altered and made true running by dressing them down against a diamond stone.

resin-bonded and rubber wheels. In a variety of settings, laboratory and clinical, the stones may be used to grind metals, enamel, resins and porcelain (Fig. 3–18).

Their classification is difficult because their sizes have not been standardized but vary with the manufacturer. In an attempt to provide some form of classification, the stones are shown along with their common names in Figure 3–17. The shape of a stone can be customized, or a worn corner can be rendered sharp again by rotating it against a diamond stone (Figs. 3–19 and 3–20).

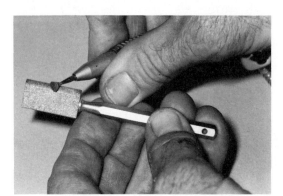

Figure 3–20. Diamond-coated block for shaping dental stones, a most effective and valuable adjunct for the office or laboratory (available from Brasseler Inc.)

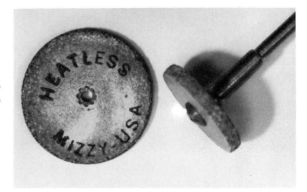

Figure 3–21. Heatless stone. Suitable for very coarse grinding but quite dirty because the surface of the stone pulverizes when being used.

Unmounted Stones

Unmounted stones are provided with a hole in the center to facilitate use with a mandrel.

Heatless Stone (Fig. 3–21). This is a very coarse stone used for grinding metal or porcelain. As a crude grinding stone it reduces material rapidly. This stone is also excellent for grinding extracted teeth. Its thickness varies from 3/32″ to 3/16″; its diameter, from 1/2″ to 1″.

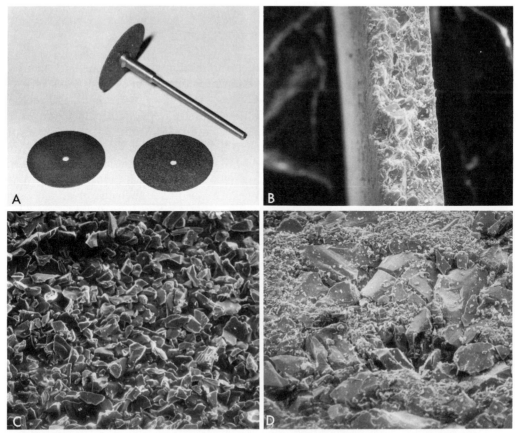

Figure 3–22. Carborundum separating disk. *A,* ⅞ disk, the basic grinding stone for the office or laboratory. *B,* Edge view of fractured disk. *C,* Fine grit side of disk (200 ×). *D,* Coarse grit side of disk (200×).

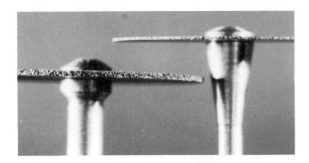

Figure 3–23. Ultra-thin disk compared to standard disk. Although very fragile these disks are very effective for sawing through gold with minimum removal of metal.

Carborundum Disk ("Joe Dandy" Disk) (Fig. 3–22). This disk is the basic tool for grinding, cutting or disking in the laboratory or chairside. Although it may be convex, it is usually flat and has a common diameter of 7/8″ and a thickness of 0.5 to 0.6 mm (0.022 inch). In its best form, coarse grit is present on one side and fine grit on the other. These disks fracture readily but are quite inexpensive.

Ultrathin Separating (Carborundum) Disk (Fig. 3–23). Diameter is 7/8″; thickness is 0.25 mm (0.010 inch). These are very fragile and must be mounted on a large-headed mandrel. When thin saw-like cuts are needed, this disk is effective in parting metal or porcelain.

Porcelain Grinding Wheel (Busch Silent Stone) (Fig. 3–24). Very fine grit stone used exclusively for grinding porcelain. Diameter is 16 mm (5/8″); thickness is 2 mm.

Unmounted Abrasive Wheels and Points

Abrasives impregnated in rubber polishing wheels are usually composed of variously sized particles of aluminum oxide or silica. They are used primarily for eliminating coarse grooves and ditches in the metal and rendering it smooth and ready for the polishing operation. Their thickness ranges from 1/16″ to 1/8″ (1.6 mm to 3.2 mm); their diameter, from 3/8″ to 1″ (9.5 mm to 25.4 mm). Wheels are used to polish flat or convex surfaces. In smaller, more delicate forms these abrasives are available as thin knife-edged wheels appoximately 1 cm in diameter or as cone-shaped polishing points, These are used to polish concave surfaces, grooves, and occlusal surfaces of metal, usually gold, either in the laboratory or at chair-side. Certain formulations can be used to polish porcelain, and where access permits, can be used directly in the mouth (Figs. 3–25, 3–26, and 3–27).

Improvements in technology have brought about cheaper manufacturing costs for diamond particles, so much so that it is now economically feasible

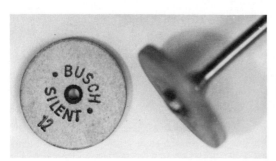

Figure 3–24. Busch silent stones. Exclusively used for grinding porcelain.

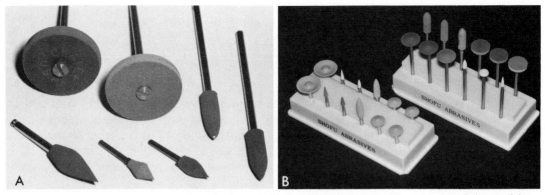

Figure 3–25. *A,* Rubber polishing wheels and points. *B,* Shofu polishing kits (porcelain and composite), containing white stones and graded rubber abrasives.

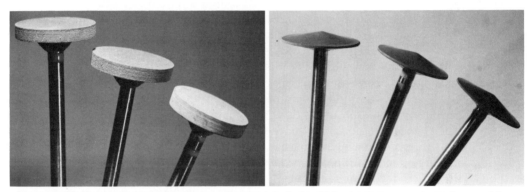

Figure 3–26. Finishing wheels. Markings on the shank indicate which wheels are coarse, medium, and fine.

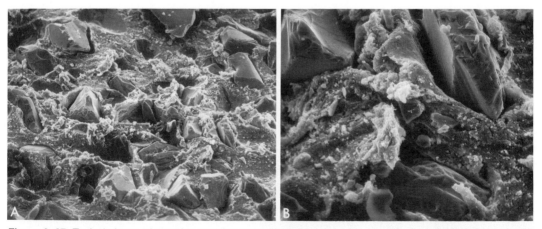

Figure 3–27. Typical picture of abrasive particles embedded within the rubber matrix of a polishing wheel. *A,* 200 ×; *B,* 1000 ×.

to impregnate rubber wheels with them. Such impregnated wheels have proven to be useful in polishing porcelain and other hard substances.

Abrasive Disks

Among the various abrasive agents for contouring, smoothing, and polishing surfaces, when used properly, the abrasive disk is without equal; the flexibility of the disk and delicate "wiping action" it can impart to produce a smoothly contoured surface are unmatched. Contouring of an irregular surface to produce a smooth flat or convex contour is usually more readily accomplished with a disk than by other methods.

Selection of an abrasive polishing disk is naturally determined by the circumstances of its application, e.g., kind of material, surface finish desired, size and shape of surface being polished, and so on. Although a wide variety of disks are available, the wise and experienced clinician will limit his selection to perhaps five or six disks that he will use in at least 95 per cent of the cases. Each operator will have his own preferences, depending upon his experience and habit patterns.

Abrasive disks are available in diamond, silicon carbide, synthetic and natural (emery) aluminum oxide, garnet, flint (sand), cuttle (powdered calcified shell of mollusk), rouge (ferric oxide), and crocus (impure ferric oxide). Backing for the diamond disks is metal. The other abrasives are cemented to a flexible backing, which is either paper, cloth, resin or some combination of these flexible backing materials.

The disks that cut best are from one of three materials: diamond, silicon carbide, and aluminum oxide. The natural abrasives (emery, garnet, flint, cuttle, and iron oxide) are more suitable for polishing than for cutting.

Aluminum oxide, which is tougher than, although not as hard as, silicon carbide, is more suitable for very hard materials than is silicon carbide. Also, there is a reaction between silicon carbide and steel that dulls the silicon carbide particles. Since alumina reacts with glass, *silicon carbide* is preferable for abrading porcelain. Gold can be cut and polished readily by silicon carbide, alumina, or garnet.

Garnet is also acceptable for acrylic resins. Although no polishing disk is particularly adaptable for the composite resins, garnet is as satisfactory as any. *Cuttle* is a softer type of abrasive and is excellent for cohesive gold, for

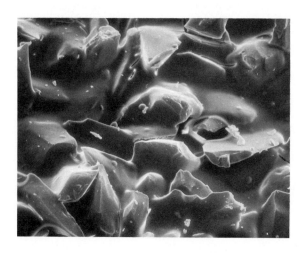

Figure 3–28. Scanning electron microscopy of a medium garnet abrasive disk (200 ×). The abrasive powders have been glued to the paper backing.

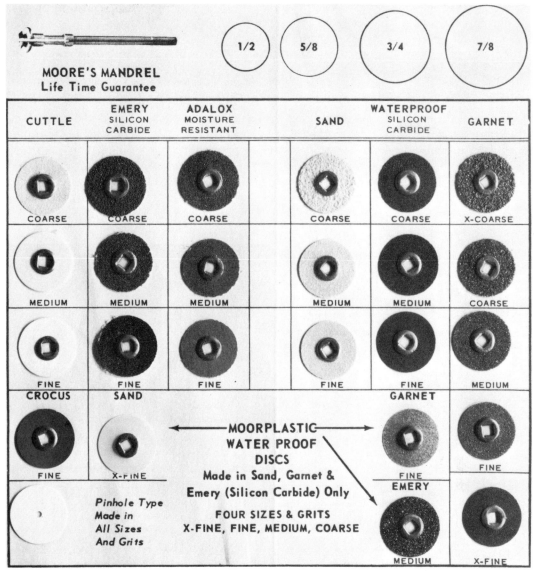

Figure 3–29. Commercial circular disks come in a wide variety of abrasive strengths, more than are actually needed. (Courtesy of E. C. Moore Co., Dearborn, Michigan 48121)

amalgam, and for imparting a polish to gold castings along the marginal areas. Other mixed abrasives* are somewhat more multipurpose, and many operators prefer them to the pure carborundum and garnet (Fig. 3–28).

Disks are available in several sizes ranging from 1/4″ diameter to 7/8″ diameter (Fig. 3–29). For sizes 1/2″ in diameter or larger, the snap-on type of mounting is desirable (Figs. 3–30 and 3–31). For the 3/8″ and 1/4″ diameters, the pinhole disk is used with the screw type mandrel (Figs. 3–32 and 3–33). Mandrels with the thin flat heads do not interfere with the working areas as do those with larger, more cumbersome heads.† (Also see Figs. 14–25 and 14–48).

---

*Adelox, a mixed abrasive, is popular among many clinicians. Available from E. C. Moore Co., P.O. Box 353, Dearborn, Michigan 48121.

†Available from E. C. Moore Co. and Miltex Corp.

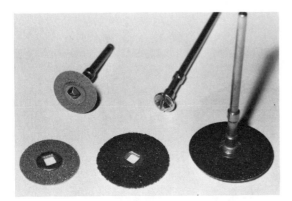

Figure 3–30. Metal center snap-on–type disks. Mandrels are available for the straight handpiece (HP) and the latch-type (RA) handpiece.

Figure 3–31. Coarse disk being used to contour some temporary acrylic crowns.

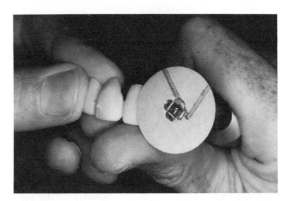

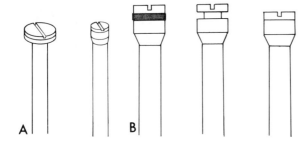

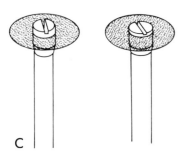

Figure 3–32. Screw-type mandrels. *A,* Large (No. 303) and small (No. 303½) sizes. *B,* Small-headed mandrels must close together without the spacer. *C,* To be effective small-headed mandrels must have a thin, not a thick, head. (Small-headed mandrels are often referred to as "Loma Linda" mandrels.)

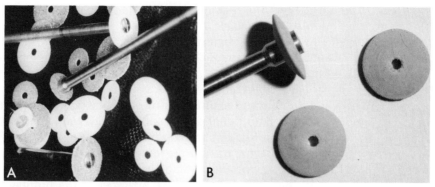

Figure 3–33. Small-headed mandrels permit effective use of ¼″ and ⅜″ diameter disks and wheels. *A,* Disks are available in cuttle, garnet, and carborundum (available from E.C. Moore Co.). *B,* Burlew wheels for intra-oral polishing.

The disadvantage of a screw-type mandrel is that rotation is limited to a forward motion only. A reverse direction unscrews the head. To offset this disadvantage innovative designs for mandrels have been developed. The "pop-on" mandrels and accompanying disks* are particularly adaptable for finishing composite resin restorations (Fig. 3–34).

The larger diameter disks have limited usage. In coarse grits they are suitable for reducing bulk of material and for shaping acrylic in temporary crowns and bridges. Smaller disks, 1/2″ diameter, are better for oral use. The 3/8″ and 1/4″ diameter disks, because of their ultra-small size, are even more useful because they permit better access for disking of proximal margins.

Suggested armamentarium for disks is as follows:

Coarse. Carborundum 7/8″ snap-on type. (Garnet is also acceptable.) Its main function is to grind and shape temporary acrylic crowns.

Medium. Carborundum (or garnet): 5/8″ diameter. It may be used for grinding temporary crowns, but is major function is to grind off humps, nodules, and sprue remnants of gold castings. Only one size is needed.

Fine. Adelox (or carborundum or garnet): 5/8″ diameter. It may be used to grind plastics; however, its major function is to impart a coarse polish to cast restorations (scratches still present).

Medium Cuttle. 5/8″ diameter. It is used to impart a medium polish to a casting (scratches still present).

---

*Pop-on mandrels and disks are available from 3M Co., P.O. Box 4039, St. Paul, Minnesota 55144.

Figure 3–34. "Pop-on" disks. These ⅜″ diameter disks are excellent for polishing composite resins. (Manufactured by 3M Co.)

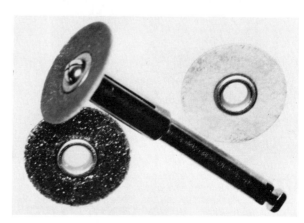

Fine Cuttle.* 1/2″ diameter. It is used to impart a velvet polish to a casting.

Naturally, the coarser disks are used before the finer grits to enable the operator to obtain a progressively finer and smoother surface. Crocus disks are recommended by some clinicians but do very little more than is possible with a fine cuttle disk.

Paper backing on abrasive disks is preferred to the stiffer plastic backing. While less durable and shorter lasting than plastic, the paper backing permits more flexibility. Additional disk flexibility with the paper backing is possible by applying a small dab of cocoa butter or Vaseline.

Sizing. Abrasive particles are most commonly sized by designating the finest mesh screen through which the particle will pass when the screen is vibrated. In the United States, sieve size means the number of openings per linear inch. Thus, a No. 100 mesh screen would contain 10,000 (100 × 100) spaces per square inch; a No. 325 mesh screen should have 105,625 spaces. Naturally the wire is coarser for the lower sieve sizes (e.g., 80 or 100 mesh) than it is for the higher numbers (270–325 mesh) (Fig. 3–35).

The finest mesh in the usual set of sieves is No. 325 (opening diameter 44 micrometers, or 0.0017 inch), but grit is graded to at least 1000. Above 240 grit, settling rate rather than a test screen is employed to grade the particles. Particles finer than 1000 grit, and larger particles also, may have their diameters stated in micrometers. For example, diamond polishing paste would be 1 micrometer or ¼ micrometer. The particle size in No. 1 polishing alumina is 5.0 micrometers; in No. 2, 0.5 micrometer; in No. 3, 0.05 micrometer.

Abrasive particles, being of irregular shape, have several diameters. Actual particle size will deviate considerably from that of the sieve openings, depending in part upon which diameter is measured. A grinding wheel or an abrasive paper of a particular grit designation will contain a range in particle size. Microscopic examination of several grits of silicon carbide paper reveals that the approximate range is 200 to 500 micrometers for 80 grit, 115 to 270 micrometers for 180 grit, 20 to 140 micrometers for 320 grit, and 12 to 40 micrometers for 600 grit.

The effective particle size range may not be as great as the measured

---

*Fine cuttle disks are optional and may be omitted in the polishing sequence.

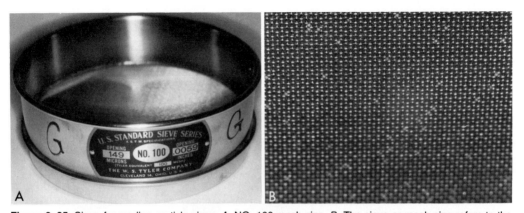

Figure 3–35. Sieve for grading particle sizes. *A,* NO. 100 mesh size. *B,* The sieve or mesh size refers to the number of spaces in the screen per linear inch. This 100 mesh screen has holes that measure 149 × 149 micrometers. Particles that can pass through this sieve but not through a 120 mesh size would be designated as 100 mesh material.

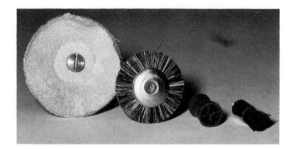

Figure 3–36. Agents for carrying polishing media: chamois, cloth, or felt wheels; brushes; rubber cups.

range, since the unmeasured third diameter, height or thickness range could be less than the range of the measured diameters.

Sharp corners or rough scratchy surfaces in the oral cavity are unacceptable; they can irritate soft tissues or the tongue. Likewise, irregularities tend to trap debris, leading to plaque accumulation, stains, and corrosion on restorations.

Smooth polished surfaces on teeth and restorations are essential. Polishing agents take on a progressively finer blend and texture, from that of a rough stone to that of a finely textured polishing compound, as the polishing process

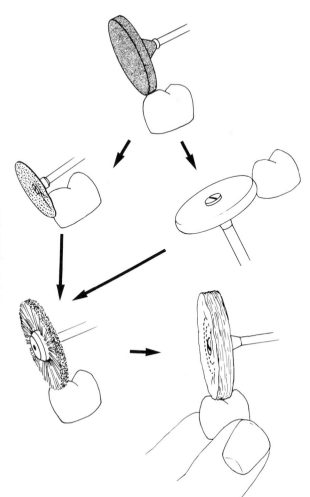

Figure 3–37. Sequence for polishing. Stone is used to remove the gross irregularities of bumps and pits. Abrasive disks and/or rubber wheels can be used to reduce the coarse surface scratches left by the stone. Brushes with Tripoli (or pumice) can be used to produce a low shine, particularly in the region of the occlusal grooves. Final polish is achieved with gold rouge or Amalgloss.

is carried out. Final polishing* is also done with a variety of compounds in the form of Tripoli, pumice, or chalk, applied with a bristle brush, rubber polishing cup, or other instrument (Fig. 3–36). (Also see Figs. 14–26 and 14–31.)

Polishing Procedure. Most dental metals are polished in a standard fashion. After shaping and fashioning them to the desired contours, the rough scratches and bumps are removed with a mounted green stone (Fig. 3–37). This is followed by a rubber wheel impregnated with an abrasive material. In delicate regions garnet disks are substituted for the abrasive wheel. In turn, the use of Tripoli polish, fine pumice abrasive, or cuttle disks changes the surface to a much finer texture in the polishing sequence. Lastly, gold rouge or pecipitated chalk is used on a thin rag wheel† to produce a high polish and luster (Fig. 3–38; see also Fig. 3–3).

Resins and porcelain are polished in a slightly different manner from metals. Rather than provide a description at this time, specific instructions in this regard will be deferred to the pertinent chapters.

Common sense and judgment must prevail in all aspects of polishing. Three specific fundamentals in this respect are:

HEAT GENERATION. Any abrasive action creates heat. On the laboratory bench, heat generation developed in polishing is of little concern, but heat

---

*A wire wheel brush is sometimes used to produce a smooth surface on gold castings, but its action is one of rubbing the surface rather than abrading away the metal.

†Fitzgerald Thins; available from Marvin H. Fitzgerald, D.D.S., 6619 N. 19th Ave., Phoenix, Arizona 85015.

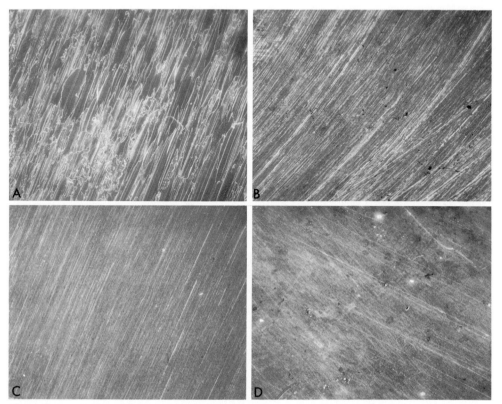

Figure 3–38. Surface finishes produced by the several sizes of abrasive particles. *A*, Green stone; *B*, Cuttle disk: *C*, Fine rubber abrasive wheel; *D*, Gold rouge.

generated from polishing in the mouth can be readily conducted to the pulp. Heat generation is particularly a matter of concern when polishing a direct gold restoration.

MARGINAL DETAIL. Preservation of certain delicate detiails in a restoration is vitally important. The use of a stiff brush to carry the abrasive, or the careless use of an impregnated wheel, can rapidly erase marginal detail that had been so carefully prepared.

COLOR. Some abrasives are dark; others are light (e.g., Tripoli is brown and pumice is white). In the mouth, where the abrasive cannot be easily cleansed from the teeth, polishing compounds are unacceptable, and only white-colored powdered abrasives should be used.

Hand Instruments

Cutting Instruments*

Most instruments are double-ended. Although a myriad of designs and shapes of hand instruments are in the dental armamentarium, the largest group consists of the cutting instruments (chisels, hatchets, and so on). This chapter will deal primarily with this group, whose major purpose is to cut substances (enamel, dentin, resins, and so on) within the mouth (Fig. 3–39). Discussion of carvers, condensors, and spatulas will be delayed to the subsequent chapters, where their application is more relevant.

Every hand cutting instrument is a miniature chisel or scraper of sorts, mounted on a ¼″ diameter octagon handle. They are used to split and plane enamel along its "grain" (enamel rods), or they are used to mortice the dentin by sculpturing the internal parts of the cavity. Ivorylike characteristics of dentin make it susceptible to carving with sharp instruments (see Figs. 11–61 and 14–40). Sizes, shapes, and angulations of the blades vary. Figure 3–40 illustrates a typical instrument blade. Except for the angle of the bevel, marked similarity exists between a dental chisel and a wood chisel. In cross-section the blade is slightly trapezoid in shape, with the base of the trapezoid forming the cutting edge. This configuration produces a blade with a dual function, one that cuts on the side edges as well as the end (Fig. 3–40).

---

*Available from American Dental Mfg. Co., P. O. Box 4546, Missoula, Montana 59801.

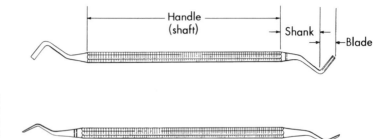

Figure 3–39. Parts of a cutting instrument. Note double circle on shank, which quickly identifies the "outward cutting" end, sometimes referred to as the contra-bevel.

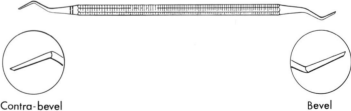

Contra-bevel

Bevel

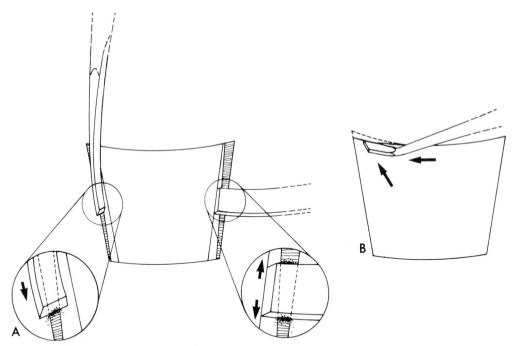

Figure 3–40. Basic elements of a hand cutting instrument. The blade is connected to the handle (not shown) by a shank. *A,* The blade has a cutting edge on its end, which is sharpened when it becomes dull. It is also slightly trapezoid in cross section, with cutting edges to be used for back and forth scraping movements. *B,* When sharpened at an angle, the blade with its acute angle tip can mortice an angular space into the dentin.

Most of these instruments are double-ended (DE) rather than single-ended (SE). In using instruments the operator imparts a thrust or a "pull" (see Figs. 6–3, 6–11, and 6–26), a "chop" (see Figs. 6–13 and 6–16), or a scraping (see Fig. 6–19) action. To achieve the desired cutting action, the shanks of the instruments have various bends and curves for placing the blade in the proper position within the mouth (see Fig. 6–26). In general, greatest control of a hand cutting instrument is gained with an instrument (1) with a large blade, (2) with a minimum number of bends, and (3) with a cutting edge in direct axial alignment with the blade. The bin-angle instrument is preferred to a mon-angle instrument when the cutting blade is long (e.g., enamel hatchets, chisels, and margin trimmers) (Figs. 3–41*B* and 3–42). This is done so the

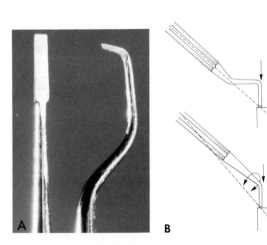

Figure 3–41. Hand cutting instruments may be absolutely simple, as typified by the straight chisel, or they may be designed with several bends to accomplish a task when access is restricted. *A,* The straightest and the widest instruments are the most effective for cutting. *B,* Hatchets: The upper instrument with an offset angle in the shank (bin-angle) permits the force to be directed in line with the handle; the lower instrument with only a single bend (mon-angle) may cause the instrument to twist in the fingers when a chopping force is applied.

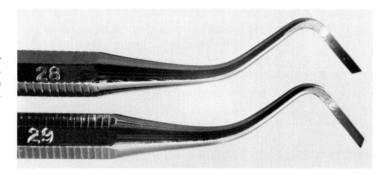

Figure 3–42. Manufacturer's or supply house identification number stamped on handle. These are the small distal and mesial gingival margin trimmers.

instrument can be held securely and not tend to rotate during use. On the other hand, short-bladed instruments (hoes and angle formers) are made with only one bend.

Left-handed operators use the same instruments as those who are right-handed. Except for a few specialized hatchets and condensors that are infrequently used, all instruments are designed for ambidextrous use. Dental manufacturers will provide these special left-handed instruments for left-handed operators when so requested. Examples of such instruments are the Jeffrey hatchets (see Fig. 6–26).

Identification of Instruments. It is expected that any artisan should be able to recognize the tools he is using by their shape and size without having to resort to identification numbers stamped on the mallet, trowel, or file.

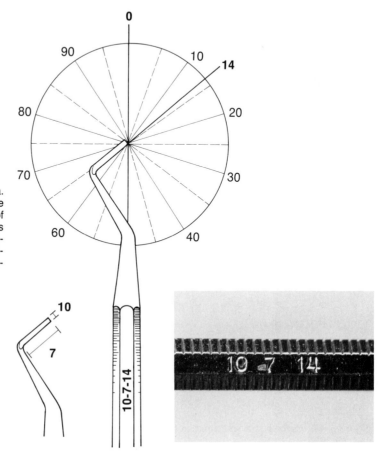

Figure 3–43. Instrument formula. The first number pertains to the width of the blade in tenths of millimeters. The second shows the length of the blade in millimeters. The third number specifies the angle formed by the handle and the blade.

Likewise, the student of operative dentistry should recognize his instruments by common name, by design formula, and for some of the common instruments, by manufacturer's number. Of the three, recognition by common name is probably most important because it provides a basis for accurate verbal communication by implying its intended usage, as for example in the names "small mesial gingival margin trimmer," and "large angle former." Throughout the text reference will be made to instruments and their usage.

To assist them in manufacturing and in filling orders, manufacturers assign numbers to instruments. Because many of these instruments have been designed by dental clinicians they are designated by an initial as well (example: Ferrier hoe: F-8). These manufacturing I.D. numbers are usually placed near one of the ends of the handle (Fig. 3–42).

Instrument formulae consist of three or four numbers stamped on the handle. Each instrument, as already observed, has a blade with dimensions, namely width, length, and thickness. With its first two numbers the design formula specifies how wide and how long the blade is (Fig. 3–43). The thickness is ignored. The third (last) number pertains to the angle the blade makes with the shaft of the instrument. If the blade is at right angles to the

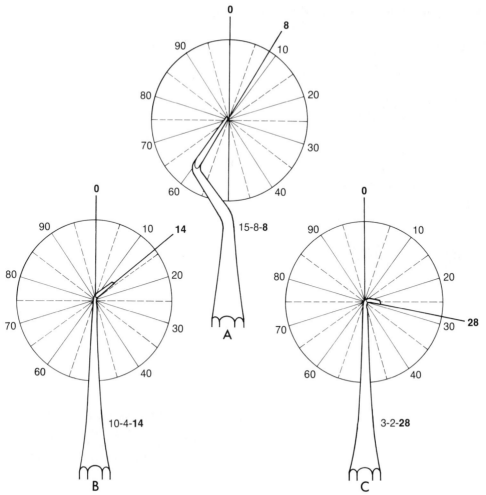

Figure 3–44. Angles of cutting instruments. *A,* Bin-angle chisel, 8°; *B,* Mon-angle hoe, 14°; *C,* Incisal hatchet, 28°.

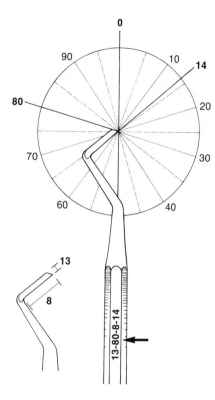

Figure 3–45. Instrument with four numbers in the formula. The second number, 80, was inserted between the width and length of the blade and specifies the angle formed by the cutting edge and the handle.

shaft, it should be 90°; and from elementary geometry one can envision angles of 30°, 45°, and 120°. The instrument shanks are bent to produce these desired angles.

Unfortunately for learning simplification, a Celsius compass of 100° was substituted for a 360° astronomical compass, so a 90° right angle, according to the Celsius compass, is only 25°; a 30° angle, 8°; and so on.

Some instruments (those sharpened to a point, such as angle formers and gingival margin trimmers) have four numbers. The additional number is inserted between those for the width and length of the blades, and it specifies the angle made by the cutting edge and the shaft of the instrument (Figs. 3–44 and 3–45).

Common Names of Instruments

Chisels (Figs. 3–46 and 3–47).
1. Straight chisel (SE) No. 15 (two widths of blades: 1.0 mm; 1.5 mm).
2. Bin-angle chisel (DE) No. 15-8-8 (two widths of blade; 1.5 mm; 2.0 mm).
3. Wedelstaedt chisel (DE) (curved chisel) No. 15-15-3 (three widths of blade: 1.0 mm; 1.5 mm; 2.0 mm).
4. Angle formers
   a. Large, medium, and small formers (DE); medium: 9-80-4-8.
   b. Bayonet angle former (DE) No. GF 17.
Hoes (Fig. 3–48).
1. Mon-angle hoe (SE).
   a. 10-4-14.

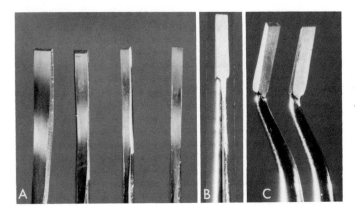

Figure 3–46. Chisels commonly used. *A,* Curved chisels; *B,* Straight chisel; *C,* Bin-angle chisels.

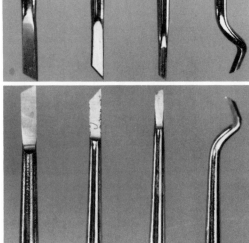

Figure 3–47. Angle formers. DE, large, medium, small. Bayonet on far right. *Bottom,* front view; *Top,* reverse side.

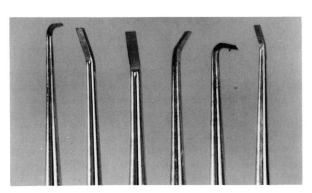

Figure 3–48. Mon-angle hoes. A hoe has a single angle, and regardless of the angle the blade makes with the handle, the hoe is used in a scraping manner—toward the operator or from side to side. Hoes are always beveled on the back side.

    b. 10-4-8.

    c. 6½-2½-9.

Hatchets (Fig. 3–49).

1. Enamel hatchet (DE) No. 15-8-14 (three widths of blades: 1.0 mm; 1.5 mm; 2.0 mm).
2. Offset enamel hatchets (DE) No. 15-8-14-7.
3. Incisal hatchet (DE) No. GF 18.

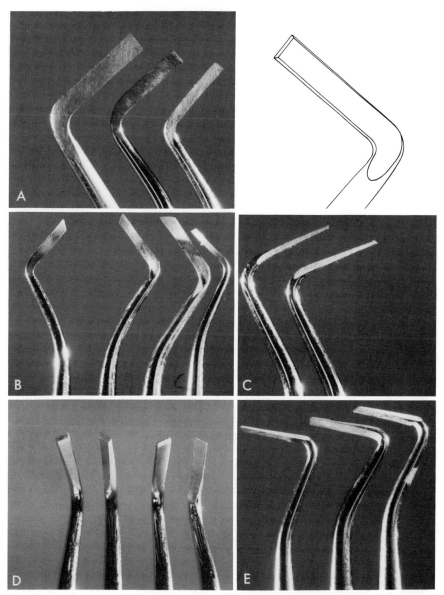

Figure 3–49. Hatchets and margin trimmers. *A,* Standard enamel hatchets: large, medium, and small. Drawing inset shows reverse side. *B,* Gingival margin trimmers. Left to right: Distal gingival margin trimmer, large; Distal gingival margin trimmer, small; Mesial gingival margin trimer, large; Mesial gingival margin trimmer, ultra-small. *C,* Off-angle hatchet. Blade is rotated at a 90° angle to the standard hatchet and double-ended for inside and outside cutting. *D,* Off-angle hatchet. Blade is rotated at a 45° angle to the standard hatchet. This angle is most convenient for planning buccal and lingual walls of posterior teeth. *E,* Jeffrey hatchets, DE, often identified as GF 13, 14, and 15. The difference between the three is the angle at which each blade is sharpened.

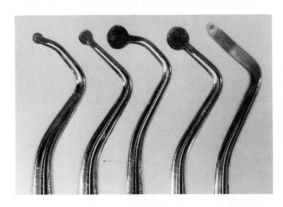

Figure 3–50. Miscellaneous excavators. A spoon-type excavator is seen on the right. A well-equipped operatory should contain several shapes and sizes of excavators in order to accommodate specific procedural needs.

4. Mesial gingival margin trimmer (DE)* No. 15-80-8-14 (two widths of blade: 1.0 mm; 1.5 mm).
5. Distal gingival margin trimmer* (DE) No. 15-95-8-14 (two widths of blade: 1.0 mm; 1.5 mm).
6. Jeffrey hatchets (also called Jeffrey chisels)†
   a. Inside cutting (DE) No. GF 13.
   b. Outside cutting (DE) No. GF 14.
   c. Square end (DE) No. GF 15.

Excavators (Fig. 3–50). (Used for removal of carious dentin.)

Excavators (DE) are available in a large variety of sizes and shapes

Miscellaneous Cutting Instruments. A wide variety of other hand instruments are used by the dentist but probably only the carvers, gold knives, and files are actually used in shaping metals or resin materials in the oral cavity. Instruments that are reasonably effective for removing hardened amalgam and composite are the gold knife, the gold file, and the discoid carver. (See Figs. 14–45 and 14–58.)

Miscellaneous Operative Instruments (Figs. 3–51, 3–52, and 3–53).
1. Spatulas for mixing cements and melting waxes.
2. Plastic instruments for manipulating cements and composite materials and waxes.
3. Condensers for packing amalgam and gold.
4. Carvers for shaping semi-hard material.
5. Burnishers.
6. Cement applicators.

---

*Used with a scraping motion, so they cannot actually be classified as hatchets.
†Must be specially ordered for left-handed operators.

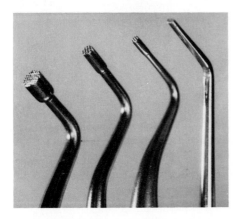

Figure 3–51. One small rectangular and three round amalgam condensers. Both large and small condensers are necessary to manipulate amalgam effectively within the cavity. Differently shaped condensers, e.g., triangular and elliptical, are important to some clinicians.

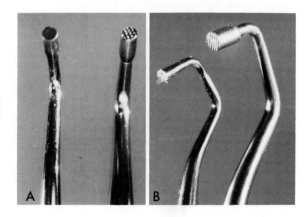

Figure 3–52. Amalgam condensers. *A,* Smooth vs. serrated faced condensers. *B,* Back action condensers. A serrated condenser can also be used as an amalgam carrier (see Fig. 12–89).

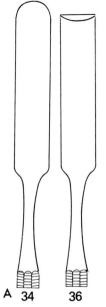

Figure 3–53. ACORDE instruments. *A,* Spatulas: *left,* flexible; *right,* stiff. *B,* Basic instruments for the ACORDE system. (Courtesy of the National Audiovisual Center, Washington, D.C.)

A   34   36

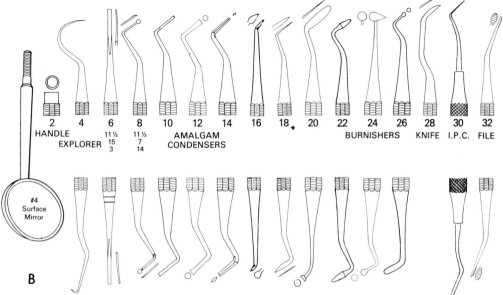

PROJECT ACORDE

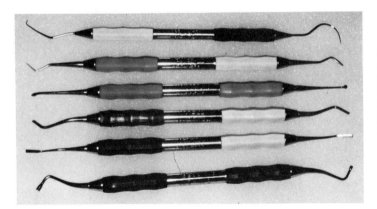

Figure 3–54. Instruments fabricated with rubberized plastic grips to prevent finger slippage and improve comfort during use. Color coding of these autoclavable plastic handles assists in easy instrument identification. (Available from Thompson Dental Mfg. Co., 1201 S. 6th St., Missoula, Montana 59801)

Instrument Variations

Over the years clinicians have been reluctant to switch from carbon steel to stainless steel cutting instruments because carbon steel is much harder than stainless steel and is less likely to dull when used on enamel. On the other hand, carbon steel instruments rust badly when subjected to autoclave sterilization. Instruments must be sterilized of course, and this has created a long-standing dilemma. The solution to this problem will probably lie in harder stainless steels, which are being developed.

A second improvement in hand instruments is illustrated in Fig. 3–54, consisting of silicone rubber coatings to provide traction for the fingers. These "grips" prevent finger slippage along the shaft of the instrument and substantially reduce the weight of the handle because of reduction in the mass of the metal. Moreover, the color coding of these non-destructible plastic covers is a distinct aid to the dental assistant in instrument identification.

Sharpening Instruments

Instruments must be kept sharp. It will be noted from the previous illustrations that the double-ended instruments have opposing directional bevels on the blades. Despite the angle of the blade to the handle, all edges are sharpened with a similar angle of the bevel.* This angle of bevel is not critical, but it should lie somewhere in the range of 60° (Fig. 3–55). If it is more blunt, it tends to crush the material than cut it; if it is too tapered, the edge dulls too rapidly. Sharpness in an instrument cannot be overemphasized. Sharpness is easily recognized by lightly thrusting the edge of the blade directly into the thumbnail (Fig. 3–55; see also Fig. 6–24). If it gouges or digs into the surface, it is sharp; if it skids along the nail surface, it is dull.

Sharpening can be accomplished by a motorized grinder (Figs. 3–56 and 3–57) or by a hand sharpening stone. The student is encouraged to become adept with the latter, not necessarily because he will use it in his office, but because hand sharpening is a good training procedure in instrument control as well as in recognizing proper bevels, cutting edges, and so on. Beneficial side effects gained by hand sharpening will be especially helpful during cavity preparations (Fig. 3–58).

---

*The incisal hatchet, a delicate and seldom used instrument, is sharpened with a double bevel like an axe instead of a wood chisel.

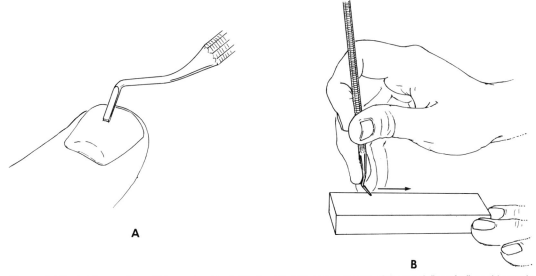

Figure 3–55. *A,* Sharpening of bin-angle chisel. Most cutting instruments are sharpened (beveled) at this angle (see Fig. 6–22). *B,* Testing an enamel hatchet for sharpness.

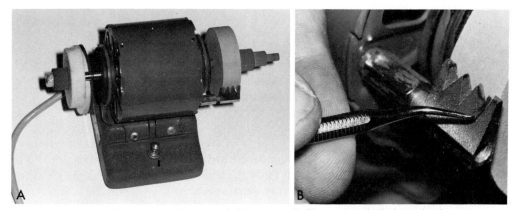

Figure 3–56. Rotary-type sharpener. *A,* Front view. *B,* Sharpening gingival margin trimmer.

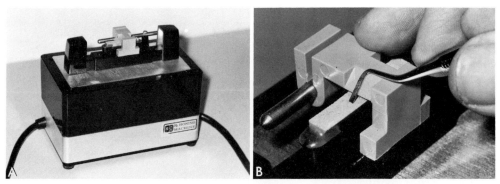

Figure 3–57. Oscillating-type sharpener. *A,* Front view. *B,* Sharpening an enamel hatchet. (R Honing Machine Corp., 1301 E. 5th St., Mishawaka, Indiana 46544)

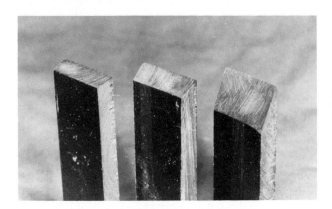

Figure 3–58. Correct and incorrect bevels at the cutting edge. *Left,* too blunt; *center,* correct; *right,* too steep and will dull rapidly.

Sharpening Procedures for Cutting Instruments (Chisels, Hatchets, Hoes, Trimmers, and Angle Formers). First and foremost in a sharpening operation is the need to position the instrument over the stone so that the bevel is exactly parallel with and flat against the surface of the stone. In conjunction with this, the instrument must be held absolutely rigid with respect to the surface of the stone. Any tipping or deflection of the handle results in a tapered or rounded bevel.

The cutting edge is thrust forward into the stone. Because of the heavy pressure exerted and because of the tiny size of the blade, one might expect the blade to gouge a furrow into the stone. This is unlikely because a hard India or Arkansas stone is used. For lubrication and to prevent metal from clogging the pores of the stone, it is soaked with a light machine oil. Soaking is used for new stones only until their pores have become impregnated with oil. As metallic markings collect on the stone they are wiped away with a cloth dampened in oil (Fig. 3–59).

Four or five scrapes or thrusts will place a keen edge on a dull instrument. Depending upon the angle of the bevel to the handle, a "thrust" or "pull" stroke is used to maintain rigidity of the instrument, and best results can be obtained when the ring finger and little finger rest and glide against a corner of the stone (see Fig. 6–22). Only the end of the blade is sharpened; the sides of the blade are left intact. With the use of auxiliaries in a modern office setting, it is expected that motorized instrument sharpness should fulfill most of the needs (Fig. 3–60). Precaution: When using a mechanized sharpener for the first time beware lest radical reduction of the metal reduce the life expectancy of the instrument.

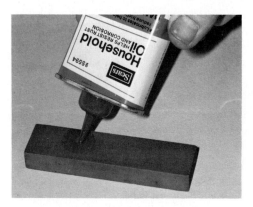

Figure 3–59. To prevent the pores from becoming clogged, oil is applied to the stone. The surface is wiped with an oil-soaked cloth after usage. Mechanical sharpeners are also treated with oil.

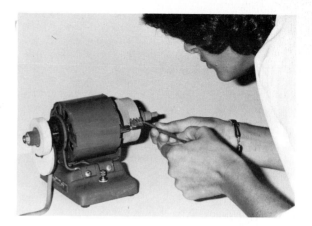

Figure 3–60. Dental assistant sharpening an instrument.

Sharpening Procedure for Excavators. An excavator is not shaped like a chisel nor can it be sharpened similarly, and mechanical instrument sharpeners do not effectively sharpen excavators. Best results are obtained when an abrasive stone of medium grit, approximately 6 to 8 mm in diameter, is mounted in the slow-speed handpiece. The stone and instrument are held rigidly, and grinding is done on the face (flat side) of the blade (Fig. 3–61; see also Fig. 6–21). Care is exercised to develop a sharp acute angle at the edges and to maintain a flat or concave surface on the face of the blade. Inasmuch as excavators are for the removal of soft dentin, it is axiomatic that they should be as sharp as possible, with a thin knifelike, rather than blunt, cutting edge. If this sharpness is not maintained and the angle is not acute, the excavator will tend to crush the rubbery infected dentin rather than shave it out of the cavity. The sharpness of the excavator becomes of vital importance when the cavity approaches the pulp (see Fig. 8–2). Many a tooth has been lost because a dull cumbersome excavator was used to remove microbe-laden carious dentin and the dull edge mashed the carious material into the pulp cavity instead of neatly severing and scooping it out.

Sharpening Procedure for Twist Drills. Although burs cannot be sharpened by the dentist, dull twist drills can readily be fitted with a new keen

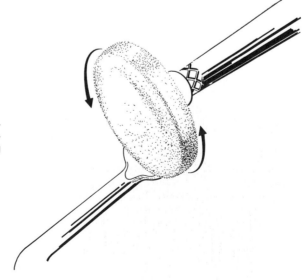

Figure 3–61. Sharpening a small spoon excavator. With suitable bracing the face of the excavator is hollow ground to produce a new cutting edge.

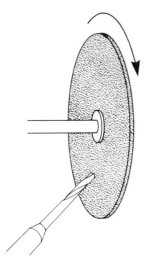

Figure 3–62. Drill being sharpened by "safe side" of carborundum disk.

edge using a "safe-sided" carborundum disk. The fine grit exposed on the "safe-side" is best for this purpose (Figs. 3–62 and 3–63; see also Fig. 13–5). Because the drills are so tiny, it is customary to sharpen the two cutting edges with the aid of a hand magnifying glass or binocular loupes. Seldom do dentists sharpen their twist drills once they become dulled; however, it is a good economic practice and can be done very quickly. Establishing in the mind's eye the correct bevels and slopes from the two cutting edges is the major accomplishment. Once these have been conceived the drill is positioned and then held against the slowly revolving disk. Contact for only an instant is needed to reproduce a sharp cutting edge. It is suggested that two 1/16" diameter twist drills be procured from a hardware store. One can be used for repeated practice sharpenings; the other, as a guide.

Another suggestion is to procure a masonry drill from the hardware store. The flat tungsten carbide tip soldered to the drill shank is beveled and sharpened in the same configuration as the twist drill. If used as a guide, this drill can be of help in perceiving the proper angles of the two cutting edges (see Fig. 13–3).

Helpful Hints in Instrument Management. The following illustrations summarize briefly some worthwhile hints that can be used to make operating conditions more pleasant and effective. As mentioned earlier, the carborundum disk is the basic grinding tool in the dental office. Another valuable cutting

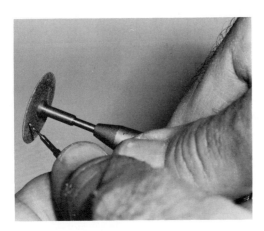

Figure 3–63. Hand position of drill and disk for sharpening. Notice bracing of the thumbs together for better control.

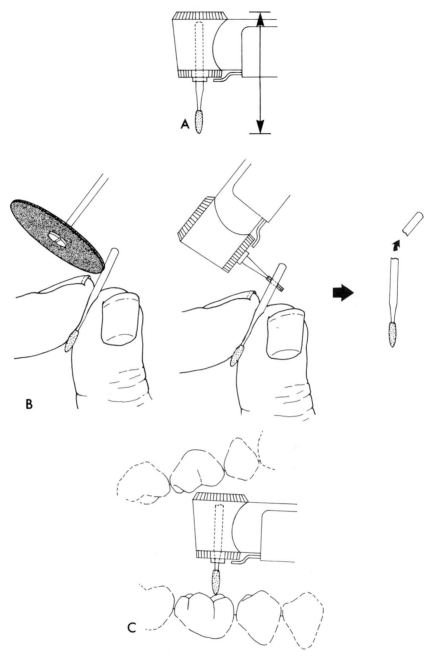

Figure 3–64. Method for shortening a bur (stone) to gain access in molar areas.

instrument for miscellaneous use is the No. 57 bur in the high-speed hand-piece. Serving as a miniature saw, this bur can alter the shapes of various instruments. When lack of operating space prevents the use of a standard length bur or diamond stone, 3 to 5 mm can be cut off the end of the bur so that it can fit farther into the handpiece (Fig. 3–64).

Using a diamond stone as an abrading tool, a standard size carborundum disk is dressed to a "V"-shaped cutting edge. This special shape can be used to cut grooves to shape embrasures (Fig. 3–65).

As the blade of an instrument wears down it becomes thicker, which

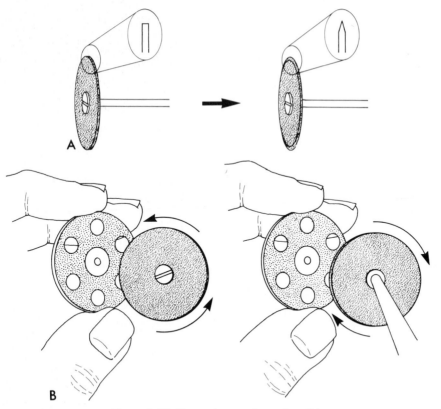

Figure 3–65. Sharpening a carborundum disk.

makes its entry into the cavity cumbersome and difficult. Rather than discard a worn-out instrument, additional use can be obtained from it if the "heel" or backside is cut away to render the blade thin again (Fig. 3–66).

Occasionally, in an emergency, a bur is needed for the straight handpiece when none is available except the corresponding bur for the contra-angle handpiece. Although it will stress the chucking mechanism of the handpiece

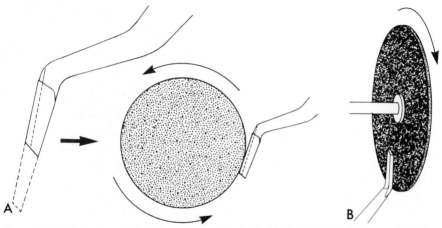

Figure 3–66. Reducing metal on the reverse side of (A) chisel and (B) angle former, to make them thin and usable again.

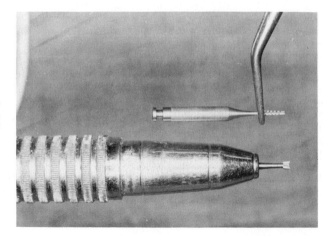

Figure 3–67. RA bur being used in the SHP. This should be done only in an emergency, as the chucking mechanism of the handpiece may become damaged.

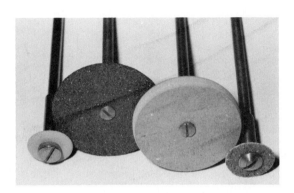

Figure 3–68. How *not* to mount wheels and disks in the mandrels. Large disks should be mounted in large mandrels; small disks, in small-headed mandrels.

Figure 3–69. Multiple disks make a wider grinding surface.

 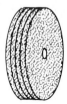 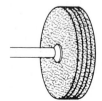

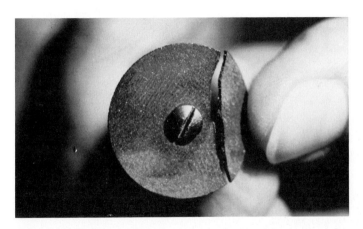

Figure 3–70. A piece of a carborundum disk is deliberately broken away.

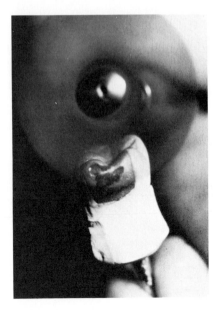

Figure 3–71. Disk shown in Figure 3–70 in use disking the contact point of a gold casting. Open space created by the fracture permits visibility without hampering the grinding capability of the carborundum disk. (Courtesy of Dr. William J. Roberts)

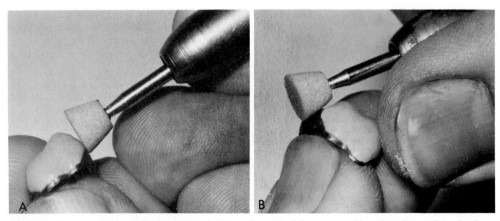

Figure 3–72. Use of inverted cone stone. *A,* Using the end of the stone with a thrusting action, the face of the stone serves well for surfaces sloping toward the operator. *B,* Using the reverse slope with a pulling action, the stone serves well for surfaces sloping away from the operator. These stones have little value when used in a contra-angle handpiece.

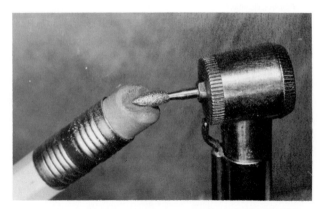

Figure 3–73. Diamond stones readily cleaned against a rubber abrasive wheel or pencil eraser.

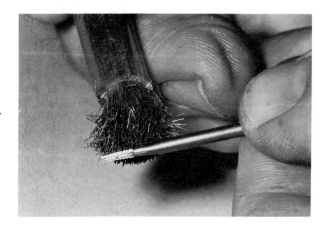

Figure 3–74. Scratch brush for eliminating debris that has clogged the flutes of a bur.

and barely protrude beyond the nose cone, the RA bur can usually be made to fit as a substitute for the HP bur (Fig. 3–67).

As observed earlier, screw-type mandrels come in two sizes. Selection of mandrel size should correspond to the size of the item being mounted (Fig. 3–68).

Another innovation involving carborundum disks and mandrels is to mount them as a short stack to form a thicker grinding wheel (Fig. 3–69).

A carborundum disk is the most commonly used grinding wheel in the laboratory. Because its larger diameter (7/8 inch) obstructs vision of the working area, fracturing away a portion (Figs. 3–70 and 3–71) makes it a "see-thru" disk without reducing is effectiveness as a grinder.

To those unaccustomed to its use, the inverted cone stone is a most awkward grinding stone. Experience and practice will reveal it to be a truly valuable instrument (Fig. 3–72).

Twist drills are intended for cutting only dentin. If by chance some metal, e.g., gold casting, must be penetrated, Vaseline can be applied to the drill as a lubricant so it will not bind or gall in the metal.

Bur and diamond stones are readily cleaned if they become clogged with debris. Diamond stones can be quickly cleaned by running them against a rubber wheel or pencil eraser. If blood from the gingivae has dried on the surface, simple immersion of the diamond stone into a 3 per cent peroxide solution will rapidly boil it off. If clogged, dental burs can be easily cleaned with a scratch brush, an item available from most dental supply houses (Figs. 3–73 and 3–74).

4

BIOLOGIC ASPECTS OF OPERATIVE PROCEDURES

Teeth are vital organs. Therefore, they must be treated with consideration when subject to operative procedures.

Although an entire book could be devoted to this subject, only a brief resumé will be presented in this short chapter. Information with respect to the physiology of oral tissues will be omitted; concentration will be upon the operative procedures that influence the health and integrity of the teeth and periodontium. Likewise in the following chapters biologic considerations involved in the selection and use of various restorative materials will be emphasized.

As was mentioned earlier, the objectives of the operative dentist are to provide oral function, esthetics, health, and comfort to the patient by restoring teeth. Frequently, the efforts of restoration may in themselves transform a comfortable tooth into one that is sensitive or pathologic. Damage caused by improper procedures is a distinct possibility and should always be guarded against, particularly by the operator who has limited experience.

Periodontium

The gingival tissue should receive careful consideration when placing restorations. Inasmuch as the contour of the restoration either enhances the good health of the gingiva or serves as a potential irritant, it should closely approximate that of the tooth involved. The interface of the enamel with the restoration, when adjacent to the gingiva, should be smooth and without ledges.

All teeth have a tendency toward mesial drift, a phenomenon counterbalanced by contact points of adjacent teeth. Failure to maintain or to reestablish physiologic contact between adjoining teeth can result in food impactions, which encroach upon the periodontal fibers between the teeth. Contact between cuspal inclines can spread the teeth apart slightly during closure, and with a plunger-like action, drive fibrous food downward into the space. Meticulous care must be taken, therefore, to insure proper contact during the fitting of castings and the placement of amalgams and other restorations.

Injury can occur from direct damage by a hand instrument or dental bur. Generally, these injuries will heal. However, severely torn periodontal fibers, especially in the interproximal regions, can lead to irreparable damage (Fig.

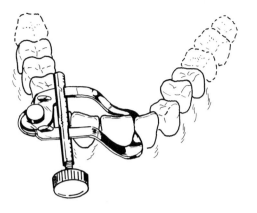

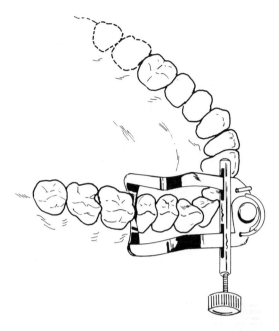

Figure 4–1. Instruments having a potential for periodontal injury, as an Elliot separator, must be used with care.

4–1) and subsequent periodontal pocket formation. Likewise, special care should be exercised when operating on the facial side of the gingival sulcus, especially if the preparation of the tooth is to be followed by an impression for a crown. To avoid unnecessary denuding of the marginal gingival epithelium, an instrument is often inserted into the sulcus to pry the tissues away in order to save them from undue abrasion from the diamond stone (Fig. 4–2).

Figure 4–3 shows a case in which the facial gingival attachment is movable. If it is necessary to operate on the tooth in this particular region, one should exercise extreme care or provide periodontal therapy such as a free gingival graft prior to the operative procedure.

To eliminate excess gingival tissue in order to gain access to operate on a lesion, the dentist frequently utilizes an electrosurgical unit to cut away unwanted tissues (Fig. 4–4). The cutting tip is the contact where the high-frequency current oscillates between the machine and the grounded patient. When deftly and properly used, this technique enables the operator to make cauterized cuts in gingival regions. Carelessness or incompetence of the operator when using the machine can result in gingival recession, and under no conditions should the electrode make contact with a metallic restoration.

Figure 4–2. A plastic instrument is used to deflect tissue when adjacent to the gingiva.

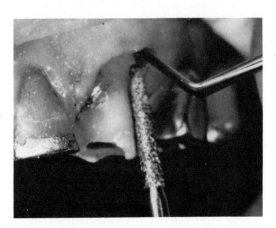

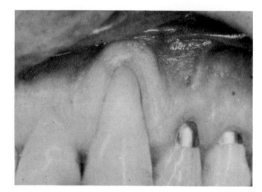

Figure 4–3. This tissue adjacent to the cuspid is easily movable.

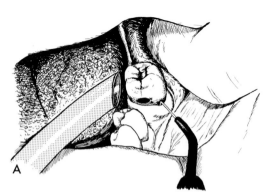

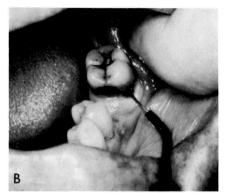

Figure 4–4. *A,* An electrosurgery tip in position, with vacuum for odor control. *B,* An electrosurgery tip in position but without vacuum, which allows for excess odor. Also beware of contact with a metallic restoration.

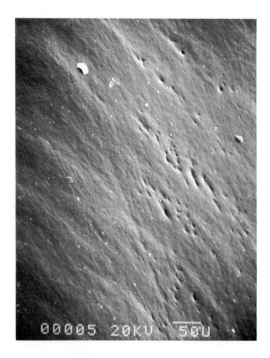

Figure 4–5. A 200× SEM of enamel surface indicates the irregularities and porosities that are natural to its surface. (Courtesy of R. Blumershine)

During operative procedures it is necessary to isolate the area with a rubber dam, thereby keeping it dry and free of saliva and blood. This often requires the placement of gingival retraction clamps, which should be used with care if they restrict circulation to gingival tissue for a prolonged period of time.

The supportive role of the periodontal ligament is provided by connective tissue, which is organized to support, provide nutrition to, and mediate sensory functions between the alveolar bone and cementum. This tissue protects the bony tissue against applications of pressure. The periodontal tissue will undergo structural changes as a result of variations in occlusal patterns. If a tooth loses function, the ligament will become smaller, and when a restoration is placed on such a tooth it may take several days before the tooth will feel comfortable during functional use.

Enamel

Enamel has been studied extensively, as it provides the initial major barrier to the caries process. It is composed of 92 per cent mineral and 8 per cent organic material and water, as measured by volume. It is recognized as the hardest human tissue. In spite of its hardness a fluid penetration through the enamel may be demonstrated (Fig. 4–5). The basic structure of enamel is the mushroom-shaped enamel rod, which begins at the dentinoenamel junction and ends at the enamel surface. Usually the enamel originates at right angles to the dentin surface and follows a spiral pattern toward the surface, ending

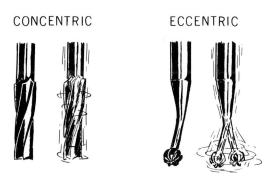

CONCENTRIC   ECCENTRIC

Figure 4–6. An eccentric cutting instrument has the potential of damaging enamel.

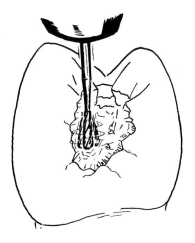

at near right angles to the surface. Cavity preparation bevels are based on this knowledge.

It is important to understand the structural features of enamel when planning cavity preparations, as this understanding provides the operator with basic knowledge regarding the strengths and weaknesses of the enamel surface and cavity margins. Operative preparations should be designed so as to preserve enamel but at the same time provide mechanical stability and good biologic acceptance.

Because of the high mineral content the enamel surface may be modified by etching the surface with phosphoric acid; this property is important when using resin systems as a means of restoration.

Eccentric burs that do not run true in the high-speed handpiece can produce crazing of the enamel (Fig. 4–6). Crazing can also be brought about by internal stress, such as might be induced by thermal changes or a retentive pin that is angled outward and that has been forced into the enamel. Crazing, per se, apparently is not serious, and although the enamel is cracked microscopically, it does not become detached from the dentin. (See Fig. 13–20.)

More damaging, however, is the unnecessary undermining of enamel. If dentin is removed unduly, the enamel can easily chip and break away. As mentioned, dentin provides a semi-elastic base to which enamel is securely attached. As long as it is present, the enamel will remain intact. When it is missing, as from caries or by the dental bur, enamel is like a ledge of glass forming a roof over a cavern, and pressure brought to bear upon it will result in fracture. This explains why a patient may have a gradually developing large cavity in his tooth and be unaware of its presence until the enamel roof caves in when he bites on a hard piece of food. Therefore, it is the intent of the operative dentist to strengthen the patient's cavity walls by carefully cutting back the unsupported enamel until the edges are resting upon solid, healthy dentin.

Dentin

Dentin is composed of 65 per cent inorganic material. The remaining 35 per cent is organic matter and water, which allows it to be cut more readily than enamel with a dental bur. Dentin is organized in the form of tubules that are supported by a calcified network of collagen fibers. The tubules contain the living extensions of the odontoblasts, whose cell bodies are in the periphery of the pulp and adjacent to the forming dentin. The tubule count per unit area is greater near the pulp as compared to the dentinoenamel junction. The tubules tend to be smaller at the enamel junction, as the wall of the tubule tends to calcify, leaving a smaller lumen.

The dentinal tubules are fenestrated with minute openings throughout the dentin thickness, indicating that the dentin contains a network of small channels. These channels contain the vital extensions of the odontoblasts, and normally they are so numerous that anytime the dentin is touched it is painful. The sensory mechanism of dentin is not fully understood. Among the theories given is one suggesting that movement of fluid within the tubules activates the nerve endings and that this movement is initiated mechanically by temperature change, dehydration of dentin, or the use of chemicals. Another suggests that sensation is transmitted directly through the extensions of the odontoblasts. The most sensitive area of the dentin is at the dentinoenamel

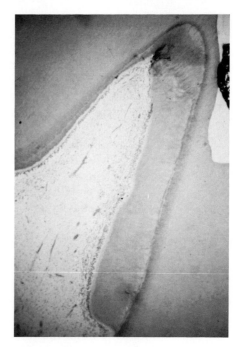

Figure 4–7. A low-power view of dentin and pulp—the odonto-blastic layer is healthy and intact. The accumulation of reparative dentin is an expected response to the adjacent cavity preparation. (Courtesy of A. Kafrawy)

junction, indicating that the greatest number of sensory receptors occur as a result of being confined by the enamel.

The formation of dentin takes place throughout life and the dentin that forms after the teeth have fully calcified and are functioning is termed secondary dentin. This becomes an addition to the original dentin and tends to occur in a pattern over the dentin at its pulpal junction.

Throughout life the dentin will respond to environmental changes, which include normal wear, caries, operative procedures, and restorations. These changes will frequently initiate a protective response by depositing reparative dentin, but this dentin formation will be limited to those tubules related to the site of irritation. The composition of reparative and secondary dentin is the same, and they differ only in location of deposition.

If the environmental insult is strong enough, it will kill the odontoblast and its tubular process, leaving the tubule empty. If there is a collection of empty tubules, they appear dark under microscopic examination and are called *dead tracts*. The pulpal end of the tubule usually is sealed with reparative dentin, and in time the tubules will calcify and the tubular pattern in cut dentin will be obliterated (Fig. 4–7). Another term used to describe the tubules that become calcified is *sclerotic dentin*.

Naturally, the degree to which dentin has become sclerotic masks out irritating elements to the pulp, elements that would be more marked and important to the permeable dentin with open communicating pathways to the pulp. In considering pulp (and dentin) damage, it must be kept in mind that references will be made to the young, permeable, non-sclerotic dentin.

Pulp

The pulp of a tooth is unique among other body tissues or organs. It is very small, but it is able to fulfill sensory and nutritional functions for a tooth. It also forms additional dentin and provides a defense against infection. The dentin, which the pulp nourishes and innervates, also acts to protect the pulp from external influence. The defensive capacity is mechanical when it lays down additional dentin because of an external response, or cellular when it produces the macrophage cells required to fight an infection. The odontoblast cells that give rise to dentin are part of the pulpal tissue.

The pulp is a highly vascular tissue and this is remarkable when we consider that the blood supply must pass through a very small non-elastic opening at the apex of the root. In spite of this restriction the arterial and venous blood flow of the pulp must stay in strict balance, otherwise there will be painful and pathologic consequences. The walls of the pulpal blood vessels are extremely thin, and bleeding easily occurs when the pulp chamber is exposed by a very small opening through the dentin.

The pulp will contain a plexus of nerves from which there arise small nerve fibers that innervate all areas of the pulp, including the odontoblastic area and the predentin.

The pulp responds very quickly to external stimuli, and the response depends on the severity of the stimulus. The preparation of cavities will bring changes to the pulp, which may be demonstrated by mild disruption of the odontoblastic layer with hemorrhage and necrosis if the instrumentation is abusive. Restorative materials will have a direct influence on the pulp, and the response will occur in a manner similar to that of the preparation. If the stimulus is mild, the response will be confined to the pulpal area next to the tubules connecting to the restoration; the response becomes more generalized as the stimulus become worse. Even through the pulpal reaction becomes severe, it does not follow that clinical symptoms will be reported by the patient.

Zinc oxide and eugenol produce mild pulpal reactions; acid-containing materials and resins cause noticeable pulpal reactions; because of their high thermal conductivity metallic restorations will influence the pulp if the distance to the pulp is minimal. Caries causes an inflammatory pulpal response; if dissimilar metals are used as restorations, galvanism may result, which is felt by the pulp; and microleakage around restorations will be an insult to the pulp. These factors, acting singly or in concert, will be damaging to the pulp if the intensity of the insult is high or if pulpal resistance is low. The intention is to minimize these factors by kind treatment and thus prevent the pulp from being overwhelmed. Some form of pulp protection is usually recommended and is accomplished by using a varnish, calcium hydroxide material, or zinc oxide and eugenol over the dentin next to the pulp. The techniques for using these materials are discussed in Chapters 7 and 8.

The pulp has the capacity to recover from injury by the formation of reparative dentin, and this is available throughout life. This includes the normal rearrangement of the odontoblastic cells to the repair of small penetrations into the pulp chamber through the dentin.

The aging process causes problems to the pulpal tissue, as is true with all tissue forms, and with age there will be a tendency toward fibrosis of the pulpal tissue, with a decrease of cellular content. It is expected that eventually collections of calcified material, resembling reparative dentin, will form in the pulp. These are called pulp stones and these have a large variation in size. The circulation within the pulp suffers the same problems as occur with aging in other parts of the body, including the loss of elasticity of the vessel walls. By comparison, the recuperating ability of a young pulp is much greater than one of advanced years. This fact is a strong influence when selecting the most desirable treatment option for a patient.

Various studies in animal and human teeth have shown a variety of biologic activity within tooth structure. Foremost in this regard is movement of fluid within the tooth. It is easy to visualize this in dentin as result of the tubular structure of dentin. Within the crystal structure of enamel there are microscopic pores that also allow for a limited flow of fluid. This fluid transport system helps maintain the health of the tooth and provides part of the defense mechanism against microbial activity. It also works to establish and maintain the mineral content of the hard tissues.

Caries activity can be predicted when several contributing factors reinforce each other. The tooth must be susceptible or lack proper defense against caries. Caries-causing microorganisms must be present and they must have an adequate food supply. An additional factor is related to the time at which it occurs, with the peak periods being childhood or until the late teen years, then late in life when root caries is prone to occur.

When a carious lesion begins in enamel it progresses slowly. It may be 3 years before the invasion reaches the dentin. A white spot signifying decalcification of enamel may be observed, following which in the normal progression of the caries process it will take 18 to 24 months before cavitation would be evidenced. The outer layer of enamel is the most caries resistant and is capable of withstanding damage. This is especially true where systemic and topical fluorides are being used effectively. However, if caries penetration does occur, demineralization takes place below the enamel surface. With the progress of caries, spaces will develop between the crystal structure, and as the structure loses its morphology it allows for the penetration of caries related microorganisms. If this process can be interrupted by a better home care regimen, including nutritional factors or more meaningful fluoride therapy, remineralization of this area is a realistic possibility. The remineralization takes place by transferring calcium and phosphorus ions from the saliva into the affected area.

Occlusal caries is related to the shape and depth of the occlusal fissures and seems most prevalent when the fissures are restrictive in size and have a tortuous morphology. (See Fig. 1–10.)

Operative Injuries to Dentin

Heat Generation and Thermal Injury

Fortunately, dentin has low thermal conductivity and diffusivity. Thus, when present in sufficient amounts it provides adequate protection to the pulp from thermal injury. However, as noted earlier, dentin can be cut very readily. Hence, there is a tendency toward continual cutting with a bur for rather long periods of time. This tends to produce a heat buildup that may produce pulpal irritation in spite of the low thermal conductivity of the dentin per se. Therefore, it is important to use cutting techniques that will minimize such undesirable thermal changes.

Also, as the tooth is being cut, surface heat generation may be produced, causing dehydration of the dentin and resulting in aspiration of moisture via the dentinal tubules. This imbalance in water content in the dentin is believed to contribute to sensitivity and pulp pathology.

Frictional heat generation is not easily recognized in a clinical setting. Masked by local anesthesia and areas of sclerotic dentin, it is impossible to depend upon patient response for determining when heat buildup is occurring. Both high- and slow-speed cutting, with either diamond stones or burs, can cause heat generation that exceeds the limits of clinical safety. If the bur or diamond is dull or inefficient, the potential for heat generation is markedly increased. It is difficult to determine the effectiveness of the rotating instrument except by experience as it is being used. Speed of rotation is probably not as important as the pressure applied to the rotating instrument.

Odor of cut tooth substance is not a reliable criterion for detecting heat generation because it is always associated with high-speed cutting but never accompanies slow-speed cutting. Unfortunately the recognition of the magnitude of heat generation, like many other entities in operative dentistry, must fall in the realm of "clinical judgment." Experience, in conjunction with a knowledge of relevant factors, will guide the operator in safely reducing tooth substance.

Coolants. Dissipation of heat is necessary when rapid gross cutting removes bulky masses of enamel and dentin and is unnecessary when intermittent cutting removes only small amounts of dentin. A coolant applied to the bur reduces the heat generated during cutting and increases its cutting rate. The chief purposes of the coolant are to reduce the temperature during cutting and to aid in the removal of debris.

There are three types of coolant available to the dentist: air, water, and water spray (air and water combined). All three forms of coolant are effective in reducing the temperature during cutting. The water stream is the most effective; water spray, second; and air alone is third.

During cutting, heat is generated by the internal friction of the material being deformed in the process of forming the chip, by the friction between the face of the tooth and the chip as it is sheared from the work, and by the friction of the blade as it moves across the work. This heat can be dissipated by conduction through the tool, by conduction through the work, by the chip itself as it is removed, and by a coolant. Although the life of the bur may be reduced markedly by the first method, the most important factor from the

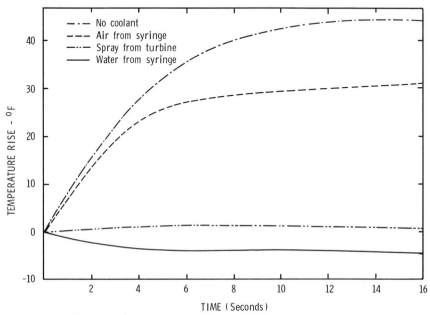

Figure 4–8. Rise in temperature at the dentin-enamel junction as related to type of coolant used. (Modified from Thompson, R.E.: Thermal effects in teeth. Thesis, University of Utah, June, 1971.)

dental standpoint is the heat absorbed by the tooth (Fig. 4–8). If the temperature of the tooth becomes too great, irreversible pulp damage may occur.

Intermittent cutting at intervals of a few seconds should be the rule. Removing the bur from the tooth intermittently for even a few seconds can reduce the heat generation considerably. Even though the temperature is kept comparatively low, a sustained application may result in greater pulp damage than would result if a higher temperature were applied for a short time.

Water coolants are universally used to dissipate heat. A fine spray of water on the cutting surface (Fig. 4–9) reduces heat and minimizes dehydration, yet also serves as a flushing medium to wash away tooth chips and to prevent clogging of the diamond stone and flutes of the bur. Water spray, if too cold, can cause thermal shock, a painful response to the patient but probably not permanently damaging to the pulp. Water spray would be ideal in all operating situations except for one detrimental factor—it drastically restricts visibility. Not only is the atomized spray distracting, but the surface layer of water deflects light rays and distorts vision.

Determining when to use or not to use a water coolant, as already mentioned, is a matter of clinical judgment. Generally the beginning part of the operation should include a water coolant (Fig. 4–10). When details of preparation refinement become important, cutting becomes more intermittent

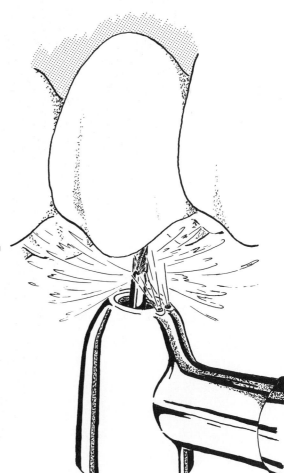

Figure 4–9. Water as a coolant directly on the tooth prevents damage due to heat.

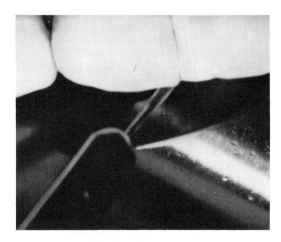

Figure 4–10. High-velocity evacuation is a necessity when using water as a means of cooling.

(allowing heat to be conducted away normally), and as visual evaluation becomes more crucial, cutting should be done without moisture. As previously indicated, high-speed cutting invariably produces an odor characteristic of burning protein. Although the odor is not necessarily associated with pulpal damage, it should not be neglected, as it is an unpleasant smell and might make the patient apprehensive. If it reaches a level of perceptibility, it is easily removed by high-velocity evacuation. (See also Chapter 9.)

Dehydration

In order to observe the progress of his tooth preparation, the operator may overly dehydrate the tooth with repeated blasts of air. Frequent application of a moist cotton pellet to the working area will minimize any problems of dehydration in this regard. (See also Chapter 9).

Thermal Conductivity in Restoration Materials

As has been mentioned, the pulp may be injured from severe temperature change induced by thermal energy passing through a metallic restoration. If a piece of ice is applied to the surface of an amalgam restoration, for example,

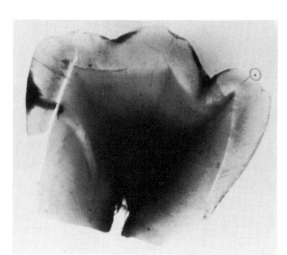

Figure 4–11. The irritation of a small lesion produces secondary dentin through the tubules and also deposits it in the pulpal chamber. (Courtesy of Dr. Wallace W. Johnson)

within approximately two seconds the temperature at the floor of the cavity will be that of the ice. Thus, wherever the cavity preparation is deep and an inadequate thickness of dentin is present for thermal insulation, protection by a cement base must be provided.

Cement bases will be discussed at length in Chapters 7 and 8. It suffices to say, however, that sclerotic dentin and a thick layer of dentin between the internal part of the cavity and the pulp reduce the thermal shock and, in turn, the need for a cement base. Shallow preparations over highly permeable dentin* may need protection against thermal stimuli (Fig. 4–11). (See also Chapters 11 and 12.)

Chemically Induced Irritation

Certain types of dental materials may produce pulpal injury from the presence of irritants or extremes of pH. When such materials are required, the dentin must be protected by the use of bio-compatible liners, varnishes, or bases. Their selection and use will be discussed at the appropriate time in Chapters 7, 8, 10, 11, and 13.

It is important to re-emphasize that pulp protection is of particular significance in the *deep* preparation. In many of these situations, one may actually have a microscopic pulp exposure without clinical evidence such as the presence of blood or an exudate.

Summary of Operative Precautions

The operative procedures that may have a deleterious effect upon dentin are:

1. Heat generated by cutting action from burs or during polishing of restorations.

2. Undue dehydration during cutting.

3. Heat transfer through metallic restorations that are thermal conductors rather than insulators.

4. Application of any restorative material that provides a toxic environment to the cut surface.

In light of these considerations and in order to minimize these effects, the cautious operative dentist will avoid things such as:

1. Prolonged application of blasts of warm air.

2. Excessive cutting of tooth substance without suitable coolants—especially to burs and diamond stones in the high-speed handpieces or under heavy loading.

3. Placement of irritating filling materials against dentin surfaces without the previous use of proper insulators and medicaments or liners to maintain the normal biologic conditions of the dentin.

Non-Vital Teeth

Non-vital teeth, those whose pulps have been previously removed, are brittle and more subject to fracture than are vital teeth, owing to organic and

---

*Anatomic areas where sensitive, highly permeable dentin is likely to be found are the facio-cervical areas of molars, especially mandibular molars.

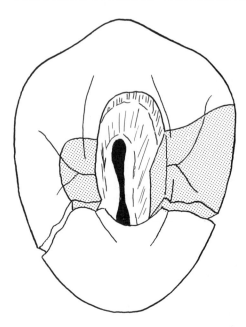

Figure 4–12. A nonvital tooth must be treated so as to prevent cuspal fracture.

biological changes occurring from death of the pulp. Therefore, restorations in non-vital teeth are usually full crowns or restorations that provide coverage of the occlusal surface with a gold casting—especially in molars and bicuspids—to prevent the tooth from fracturing. The placement of mesial, distal, and occlusal restorations weakens the crown and predisposes the tooth to fracture (Fig. 4–12). Thus crowns or other restorations that cover all of the occlusal surface are necessary as a measure to prevent a fracture that can even extend into the root. Such damage is irreparable and may require extraction of the tooth.

Occlusal Considerations

Although intricacies and intercuspation of the occluding components of the teeth are of extreme significance to the operative dentist, only a brief word of caution will be expressed in this regard. The tooth being restored should not precipitate occlusal problems. A restoration left "high in occlusion" is perhaps the most common single iatrogenic problem arising from operative procedures. As the patient is unable to close his teeth completely together because of a "high" filling, he seeks a comfortable position for his lower jaw. In attempting to adapt to this new position, stresses are placed upon the temporomandibular joint and teeth may shift or loosen because of new cusp inclines and abnormal jaw closure of the patient. Despite the use of carbon marking paper and bite wax registrations, even the careful operator is sometimes guilty of leaving a restoration too "high in occlusion."

This does not mean that overcarving so as to produce an undercontoured restoration is a desirable prophylactic measure. Teeth restored in this fashion may also precipitate occlusal problems resulting from tipping or migration of teeth.

At the same time, the careful operator will make sure that his restorations provide proper interproximal contacts. The shape of the contact points is as important as are the embrasures blending gingival, occlusal, and axial surfaces together. The operative dentist can prevent contact difficulties by the correct application and wedging of matrix materials (see Chapters 10 and 12).

In general the operative dentist must have knowledge of dental anatomy, of the restorative materials he will use, and of the engineering principles associated with their use. Lack of knowledge, lack of judgment, or carelessness in the use of materials is no excuse for the operative dentist to create, in his treatment, additional problems for the patient. These matters will be re-emphasized in the pertinent sections of the chapters that follow.

5

ESTHETIC* CONSIDERATIONS IN OPERATIVE DENTISTRY

Teeth play a major role in the beauty of a face and in the personality of an individual. Tooth size, color, contour, and alignment are all significant in the achievement of a natural beauty to the smile.

Bones, particularly the maxilla and mandible, form the contour of the lower face and provide the foundation for lips, cheek pads, and associated musculature. Underdeveloped or overdeveloped mandibles cause the most obvious departure from the normal, as can be observed in the comic strips with the Andy Gump and Dick Tracy profiles.

Bones of the face are not the only structures involved in the facial contours. The crowns of the teeth as they come together form a natural "stop," preventing the chin from approaching the nose, as well as preventing the lips from falling inward. Perhaps even more important than the crowns are the roots that support them. Embedded inside alveolar bone, they stimulate bone growth and maintain the structure and form of the alveolus. When roots are gone, bone loss is inevitable, and over the years the edentulous patient will lose unbelievable amounts of bone from the alveolar ridge. Many and varied attempts have been made to embed material in or to transplant tissue to the alveolar ridge, either to prevent resorption of the bone or to reconstruct or replace its natural form. All of us have seen the dental cripples consigned to wearing dentures, who have problems with masticating their food and esthetic problems because the facial tissues tend to "sag in."

Individuality plays a major role in dental esthetics. Wide variation in

---

*"Esthetic" is derived from "aesthete": that which is beautiful in art or nature.

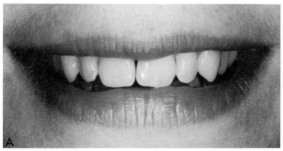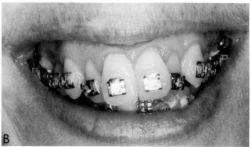

Figure 5–1. Comparative lip lines during laughter or a smile. *A,* Low lip line. *B,* High lip line.

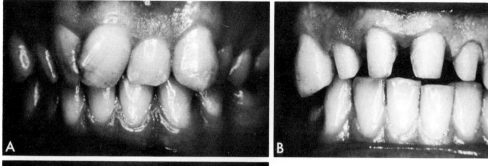

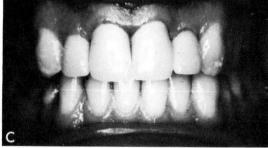

Figure 5–2. Overlapped and crowded maxillary incisors corrected by placing crowns. *A,* Tipped and overlapped central incisors; lateral incisors are in lingual version. *B,* Teeth prepared for crowns. *C,* Finished crowns; lateral incisors were over-contoured toward the labial.

such a common element as a smile is obvious once one observes it among people. The musculature of the upper lip and its size and attachment might, during a smile, show only the incisal edges of the teeth or display much of the labial gingivae as well. Occasionally the lip musculature seems to be reversed, and the individual displays only lower teeth during smiling and conversation (Fig. 5–1).

Shape and Position of Teeth

Malalignment or malpositioning of the teeth can be unsightly. Orthodontic literature is replete with illustrations and case studies of patients whose appearance has been improved following therapy. Although orthodontics as a discipline or specialty corrects oral abnormalities by tooth straightening, operative dentistry also plays a role in minor modifications of tooth shaping and contouring (Fig. 5–2). It is not unusual for a patient with crooked or

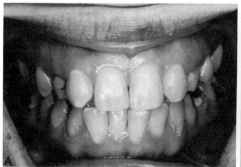

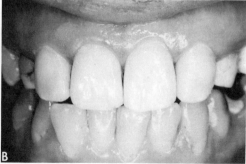

Figure 5–3. Congenitally missing lateral incisors. *A,* The pointed canines have drifted forward to occupy lateral incisor positions. *B,* The labial curvatures of the canines were flattened, and false incisal corners were added with composite resin (see Chapter 10 for acid etch technique).

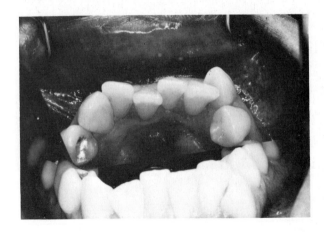

Figure 5–4. Crowded lower anterior teeth. With thin incisal edges and flattened surfaces they readily slip out of position and overlap each other. As can be seen in Figure 5–8 this marked overlapping is not as unsightly at conversational distances as the teeth appear here.

overlapped teeth to have them "capped" to correct their alignment, especially the maxillary anteriors. For cosmetic reasons many people in the entertainment field have resorted to this method to improve their stage presence. It is obvious, however, that any such corrections should be made to change rotational rather than positional abnormalities.

Another method for changing tooth shape is through selective grinding. Teeth can be shortened, narrowed, notched, or rounded, within the limits of the enamel of course, to make them appear more natural. Until recently dentists had no simple method at their disposal for reshaping teeth except to crown them. Thanks to the acid etch and bonding techniques, certain teeth can be lengthened, widened, and reshaped. It should be borne in mind, however, that bonding has its technologic limitations and composite resin is not as permanent as enamel or porcelain. Figure 5–3 illustrates the effects of combined grinding and bonding to make canines look like lateral incisors.

Compatibility must be present between the size of the teeth and the space they are to fill. Nature does not automatically produce this balance. One person may have a broad full arch but only small teeth to fill it; the next person may have a small arch with teeth too large for the space. The former creates spaces between the teeth; the latter, bunched and overlapped incisors.

Correction of this imbalance through operative dentistry is more readily accomplished with maxillary than with mandibular teeth. Moreover, lower teeth are more inclined toward incisal corner overlap, probably because their incisal edges are thinner and more likely to slip by each other from the forces of mesial drift that are directed against them (Fig. 5–4).

Correction of this condition by crowning, as mentioned earlier, is a

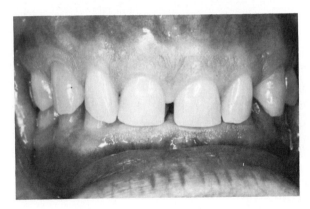

Figure 5–5. Steep overbite with inward inclination of the incisal edges of the maxillary teeth. This is in marked contrast to an open space (see Figure 5–8) between the incisors. Deep overbites are often associated with powerful musculature in the lower lip.

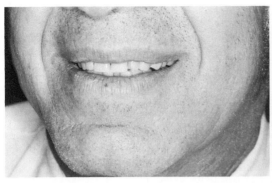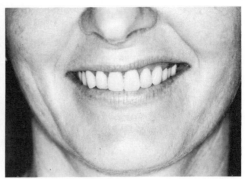

Figure 5–6. Gender is apparent in the two photographs above. Particularly note the prominent mental process of the mandible of the male. (Courtesy of Dr. Joseph A. Grasso)

common practice for maxillary overlap, but it is not commonly done in mandibulars. Lower incisors are small and delicate, with flat rather than round roots, a combination that makes tooth preparation and fitting of the crowns quite difficult. Moreover, fabrication of the crowns in the laboratory presents technologic problems, especially with regard to producing a natural-looking incisal edge.

Vertical as well as horizontal angulations of the facial surface are important in producing a harmonious appearance. Protruding teeth that are tipped outward are obvious to the viewer, as are anterior teeth with a steep vertical overlap (Fig. 5–5).

Gender Considerations

Masculine and feminine characteristics can be incorporated into the dentition in order to capture the personality of the patient (Fig. 5–6). Foremost in this regard is the character of the incisal edges. A straight line from canine to canine denotes masculinity, whereas rounded incisal corners allude to femininity. Indeed, this concept can be carried to the individual tooth where a masculine central with its worn straight edge contrasts markedly with the gentle rounded incisal corners of the feminine incisor.

Overlapping is commonly employed by the dentist to depict a hard, aggressive appearance or a soft, gentle one. Central incisors that overlap the lateral incisors show the former, whereas laterals that overlap the centrals demonstrate the latter (Figs. 5–7 to 5–9).

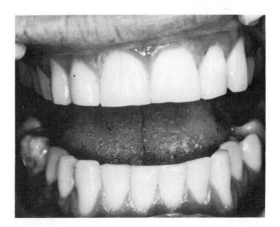

Figure 5–7. A straight incisal edge devoid of curves and rounded corners is a characteristic of masculine teeth, especially maxillary teeth. Compare this picture with the feminine incisal edges shown in Figure 5–1.

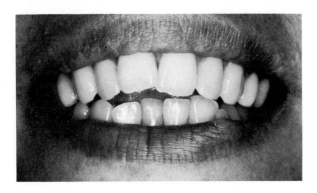

Figure 5–8. This female patient has space between her anterior teeth during closure and subjects her incisors to only minimal stress in biting. In contrast the patient in Figure 5–5 subjects his teeth to maximum stress. Restorations are designed according to the functional needs of the teeth as well as the appearance.

Discolored Teeth

Pearly white teeth are a joy to behold, yet not too many people are blessed with such a perfectly colored dentition. Blemishes in the form of stained restorations, discolored enamel, and internal discoloration are elements with which the operative dentist must contend. Discoloration may involve only one tooth, a filling, or many teeth. Moreover, discoloration may be a surface stain or it may be embedded deep within the structure.

Two factors about enamel must be recognized as one considers the study of tooth color. One factor is the actual color of the tooth; the other is its degree of transparency (translucency).* A piece of paper may have a light blue color, but it will appear markedly different from a stained glass window with the same light blue color. Structural lamination of glasslike enamel supported by opaque dentin creates a most unique arrangement in which shading and color are blended with transparency. Because enamel is thinner toward the root a tooth appears more glassy toward the incisal edge. Because enamel is whiter than underlying dentin, the crown of the tooth is likely to appear darker toward the gingival border than it does at the incisal edge.

In actuality some of the light rays will contact the tooth and be reflected back to the viewer; other rays will pass through the enamel and be reflected off the dentin; and some rays will pass part way through the enamel and be

---

*Translucency: letting light pass through but diffusing it so that objects on the other side cannot be distinguished.

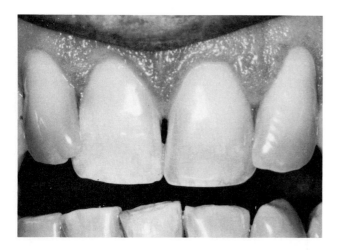

Figure 5–9. Lateral incisors that slightly overlap the centrals provide a soft gentle appearance. Conversely, if central incisors overlap the laterals a harsh severe appearance results.

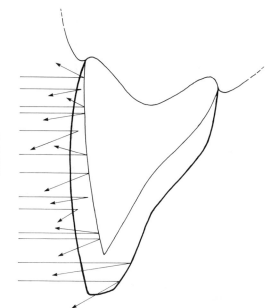

Figure 5–10. Translucency is the ingredient that gives a tooth its lifelike appearance. Because light rays can both pass through and reflect off of the enamel (translucent implies semi-transparent), the overall color blend can yield a pearly white, lifelike color to the dentition.

reflected back to the viewer. The number of rays that are reflected from the enamel in contrast to the dentin, and the surface depth from which they are reflected, determine the relative opacity or translucency of the tooth (Fig. 5–10).

Surface Stains. Surface staining of enamel can be diffuse or it can involve only certain teeth. A very common surface stain is mottled enamel, a defect that causes the enamel to lose its translucency and become opaque. Moreover, its surface texture is rendered soft and capable of absorbing foreign material, which discolors the enamel. The person severely afflicted with fluorosis gradually develops a mottled appearance, with a chalky white color mixed with brown blotches. The cause of mottled enamel is an excess of fluoride in the drinking water of the child during early periods when enamel was being formed (Fig. 5–11).

Another surface stain is observed after or during the carious process. Acid action from plaque, if caries is quite active, leaves the enamel somewhat porous, soft, and chalky white. Porosity in the course of time attracts foreign matter, which becomes embedded therein, causing subsequent dark discoloration. Effective treatment of this stained enamel, whether mottled or carious,

Figure 5–11. Staining of the enamel caused by fluorosis. Although the enamel may actually be softer, it is equally as immune to caries as hard normal enamel. (Courtesy of Dr. Ellen Eisenberg)

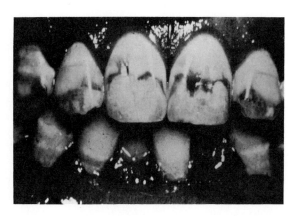

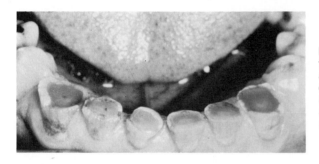

Figure 5–12. Patient with dentinogenesis imperfecta, often called opalescent dentin. Patients afflicted with this congenital abnormality have dentin that is amber colored, insensitive to stimuli, and softer than normal. Notice how badly abraded and shortened the incisors have become at the age of 22.

requires its removal and replacement. This can be done by crowning the tooth with porcelain or by selective replacement with composite resin. Some patients—or patients' mothers—may feel very strongly about the elimination of stained enamel; others, after realizing the difficulty and expense involved in replacement, elect to leave it as it is and ignore the cosmetic deficiency.

Internal Stains. Internal staining is more complex, and treatment requires equally as drastic means as does mottled enamel. Internal staining as a general problem afflicting all the teeth is usually manifested in one of two forms: (1) dentinogenesis imperfecta, a congenital defect in tooth formation characterized by a brownish dentin, or (2) tetracycline staining, a condition brought about by the administration of tetracycline as an antibiotic during tooth formative periods. The enamel and dentin formed during this period, although still sound and intact, acquire a dark gray shade that is quite unsightly (Figs. 5–12 and 5–13).

Internal discoloration is also observed with age. Teeth that have been in service for many years are bound to become darker, owing to a change in color of both the enamel and the dentin.

Internal discoloration of an individual tooth is usually associated with pulp death (Fig. 5–14). Dentin, being the viable structure that it is, is composed of living processes, which degenerate when deprived of their source of nutrients (pulp). The major discoloration that might result from a degenerated pulp occurs from by-products of the pulp that tend to diffuse through the dentin. Depending upon the time lapse between pulp injury (death) and therapy, the dentinal tubules may or may not be infused with by-products from pulp necrosis. Prolonged time before treatment permits irreversible staining of the dentin; early treatment permits effective bleaching to render the tooth white again.

Bleaching is done by opening the pulp chamber from the lingual and exposing the dentin internally to a very strong (30 per cent) solution of H_2O_2.

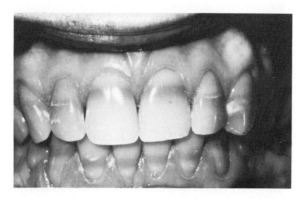

Figure 5–13. A set of beautifully formed and arranged anterior teeth. Unfortunately these teeth during their formative period were stained by systemic administration of tetracycline. This intrinsic staining factor extends deep into the dentin and is characteristic of this particular antibiotic. (Courtesy of Dr. Fred F Simmons)

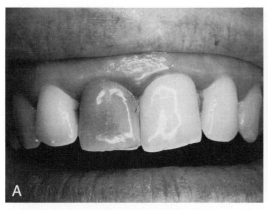
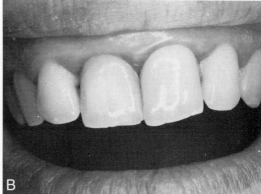

Figure 5–14. *A,* Right central incisor badly stained from decomposition products following pulp death. *B,* After bleaching with H_2O_2 the tooth looks white again.

To augment the oxidation of these organic compounds and render them colorless a high-intensity lamp is often applied from the labial. Although bleaching effectiveness is somewhat unreliable, serial treatments can often produce lasting results if treatment is initiated soon after pulp death and if Fe^{++} ions from hemorrhage (red blood cells) have not permeated the dentinal tubules.

One of the cosmetic problems associated with composite resin pertains to staining. Discoloration of composite resins (see Chapter 10) may occur over a prolonged time period and manifests itself as surface staining and/or as a dark line along the enamel-resin interface (Fig. 5–15). Often this requires replacement of the restoration, depending to some extent upon the wishes of the patient. Reduction in discoloration along cavity margins can be made by the use of acid on the enamel. This process is one whereby acid applied to the enamel dissolves away the smooth polished surface, replacing it with rough microcraters into which unpolymerized resin can flow. Surface adhesion produced by this resin serves as an interlocking enamel glue which, to a degree, resists its dislodgment. This modality, the "acid etch technique" (see Chapter 10), provides the dentist with the means for using resin to cover color blemishes or irregular contours on the facial surface of the enamel.

Spaces Between Anterior Teeth

Many patients resent the appearance that results from spaces frequently created as the permanent teeth assume their position in the dental arch. This

Figure 5–15. Stained composite resin.

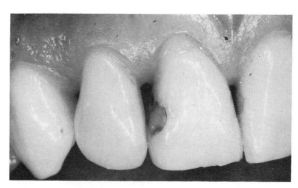

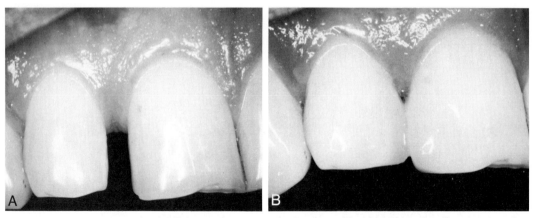

Figure 5–16. The diastema is closed by treating one tooth at a time with acid etching, bonding agent, and a hybrid resin.

occurs most frequently with the upper anterior teeth. Many patients will seek an orthodontic solution to the problem, but many will ignore it for reasons of convenience or economy.

The acid etch and bonding procedures described in Chapter 10 are useful in resolving some of these problems. Although not as durable as ceramic crowns it does provide a reasonable method for improving individual esthetics (Fig. 5–16).

In treatment planning it is determined how and to what extent the space is to be closed or modified. The selected teeth will be enlarged by resin addition to overcome the space problem, and usually the teeth on each side of the space will be expanded equally so as to maintain symmetry.

Following isolation by rubber dam the appropriate portion of the tooth is acid etched and bonded followed by the application of a visible light-activated resin. This allows the operator treating one tooth at a time to place and adapt the resin so as to secure the desired contour and size before exposing it to a visible light system for polymerization. The finishing procedures are the same as those described in Chapter 10.

Metallic Restorative Materials

A half century ago gold, silver, and porcelain composed the "permanent" filling materials for teeth. Today the profession is without great change from yesteryear except that tooth-colored resins are an improvement over the siliceous cements. Metal such as amalgam is more durable and to date has physical properties superior to the tooth-colored materials. Where masticatory forces subject the restoration to greater stresses, e.g., along occlusal and marginal ridges, it is axiomatic that metallic restorations be used. In our culture most people prefer to have teeth restored without the display of metal, e.g., amalgam or gold, so efforts should be made when possible to camouflage metal where it may be unsightly.

Certain locations in the mouth attract attention, whereas other places are very obscure. In descending order of esthetic importance these locations are as follows:

1. Facial surface of maxillary incisors and canines.
2. Incisal edge of mandibular incisors and canines.

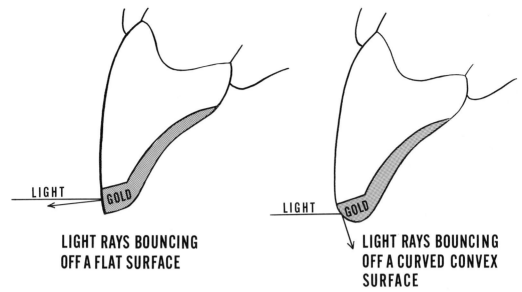

LIGHT RAYS BOUNCING OFF A FLAT SURFACE

LIGHT RAYS BOUNCING OFF A CURVED CONVEX SURFACE

Figure 5–17. Light deflection to reduce the prominence of a gold incisal edge. Light rays are deflected away from the viewer and the gold border appears narrower.

3. Facial surface of maxillary premolars. Facial surface of mandibular anteriors.

4. Occlusal surface of mandibular premolars. Facial surface of maxillary 1st molars.

5. Buccal surface of mandibular premolars. Occlusal surface of mandibular molars.

6. Occlusal surface of maxillary posteriors.

7. Lingual surface of anterior teeth.

8. Lingual surface of posterior teeth.

Like a mirror, polished gold tends to reflect light back to the viewer, who, at conversational distance, faces the patient. In contrast to anterior teeth, whose facial surfaces are clearly visible, posterior teeth are somewhat hidden, as they are farther away and facing outward. Mesial slopes of buccal surfaces and mesial ridges of buccal cusps are more visible, naturally, than are distal slopes. A large mesial restoration in gold that is displayed in the buccal embrasure is less acceptable than a distal restoration of comparable size. It behooves the operator therefore to design cast gold restorations with this in

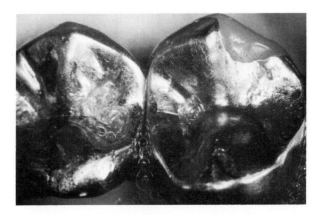

Figure 5–18. Close-up occlusal view of maxillary right first premolar. In an effort to minimize the amount of gold that will be displayed, the mesial cusp ridge of the buccal cusp was left intact and the gold margin finished lingual to it.

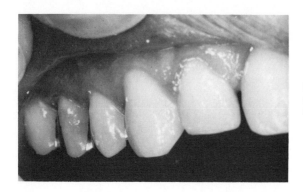

Figure 5–19. Buccal view of same tooth. Aside from a thin strip in the buccal embrasure, the conservative casting for this tooth is virtually invisible.

mind and to be most cautious in removing enamel unnecessarily in these srategically esthetic areas (Figs. 5–17, 5–18, and 5–19).

Light reflected against polished metal surfaces (gold) under certain conditions in the mouth presents optical illusions. A gold restoration, for example, replacing only one of the surfaces forming a buccal embrasure, will appear to be a gold color because much of the light striking it is white light reflected from the white enamel of the adjacent tooth. However, when two gold restorations, placed back to back, form the embrasure, the light rays are absorbed by the first restoration, leaving no light rays to be reflected back toward the viewer. The end result is a dark spot, appearing to the viewer as a hole between the teeth (Fig. 5–20).

On occasion the operative dentist is called upon to place a metallic (amalgam) restoration directly underneath some translucent enamel. To prevent a dark or gold metallic cast from shining through the enamel, the operator may coat the inside of the enamel with a thin layer of a white cement, thereby masking the unsightly effects from metal (see Fig. 13–45).

A fractured incisor, as mentioned in an earlier chapter, is an esthetic blemish that should be corrected. Ordinary methods of restoration of a fractured incisor are (1) radical replacement with a full crown or (2) acid etching of the enamel and replacement of the missing part with a tooth-colored resin (Chapter 10). Because of insult to the pulp required in placing a full crown and because of the cost involved in fusing porcelain to a metal crown, the dentist generally uses the second option. A third method, although not often employed, is the use of a gold casting with an esthetic window. The strength and support of a gold casting is comparable to porcelain; it is more conservative than a full gold crown; and it is somewhat less expensive than the porcelain crown. Anchored to the tooth with grooves and pins, the gold

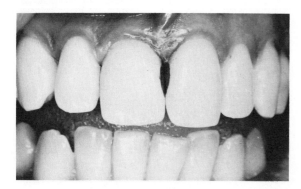

Figure 5–20. Gold restorations facing each other. Despite the degree of polish imparted to these restorations, they will appear dark, as though a berry seed were caught between the teeth.

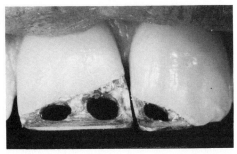

Figure 5–21. Pin-retained casting cemented to a tooth. Open space that remains will receive composite resin of the proper color.

restoration is cemented, after which the open area is filled in with a properly colored composite resin (Fig. 5–21).

Absence of Teeth

When a tooth is lost, the gingiva recedes, producing a saddle-shaped ridge between the adjacent teeth. On observation the loss of the tooth is obvious, but the loss of the two gingival papillae mesial and distal to the space escapes unnoticed. In replacing this tooth with a fixed bridge this papilla loss often becomes apparent and makes natural-looking replacements most dfficult. What formerly appeared as pink interseptal gum tissue now appears as open spaces (Fig. 5–22). The unnatural appearance, as it catches the eye, is not interpreted as open spaces; it is viewed by the eye as dark spots, especially in mouths in which they contrast with large pink gingival papillae adjacent to them.

Replacement of the missing tooth to mask out this illusion is possible with some discrete manipulation in fitting the replacement tooth (pontic). Instead of utilizing a normal contact point relationship, the convex contacting surface is altered to make it concave so the mesio-distal dimension of the tooth is broader in its gingival half. The gingival embrasures are thereby reduced in size, and the absence of the papillae goes by unnoticed (Fig. 5–23).

Esthetics for Operative Procedures

The operative dentist must consider the esthetic result when designing preparations. The operator should give close attention to the natural contours and angulations that exist in all teeth and when possible place margins so as to complement the esthetic sense.

The class III restoration with limited facial extension but with a reasonable

Figure 5–22. Problem in esthetics caused by missing gingiva. Teeth with narrow necks show more gingiva than teeth that are more square. This patient had some recession following the loss of her left central.

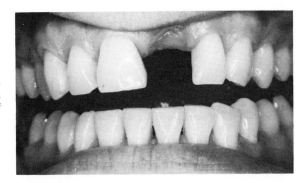

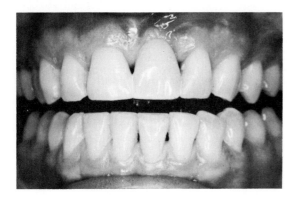

Figure 5–23. To offset these open spaces the false tooth (pontic) was made wider, especially at the gingival end. Although a wider tooth does camouflage these two "holes," they still appear as a blemish to the smile.

gingival-to-incisal length that conforms to the natural coronal inclinations and angles is frequently not as conspicuous as a much smaller restoration that has the same facial extension (Fig. 5–24).

When placing gingival metallic restorations that are confined below the cervical height of contour, esthetics are better when the mesial and distal margins are covered by the marginal gingiva, as compared with those that barely escape marginal coverage.

The design of castings should reflect the best possible esthetics. The mesial and most of the facial margins are obvious and should be placed so as to minimize display of metal if it can be done with minimal risk to the security of the restoration. In contrast, the margins that occur distal to the facial height of contour can be placed with greater esthetic freedom. These considerations will influence all preparations that will be considered.

Cosmetic factors are personal and may mean much more to one person than to another. Many patients are willing to sacrifice durability, strength, and economics in order to achieve the utmost in esthetics. On the other hand, many patients are more concerned with strength, function, and cost, with esthetics playing a secondary role. Thus, the dentist arrives at the appropriate restorative procedure after weighing the priority of these considerations.

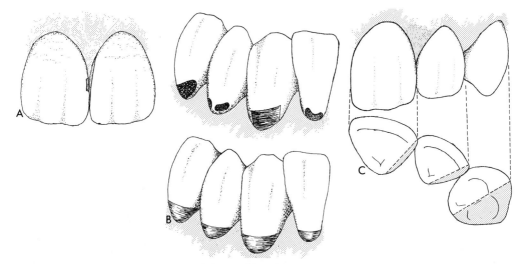

Figure 5–24. *A,* With equal facial extension and color mismatch, a short gingival-to-incisal restoration may not be as esthetic as a restoration with greater length. *B,* Gingival restorations with a continuous incisal or occlusal line with the remaining margins covered with the free gingiva are more esthetic when compared to restorations with ad lib margins. *C,* As the preparations move distally there is greater leeway for margins and good esthetics on the facial segments of teeth.

6

INSTRUMENT GRASPS AND OPERATING CONSIDERATIONS

As observed in Chapter 2, the method of tooth reduction and cavity preparation is largely mechanical in nature. Besides being a physician of the mouth, the operative dentist must also be a biologically oriented engineer and machinist. Accuracy and delicate skills are particularly important for the operative dentist. Whereas bone and soft tissue can regenerate from crude or inaccurate cutting, dentin and enamel will not regrow. The dentist therefore must be very conscious of the protection of his patient from poorly directed movements from cutting instruments and rotating burs. Although a dentist can be forgiven many mistakes, few patients are willing to be charitable toward a careless dentist whose hand slips while operating and permits the instrument to gouge the gingiva. Moreover, apparent carelessness can result in a lack of confidence by the patient. Patients can readily detect such an operator, and many a patient has defected to another dentist solely for this reason. Control, therefore, is the basic issue and the essential ingredient of a good operator.

In a machine shop, the metal part or the cutting tool would be clamped rigidly in a vise or in a chuck. In the mouth or in the dental laboratory this is not possible. The dentist with his hands and body must provide the rigidity and bracing so necessary in achieving control against unwanted movement. In the mouth the hands or fingers of an operator should be firmly braced against the teeth (Figs. 6–1, 6–2, and 6–3). Maxillary teeth, incidentally, provide better support than mandibular teeth because they are attached directly to the skull rather than a moveable bone (mandible).

Most prior experiences in school that require digital expertise, e.g., writing with a pen or using a typewriter or a computer, require only light forces of barely an ounce of pressure. Operative dentistry, on the other hand, requires controlled pressure of six to eight pounds in many procedures. Moreover, these forces must be applied repeatedly without tiring the hand. Therefore, it behooves one to know what forces his hands can generate and be able to apply this force to a dental instrument in a manner so that the force will be under perfect control. Figure 6–4 illustrates a pressure gauge for measuring a force applied through an instrument.

Strengthening the hand and fingers so these forces can be developed is an individual responsibility. Squeezing a rubber ball and other hand-strengthening exercises can, over a period of time, develop the muscles toward this end.

Movements are more easily controlled if the bracing point is as close to

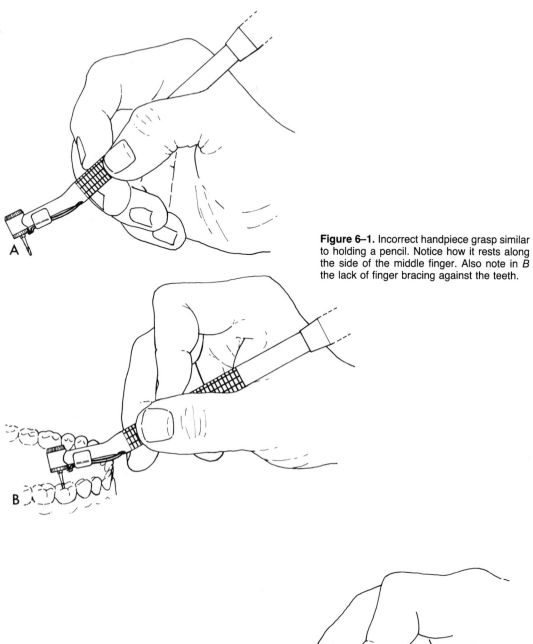

Figure 6–1. Incorrect handpiece grasp similar to holding a pencil. Notice how it rests along the side of the middle finger. Also note in *B* the lack of finger bracing against the teeth.

Figure 6–2. Ring finger braced against the teeth. Note correct grasp of handpiece with the end, not the side, of the middle finger engaging the handpiece.

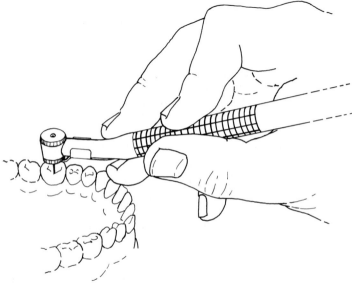

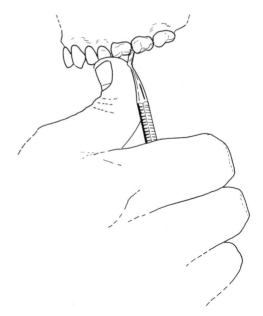

Figure 6–3. Cutting chisel in use. Note bracing against the teeth with the thumb.

the actual site of the operation as possible. Moreover, the teeth should be dry lest the bracing fingers slip on the coating of mucinous saliva. To accomplish bracing one can frequently use two hands more effectively than one. While holding the handpiece to operate on the opposite side of the mouth, a right-handed dentist may reach his left hand around the patient to stabilize the head of the handpiece with his left hand (Fig. 6–5).

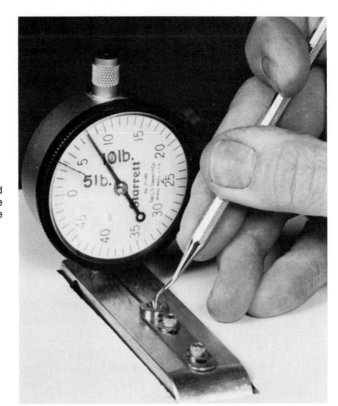

Figure 6–4. Thrusting force being registered on a dial gauge. (Pressure gauges available from George Seifert, 22965 Vista Grande Way, Colton, California 92324.)

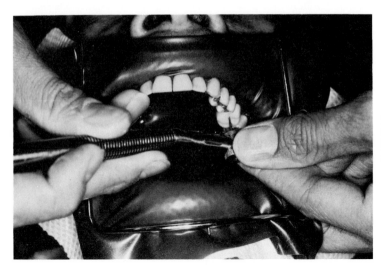

Figure 6–5. Handpiece being held with two hands to enhance bracing. Use of this method for bracing relies on direct vision.

From childhood one becomes accustomed by everyday experience to grasping handles, pencils, or knobs in the most convenient manner. However, past experience and habit patterns do not always lead one to the correct grasp in a new situation. The golf club is a case in point. A novice who has never observed or played the game will invariably hold the club as he would a baseball bat. Similarly, a beginning dental student will be inclined to grasp a dental instrument as he would a pencil (see Fig. 6–1).

As the grasp and swing of a golf club are essential in achieving success on the fairway, dental instrument grasps must be learned and used to achieve success in the operatory. If they are practiced repeatedly, they will soon become second nature to the operator. Correct instrument grasps therefore are important to learn before bad habits are formed. Unfortunately, many dentists in practice today have never learned to hold and use instruments correctly. Like the "hacker" on the golf course, who eventually gets around the course, the dentist does "get the job done," but without the finesse and skill that make him proud of his results or happy and relaxed at the end of a day in the office.

Palm Grasp

The operator can provide himself with two basic instrument grasps: (1) the "pen" grasp, which provides him with more flexibility of movement but less power and (2) the "palm" grasp, which provides only limited movement but with controlled power.

The palm grasp should be cultivated and used whenever possible. As can be seen in Figure 6–6, the instrument is grasped with the thumb serving as a brace. A forward thrust with the arm or wrist can be controlled by the opposing action from the thumb, which is braced against the teeth. Simulating a pair of pliers, the instrument can also be moved laterally with considerable force as it is squeezed toward the thumb.

Unfortunately the power obtained in these two actions, thrust and compression, does not accomplish all the rotating, pulling, and other necessary actions required in instrumentation. A modified palm grasp does help in this regard, however, and should be learned after the palm grasp has been mastered.

While it does not provide as much power as the true palm grasp, it does permit more versatility of movement (Figs. 6–6 through 6–11). While it may seem difficult to learn, once mastered, the modified palm grasp is the most valuable aid in operating inside and outside the mouth.

Pen Grasp

The pen grasp is somewhat misnamed because the dental instrument should not be grasped as one would a writing pen. Figures 6–12 and 6–13 illustrate the difference. It will be noticed that the middle finger must engage the instrument through the fleshy portion (end) rather than the side of the finger. This is necessary in order to obtain the greatest purchase of the instrument, a factor that is not important when writing with a pencil. With the typical pen grasp the instrument is pinched between the thumb and forefinger. The third finger then engages the instrument, care being taken to

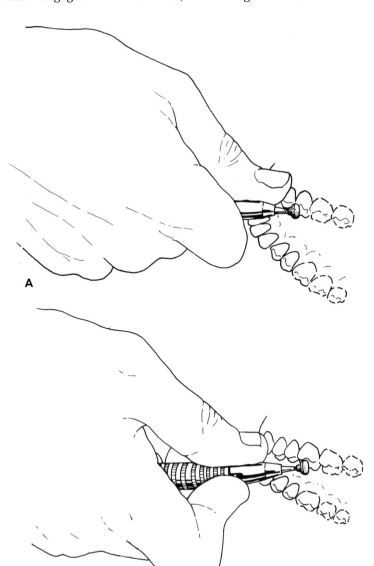

Figure 6–6. *A,* Palm grasp of handpiece with bracing accomplished through the thumb. *B,* Thumb resting against the facial surface or the incisal edge.

A

B

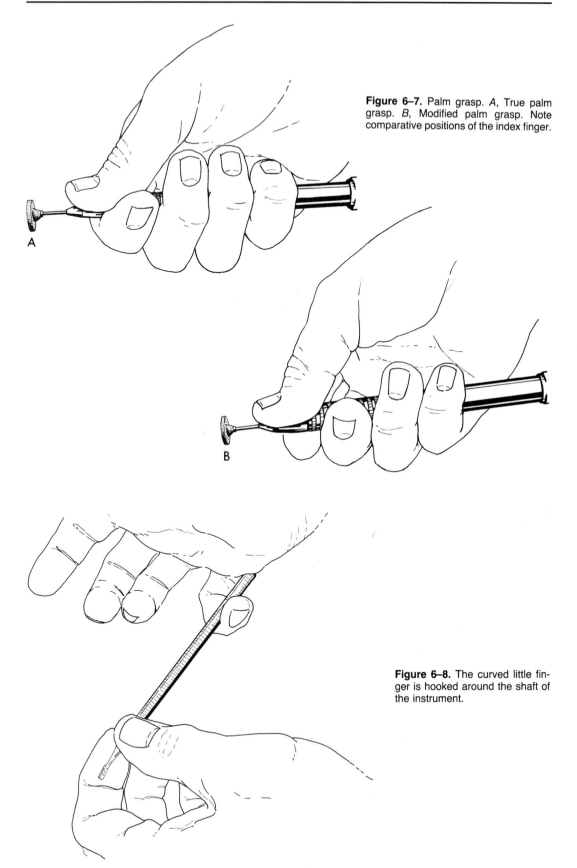

Figure 6–7. Palm grasp. *A,* True palm grasp. *B,* Modified palm grasp. Note comparative positions of the index finger.

Figure 6–8. The curved little finger is hooked around the shaft of the instrument.

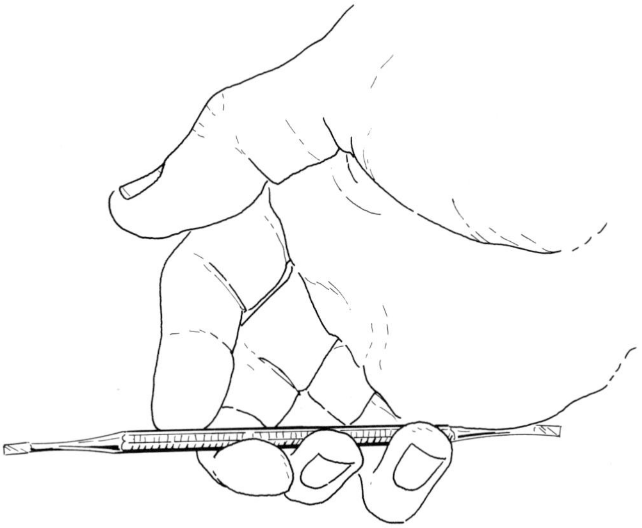

Figure 6–9. The index finger pushes the instrument outward while the ring and little fingers grasp it tightly. The middle finger serves as a stabilizer.

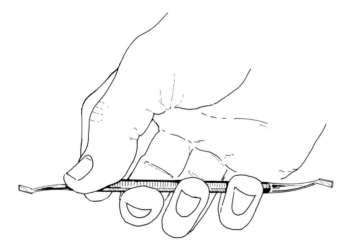

Figure 6–10. Completed grasp. The thumb need not rest heavily against the shaft of the instrument.

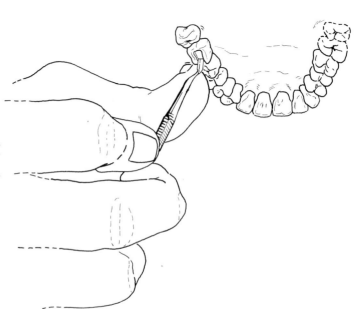

Figure 6–11. Modified palm grasp. A palm grasp, modified or true, is the standard method for grasping the bin-angle chisel for use in the maxillary arch. (See Chapter 11.)

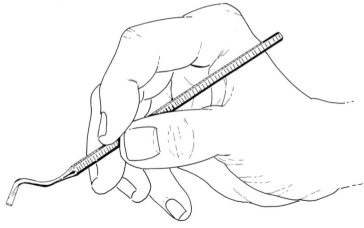

Figure 6–12. Pen grasp as might ordinarily be used for a pen or pencil. This is *incorrect* for a dental instrument.

be sure the shaft does not rest against the side of the finger (Figs. 6–14, 6–15, and 6–16).

Two distinct kinds of "pen" grasps can be identified, depending upon the arm or wrist motion the operator chooses to use. If the operator uses an "up" and "down" chopping motion with action in the wrist, the typical pen grasp is used (Figs. 6–12 and 6–17A). Contrarily, if the operator uses a rotating motion, with the action taking place in the forearm instead of the wrist (Fig. 6–17B), the modified pen grasp is employed. If the operator has strong adductor muscles in the thumb and if pronating actions are comfortable, the latter grasp is preferred. The former grasp is easily learned but the latter, when mastered, is more effective because it uses the arm to transmit controlled power to the instrument (Figs. 6–18 and 6–19).

Because the instrument shaft is small the fingers are inclined to slip during thrusting movements. The recent design of silicone-covered handles* has markedly reduced finger slippage and has improved the general comfort of handling the instruments (Fig. 6–20; see also Fig. 3–54).

---

*Available in various colors from Thompson Dental Mfg. Co., 1201 S. 6th St., Missoula, Montana 59801.

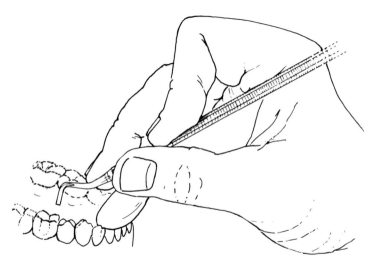

Figure 6–13. Correct pen grasp. The shaft of the instrument is engaged by the end of the middle finger. This one single difference makes the grasp more secure than that shown in Figure 6–12 and provides the operator with more finger power in its usage.

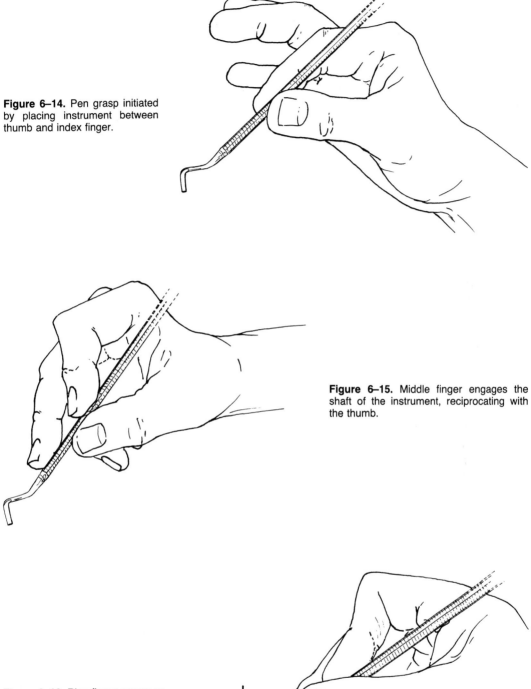

Figure 6–14. Pen grasp initiated by placing instrument between thumb and index finger.

Figure 6–15. Middle finger engages the shaft of the instrument, reciprocating with the thumb.

Figure 6–16. Ring finger serves as a brace against the teeth to permit a thrusting or "chopping" action.

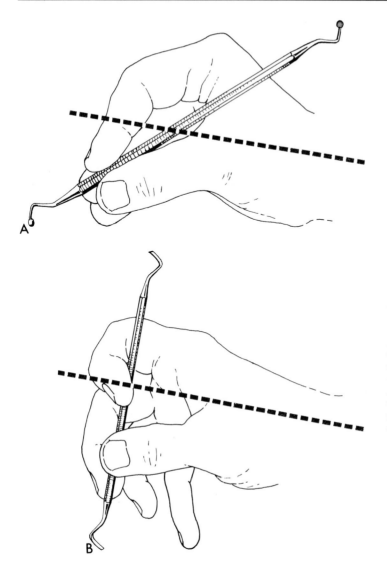

Figure 6–17. Basic difference between pen grasp and modified pen grasp. *A,* Typical pen grasp. *B,* Modified pen grasp. Note the difference in angle formed by the shaft of the instrument and the long axis of the forearm. With a modified pen grasp *(B),* the fingers and thumb engage the instrument as a grappling hook. The base of the index finger and the tip of the middle finger reciprocate, with the thumb placed midway between them. The typical pen grasp *(A)* involves wrist movement; the modified pen grasp involves the forearm, which turns inward (pronates) or outward (supinates). Depending upon the strength of the thumb and individual preferences toward forearm or wrist movement, each operator will select the grasp most comfortable for him.

With respect to the modified pen grasp (Fig. 6–17B) the two salient features are a straight wrist and a curved index finger. In many respects the instrument is held like a teaspoon. Reciprocal grasping occurs with the thumb positioned midway between the middle and index fingers. In Figure 6–17B attention is also called to the 90° angle formed by the instrument and the long axis of the arm and wrist. Because of its viselike grip the instrument is not inclined to slip.

The pen grasp gives the operator the greatest versatility of movement, but bracing is difficult because only the ring finger *and the little finger* can be used (see Fig. 6–2). These fingers can readily slip off the teeth, particularly if the surface is wet with saliva. Precautionary measures dictate, therefore, that the bracing area be dry (isolated with the rubber dam is best) and that priority always be given to bracing before any cutting is done to the teeth.

It is not possible to specify whether an operator should use a palm grasp or a pen grasp. It is possible, however, for the beginning operative dentist to discipline himself and adhere to the cardinal rules that (a) bracing with the thumb or fingers always exist whenever cutting or grinding in the laboratory or in the mouth, and (b) bracing always be moved as closely as possible to

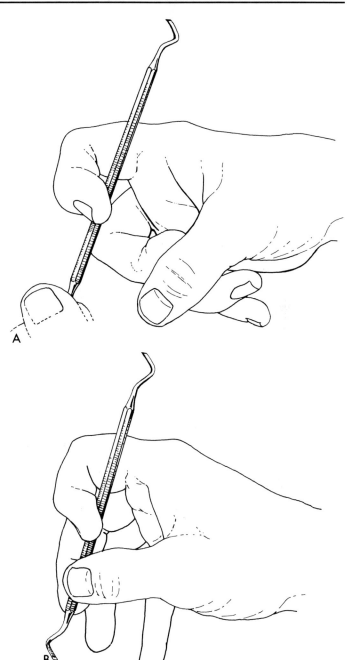

Figure 6–18. Additional stability for instrument. *A,* Certain people with supple joints can engage the shaft by locking it within the curve of the index finger. *B,* Instrument ready for use.

the point of contact between the instrument and the tooth. By initial training in this regard he will develop habits that have application in other disciplines such as oral surgery and periodontics, as well as in performing procedures outside the mouth (Figs. 6–21 through 6–26).

Mirrors

In any operating procedure clear and distinct vision is important. Direct vision should be employed wherever possible, particularly if the presence of

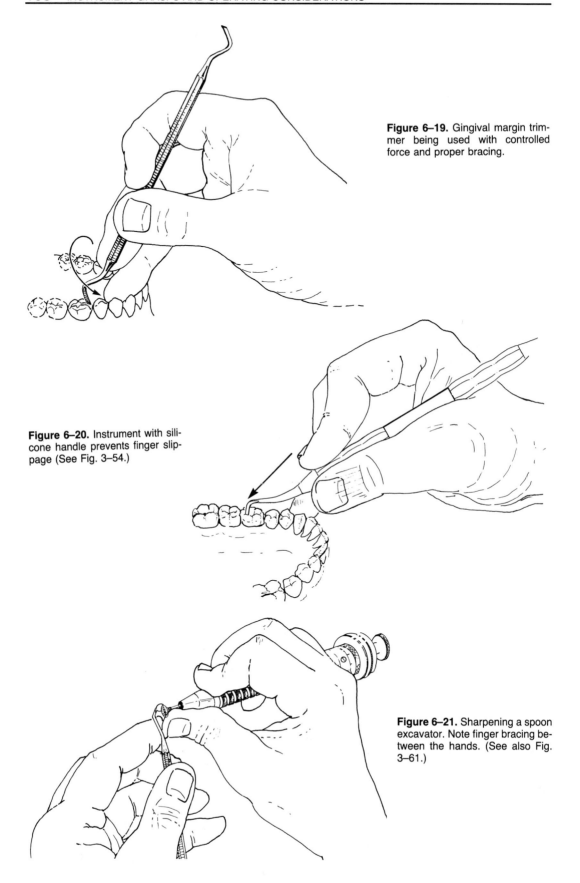

Figure 6–19. Gingival margin trimmer being used with controlled force and proper bracing.

Figure 6–20. Instrument with silicone handle prevents finger slippage (See Fig. 3–54.)

Figure 6–21. Sharpening a spoon excavator. Note finger bracing between the hands. (See also Fig. 3–61.)

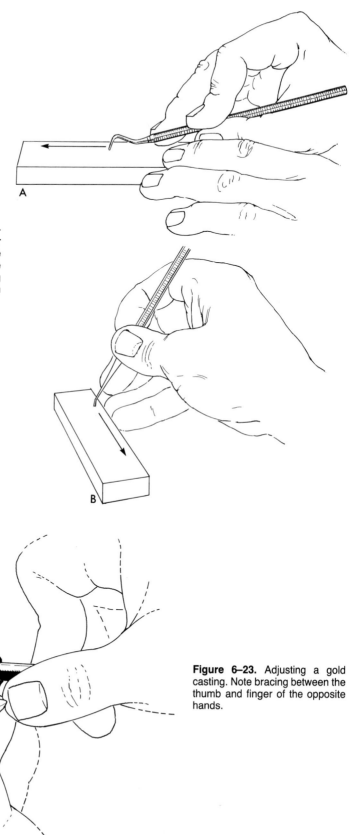

Figure 6–22. Sharpening hand instruments. Please note finger positions for grasping the instruments. *A,* Off-angle hatchet, pushing action. *B,* Mon-angle hoe, pulling action. Note the gliding support provided by the 4th and 5th fingers. (See also Fig. 3–55*A.*)

Figure 6–23. Adjusting a gold casting. Note bracing between the thumb and finger of the opposite hands.

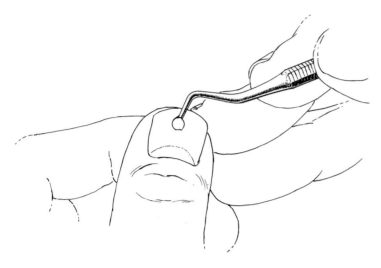

Figure 6–24. Bracing the fingers while testing the sharpness of an excavator.

the mouth mirror will obscure working access. As a dental tool or instrument the mouth mirror is quite unique. Foremost as a mirror it affords the operator an opportunity to see into obscure areas of the mouth and to observe procedures (Fig. 6–27). Nearly as important is its function as a reflector of the operating light. When the operating light enters the mouth it leaves lingual and posterior sides of the teeth in the shadows. A correctly placed mirror reflects the light to illuminate these regions, simultaneously providing vision to the operator. A third function of the mirror is as a "shoe horn." As a paddle it can reflect the tongue or the cheek for insertion of cotton rolls or for general operating access (Fig. 6–28).

In the early training of a dental student one of the most annoying procedures to master is learning to work effectively in a mirror. Hand and eye coordination must become as efficient through the mirror as by direct vision. The best way to master the mouth mirror is to practice with it repeatedly until

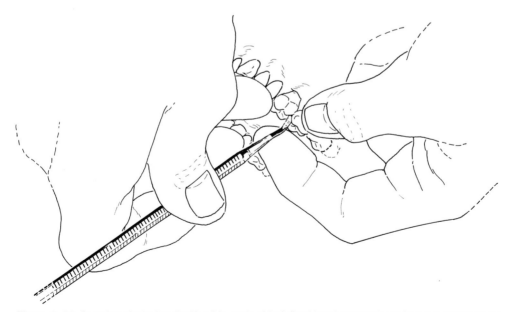

Figure 6–25. Scraping gingival wall with a bin-angle chisel. Dual hand action: the right hand stabilizes the chisel in position while the index finger of the left hand pulls the shank toward the buccal.

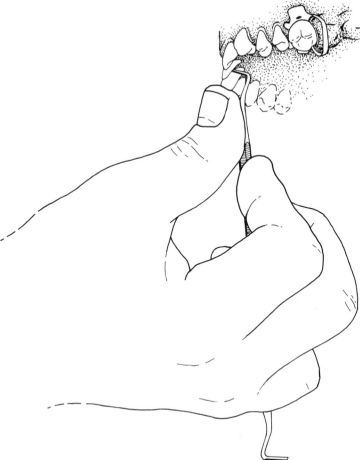

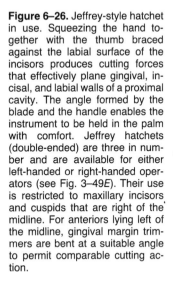

Figure 6–26. Jeffrey-style hatchet in use. Squeezing the hand together with the thumb braced against the labial surface of the incisors produces cutting forces that effectively plane gingival, incisal, and labial walls of a proximal cavity. The angle formed by the blade and the handle enables the instrument to be held in the palm with comfort. Jeffrey hatchets (double-ended) are three in number and are available for either left-handed or right-handed operators (see Fig. 3–49E). Their use is restricted to maxillary incisors and cuspids that are right of the midline. For anteriors lying left of the midline, gingival margin trimmers are bent at a suitable angle to permit comparable cutting action.

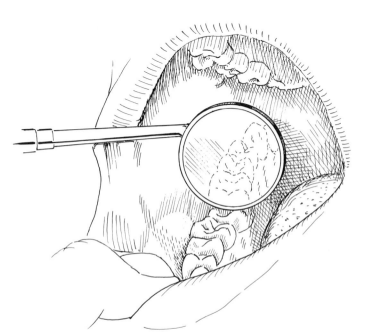

Figure 6–27. The dental mirror. Besides enhancing vision it reflects light to the operating area.

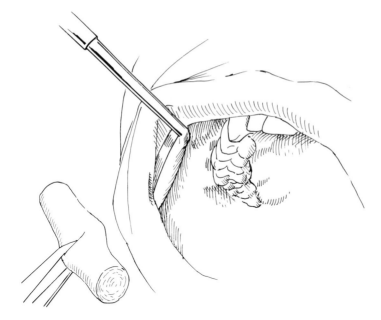

Figure 6–28. Mouth mirror being used to retract the cheek to permit insertion of a cotton roll into the maxillary vestibule.

it does not seem awkward. At some point in time the student will realize that he is effectively using the mirror, but he will not be aware of the precise time at which this learning took place.

It behooves the operator to keep his mirror clean, to avoid scratching its surface with revolving stones, and to replace it with a new one when worn. Mirrors are either regular or front surface: the latter are silvered on the outer surface of the glass; the former are silvered on the inner side. Front surface mirrors, although more susceptible to scratching, are much to be preferred over the regular type because they do not produce double images.

Mirrors come in a variety of sizes and with flat and convex (magnifying) surfaces (Fig. 6–29). The No. 4 mirror without magnification is the standard size used, although individual preferences and specific conditions may cause the operator to use larger or smaller sizes.

Tactile sense augments vision and should be learned as quickly as possible. In certain regions of the mouth, e.g., distal surfaces of maxillary left molars, lack of space frequently prevents use of the mirror while working with the handpiece. In these instances one must work as best he can with direct vision and tactile sense, stopping frequently to insert the mirror to observe progress of the procedure.

Eye-hand coordination is probably not more important in any profession than in dentistry. Without being able to see minute details in the operating area, skillful and exacting procedures are most difficult to execute.

Being able to "see" is dependent upon several factors: good light; the elimination of fluid films on the surface, which distort light rays; and a suitable working distance so small surface details can come into focus.

Recent light systems using fiber optics have become very popular, particularly those that illuminate the bur and working area through the handpiece (Fig. 6–30). These should be used in conjunction with the traditional operating light to avoid dark peripheral intra-oral shadows, which can be very tiring to the eyes of the operator.

A washed field technique has been most valuable for bulk reduction in tooth preparation. However, the time comes when one must dry the tooth and

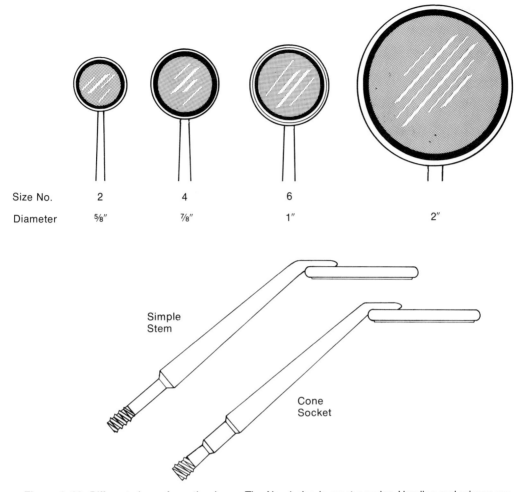

Size No.   2   4   6

Diameter   5/8"   7/8"   1"   2"

Simple Stem

Cone Socket

Figure 6–29. Different sizes of mouth mirrors. The No. 4 size is most popular. Handles and mirrors are sold separately because of the short life span of the mirrors. "Simple stem" or "cone socket" mirrors must match the same type of handle. They are not interchangeable. The largest size (2"diameter) is used for viewing parallelism in multiple crown preparations.

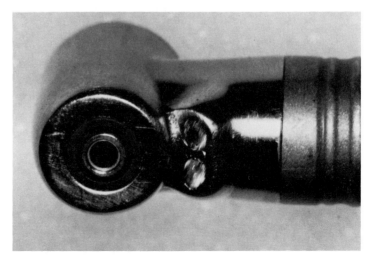

Figure 6–30. Self-illuminating high-speed handpiece. Note two bundles of fiber optics, which disseminate the light over the working area.

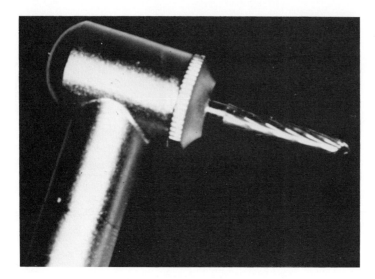

Figure 6–31. Multi-bladed carbide finishing bur in a slow-speed handpiece. This gear-driven handpiece requires more pressure to cut dentin, which in turn provides better tactile sense and better visibility for greater accuracy.

with deft movements delicately refine surface details on margins and elsewhere in the tooth preparation. For this refinement a dry field is essential and, where crown preparations are concerned, a proper instrument driven by slow speed under close visual scrutiny is extremely important (Fig. 6–31).

Working distances are of little consequence to the young operator who still has good focal accommodation. For those who reach the 40s, however, magnification becomes necessary for many in the profession. Several types of magnifiers are helpful. Many who wear glasses prefer a kind of headband to support magnifying lenses (Fig. 6–32), whereas a magnifying attachment that clips to the glasses themselves is also quite popular (Fig. 6–33). If the operator is not comfortable working at a distance of 16 inches or less, he should seriously consider obtaining one of these auxiliary aids.

Eye protection is becoming more and more important as sophisticated techniques come into the dental office. Water sprays and infectious foreign elements are hazardous when working around the mouth. Plastic protective glasses are definitely indicated for both the operator and dental assistant who are not already wearing corrective lenses. These along with the protective face mask should be available for use when needed.

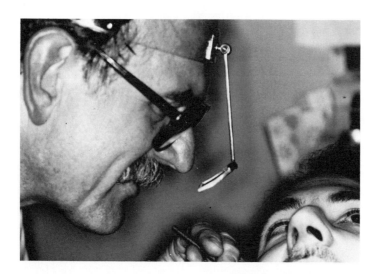

Figure 6–32. Magnifying lenses supported by a headband (available from Atwood Industries, P.O. Box 655, Tarzana, California 91356).

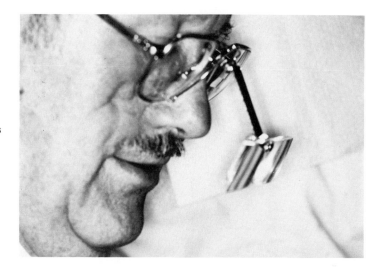

Figure 6–33. Magnifying glasses that clip onto existing glasses.

There is an increase occurring in the use of visible light as a means of curing composite resins. Normal preventive precautions are required as would be expected with any bright source of light. Those who find themselves utilizing visible curing lights several times in the course of a day should consider the added precaution of wearing suitable glasses; this includes both operator and assistant (Fig. 6–34). These tinted glasses are available from a number of sources.*

Operating Positions

Needless to mention, the operator must be in a comfortable position in which he can manipulate instruments properly. Patients are usually reclined in a supine position so that both operator and assistant can be seated comfortably on each side of the patient. The right-handed operator seats himself on the right side of the patient with the dental assistant on the left

---

*Buffalo Dental Mfg. Co., 575 Underhill Blvd., Syosset, New York 11791; Dioptics Professional Products, 10015 Muirlands Parkway Suite "E," Irvine, California 92714.

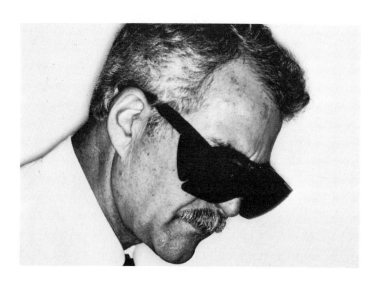

Figure 6–34. Dark glasses (with side panels) made from plastic. These may be worn by dentist and assistant when using the high-intensity visible light for curing composite resin.

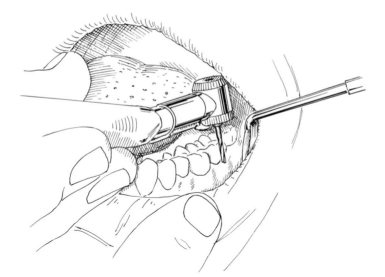

Figure 6–35. Operating in the lower left quadrant, right-handed operator. Operator is on the patient's right side just behind the head. Operator's right hand holds the handpiece with a direct frontal approach. Notice fingers braced on the left anterior teeth. This position is good for preparing most of the tooth surfaces.

side; the left-handed operator and his assistant are seated in the reverse positions. Literature and audiovisual material freely describe work simplification concepts and effective dental assistant utilization. Consequently, these topics will not be covered in this chapter.

Despite the need for improved efficiency, nothing should be incorporated into the procedure that will hamper the operator as he controls his instruments and manipulates instruments with precision. Figures 6–35, 6–36, 6–37, 6–38, 6–39, 6–40, and 6–41 illustrate a variety of hand and mirror positions for the four posterior quadrants of the mouth. One should observe the bracing and support that can be achieved with these respective positions and practice them on a manikin or a fellow student.

The dentist operates alone or with a dental assistant. Wherever possible he utilizes a dental assistant to perform functions such as passing instruments, mixing amalgam, aspirating saliva, and so on. His working methods should enable him to operate effectively alone if necessary (Figs. 6–42 and 6–43).

The operator should be able to operate in either a seated or a standing position. Of foremost importance in any operation is that the body should not be wrenched out of its physiologic form. Musculoskeletal problems can develop after years of bad postural practices. In this regard it is necessary for the operator and his assistant to feel comfortable, regardless of the task they are performing (Figs. 6–44, 6–45, 6–46, and 6–50).

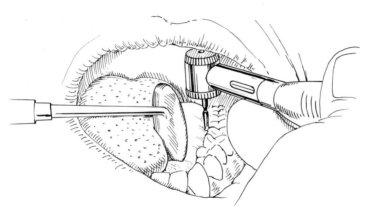

Figure 6–36. Operating in the lower left quadrant, right-handed operator. Operator is seated in front of the patient and the approach is from the side as the patient's head is turned toward the operator. Note the bracing in the region of the first molar. This position is good for instrumenting lingual surfaces. Another advantage is that it permits better direct vision of the operating area. In this position and that shown in Figure 6–35 the tip of the high-velocity evacuator can substitute for the mirror to control the cheek and the tongue.

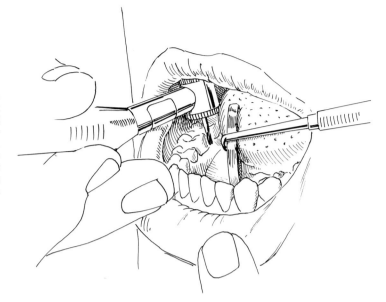

Figure 6–37. Common position for operating in the lower right quadrant is comparable to that shown in Figure 6–36. This drawing illustrates another approach. The operator is seated behind the patient. The ring finger can be moved backward as far as the molars to provide bracing and lip retraction.

If he is right-handed, the operator will operate on the right side of the patient from a 7:00 o'clock to an 11:00 o'clock position. (Conversely, a left-handed operator will do likewise but on the patient's left side.) Most of the time the dentist will be operating alongside (9:00 o'clock position) or to the rear (11:00 o'clock position) of the patient because most maxillary procedures and many mandibular ones are done from these operator locations (Fig. 6–47).

Frequently a frontal operating position includes the elevation of the patient's head (Fig. 6–43). Seated somewhat behind the patient using a mouth mirror is the most universal position from which the dentist operates, however (Fig. 6–48).

Another variable with regard to chair position is the chair adjustment. As can be observed in Figure 6–42 the patient is in a supine position. In many

Text continued on page 122

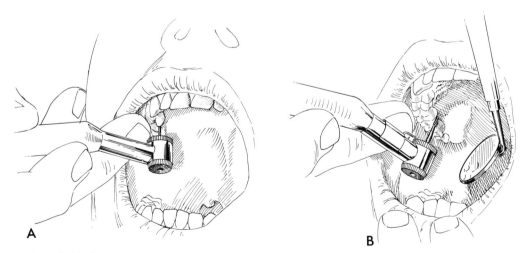

A   **B**

Figure 6–38. Operating position in maxillary right quadrant, right-handed operator. *A* and *B,* The operator is seated behind the patient, working entirely with a mirror. Bracing occurs as far posteriorly as possible. The ultimate in bracing occurs when the ring finger rests on the tooth adjacent to the one being operated on and the handpiece in turn rests on the fingernail. A modified pen grasp is used for this position.

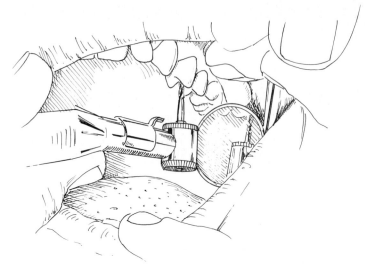

Figure 6–39. Operating position for maxillary left quadrant, right-handed operator seated behind patient's head, with the patient's head turned toward the operator. Bracing is located as close as possible to the operating site. Standard pen grasp is used. On occasion, cross-arch bracing can be accomplished by stabilizing the head of the handpiece with the left hand while primary bracing is done on the occlusal surface of the right premolars. Without obstruction from equipment and knuckles direct vision is now possible. (See Fig. 6–5.)

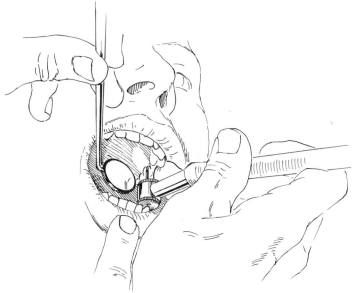

Figure 6–40. Operating position for maxillary posteriors, lingual surfaces. Operator is seated in front of the patient, whose head is tipped back, and direct vision is used. The primary function of the mirror is to reflect light. A modified pen grasp is used and bracing is accomplished by placing the tip of the ring finger on the buccal surface of the tooth being operated on.

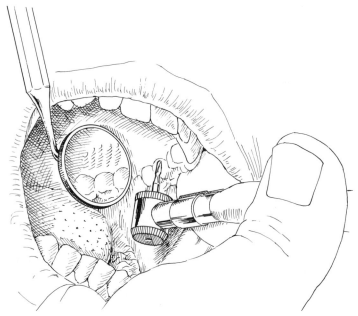

Figure 6–41. Closeup of Figure 6–40. There is very little, if any, movement in the wrist or fingers. Pronating and supinating movements of the forearm cause the hand and handpiece, as a fixed unit, to rotate (pivot) around the tip of the ring finger and the long axis of the tooth.

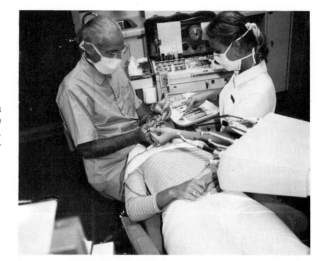

Figure 6–42. Operator and assistant work as a team with the patient in a supine position. The maxillary left quadrant is receiving attention. (From Kilpatrick, H. C., Functional Dental Assisting. W. B. Saunders Co., 1977)

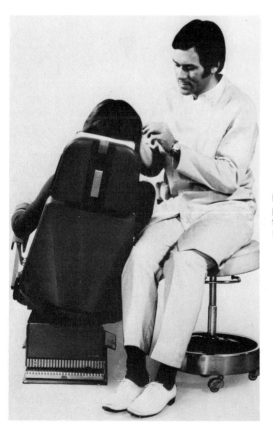

Figure 6–43. Operator is working alone from the 8 o'clock position. Mandibular teeth are receiving attention. Notice the semi-upright chair position. (From Kilpatrick, H. C., Functional Dental Assisting. W. B. Saunders Co., 1977)

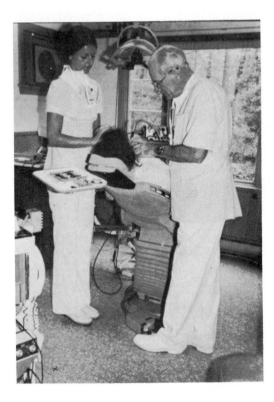

Figure 6–44. Dentist and assistant standing comfortably while operating in the lower left quadrant from a 7 or 8 o'clock position. (From Kilpatrick, H. C., Functional Dental Assisting. W. B. Saunders Co., 1977)

Figure 6–45. Typical use of "four-handed dentistry." The operator controls the handpiece and mouth mirror; the dental assistant controls the high-velocity evacuation system and the air-water syringe. (Courtesy of Jonelle Self)

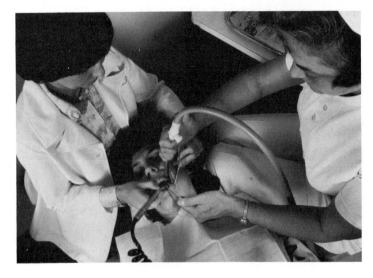

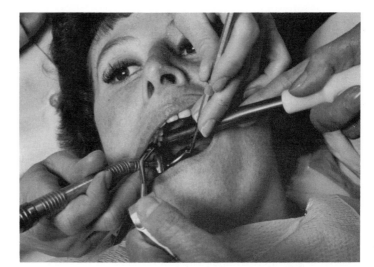

Figure 6–46. Close-up view of "four-handed dental operation." (Courtesy of Jonelle Self)

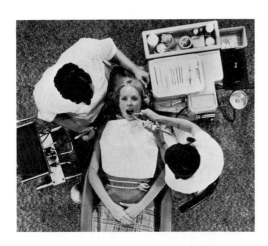

Figure 6–47. In this supine position of the patient, notice the 10 o'clock position of the operator. (From Kilpatrick, H. C., Functional Dental Assisting. W. B. Saunders Co., 1977)

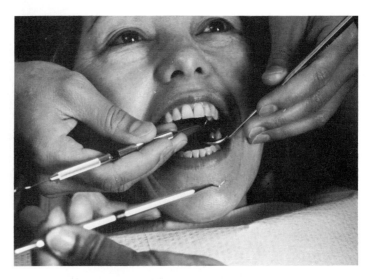

Figure 6–48. Examining the maxillary left teeth from behind the patient (11:00 position). Notice the ring finger is braced against the tip of the right cuspid. (Courtesy of Jonelle Self)

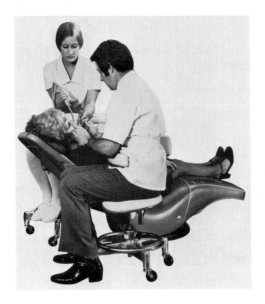

Figure 6–49. Patient seated in a 45 degree position. The mandibular right quadrant is receiving treatment. Notice how the thighs are parallel with the floor and the dental assistant is working from a higher elevation than the dentist. (From Kilpatrick H. C., Functional Dental Assisting. W. B. Saunders Co., 1977)

respects this is an ideal position, except for easy aspiration of foreign bodies. Also, in this position impression material is more likely to run out the end of the tray and down the patient's throat, whereas an impression taken with the occlusal plane more level with the floor is less likely to be affected by gravity (Fig. 6–49).

Figure 6–50. Incorrect and uncomfortable operating position. Notice how the operator is hunched over the patient and probably not very comfortable. (Courtesy of Jonelle Self)

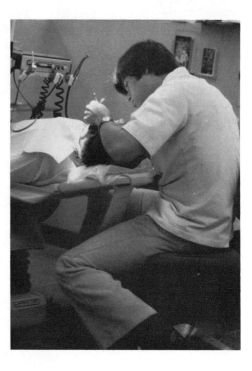

7

LINERS AND CEMENTS
(Bases and Luting Materials)

Cleansing the Preparation Surface

Following cavity preparation the enamel and dentin surfaces are generally covered with a thin layer of tenacious debris. This debris is referred to as the "smear layer" (Fig. 7–1). Also the cavity preparation may be covered with a thin film of cement such as zinc oxide–eugenol, if a temporary restoration was placed. Unless this film of debris is removed it may interfere with the physical characteristics of some materials or with the quality of their adaptability or adhesion to cavity walls. Optimum behavior of a dental cement, particularly the polyacrylic acid systems, is markedly influenced by the surface cleanliness of tooth structure at the time of placement.

A primary consideration in the selection of a cleansing agent is its biologic character. It must cleanse without producing irritation to the pulp. From this standpoint, irrigation with water is a common procedure, as it is safe and convenient and will cleanse reasonably well. Actually, the best means of removing the smear layer is by scrubbing the surface with a pumice wash. If water does not seem adequate, a solution of 2 or 3 per cent hydrogen peroxide may be used on a pellet of cotton to scrub the cavity walls (Fig. 7–2). Following this, the preparation is rinsed with water and gently air dried. If the highspeed instrument emits oil with the water spray, it may be necessary to use a commercial solution in order to remove traces of oil from a preparation or temporary restoration.* Another effective means is a 15-second swabbing of the surface with the polycarboxylate cement liquid. This is a biocompatible medium, as will be noted later, and is an effective cleanser. At least one manufacturer supplies a solution for that purpose. In summary then, particularly when cements are used where a potential adhesion to tooth structure is possible, a meticulously clean surface is essential. However, this must be accomplished without disturbing the living process in the dentin.

Historically, it was recommended that the dentin be sterilized before placement of any restorative material. The rationale prevailing then was that any residual micro-organisms should be eliminated in order to prevent the potential propagation of the caries. Among the chemicals suggested for this purpose were silver nitrate precipitated with eugenol, phenol, thymol, and potassium ferrocyanide.

---

*Cavilax, Premier Dental Products Company, 1710 Romano Dr., Norristown, Pennsylvania 19401.

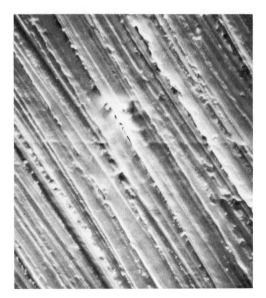

Figure 7–1. "Smeared layer " of dentin.

There is no evidence that any one chemical was superior to the others in this regard nor has the need for cavity sterilization been established. Furthermore, in recent years it has become known that agents such as those mentioned may be irritating to the pulp when applied to dentin surfaces. Thus any chemical that is capable of destroying micro-organisms may also have a detrimental influence on the pulp.

However, as was noted earlier, infiltration of micro-organisms at the tooth-restoration interface can produce microbial activity and acid production. This may then contribute to continuing pulpal irritation. Therefore, in the chapters to follow, care will be given to matters that influence microleakage and thus the health of the tooth.

Liners and Bases

When the preparation is completed, usually some intermediate material will be placed over the dentin before inserting the permanent restoration. The selection of this material is influenced by the proximity of the pulp following

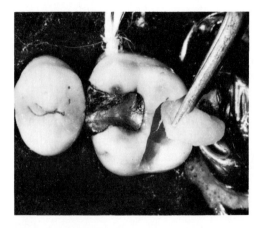

Figure 7–2. Hydrogen peroxide being used to cleanse preparation. (Also see Fig. 8–6.)

caries removal. The terms liners and bases need definitions and they are loosely related to the way the materials function.

Liners. Liners are materials that are placed as thin coatings, and their main function is to provide a barrier against chemical irritation. They do not function as thermal insulators. They are not used to produce a structural form for the preparation. Examples of liner materials are varnish-type materials to which calcium hydroxide or zinc oxide powder is added.

Bases. Base materials function as barriers against chemical irritation, provide thermal insulation, and resist forces applied during condensation of the restorative material. They are capable of being shaped and contoured to specific preparation forms. Examples of these materials are zinc oxide–eugenol, zinc phosphate, polycarboxylate, and glass ionomer cements, and some of the commercial preparations containing calcium hydroxide (Fig. 7–3).

The base materials are conventionally used with the carious lesion, as will be discussed in Chapter 8. There are times when a cement base material such as zinc phosphate, polycarboxylate, or glass ionomer will be needed to line a moderate lesion. A good example is when a defect needs correction before placing a direct gold restoration. The cements mentioned are the only ones that are able to support the condensation of direct gold.

An intermediate material is used for several reasons. Ideally it should stimulate pulpal repair, by the production of secondary or reparative dentin near a site of irritation. It should provide protection to the pulp from injurious toxic agents found in some restorative materials. The intermediate cement

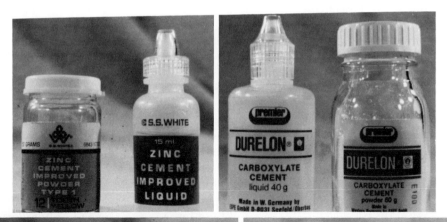

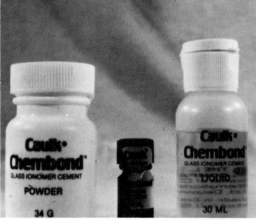
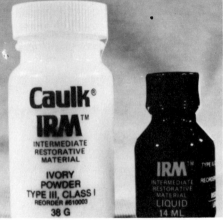

Figure 7–3. Cements useful for bases.

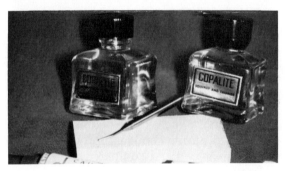 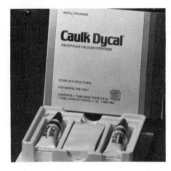

Figure 7–4. A varnish *(left)* and a calcium hydroxide liner *(right)*.

base is also used to block thermal diffusion through a metallic restoration material. To be effective a thickness of approximately 1.0 mm is needed. Likewise, in many preparations the base provides a firm foundation for the support of the forces required to condense direct gold and large amalgam restorations.

Varnish

If amalgam or direct gold is to be used, the preparation is coated with a cavity varnish* (Fig. 7–4). Cavity varnishes are natural rosins or synthetic resins dissolved in a solvent such as ether or chloroform. The solvent evaporates, leaving a thin film on the cavity preparation. In essence, this film provides a bandage over the fresh cut dentin. One of its principal functions is to reduce microleakage that occurs in conjunction with the amalgam restoration. Since dental amalgam is not adhesive to tooth structure, microleakage normally occurs around the freshly placed restoration. In time corrosion products form at the amalgam-tooth interface, but the microleakage that takes place during the first few months is a potential source of pulpal irritation and sensitivity. The cavity varnish inhibits microleakage during the first few weeks until the corrosion products form. Sensitivity, as induced by the penetration of deleterious fluids or debris, is markedly reduced.

A film of varnish placed under a metallic restoration is not an effective thermal insulator. Although varnishes have a low thermal conductivity, when properly applied the thickness of the film is in the range of only 4 μm; hence it is too thin to provide thermal insulation.

If the restorative material is in itself irritating, an example being zinc phosphate cement, varnish is applied to prevent penetration of the acid into the dentin and pulp. Such protection reduces the possibility of postoperative sensitivity. In the case of a silicate cement (Chapter 10), the varnish should be removed from the enamel in order to permit the fluoride present in the cement to interact with it.

Calcium Hydroxide

A varnish is not used when the restoration is either a composite or an unfilled resin. As the resin comes in contact with the varnish, polymerization

---

*Distributed by Harry J. Bosworth Co., 7227 N. Hamlin Ave., Skokie, Illinois 60076.

of the resin may be inhibited, producing a softening at the varnish-resin interface. However, it is essential to provide a barrier of some type between the resin and dentin to block any potential irritants in the resin from diffusing through the dentin into the pulp.

A material used extensively for pulp protection under not only resin but virtually all restorative materials is a calcium hydroxide cement (Fig. 7–5). Calcium hydroxide is particularly effective in promoting the formation of secondary dentin. Secondary dentin is an important aid in the repair of the pulp. Likewise, it provides a thicker layer of dentin, which assists in protecting the pulp from irritants, such as toxic products from restorative materials or deleterious agents that may penetrate from microleakage.

Commercial calcium hydroxide cements* are generally supplied as a two-paste system. Invariably they contain six or seven other ingredients added to improve certain properties. Nevertheless, generally they do provide the typical calcium hydroxide type of pulpal response. These materials have adequate hardness and strength to allow them to be used as a foundation for the placement of a restorative material (Fig. 7–6). Thus they are effective materials for rebuilding the defect produced by a moderate carious lesion.

Procedure for Placement of Liners and Bases

Varnish

Selection of the brand of varnish is based on personal preference and the handling characteristics of the material. There are no significant differences

*Dycal, L. D. Caulk Co., Box 359, Milford, Delaware 19963. Life, Kerr Co., 28200 Wick Road, Romulus, Michigan 48174. Pro-cal, 3M Company Dental Products, 2501 Hudson St., St. Paul, Minnesota 55119.

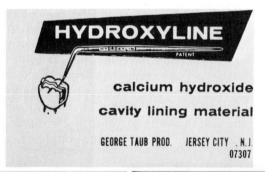

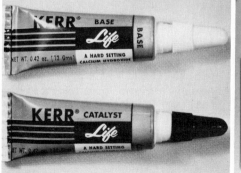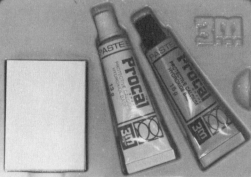

Figure 7–5. Calcium hydroxide liner materials.

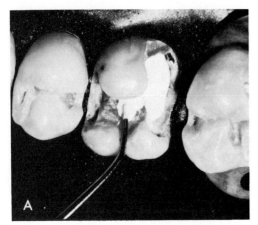

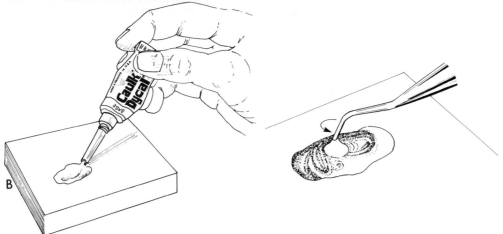

Figure 7–6. *A*, Calcium hydroxide being applied to a preparation for dental amalgam. *B*, Small amounts of calcium hydroxide base and catalyst are mixed on a paper pad until homogenous. (Courtesy of Dr. Michael T. Hanst.)

in the properties of the various varnishes and selection should be made on the basis of properties such as viscosity, visibility, and ease of application.

It is important to develop a uniform and continuous coating over all surfaces of the prepared cavity (Fig. 7–7). A minimum of two thin layers should be applied. As the initial layer dries it leaves small pinholes, and the second coating fills in the voids and produces a more continuous coating. The varnish should have a thin viscosity. If the varnish becomes too viscous, it will not properly wet the tooth, permitting microleakage to occur between the varnish and the tooth. Therefore, the top should be kept on the bottle whenever

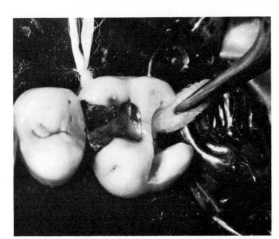

Figure 7–7. A cavity varnish being applied to a cavity preparation. (Also see Fig. 14–42.)

the varnish is not being dispensed. Thinner should be used whenever the varnish becomes too thick. The thinning agent is generally ether or chloroform and is supplied by the manufacturer.

The size of the preparation should be evaluated. Small pellets of cotton may be formed to paint the walls of the preparation with the varnish. After they have been moistened in the varnish the pellets may be carried to the preparation by cotton pliers. The preparation walls are quickly coated with varnish and dried carefully using air.

At times the preparation outline is too small to allow the use of cotton pliers so the varnish-covered pellet is brought to the cavity opening and maneuvered through the preparation with an explorer. Gravity permitting, the varnish can also be carried to the cavity with a plastic instrument.

The varnish can also be effectively applied by using root canal reamers as carriers. With this method the reamer is dipped into the varnish and a pellet of cotton of appropriate size is formed on the reamer, following which the varnish is applied as described above. Varnish also may be applied by using a camel's hair brush. A wire loop for the same purpose is supplied by one manufacturer.

Cements

Although a variety of materials and techniques for using bases and dressings could be described (Table 7–1), four will be discussed: (1) zinc oxide–eugenol cement, (2) zinc phosphate cement, (3) polycarboxylate cement, and (4) glass ionomer cement. (See Fig. 7–3).

ZINC OXIDE–EUGENOL CEMENT (ZOE)

Zinc oxide–eugenol cement is a soft sedative-type cement. It is usually dispensed in powder and liquid form and is useful as an insulative base. It is also the material most often used for temporary dressings. The pH is near 7, which makes it one of the least irritating of the dental cements.

Eugenol has a palliative effect upon the dental pulp and this is one of the advantages of this type of cement. Another advantage is the ability of the cement to minimize microleakage, an added protection for the pulp. This material is used mostly when treating large carious lesions.

A conventional mixture of zinc oxide and eugenol is relatively weak. In recent years "reinforced" or "improved" zinc oxide–eugenol cements have been introduced. One popular reinforced ZOE product* makes use of a polymer for reinforcement (Fig. 7–8). In addition, the particles of the zinc oxide powder have been surface-treated to produce better bonding of the particle to the matrix. This results in greater toughness and longer durability when used as a temporary holding type of material. A number of other ingredients, such as hydrogenated resin, may also be present in some products.

Armamentarium
1. Zinc oxide–eugenol cement (powder and liquid)†
2. Paper mixing pad and metal spatula
3. Long pointed explorer (No. 6 or 23 type)
4. Small cotton pellet and cotton pliers

---

*IRM[R], L. D. Caulk Co., Box 359, Milford, Delaware 19963.

†A pure zinc oxide powder and pure eugenol mixture is prone to a prolonged slow set. Setting time can be shortened by the addition of approximately 0.5 ml glacial acetic acid to 1 ounce of eugenol liquid.

Table 7–1. COMPARATIVE PROPERTIES OF CEMENTS

Material	Time of Setting	Compressive Strength at 24 hrs.		Film Thickness	Solubility and Disintegration (By Weight)	Diametral Tensile Strength at 24 hrs.		Pulp Response
	min	MPa	psi	micrometers	per cent	MPa	psi	
ADA Spec. No. 8 Type I (cementing)	5 min. 9 max.	68.7	9956	25 max.	0.2 max.	No specification		Severe*
Zinc Phosphate	5.5	103.5	15000	18	0.2	5.5	800	Moderate
ZOE	4–10	27.6	4000	25	0.04	—	—	Mild
ZOE + EBA and Alumina	9.5	55.2	8000	26	0.05	4.1	600	Mild
ZOE + Polymer	6–10	48.3	7000	32	0.08	4.1	600	Mild
Silicophosphate	3.5–4	144.8	21000	42	0.4	7.6	1100	Moderate
Resin Cement	4–10	65.5	9500	10–60	0.0–0.4	Not available		Severe
Polycarboxylate	5.5	55.2	8000	21	0.6	6.2	900	Mild
Glass Ionomer	6.5	86.2	12500	24	1.25	6.2	900	Mild

*Based on a comparison with silicate cement.

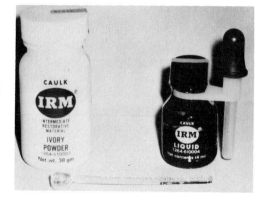

Figure 7–8. A reinforced zinc oxide–eugenol material that is used as a base or temporary restoration.

Procedure for a Base. In mixing the cement a paper pad is chosen rather than a glass slab. Sufficient powder is added to a few drops of eugenol and mixed until it reaches a thick puttylike texture that can be handled without sticking to the fingers (Fig. 7–9). A *small* piece about the size of a sesame seed is attached to the tip of the explorer and deposited carefully within the cavity. Avoid smearing the cement on the edges of the cavity walls.

An ultra-small pellet of cotton is grasped in cotton pliers and used as an instrument to "pat" the material and mold it within the cavity. The newly mixed cement will adhere to any metal or plastic instrument, hence the need for dry cotton. Additional increments can be added in a similar fashion until sufficient bulk is present.

Cementation. Some zinc oxide–eugenol formulations are used as luting agents for the cementation of castings.

In order to improve the compressive strength of the cement various additives are used. Polymers and inorganic compounds, such as alumina, may

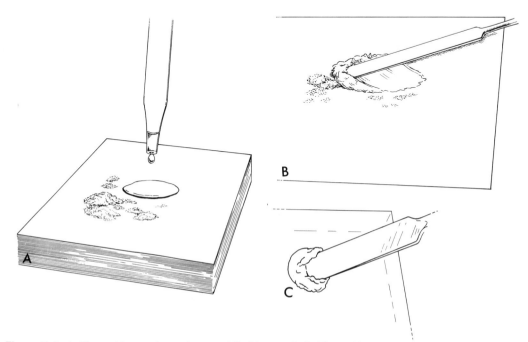

Figure 7–9. *A,* Zinc oxide powder and eugenol liquid on pad. *B,* Zinc oxide and eugenol being mixed on a paper pad or glass slab. *C,* For a base the cement should be mixed to putty-like consistency.

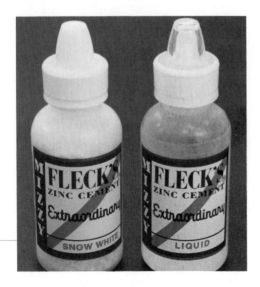

Figure 7–10. An example of a zinc phosphate cement.

be added to the zinc oxide powder in order to produce a composite structure and thereby greater strength. Another popular additive is o-ethoxybenzoic acid (usually referred to as EBA), which is placed in the eugenol.

These newer formulations have been referred to as "fortified," "reinforced," "modified," or "improved" zinc oxide–eugenol cements. Commercially, some are often called EBA cements when the product contains o-ethoxybenzoic acid as a partial replacement for the eugenol. These cements are designed particularly for the permanent cementation of inlays, crowns, and bridges. Their physical properties (e.g., strength) are superior to the conventional or non-reinforced zinc oxide–eugenol cements.

The use of EBA cements as luting agents for the permanent cementation of fixed restorations is somewhat debatable. Only long-term clinical observations will establish whether the somewhat reduced strength of this type of cement, as compared to zinc phosphate cement, will lead to a loss of retention and the dislodgement of the restoration. Also, the degree of solubility of these cements remains controversial.

The advantage of these "improved" zinc oxide–eugenol cements is principally a biologic one. In certain situations in which the dentist knows that the restored tooth will probably be sensitive, because of factors such as cavity depth and pulpal condition, such a cement is indicated. In such cases, the biologic considerations are more important than any other.

ZINC PHOSPHATE CEMENT (ZP)

Zinc phosphate cement is hard and strong but irritating to the pulp. It is a powder-liquid system; the powder is mostly zinc oxide and the liquid is ortho-phosphoric acid, metallic salts, and water. The primary and traditional use for this material is to lute cast restorations to the teeth. It is also used as a base material when high compressive strength is required.

The initial cement mixture is highly acidic, because of phosphoric acid, although the pH approaches neutrality in a short period of time. Newly mixed phosphate cement is highly irritating to the pulp, and without the protection of a varnish or other type of base material, it may produce irreversible pulpal damage.

This type of cement is the oldest of all those used in dentistry (Fig. 7–10).

It is easy to manipulate, has the high strength necessary for a base, withstands mechanical trauma, and, as with other types of base materials, provides good protection against thermal shock. It is quite brittle, however, and does not serve well for temporary restorations.

Proper care of the powder and liquid is essential. The concentration of the phosphoric acid is carefully regulated by the manufacturer. Even slight changes in that concentration can have a marked effect upon setting time, strength, and solubility. Therefore the top should be placed back on the bottle immediately after dispensing the liquid. Likewise, the ingredients should not be placed on the mixing slab until just before the mix is to be made. It is also a good policy to discard a bottle of liquid when it is 4/5 used, as the remaining liquid in the bottle will probably have become adulterated from repeated openings.

If used for the purpose of luting castings, the film of cement should be thin enough so as not to interfere at the tooth-casting interface. The particle size of the powder is directly related to the film's thickness. However, the particle size is reduced by mixing the powder into solution with the cement liquid and by the pressure induced during seating of the casting. The particles that are squeezed between the walls of the restoration and the tooth are eventually able to withstand the pressure exerted by the dentist upon the casting. Generally, the finer the original powder particles of the cement, the smaller is the effective grain size of the cement and the lower its film thickness. The thinner the thickness of the film, the greater is its retentive capability.

Solubility. Probably the one property of greatest clinical significance is the solubility and disintegration of the cement. In fact this property is one of the most important considerations in the use and selection of any dental material. In the cemented cast restoration, solubility of the cement is of particular significance. As noted, a thin line of cement is always exposed to oral fluids at the margins, even though this cement line may not be readily visible to the naked eye. Visual acuity under oral conditions is approximately 50 μm. Thus, whenever any cement line is visible in the mouth it is probably greater than 50 μm. In the cervical region where visibility is difficult, marginal discrepancies several times this magnitude will pass unnoticed. This exposed layer of cement gradually dissolves, so that the inlay eventually may loosen or secondary caries may develop.

In view of the fact that the water content of the cement is critical, it is imperative that the area near the cement be kept dry while the powder-liquid mixture is being prepared, while it is being placed on the tooth, and during its hardening. If allowed to harden while in contact with saliva, the surfaces of most types of cements become dull and soft and are easily dissolved by the oral fluids.

Armamentarium for Bases and Luting
1. Cool clean glass slab and spatula
2. Zinc phosphate cement, powder, and liquid
3. 95 per cent alcohol in dappen dish (to keep cement from adhering to the instruments)
4. Two plastic instruments of choice: one to mold the material on the axial wall; the other to form the pulpal wall
5. Explorers No. 6 and No. 23

Procedure for Cementation. The amount of cement needed will dictate the amount of liquid that is placed on the slab. It is best to provide for a noticeable surplus to make sure there will be an adequate supply and that it can be properly mixed.

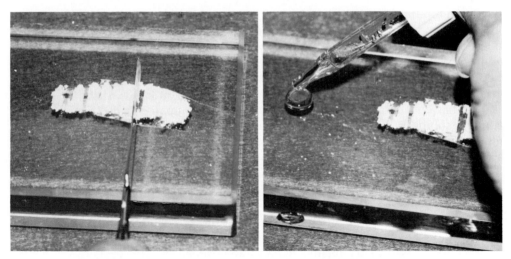

Figure 7–11. Zinc phosphate powder and liquid being placed on a glass slab.

1. Three to six drops of liquid, along with some powder, are placed on the glass mixing slab (Fig. 7–11). It is not necessary to use a measuring device for proportioning the powder and liquid, as the desired consistency may vary according to the clinical conditions. However, the maximal amount of powder possible for the operation at hand should be used in order to reduce the solubility and to increase the strength of the cement. Solubility and strength are markedly influenced by the powder to liquid ratio. The higher the ratio, the better the properties.

2. A cool mixing slab should be employed. The temperature of the slab should not be below the dew point of the room, lest moisture condense on the surface and dilute the cement. The cool slab delays the setting and allows the operator to incorporate the maximal amount of powder before the crystallization proceeds to a point at which the mixture stiffens.

3. Mixing is initiated by the addition of a small amount of powder at the start, as shown in Figure 7–12. This procedure assists in neutralizing the acid. After waiting about 30 seconds, the buffering action of the salts in the acid is completed. Larger quantities of powder are now incorporated, using a brisk, rotary motion of the spatula (Fig. 7–13). In mixing the cement a large area of the slab is used. A good rule to follow is to spatulate for about 15 seconds after adding each increment. The mixing time for this type of cement is not unduly critical, and completion of the mix usually requires approximately one and a half minutes.

4. The actual consistency varies with the purpose for which the cement is to be used (see Chapter 18). The desired consistency is always attained by the addition of more powder and never by adding new liquid to the mix.

5. Good consistency for luting is an arbitrary determination and a suggested test is to concentrate the freshly mixed cement and touch the side of the spatula to the cement and lift up a strand of cement (Fig. 7–14). For good consistency, a strand of cement should extend upward for 1/2 to 3/4 inch. If it is less than 1/2 inch, more powder should be added; if it is in excess of 3/4 inch, it would be best to start again.

6. For use as a base, the consistency should be of a puttylike mixture (Fig. 7–15). This is achieved by rapidly adding powder after the slowly mixed cement has reached a thick, creamy texture. After this stage, if the operator

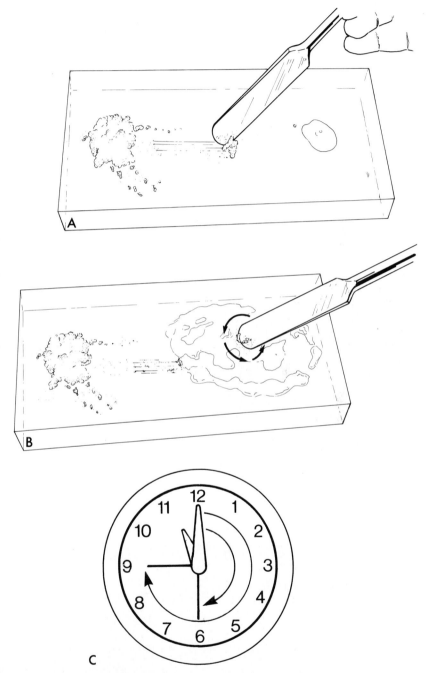

Figure 7–12. *A,* A small amount of powder is used to begin a mix of zinc phosphate cement. *B,* The initial increment of powder is thoroughly mixed into the liquid. *C,* Allow a 30-second delay before succeeding increments are added.

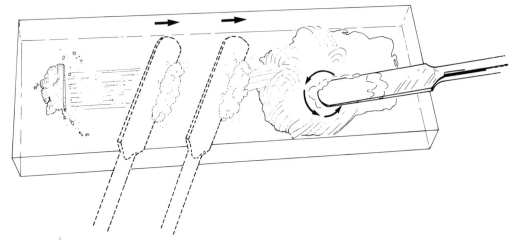

Figure 7–13. Added increments of powder are folded into the mix using a circular motion with the spatula.

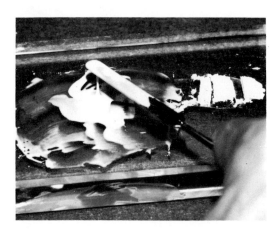

Figure 7–14. For the purpose of cementation, a 1/2 inch strand of cement should extend from spatula to glass slab to indicate proper consistency.

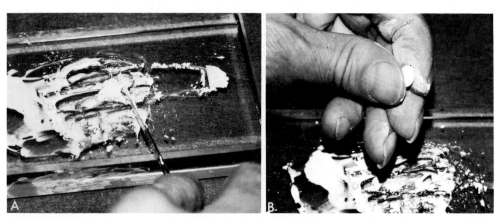

Figure 7–15. *A,* For the purpose of mixing a base, powder is added to provide a thick texture. *B,* The base should be thick enough to allow it to be picked up by one's fingers.

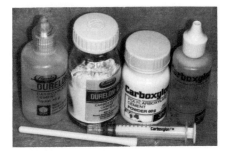

Figure 7–16. Examples of polycarboxylate cement.

desires, he may dust his fingers with cement powder and manipulate the cement in his fingers. When mixing this cement for a base, a small tag of "creamy mix" material is placed on the corner of the slab and retained for attaching the base.

POLYCARBOXYLATE CEMENT

This is one of the recent dental cement systems, and it gives evidence of adhesion to at least the calcium component in the tooth structure (Fig. 7–16). Although somewhat difficult to manipulate, it does have a potential for chemical adhesion to the calcium ions in enamel and dentin. As with zinc phosphate cement, its primary use is as a luting agent (Chapter 18), but it is used also as a base material, as an insulating liner, and as a masking agent underneath thin enamel to prevent metallic-colored materials from shining through. Inasmuch as it tends to harden quite rapidly, no effort is made to mix it to a puttylike consistency as with zinc phosphate cement.

The powder of this cement is similar to that of zinc phosphate cement. It contains zinc oxide and originally a small amount of magnesium oxide. Some products now substitute stannic oxide, as well as stannous fluoride, for the magnesium oxide in order to modify setting time and to improve the strength and handling characteristics. (Perhaps it should be mentioned that in this case the added fluoride seems to afford little potential for anticaries protection.)The liquid is polyacrylic acid and water. The manufacturers are able to vary the viscosity of the liquid by changing the molecular weight of the polyacrylic acid.

The pH of a polycarboxylate cement is initially comparable to that of zinc phosphate cement, but the pulp response is comparable to that of the zinc oxide–eugenol cements. A possible explanation for the low level of irritation is the large size of the polyacrylic acid molecule, which restricts penetration through dentin, and/or its attraction to protein, which may limit its diffusion through the dentinal tubules. The major reason for the popularity of this new cement is the favorable biologic acceptance by the pulp and therefore the low incidence of postoperative sensitivity.

Its use as a luting agent is of interest because of its excellent biologic characteristics and, as noted, because it forms an adhesive bond to the calcium in the tooth structure. This bond is stronger with enamel than it is with dentin, which is expected because enamel has a higher percentage of calcified material. In addition, it has an advantage over zinc phosphate cement in that *small* deviations in the powder-liquid ratio are not as critical to its physical properties.

Despite the adhesion of the cement to tooth structure, polycarboxylate cements may not be superior to zinc phosphate cement with respect to

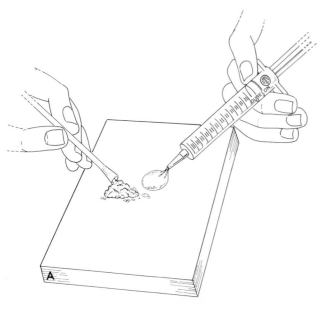

Figure 7–17. *A,* Care is taken to place the proper amount of polycarboxylate powder and liquid on the mixing pad, or *B,* the glass slab.

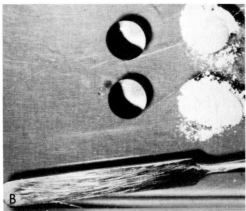

retention of cast gold restorations. A comparable force is required to remove castings that have been cemented with either of these materials. With zinc phosphate cement, failure usually occurs at the cement-tooth interface. In the case of polycarboxylate cements, the failure usually occurs cohesively or at the cement-metal interface. Apparently the cement is unable to bond to the metal in the chemically dirty "as cast" or pickled condition. The best means of cleaning the casting is with an air-abrasive device, which improves the retention of the cement to the metal. Before cementation both casting and preparation must be devoid of any contamination. Since retention of the cement is dependent upon achieving an adhesive bond between the cement and the calcium in the apatite structure of the tooth, a meticulously clean tooth is essential, as was discussed at the beginning of this chapter.

Armamentarium
1. Clean paper pad or glass slab and mixing spatula
2. Polycarboxylate cement and liquid
3. Instruments of choice for handling the cement (should include a ball burnisher)
4. Explorers No. 6 and No. 23

Procedure for Base. The instructions supplied by the manufacturer should be observed and followed very carefully. The powder-liquid ratio required to produce a cement of suitable base consistency varies among different brands, but it is in the general range of approximately 2 to 3 parts of powder to 1 part of liquid by weight. Somewhat lower powder-liquid ratios (approximately 1.5 to 1) are preferred when using a polycarboxylate cement as a luting agent.

The material should be mixed on a surface that will not absorb liquid (Fig. 7–17). A glass slab may afford some advantage over the treated paper pad that is generally supplied, as it can be cooled. Cooling slows the chemical reaction to some extent and thus provides a somewhat longer working time.

The liquid should not be dispensed until just prior to the time that the mix is to be made. Exposure of the cement liquid to the atmosphere for even a short period (e.g., 60 seconds) results in sufficient evaporation of water to cause a significant increase in the viscosity. Changes in the concentration of the polyacrylic acid also result in definite decreases in strength and higher solubility.

The powder is rapidly incorporated into the liquid in large quantities (Fig. 7–18). The mix should be completed within 30 or 40 seconds in order to provide sufficient working time to carry out the basing operation (Fig. 7–19). It should be noted that the mixing procedure is entirely different from that used for zinc phosphate cement. During placement and when molding the material in the cavity, dry powder, rather than alcohol, is used to prevent cement from sticking to the instruments. Otherwise the procedure for placing the base is very similar to that described for zinc phosphate cement, as is the procedure for completing the surface of the hardened cement.

Procedure for Luting. Observe carefully the instructions by the manufacturer for measurement of the powder and liquid. The liquid is best measured using a calibrated syringe provided by some manufacturers.

1. With the cement spatula incorporate the powder into the liquid to form a homogeneous mass as quickly as possible— the mix *must* be completed within 30 seconds. There then follows about 3 minutes of working time to allow the casting to be fully seated. When the cement is mixed properly the mix appears quite viscous. Despite this viscous appearance, if handled correctly the film thickness will be 25 μm or less.

2. The mix of cement must have a glossy appearance at the time the casting is seated. If during mixing a stringy texture develops or if the cement takes on a dull appearance, the set has progressed too far or too high a ratio of powder to liquid was used (Fig. 7–20). Such a mix must not be used for

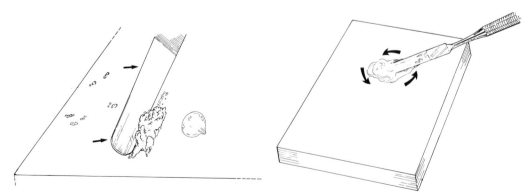

Figure 7–18. Polycarboxylate cement is mixed as quickly as possible.

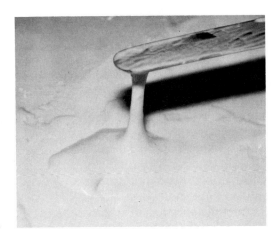

Figure 7–19. In preparing a base the polycarboxylate cement is mixed to a thick consistency.

cementation. The glossy appearance indicates that liquid is still available to bond to the tooth. Otherwise, no retention will occur.

3. Clean the instruments as quickly as possible after mixing the cement.

SILICOPHOSPHATE CEMENT

A cement that may be considered for cementation, silicophosphate cement is one in which considerable amounts of zinc oxide are added to the usual constituents of a silicate cement powder. These cements are hybrids in that they are combinations of zinc phosphate cement with silicate cement and are often referred to as silicophosphate cements. One of the most popular silicophosphate cements is composed of 90 per cent silicate cement powder and 10 per cent zinc phosphate cement powder. By virtue of the fluoride contained in the silicate portion of the powder, the cement affords protection against secondary caries.

Early formulations were inferior with respect to manipulative properties, and the film thickness was unduly high. Because of the high film thickness, it was not suitable for cementation of precision cast gold restorations. Recent formulations* have been developed with improved handling characteristics and reduced film thickness. These improvements have extended the usefulness of the material to include cementation of gold castings. In view of the anticariogenic properties, zinc silicophosphate is often the luting agent of

*Fluoro-Thin, S. S. White Co., 3 Parkway, Philadelphia, Pennsylvania 19102.

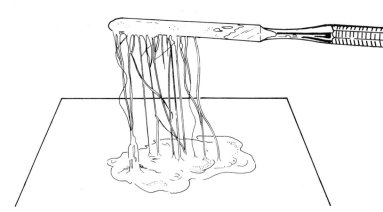

Figure 7–20. When polycarboxylate cement is used for luting it must possess a surface gloss but no evidence of a web formation when the spatula is lifted from the mix.

choice in mouths with a high caries rate. The same precautions for pulp protection are followed as for zinc phosphate cement.

GLASS IONOMER CEMENT (GI)

Another newer type of cement that is also based upon polyacrylic acid is the glass ionomer cement. Because of its biologic kindness and potential for adherence to the calcium in the tooth (as with the polycarboxylate system), the glass ionomer cement is used primarily as a restorative material for treatment of the eroded area and as a luting agent. It can also be employed as a base material, even though the material is very water sensitive and a dry field is imperative.

The glass ionomer cement is an extension of the zinc polycarboxylate cement. The liquid is essentially polyacrylic acid with additives of certain other acids, e.g., itaconic, to improve certain properties. Thus the acid has the potential for chelation to certain ions in tooth structure, particularly the calcium. This primary chemical bond then provides for the retention of the cement to the tooth. As noted earlier, this particular liquid is also very kind in terms of tissue response.

The powder is an alumino-silicate glass. Being largely a silicate cement, it displays the typical fluoride leaching pattern as that type of material, and

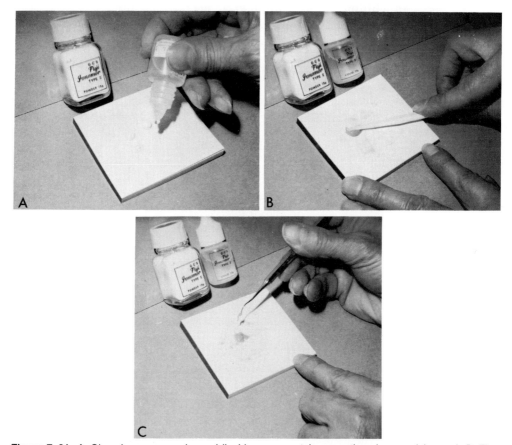

Figure 7–21. *A,* Glass ionomer powder and liquid are accurately proportioned on a mixing pad. *B,* The glass ionomer powder and liquid are mixed in a rapid manner to a luting consistency. *C,* Additional powder provides a base consistency.

possibly the same resistance to caries. One can thus see the attraction of the basic system: it is one that has a potential for adherence to tooth structure, is biologically kind, and as a result of the fluoride content possesses some anticariogenic characteristics.

The material is usually supplied as a powder and liquid. In a few cases the manufacturer has freeze-dried the acid and placed it in the powder. The mix is made with distilled water but the setting reaction is the same. The mix can be made either on a disposable paper pad or on a glass slab. A plastic or agate spatula is preferred to a metal one in order to minimize possible contamination of the mix from abraded metal. As with polycarboxylate cement, the polyacrylic acid–based liquid is not dispensed until just prior to the start of the mix. The glass ionomer cements are mixed in a manner similar to that used for other polyacrylate cements: large increments of the powder are rapidly incorporated into the liquid (Fig. 7–21), and the mix should be completed within 40 seconds. In general, the working time is somewhat shorter than for zinc phosphate cement and is usually not longer than 3 minutes following the start of the mix. In no instance should the material be used if the mix has lost its gloss or if a skin has formed, as was noted for the polycarboxylate cement. Rubber dam isolation is advocated to maintain dryness during placement.

After setting, the material is more brittle than a polycarboxylate cement. It can be trimmed and finished in much the same manner as zinc phosphate cement. Before the patient is dismissed, all of the accessible margins are covered with the varnish supplied by the manufacturer. This is to protect the cement from oral fluids during the next few hours when the setting process continues.

8

TREATMENT OF THE CARIOUS LESION

Treatment of enamel and dentin that have become softened by the carious process is the subject of this chapter. As might be expected, shallow lesions are treated differently from deep lesions, and deep lesions are treated differently when they encroach upon or expose the pulp. Consequently this chapter has been divided into treatment of (1) the shallow or moderate carious lesion, (2) the deep carious lesion, and (3) the exposed pulp.

Steps in Cavity Preparation

Dr. G. V. Black outlined the steps* that should ordinarily be followed for caries removal and the preparation of the tooth to receive a restoration. Despite the advent of the air turbine handpiece and other technological improvements (newer amalgam and composite formulations) during the last years, this systematic approach is still recommended to the operative dentist as a reliable guideline for today.

Step 1: Outline of the Proposed Restoration. As the sculptor envisions the finished statue in his block of uncut marble, so the operative dentist should envision the finished tooth preparation with regard to its borders. It may be necessary to alter the prepared cavity as unseen internal problems arise; however, a mental image of the finished preparation should be conceived before any cutting is done.

The bur is used to penetrate and make entry into the cavity. After the desired depth has been reached, lateral cutting is done in several directions to rough out the cavity to its desired form. The most efficient results are achieved if the depth cut is first established before the cavity is enlarged to its final form.

Step 2: Resistance and Retention Considerations. While still ignoring carious dentin, the operator with his bur or hand instruments makes necessary modifications in the roughed out preparation to accomplish two results: (1) Pulpal and gingival walls should be flat in order to resist occlusal forces squarely. Conjointly, adjacent walls are to be placed at right angles to the occlusal walls so that the finished restorations will not skid or rotate (see Fig. 11–25). (2) Sufficient undercuts are incorporated into the cavity in order to keep the restoration from being dislodged when subject to masticatory forces.

---

*These steps are routinely followed except for some deep carious lesions.

Ordinarily these structural needs will be met during the initial stages of the preparation. A third structural consideration, which may not be obvious to the operator, is resistance to shearing forces in preparations involving the proximal segments of posterior teeth. Occlusal portions of the restoration may be adequately stabilized, while the proximal portion may be poorly supported. Occlusal forces (see Figs. 11–28 and 11–47) may cause dislodgement or fracture if precautions are not taken to mechanically secure the proximal segment of the restoration.

Step 3: Access for Removal of Carious Dentin and Placement of the Restoration. During the "rough-out" stage, the operator will automatically have sufficient access. Exceptions occur when teeth are malpositioned, in which case it may be necessary to remove additional enamel so as to facilitate removal of caries and placement of a restoration. Sometimes it is actually necessary to cut off a cusp in order to see and to operate inside an inaccessible cavity.

Step 4: Carious Dentin Removal. The mechanics of this step are explained later in the chapter (Fig. 8–1).

Step 5: Refinement of the Internal Part of the Cavity. This step transforms the initially rough preparation to one with precise and clean-cut surfaces. This is accomplished with burs and sharp cutting instruments. The placement of a cement base might also be considered as part of this step.

Step 6: Refinement of Preparation Margins. Ripples and irregularities left by the bur are reduced so as to leave smooth margins, which are usually produced with hand instruments or enamel finishing burs. The gingival wall requires special consideration, because recurrence of caries frequently occurs at this location. Debris tends to accumulate at the gingival margin and to obstruct visibility. In areas where hemorrhage and debris are a problem, the matrix band is often applied prior to this step so it can serve as a barrier against contamination while planing the gingival floor.

Treatment of the Moderate Carious Lesion

The diagnosis and treatment of the moderate carious lesion is required in those situations in which caries has penetrated through the enamel or has involved the dentin, but not to the extent of endangering the pulp. A moderate lesion is defined as one in which caries penetration is easily observed in the

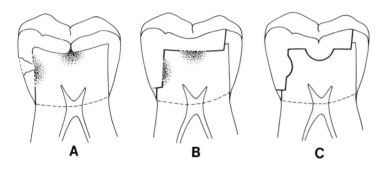

Figure 8–1. Carious dentin is removed *after* (not before) the cavity is prepared. *A,* Simulated carious lesions, mesial and occlusal, on a mandibular second molar. *B,* Steps 1, 2, and 3 have been completed while the carious dentin has been ignored. *C,* Step 4, carious dentin is now identified and removed.

A   B   C

dentin and may involve up to one half the dentin thickness between the dentino-enamel junction and the pulp. As a therapeutic measure the restorative process is aimed at arresting the progress of the disease and replacing structural components of the dentin and enamel. There are occasions when caries should be treated prior to the point at which it reaches the dentin. For example, when a posterior tooth requires a distal surface to be restored and radiographic evidence also reveals a beginning lesion on the mesial surface, clinical judgment would dictate the restoration of the mesial surface as well inasmuch as the tooth is already receiving surgical reconstruction.

The shallow or moderate "carious" lesion is differentiated from the deep lesion by its clinical penetration into dentin and its proximity to the dental pulp. A "deep" lesion in the cervical area of a premolar may actually be more shallow than a "moderate" lesion on the occlusal surface of a molar.

The majority of teeth having minimal caries penetration will exhibit no sensitivity or adverse postoperative effects following any ordinary dental treatment. Surgical treatment of hard tissue in the mouth should not be taken lightly, as minimal irritation in some teeth can cause severe postoperative sensitivity. In view of the multiple possible causes of pulpal irritation, it behooves each dentist to operate with care and caution to minimize injury during treatment.

Mechanics of Caries Removal

The depth of the carious penetration of a lesion does not exert a significant influence on the final outline of the cavity preparation. When the proposed outline of the preparation (Step 1) is near completion, an evaluation is made to determine the lateral penetration of the caries. This is done by probing with the explorer. Essentially all enamel unsupported by sound dentin is removed, which in turn influences the final outline of the preparation. During this exploratory and probing process it is acceptable to remove carious dentin underneath the enamel (Figs. 8–2 and 8–3).

When considerable carious dentin is present, excavation of which would probably not involve the pulp, it is removed with either a round bur or a hand excavator. When using a bur, slow speed is preferred, as it will minimize the possibility of overcutting. The bur size should be large and should harmonize with the size of the tooth and the amount of remaining carious dentin, i.e., sizes No. 4, 6, or 8. When removing carious dentin of this amount, both the color and texture of the remaining dentin may be used as a guide to indicate proper removal (Fig. 8–4).

Many times discolored dentin should not be removed. The hardness and texture of the dentin at the base of the cavity serve as indicators of caries penetration. Tactile sense with a hand excavator is more reliable than a dental bur in detecting the difference between diseased and healthy dentin (Figs. 8–2 and 8–3). When the carious dentin is gone, the remaining surface will appear smooth and semi-polished, even though the dentin may still be discolored. The healthy dentin will be very resistant to the excavator, as compared with carious tooth structure.

Carious dentin in the depth of the cavity is readily recognized and easily removed. Not so obvious, however, are small fragments of carious dentin underneath occlusal enamel ridges. Close scrutiny along the edges just underneath the enamel is important in the excavation process (Fig. 8–5).

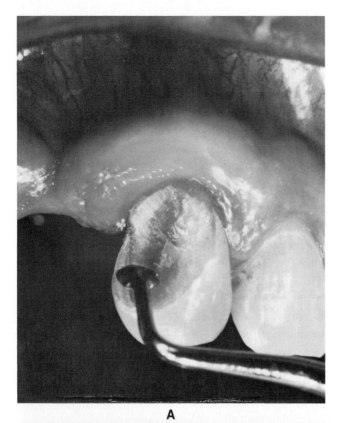

A

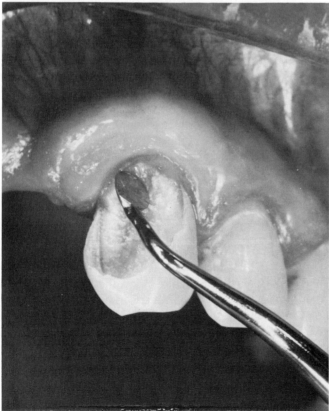

B

Figure 8–2. Peripheral caries removed with large excavator. Notice how the carious dentin tends to fragment as it nears the base of sound dentin. *B,* Regardless of the closeness of the lesion to the pulp, *all peripheral* carious dentin is removed until hard dentin is reached. This applies to the peripheral area of all lesions regardless of where they are located.

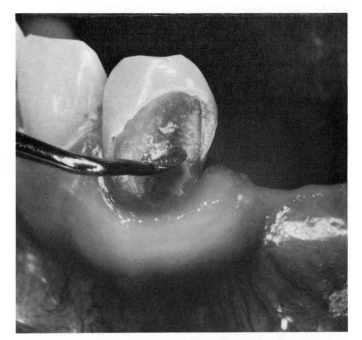

Figure 8–3. Removal of carious dentin over the pulp is done last. Excavator must be inspected for sharpness prior to this final stage of caries removal.

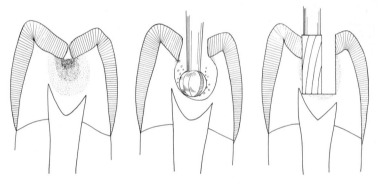

Figure 8–4. Removal of carious dentin with a bur. Round steel burs (size 4 or 6) operating at slow speed are more inclined to shave away the dentin than carbide burs. At no time should one resort to using a bur with sharp corners for removing carious dentin, old cement, or old amalgam. Inadvertent pulp exposure is one of the potential dangers accompanying the use of sharp-cornered burs in deep lesions.

Figure 8–5. Removal of carious dentin that escapes detection by larger excavators or round burs. Fragments of carious dentin often escape notice under occlusal and incisal shells of enamel.

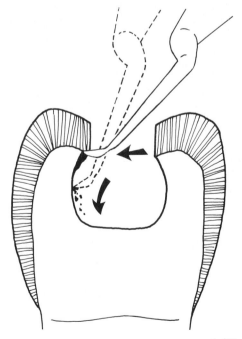

Cleansing the Prepared Surface

Following cavity preparation, the enamel and dentin surfaces are generally covered with a thin layer of tenacious debris. The removal of this microscopic film, or of remnants of a temporary filling material, may interfere with its adaptability to the cavity walls. This may be detected at the time of insertion of the restoration, or, even worse, may not be apparent until some time later. Likewise, optimum behavior of a dental cement, particularly the polycarboxylate system, is markedly influenced by the surface cleanliness of the preparation at the time of insertion.

Hydrogen peroxide is the all-purpose cavity cleanser. Wherever debris occurs within the tooth preparation, blood seems to be inevitably present. A 3 per cent solution of hydrogen peroxide in contact with blood (fresh or dried) immediately releases bubbles of oxygen, which seem to dislodge the debris and make it an easy target for removal with the air/water syringe and high-velocity evacuation (Fig. 8–6).

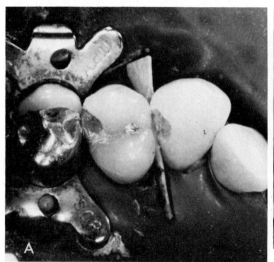
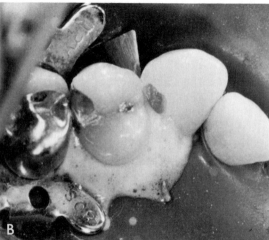
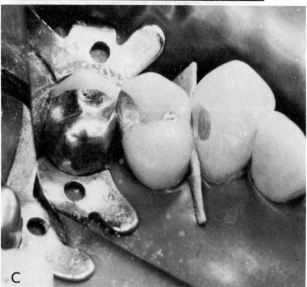

Figure 8–6. Hydrogen peroxide (3 per cent) bubbling debris out of a cavity. H_2O_2 is very effective in cleansing a cavity of dried blood. *A,* before; *B,* during (note oxygen bubbles); *C,* after.

Table 8–1. TREATMENT OF THE CARIOUS LESION
WITH MEDICAMENTS AND CEMENTS

Material	Moderate	Deep	Definite Pulpal Penetration (Exposure with Bleeding)
Cavity Varnish	Yes	No	No
Fluoride Solution	Yes	Yes	No
Cavity Cleansers (de-greasing or oil removal agent)	Yes	Yes	No
H_2O_2	Yes	Yes	No
Eugenol	Yes	Yes	No
Corticosteroids	(Yes)	(Yes)	(Yes)
Calcium Hydroxide (any form)	Yes	Yes	Yes
ZnO and Eugenol Cement	Yes	Yes	No
Zinc Phosphate	Yes	No	No
Polycarboxylate Cement	Yes	Yes	No
Air Syringe	Yes	Yes	No

Placement of Calcium Hydroxide Liner

As shown in Table 8–1, most cleansing agents, medicaments, liners, and bases can be used at will in the moderate carious lesion. A common practice is to employ calcium hydroxide as a kind of liner within the cavity. Supplied as an aqueous suspension, as a powder, or as a paste, calcium hydroxide serves as a calcium-rich liner over freshly cut dentin or as an insulator over deeper portions of the cavity. The paste form* is the most popular because it is easily applied and because it hardens so rapidly (see Fig. 7–6). Dycal can be applied with the same instrument used to mix it. Before placing the material the instrument is wiped clean, as the liner material must be placed very precisely where it is needed in order to avoid random smearing of the general area (Fig. 8–7).

*Dycal, L. D. Caulk Co., Box 359, Milford, Delaware 19963.

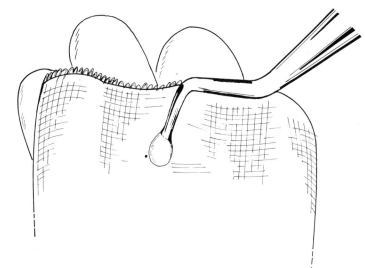

Figure 8–7. Ball burnisher wiped clean after mixing of calcium hydroxide liner. (See also Fig. 7–6.)

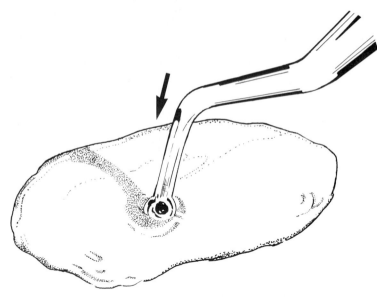

Figure 8–8. Only the terminal half of the spherical ball is dipped into the paste to enhance control of the material and prevent it from running down the shank.

A number of instruments may be used, depending on handling convenience. The size and location of the preparation dictate which instrument is the most convenient. The back side of a small excavator can be useful in placing the cement. One instrument that is effective is an applicator shaped like a probe with a small ball on the end (Fig. 8–8). Dipping the ball only halfway into the mixture is desired when placing the paste in an upper tooth (or "uphill" surface) (Fig. 8–8). If more than the terminal half of the ball is wetted, the material will not remain on the end of the ball but will run down the shaft toward the instrument handle (Figs. 8–9 and 8–10).

Amalgam and resin preparations will have retentive undercuts in dentin. There is a strong tendency for a liner material, such as Dycal, to flow into and fill these undercuts, which would leave the restoration without the required mechanical locks for retention. When this occurs, an explorer or cutting instrument is used to remove the material from the retention sites after it has hardened.

Liner materials harden very rapidly after mixing, so they must be placed promptly after mixing. The temperature of the mouth causes an acceleration of the setting reaction. Increasing the humidity will also decrease the setting

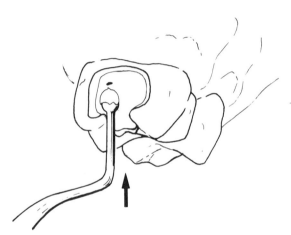

Figure 8–9. Paste is carried to difficult areas. The same technique is employed for applying calcium hydroxide paste either as a liner or as a pulp-capping substance.

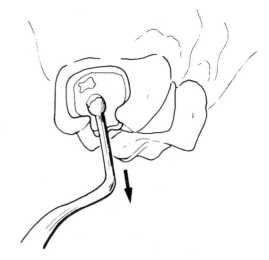

Figure 8–10. Paste adhering to the dentin where it dries and hardens to form a hermetic seal.

time, a consequence if the rubber dam is not present. Following the placement of the liners or bases of choice, the permanent restoration is placed.

Treatment of the Deep Carious Lesion

In contrast to the shallow lesion, the deep cavity can destroy the structural components of the tooth, as well as encroach upon the pulp. Because of technological problems brought on by undermined enamel and because of postoperative pulpal response, the treatment of the deep carious lesion requires special consideration, particularly by the budding operative dentist.

Defense against an advancing lesion takes the form of reparative dentin deposits within the pulp chamber and within the tubules. If the rate of the carious process exceeds the speed of the pulpal response, this base of hard dentin may not be present. Or, if the condition is severe, the softened dentin communicates with the pulp itself.

A tooth with a deep cavity will reveal, upon excavation of the caseous and necrotic dentin, an interface (approximately 0.5 mm thick) of decalcified and softened, but still intact, dentin. If this layer of semi-solid dentin is removed and if the pulp has been successful in coping with the onslaught of the carious process, one may encounter a layer of solid hard dentin, often with a shiny glossy surface. However, all carious dentin directly adjacent to the pulp is not necessarily removed, as will be discussed later in the chapter.

Ravages from the carious process, aside from their effect on the pulp, may have a great impact upon the structural integrity of the tooth. A large portion of enamel may unexpectedly break away while chewing hard food, the first symptom of a cavity that the patient might experience. If the fracture involves a marginal ridge, an open funnel is formed whereby food can wedge between the teeth, causing discomfort and gingival irritation. Loss of proximal contact also permits mesial drift with subsequent migration of the teeth.

If a cusp is broken off, food may impact directly into the tooth, causing pain and discomfort. Moreover, loss of occlusal contact from the opposing tooth allows it to erupt into the space, interfering with the occlusal plane. Also, fractured teeth, particularly lower molars, often leave sharp jagged edges, which may lacerate the tongue.

Treatment Alternatives

The biologic and structural features mentioned above are among the problems with which the operative dentist must cope as he seeks to functionally restore the tooth. Faced with a deep carious lesion, the operator has several options. In descending order of severity they are as follows:

1. The tooth can be removed.

2. Endodontic therapy* can be followed by structural reinforcement of the root and crown (see Chapter 19).

3. If the lesion approximates the pulp, the pulp can be treated and a temporary restoration placed. At a later period, pulp health permitting, a permanent restoration can be placed.

4. With favorable prognosis the tooth can be permanently restored as though it were a moderate lesion.

5. For emergency care, superficial carious dentin can be excavated and a temporary restoration placed. Jagged edges of enamel can also be reduced with a diamond stone so they do not abrade the tongue or cheek.

Diagnosis and Treatment Planning

If one follows option 3 or 5 it must first be decided whether the temporary restoration is to function for only several days or for three or four months. Although the state of the pulp has some influence on this decision, mutual convenience to both dentist and patient is also a concern in this regard.† (See Table 7–1.)

Failure to plan for a strong and durable temporary cement restoration is the cause of many pulp deaths, because the patient chews it out and the cavity is re-exposed to saliva and contaminants. Common sense and clinical judgment should prevail. As a highway detour provides a serviceable roadway for automobile traffic, so the temporary cement restoration must provide reliable protection for the tooth and comfort to the patient until such time as it can be replaced.

If structural components of the existing enamel can be retained to provide support, cement alone will usually suffice for the required time of service. If not, an aluminum crown is often an option (Figs. 8–11 and 8–12). Fitting such a crown requires some reduction of enamel so the edges will approximate the tooth surface.

The crucial factor in this regard is the buccal and lingual plates of the tooth. If these are left intact, they can often support a cement restoration sandwiched between them (Fig. 8–13A and B). If insufficient buccal and lingual tooth structure remains, a crown is indicated. Fitting a crown often requires the removal of some peripheral enamel. Otherwise, an oversized aluminum crown is required that will have overhanging edges that will be very irritating to the gingiva. If the bulges of buccal and lingual enamel are cut away to permit a crown to fit around the neck of the tooth, the buccal and lingual supporting components will have been sacrificed in the process. It is incumbent upon the operator to know *before* rather than *after* the enamel is

---

*Pulpotomy, the removal of the coronal portion of the pulp as an emergency treatment, will not be discussed in this chapter.

†For example, if the patient is planning a trip or if the dentist's schedule will not permit permanent treatment as soon as desired, a long-term temporary restoration is indicated.

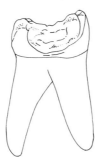
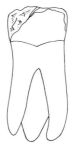
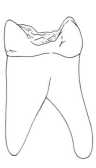

Figure 8–11. Three views of a badly broken down molar. Notice the buccal and lingual contours of the crown, which can be easily reduced so the aluminum cap will fit better.

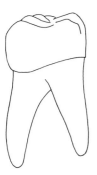
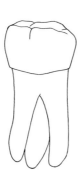
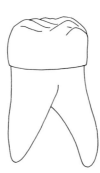

Figure 8–12. Aluminum cap serving as temporary protection for the sedative cement. Note the close fit around the neck of the tooth, a most important feature for gingival comfort.

Figure 8–13. *A,* Extensive and deep carious lesion within the shell of bell-shaped molar. *B,* A temporary crown is contraindicated for this tooth. Buccal and lingual plates can adequately retain the sedative cement instead.

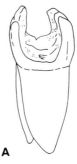
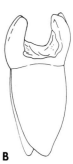

A   **B**

removed which modality he intends to employ to hold the cement—a natural remaining tooth structure or an artificial crown of metal or plastic* (see Fig. 16–30).

A second decision that bears distinctly upon therapy is whether or not the pulp has been penetrated by the lesion and, if so, to what extent. History of dental pain, radiographs, and other clinical diagnostic tools are helpful in predicting whether or not the dentist will find an exposed pulp when the carious dentin is removed.

Lest it be assumed that all teeth with exposed pulps should be treated and salvaged, the dentist should ask himself the following questions: "Is the tooth strategic for maintenance of oral health, and should it be saved at all costs?" "If the pulp capping is not successful, will the expense of endodontic therapy and crown placement be economically feasible to the patient?" "Are there other options in the treatment plan (e.g., placement of a fixed bridge) that might be equally attractive?" "If the pulp capping and/or endodontic therapy fails and the tooth is subsequently removed, what effect will it have on treatment planning?" Discretion is often the better part of valor, and optional treatment plans should always be considered.

Caries Control. For a mouth with many carious lesions rapid emergency treatment can often be provided because it is so easily applied by simply initiating caries control procedures, namely, by replacing carious dentin with zinc oxide–eugenol cement (option 5). This changes the oral flora and arrests the advance of caries on the teeth so treated. Although not a permanent treatment, it can serve as a therapeutic measure for the patient who is prone to caries. It provides a holding pattern until the dentist can place permanent restorations at his and the patient's convenience. When placing the permanent restoration the operative dentist can leave the cement dressing in the deeper portion of the cavity as a cement base† providing, of course, that all carious dentin has been removed.

With the moderate carious lesion the operator may choose to use a liner and/or a cement base prior to placement of the permanent restoration. With the deep carious lesion, a zinc oxide–eugenol type of base can be used alone, or a thick calcium hydroxide liner may be placed into the deeper portions of the cavity (Fig. 8–14).

Zinc Oxide–Eugenol Cement. Zinc oxide–eugenol cement (see Chapter 7) is very popular and can be handled with ease if it is mixed to a thick puttylike consistency. A *small* piece about the size of a sesame seed is attached to the tip of the explorer and deftly carried to and deposited within the cavity (Figs. 8–15 and 8–16). Care is taken to avoid smearing the cement on the edges of the cavity walls.

An ultra-small pellet of cotton is grasped in cotton pliers and used to "pat" the material and mold it within the cavity. Any metal or plastic instrument will adhere to the cement, hence the need for dry cotton as the manipulative instrument (Fig. 8–16). Additional increments can be added and molded in a similar fashion until sufficient bulk is present.

---

*Polycarbonate crowns are often used instead of metal when esthetics is a matter of concern.

†One reason for using a cement base under amalgam is for insurance against the day when the amalgam restoration may need to be removed. Amalgam and stained dentin are dark colored and have similar cutting textures. In removing a previously placed amalgam (see Fig. 11–81), penetration of the bur beyond the amalgam-dentin interface can unwittingly occur. Particularly in deeper areas of the tooth, pulpal penetration by the bur is a hazard. The presence of a softer and white material is a distinct guide to the operator and assists him in safely removing only the old amalgam restoration.

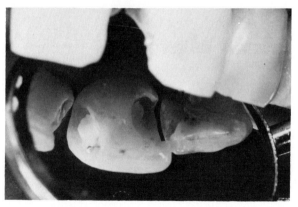

Figure 8–14. Maxillary central incisor with deep lesions from previously placed restorations. Dycal has been placed as a thick liner over the pulpal areas. Composite restorations will be placed in this tooth.

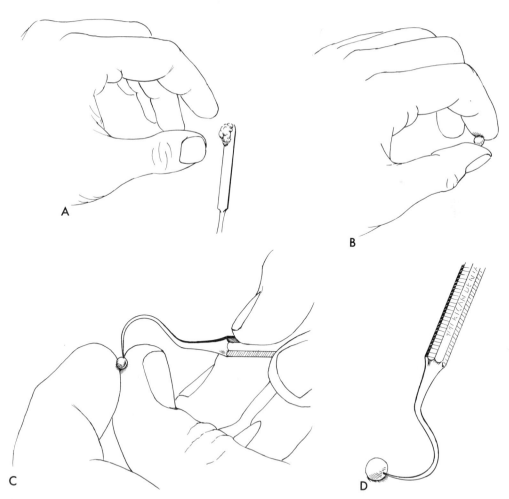

Figure 8–15. Zinc oxide–eugenol cement. *A,* Mixed to a thick consistency. *B,* If the cement adheres to the fingers, more powder should be added. *C,* A pellet of cement is picked up with an explorer and carried to the cavity *(D).*

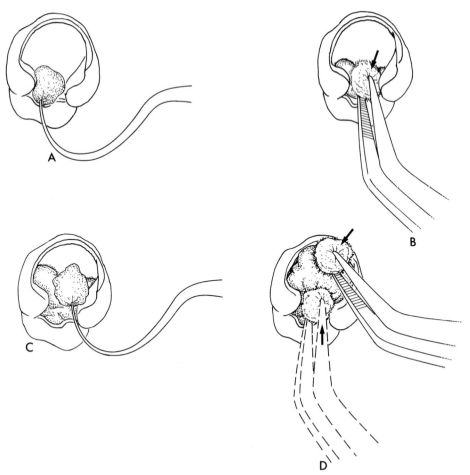

Figure 8–16. Placement of zinc oxide–eugenol cement. *A,* The cement is transferred to the cavity site. *B,* A small dry cotton pellet is used for manipulating cement inside the cavity. *C,* Additional increments of cement are added. *D,* The cement is shaped with a cotton pellet.

This kind of base can be placed to rebuild the entire internal form, or it can be placed as only a thin layer to be covered with a harder base such as zinc phosphate cement. As will be observed from experience, the clue to successful and easy use of ZOE cement is a thick mix that is deftly and cleanly inserted into the cavity. With only a little practice the operator will discover that this modality of placement is exceptionally easy, especially in maxillary or distal areas where a less viscous material, because of gravity, will flow over unwanted areas.

After the cement has set, a bur with light pressure at slow speed can be used to smooth the pulpal floor of the cavity (Fig. 11–17). Utilizing the light tactile sense, a bur such as a large inverted cone can act as a miniature floor polisher, to render the surface clean and smooth at the desired depth. Axial walls may often be made smooth with a chisel or hatchet, excess cement being removed from retentive grooves with an explorer tip or with the No. 700 bur (see Fig. 8–24). As a base it is now ready for the permanent restoration.

If the intent is to utilize the cement for a temporary restoration instead of a base, it is mixed and applied similarly to fill the cavity. It is checked for occlusion before dismissing the patient. A matrix band is not used, and a dry

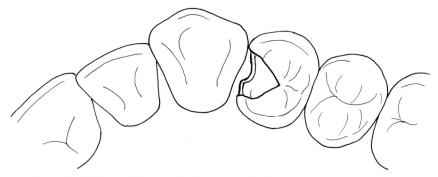

Figure 8–17. Proximal lesion to be "temporized" with zinc oxide–eugenol cement.

cotton pledget is employed to press the material into the cavity and quickly mold it to shape (Figs. 8–17, 8–18, and 8–19).

Another popular material, a reinforced zinc oxide–eugenol cement, is IRM (see Chapter 7). Its superior hardness and resistance to abrasion along with its ease of handling is largely responsible for its popularity. Possibly because of the polymer filler particles it cannot be mixed to the same plastic consistency as non-altered zinc oxide–eugenol cement.* It is placed into the cavity with a plastic instrument and patted to place with a dry pellet of cotton or a burnisher as it approaches hardness (Figs. 8–20, 8–21, and 8–22).

Zinc Phosphate Cement. In lesions, large or small, the operator may wish to use zinc phosphate cement or other "liner," thereby providing the tooth with a stronger and harder base. It is presumed, of course, that a suitable liner has already been applied. In using zinc phosphate cement as a base, the consistency should also be very thick and puttylike except for a small tag of "creamy mix" material that is placed on the corner of the slab and retained

---

*If the operator wishes to dilute or thin out a stiff mix of the zinc oxide–eugenol cements, he can dilute it with more liquid. This is not possible with zinc phosphate and most of the other cements.

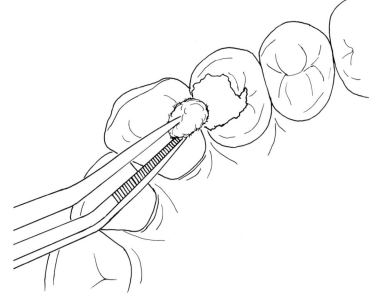

Figure 8–18. Cement is inserted into the cavity. It is not necessary to use a matrix band.

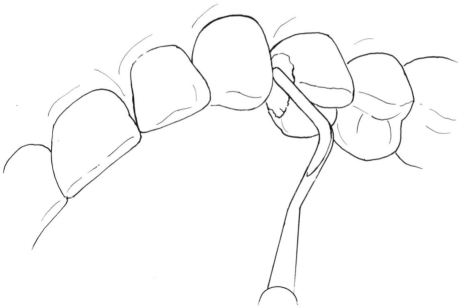

Figure 8–19. Thin-bladed instrument is used to re-establish embrasure form.

for attaching the base. With a small plastic instrument or ball burnisher, some of the creamy material is picked up and placed in the retention areas of the cavity (Fig. 8–23A). Then with a clean plastic instrument, the needed amount of thick base is carried into proper position and molded to form (Fig. 8–23B). Desirably only a slight excess of cement is carried into the cavity because unwanted excess only smears up the tooth surface. Cavity varnish applied as a liner prior to the cement serves as an adherent to hold the cement securely against the dentin and also serves as a barrier against irritation from the unset cement.

Zinc phosphate cement sets rapidly, making it difficult to place additional increments. Plastic instruments may be dipped in 95 per cent alcohol to prevent the cement from sticking to them while the pulpal and/or axial walls

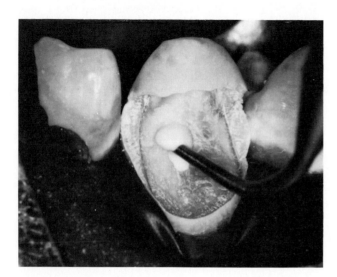

Figure 8–20. Applying Dycal over the pulpal area. (Courtesy of Dr. Michael Hanst)

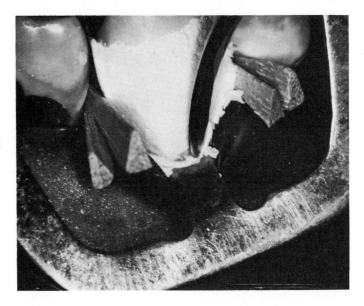

Figure 8–21. Filling the cavity with a stiff mix of IRM cement. (Courtesy of Dr. Michael Hanst)

are molded to shape. Cement powder also helps prevent cement from adhering to instruments and fingers. Two types of instruments are needed for this purpose: a smooth-faced plugger for the pulpal wall and a flat or cylindrically shaped instrument for the axial wall (Fig. 8–23).

After the base has hardened, slow-speed steel burs are used to smooth pulpal, axial, and gingival walls (Figs. 8–24 and 11–17). As soon as the cement has been placed in the cavity the glass slab should be placed in water as an aid in cleaning.

Polycarboxylate Cement. Polycarboxylate cement may also be used as a cement base. The zinc phosphate cements are routinely used after application of a cavity varnish; the polycarboxylate cements are placed directly against tooth structure.

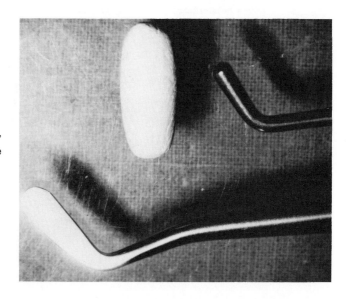

Figure 8–22. Proper consistency of "stiff" mix, with plastic instruments to manipulate it. (Courtesy of Dr. Michael Hanst)

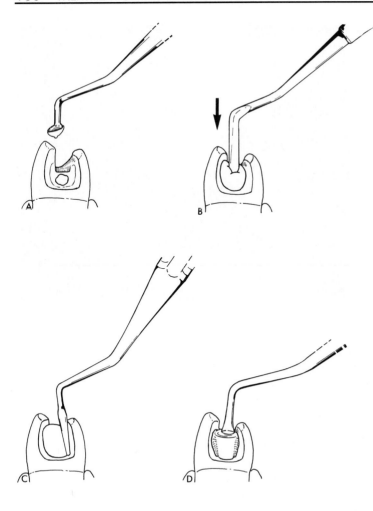

Figure 8–23. Placement of zinc phosphate cement. *A,* Creamy mix of zinc phosphate cement being applied to "wet" the surface of the dentin. Notice retentive areas in the preparation to stabilize and fasten the cement. *B,* Putty-like mixture of zinc phosphate cement added and molded to form. The earlier application of thin cement serves as glue to enhance adhesion. *C,* Plastic instruments in use. Ethyl alcohol, 95 per cent, prevents cement from adhering to the instrument. *D,* Smooth-faced condenser to shape the pulpal floor. *E,* Plastic instrument (Mortenson's No. 2) to mold and shape the axial wall.

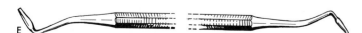

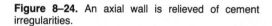

Figure 8–24. An axial wall is relieved of cement irregularities.

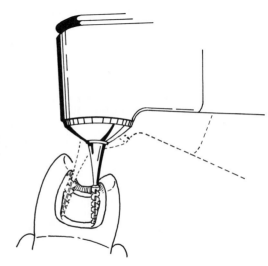

The super-stickiness of the polycarboxylate cement is a single factor that makes it quite difficult to handle. No substance to coat the instruments seems to prevent the cement from sticking to them,* which makes molding and shaping quite difficult.

Because of its superior stickiness, polycarboxylate cement is an excellent material to place underneath a thin enamel plate to prevent a metallic restoration from showing through. If, for example, the carious process has undermined the mesio-buccal plate of enamel in a maxillary first premolar, the cosmetic effect would suffer if amalgam were placed directly against the inside of the enamel, where it would appear as a dark gray stain. Painting the inside of the enamel to mask the amalgam is in order; polycarboxylate is an excellent "paint" for this purpose (Fig. 8–25).

Treatment of the Exposed Pulp

Clinicians are not always in agreement as to how deep carious lesions should be handled, especially those that approach the vicinity of the pulp. In a shallow or moderately deep cavity, all carious dentin should be removed, leaving a glassy-hard dentin surface. Even in deep lesions all carious dentin at the periphery of the cavity should be excavated to establish a clean hard junction with the restorative material. Removal of carious dentin along the gingival floor is often overlooked in the removal of peripheral decay (Fig. 8–26).

Attention is now directed toward the carious dentin in the central (pulpal) area of the lesion. A question arises with regard to the excavation of the semi-hard dentin adjacent to and directly overlying the pulp. Should all carious dentin be removed (thereby exposing the pulp) or should the semi-hard interface material be retained and treated, thereby avoiding an actual exposure? If one follows the former method, he treats the pulp as an open wound, free of debris and contaminants (direct pulp capping); if he follows the latter, he delays removal of the very deep carious dentin (indirect pulp capping) until a later appointment.

*Dry powder is somewhat helpful.

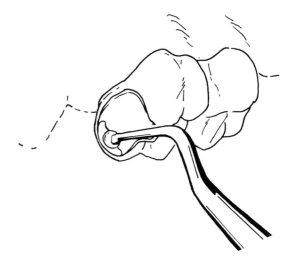

Figure 8–25. Polycarboxylate cement being painted inside the enamel plate to mask out the underlying amalgam restoration.

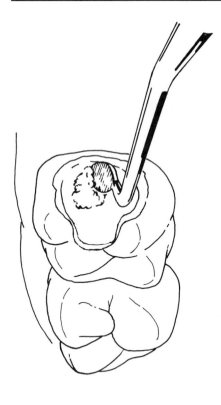

Figure 8–26. Caries removal along gingival floor with a large sharp excavator. Peripheral carious dentin along the gingival floor is *completely* removed *before* inspecting the pulpal area.

Direct Pulp Capping

Direct pulp capping is a one-appointment procedure. Following local anesthesia and application of the rubber dam, the carious dentin is completely excavated. The pulp will bleed when cut with the excavator. After the bleeding has stopped, calcium hydroxide in a paste or powder form is applied to the pulpal opening and securely attached to the internal walls of the lesion with cement.

Initial bandaging of the pulp with calcium hydroxide and a cement dressing is followed by a three- or four-month time interval to permit healing of the pulp and formation of secondary dentin. After the time has elapsed and the tooth has been free from pain or discomfort, a favorable prognosis can usually be made and a permanent restoration placed. Whether the restoration takes the form of an amalgam or a cast gold crown, the internal part of the cement dressing in the depth of the cavity is left undisturbed* to serve as a protective base.

The need for providing a hermetic seal and a strong, intact, non-dislodg-able cement restoration over the exposure site during the healing period cannot be overemphasized. If the dressing is not secure and breaks loose from the tooth during mastication, the pulp comes in direct contact with oral contaminants, and hopes for successful healing obviously must be abandoned.

So important is structural integrity in retaining a reliable hermetic seal over the pulp that many operators gamble on the pulp's healing ability and

*After this waiting period some clinicians prefer to completely remove the cement and inspect the exposure site for secondary dentin formation. If the pulp has manifested sufficient vitality to build a secondary dentin bridge over the orifice of the exposure site, a favorable prognosis is rendered. If not, the pulp is condemned and endodontic therapy initiated.

place a permanent restoration (e.g., amalgam) over the calcium hydroxide and cement at the same appointment. If the pulp does not heal but becomes necrotic, he can always gain access through the restoration to initiate endodontic therapy. In the meantime the patient has had the comfort of a hard strong restoration rather than a softer temporary cement.

Armamentarium
1. Round burs C. A. Nos. 2, 4, 6, 8
     F-G bur: No. 245
2. Large excavator
3. Enamel hatchet or bin-angle chisel
4. Medicaments (calcium hydroxide: powder or paste)
5. Paste applicator
6. Cotton pliers and pledgets of cotton
7. Cement: zinc oxide–eugenol
8. Plastic instrument

Procedure
Excavation. Enamel is cut away to permit access, but not so much that the integrity for retaining the cement is jeopardized. When an exposure might be anticipated, the peripheral carious dentin is removed first (Figs. 8–2, 8–2B, 8–27, and 8–28). Having eliminated 90 per cent of the carious material, the operator now directs his attention to the dentin overlying the pulp. Because of anatomic configurations of the pulp horns and patterns of caries activity, this "pillow" of carious dentin is usually on the side rather than at the bottom of the cavity. The *larger* excavator is now inspected for sharpness (see Fig. 6–21) and resharpened if necessary (see Fig. 3–61). With deft and careful

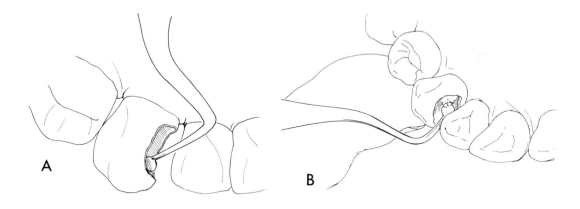

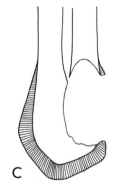

Figure 8–27. Removal of carious dentin in a deep lesion of a canine (probably a pulp exposure). *A,* Removing incisal carious dentin. A very small sharp excavator is necessary to eliminate final remnants of debris wedged between enamel plates at the incisal edge. *B,* All peripheral dentin has now been completely removed. Remaining carious dentin alongside the pulp is now carefully curetted away with a large sharp excavator. *C,* Contrary to what might be expected, the exposure site is invariably on the axial wall (on the side rather than the bottom of the cavity).

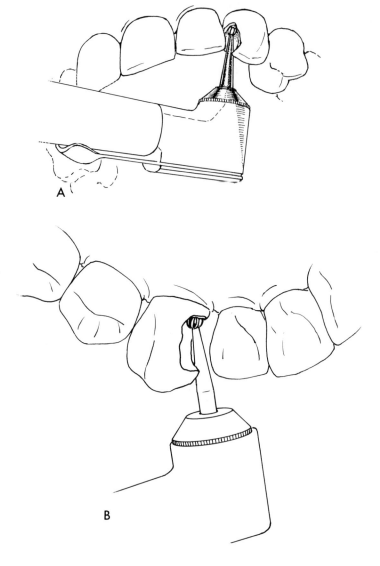

Figure 8–28. *A*, Large round bur riding against the enamel is an acceptable instrument in removing peripheral carious dentin. *B*, Bur removing peripheral carious dentin in the cingulum area.

strokes this soft carious dentin (usually on the axial wall) is carefully shaved away (see Fig. 8–27). Extreme care is exercised not to force carious dentin into the pulp chamber with a careless movement of the excavator, especially with a dull blunt-edged excavator. Obviously, a bur should not be used for this purpose, as it, like a dull excavator, would inoculate the pulp with debris.

As an agent to eliminate traces of blood in various clinical procedures, H_2O_2 is quite effective, but it should NEVER be used over an open pulp. In contact with the blood, H_2O_2 causes oxygen bubbles to develop in the chamber, which strangulate the vessels and impede circulation. Clean fresh water (preferably distilled) or saline solution is an acceptable cleansing agent. In this regard some operators feel that the use of the air syringe around an exposure site should be guarded lest air enter the pulp chamber.

The degree and kind of hemorrhage experienced during the exposure of the pulp is a valuable diagnostic aid for prognosis. Generally, if the blood is red, if it flows freely, and if clotting time is normal, the prognosis for a successful pulpal healing is good. If the blood is pale and is associated with serum exudate, the prognosis is poor.

Capping. If bleeding at the exposure site is arrested and the area is dry, calcium hydroxide paste is the capping material of choice. It is applied in the same manner as shown in Figures 8–8, 8–9, and 8–10, with the paste extending on the sound dentin only 1 to 2 mm peripheral to the exposure.

If bleeding is stubborn, calcium hydroxide powder is preferred to a paste because of its blotting and coagulating effects upon blood. After cleansing the area to eliminate as much blood and debris as possible, the cavity is dried with cotton pellets (Fig. 8–29). A small pellet of cotton is moistened, blotted free of excess water, then dipped into the dry calcium hydroxide powder to pick up a tuft of calcium hydroxide powder. This is carried to the cavity and placed over the exposed area. The powder, now somewhat dampened from the cotton pledget, is transferred from the cotton to the wet pulp. A second and larger pellet of dry cotton is then pressed over the area to blot the powder dry and to stabilize it over the exposure site (Figs. 8–29 and 8–30).

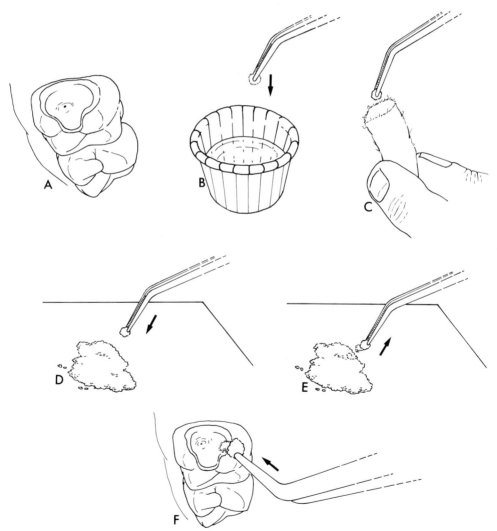

Figure 8–29. Direct pulp capping procedure using calcium hydroxide powder. *A,* Exposure site is clean but may still be oozing blood. *B,* A pellet of cotton is moistened with water. Pellet must be very small and rolled into a tight ball. *C,* The pellet is blotted free of excess moisture. *D,* Calcium hydroxide powder. *E,* Picking up a tuft of powder. *F,* Carrying it to the exposure site.

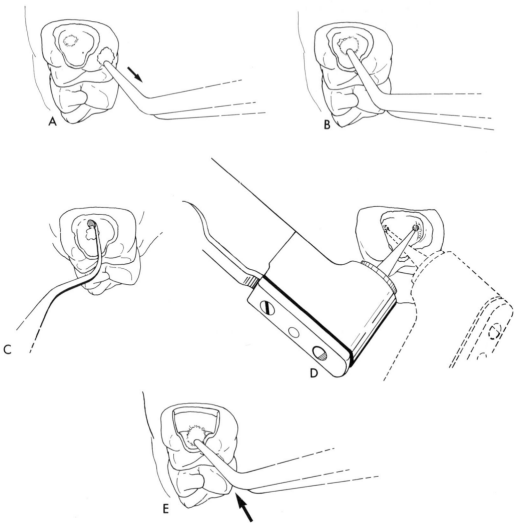

Figure 8–30. Direct pulp capping procedure *(continued). A,* Depositing powder over the pulp. *B,* Larger pellet of dry cotton adapts powder to close the orifice and arrest bleeding. *C,* Excess fragments of powder are flaked away so the zinc oxide–eugenol cement can adhere to the surface. *D,* Grooves are prepared well out to the edges of the cavity. They are usually best placed toward the buccal and lingual and serve as mechanical interlocks to retain the zinc oxide–eugenol cement. A No. 2 steel round bur operated at slow speed is best for this purpose. *E,* The cavity is based with zinc oxide–eugenol cement. The cement forced into the grooves provides a stable and secure covering for the calcium hydroxide.

Bleeding is immediately arrested, and an excavator is used to scrape excess fragments of calcium hydroxide from the periphery of the area. The calcium hydroxide need not extend more than 1 mm beyond the edges of the exposure site lest it occlude retentive areas intended for the cement (Fig. 8–30C). As mentioned earlier, cement does not readily adhere to dentin. It is usually wise, using a No. 2 round bur, to place groovelike interlocks or undercuts toward the buccal and lingual to retain the cement and prevent its dislodgement (Fig. 8–30D).

Sealing. Attention is now directed to the task of sealing the calcium hydroxide in place with zinc oxide-eugenol cement. A small ball of cement is selected, placed on the tip of an explorer (Figs. 8–15 and 8–16), and carried to the exposure site. Sticking to the dentin, it now frees itself from the explorer and is ready to be molded into the undercuts with a small dry pledget of cotton. Naturally pressure from the cotton pledget should be gentle over the pulp area to avoid forcing it into the pulp chamber.

At this stage the pulp has been protected by an internal coating of calcium hydroxide and covered by a hardened patty of zinc oxide–eugenol cement. If the cement has been securely anchored within the interlocks, it forms an integral restoration that is secure, that forms a seal over the pulp, and that protects the exposure site from pressure. The operator can now wash the area and make cavity refinements without fear of dislodging the pulp capping material and re-exposing the pulp.

At the wishes of the operator the tooth can now be restored permanently with a cement base and amalgam or temporarily with an aluminum crown.

Indirect Pulp Capping

Indirect pulp capping is a two-or-more appointment procedure.

Preferred by many clinicians, the indirect pulp capping procedure is felt to be more conservative and more likely to yield favorable results than the direct method. The supporters of this approach prefer not to traumatize the tooth by subjecting it to an exploratory procedure to determine whether they are dealing with an actual pulp exposure or whether they are dealing with only a deep carious lesion.

Giving the tooth the benefit of the doubt they leave some of the questionable carious dentin over the pulpal area and seal it over. Sometime later after remineralization has had opportunity to take place, the lesion is re-opened, all cement and carious dentin is removed, and the cavity is then treated as a deep carious lesion.

Procedure. The field must be isolated from moisture and use of the rubber dam is advised. All peripheral carious dentin is removed with large round burs or an excavator. The internal portion directly adjacent to the pulp is debrided of only the soft carious dentin. The cavity is then washed clean and dried and a thick mix of ZOE-type cement is placed. The patient is dismissed, and the tooth is left undisturbed for three months or longer.

At a subsequent appointment the tooth is again isolated, the cement removed, and the internal surface of the cavity inspected. During the interim period the dentin undergoes remineralization* and it becomes harder. With this added protection from remineralization and from additional secondary dentin formation inside the pulp, the operator can now remove any residual soft dentin. It is now receptive to a permanent restoration.

If, after the interim period, inspection reveals no change in dentin structure and remineralization has not yet taken place, the operator may elect to re-treat the tooth with another cement restoration.

Direct Versus Indirect Pulp Capping

What factors should determine the use of direct pulp capping in contrast to indirect pulp capping? Despite the differences between these two modalities, let us concentrate on the similarities between the two. The foremost similarity is the removal of *all* carious dentin peripherally in the lesion. This trough of

---

*In an effort to stimulate remineralization it is a common practice among many clinicians to apply calcium hydroxide or fluoride solution to the cavity after the initial caries removal.

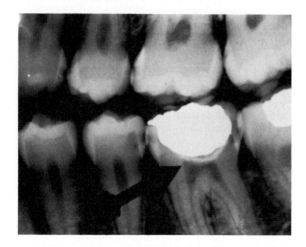

Figure 8–31. Indirect pulp capping of lower first molar. Note the remineralization that has taken place over the pulp chamber. Had all the softened carious dentin been removed a pulp exposure would have occurred. (Courtesy of Dr. Wallace W. Johnson, U. of Iowa)

clean cut dentin (carious dentin removed) is 2+ mm wide as it completely encircles the center of the lesion. Both the direct and indirect methods provide a seal to the lesion so that fluid leakage will not occur (minute marginal percolation notwithstanding). Both methods require a clean dry field and very sharp excavators.

The issue of whether to use a direct or indirect procedure is dependent upon factors other than only the health of the pulp. Placement of a stable temporary restoration without any occlusal and periodontal interferences is not always easy to achieve. Moreover, patient and operator availability to replace the temporary restoration with a permanent one at the end of the waiting period cannot always be taken for granted. To complicate the selection of the treatment plan is the factor of not knowing whether there is communi-

Table 8–2. DIAGNOSIS AND TREATMENT OF A *DEEP* CARIOUS LESION
NOT PENETRATING THE PULP

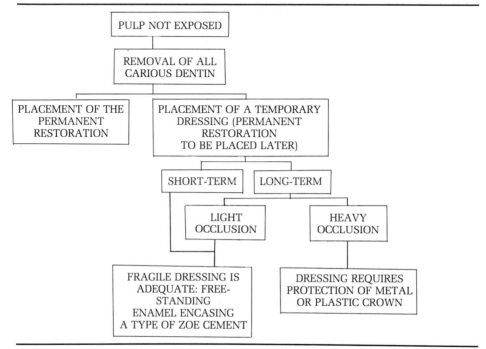

cation between the lesion and the pulp until the carious dentin is actually removed (Fig. 8–31).

For example, a busy office executive may experience a deep carious lesion on the distal surface of the maxillary second premolar. To undergo an indirect pulp capping to permit secondary dentin formation to occur seems to be a small benefit when considering the "price," which includes (a) an additional appointment for the patient and (b) at least three months of discomfort wearing a soft "temporary filling," which is subject to erosion, contact point breakdown, and possible food impaction. This patient, knowing the facts of the case, would probably choose to have all carious dentin removed and risk the success of a direct pulp capping if an exposure of the pulp occurs in the process of treatment. If the gamble proves favorable, no further treatment will be necessary. If the gamble proves unfavorable, simple endodontic therapy can probably be performed.

On the other hand, a patient in her early 20's may present herself with three or four deep lesions as determined by clinical and radiographic examination. Arresting the carious process and sealing the lesions with a zinc oxide–eugenol cement appears to be prudent. During the ensuing three-month period, or longer, other restorative procedures can be completed. The indirect pulp capping is now completed and the tooth is ready for a permanent restoration.

Table 8–3. DIAGNOSIS AND TREATMENT OF DEEP CARIOUS LESION
THAT MAY OR MAY NOT PENETRATE THE PULP

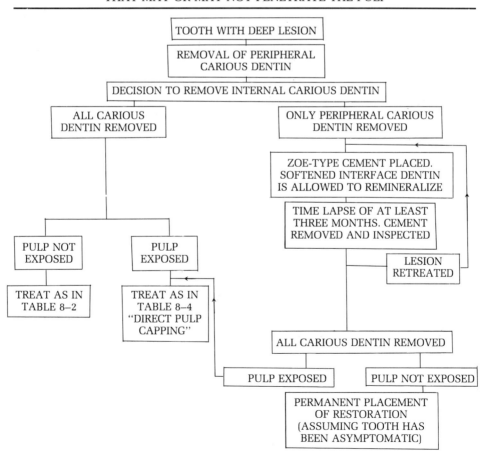

It is not the intent of this chapter to discuss clinical symptoms, e.g., tooth sensitivity to heat and cold, which obviously could have a bearing on the treatment of choice (direct vs. indirect pulp capping). In the final analysis the judgment of the experienced clinician should prevail. In an effort, however, to clarify the options of treatment, Tables 8–2, 8–3, and 8–4 are provided for study.

Fluoride Therapy in the Operatory

Requiring only minimal time, effort, and expense, fluoride application can become a part of the routine of operative dentistry. Two substances, a thixotropic acidulated phosphate fluoride gel and a stannous fluoride crystal, serve the need of ordinary procedures; the former is stable and may be used in impression trays or in a syringe; the latter is unstable and must be mixed daily to form a 10 per cent (saturated) solution (Tables 8–5 and 8–6). SnF_2 solution is watery and is applied with a cotton pellet to the cavity prior to placing the restoration.

Stannous fluoride treatment is recommended for those preparations that are influenced by a rapid caries activity or decalcification. If resins are to be placed in these preparations *sodium* fluoride is applied following its restoration, as stannous fluoride may lead to discoloration of the resin.

Table 8–4. DIAGNOSIS AND TREATMENT OF DEEP CARIOUS
LESION PENETRATING THE PULP

Table 8–5. APPLICATION OF STANNOUS FLUORIDE (10 PER CENT) DURING
OPERATIVE PROCEDURES

**Small/Moderate Cavities Direct Pulp
Capping, Cementation of Castings**
1. Dry surface
2. Apply fluoride to prepared dentin*
3. Wait 30 seconds
4. Dry surface
5. Apply copal varnish
6. Continue with operative procedure

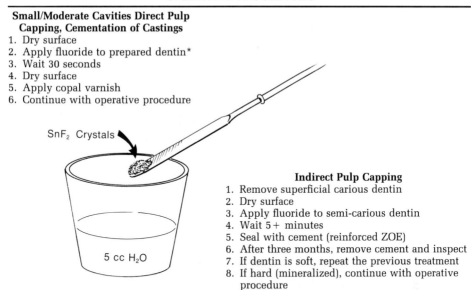

SnF$_2$ Crystals

5 cc H$_2$O

Indirect Pulp Capping
1. Remove superficial carious dentin
2. Dry surface
3. Apply fluoride to semi-carious dentin
4. Wait 5 + minutes
5. Seal with cement (reinforced ZOE)
6. After three months, remove cement and inspect
7. If dentin is soft, repeat the previous treatment
8. If hard (mineralized), continue with operative
   procedure

*Opening to pulp should be sealed.

Table 8–6. FLUORIDE GEL APPLICATION DURING OPERATIVE PROCEDURES

**Root Sensitivity, Shallow Root Caries
No Restoration Indicated**
1. Clean with pumice slurry
2. Remove superficial caries
3. Dry thoroughly
4. Apply gel (trays O.K.)
5. Wait four minutes
6. Have patient expectorate and rinse

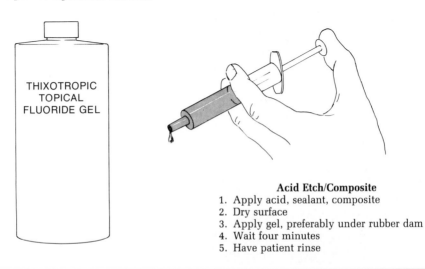

THIXOTROPIC
TOPICAL
FLUORIDE GEL

Acid Etch/Composite
1. Apply acid, sealant, composite
2. Dry surface
3. Apply gel, preferably under rubber dam
4. Wait four minutes
5. Have patient rinse

ISOLATION OF THE WORKING FIELD

9

Needs for isolation of the oral working area are rather obvious. A tooth bathed in saliva, a tongue that insists on obstructing vision, and a bleeding gingiva are but a few of the obstacles that must be overcome before delicate and accurate workmanship is possible. Several methods can be employed for isolating the working area: high-velocity evacuation (an oral vacuum cleaner), saliva ejectors, cotton rolls, and the rubber dam (Fig. 9–1).

The saliva ejector and high-velocity evacuation differ primarily in the size of the tip that is placed in the mouth; the former, with a diameter of 4 mm, is used to aspirate saliva that collects in the floor of the mouth; the latter, with a diameter of 10 mm, whisks away moisture and debris from the working

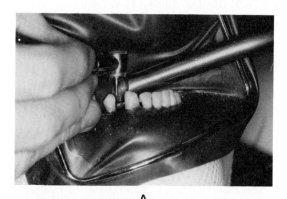

A

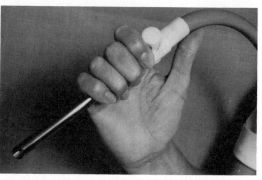

B

Figure 9–1. High-velocity evacuation. Inside diameter of tip is ⅜″ contrasted to 5/32″ for a saliva ejector. *A,* HVE is very effective with the rubber dam. *B,* Proper grasp of the evacuator by the dental assistant.

area. Ordinarily, high-velocity evacuation (H.V.E.) is operated by the dental assistant (Fig. 9–1), whereas the saliva ejector hangs unattended in the floor of the mouth (Fig. 9–2). H.V.E. is very effective when both the dentist and the assistant operate as an experienced and skillful team.

The most critical part of a saliva ejector is its tip. Resting in the floor of the mouth, under constant negative pressure, it can draw delicate soft tissue into its orifice resulting in an ugly lesion. Frequent inspection of the ejector should be a habit to insure against occlusion of the tip, particularly when a local anesthetic has deprived the patient of sensory responses in the floor of the mouth (Fig. 9–2C).

Cotton rolls to absorb saliva are quite effective in providing short-term isolation. Naturally they must be changed frequently as they become saturated with saliva. Cotton rolls come in a variety of lengths and sizes, but No. 2 cotton rolls, 1½" long and ⅜" in diameter, are the most popular. Location and method for placement of cotton rolls are shown in Figure 9–3.

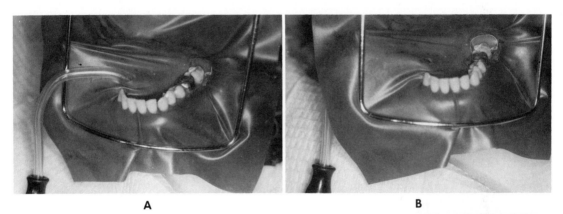

A   B

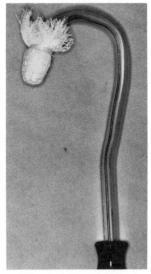

C

Figure 9–2. Saliva ejector in position where it is comfortable for the patient and convenient for the dental assistant and least obstructs the operating area. *A,* Inserted through a hole in the dam. *B,* Inserted under the dam. Frequently the patient prefers to hold the aspirator himself during the procedure. After the dam has been applied many patients prefer to forgo the inconvenience of the ejector and swallow instead. *C,* Piece of 2″ × 2″ gauze tied around the tip of the saliva ejector to prevent aspiration of mucosa from the floor of the mouth. (Courtesy of Dr. Jay Gaeman)

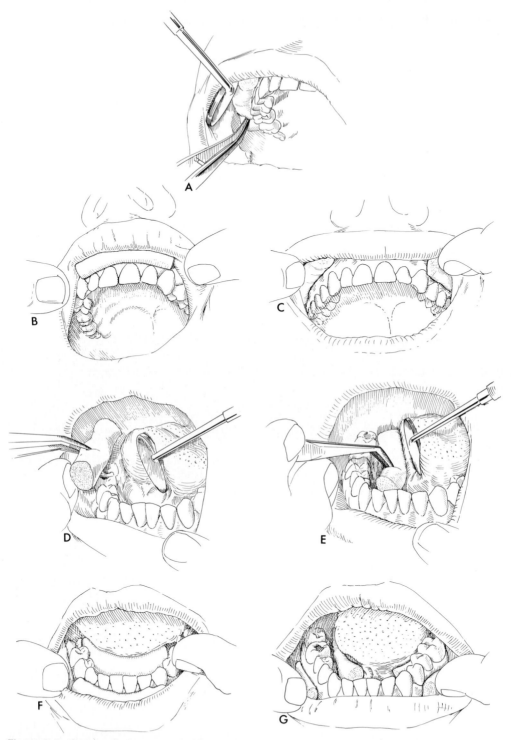

Figure 9–3. Cotton roll placement. *A,* Mirror reflects lip and cheek to make space available in the vestibule for the cotton roll. *B,* Incorrect. Cotton rolls should not be placed in the midline. In this position they are readily dislodged. *C,* Correct isolation for maxillary anteriors. Adequate space is available from the canine posteriorward to receive and retain cotton rolls. Because no salivary ducts are in the labial vestibule it is not necessary to place a cotton roll underneath the upper lip. *D,* A muscular tongue being reflected to receive a cotton roll in the floor of the mouth. *E,* Correct location for cotton roll. Where space permits two cotton rolls are used instead of one. *F,* Incorrect. Frenum attachment and tension from the lip make this type of isolation relatively impractical. *G,* Preferred isolation for mandibular incisors. Bilateral rolls absorb more moisture and are not as readily dislodged. Cotton rolls should be thoroughly wet before removal lest soft tissue surfaces adhere to the fibers and the outer layer of epithelium be stripped away.

Another popular absorbent medium is the Theta "Dri-Angle."* Inserted in the right or left vestibule, it is effective in absorbing secretions from the parotid ducts (Fig. 9–4).

Rubber Dam to Isolate the Working Area

Of all techniques and methods for isolation of the working field, none is quite as effective as the rubber dam, and it is considered the standard device for isolating the working area during operative procedures. This rubber sheet, with the teeth projecting through it, provides positive, long-lasting dryness of the teeth requiring treatment. Because it has no substitute and because its mastery is an absolute "must" for operative procedures, the balance of the chapter will be devoted to its use (Fig. 9–5).

Selection of Materials

Rubber Dam. The rubber dam material should be reasonably fresh. After 2 or 3 years on the shelf, it deteriorates and tears readily when stretched over the teeth. Because of its contrast against the white teeth, a dark color is chosen as being most effective. Although available in rolls or precut sheets, the standard selection for size is 5″ × 5″ for children and 6″ × 6″ for adults.

Rubber is available in a variety of thicknesses†: thin, medium, heavy, and extra heavy. It is also available in colors: green (heavy) and blue (medium).

---

*Theta: "Dri-Angle" available from Dental Health Prod. Inc., P.O. Box 884, Niagara Falls, New York 14302.

†Approximate thickness of rubber dam (Hygienic Dental Mfg. Co.):

thin	0.15 mm
medium	0.20 mm
heavy	0.25 mm
extra heavy	0.30 mm
special extra heavy	0.35 mm

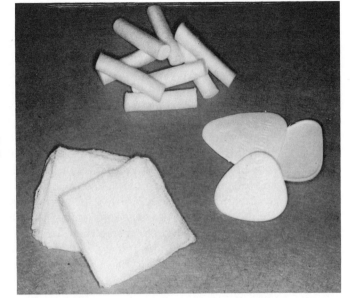

Figure 9–4. Absorbent media. Cotton rolls, 2″ × 2″ gauze pads, and alpha cellulose wafers.

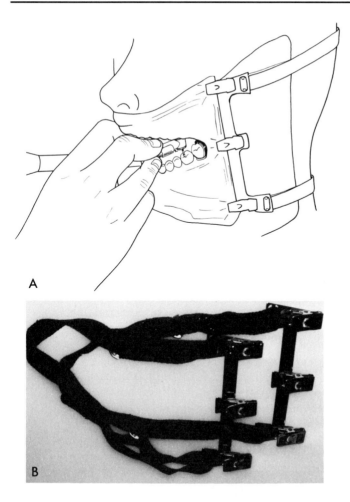

A

B

Figure 9–5. Strap type holder. *A,* Straps hold the rubber against the face for better bracing. *B,* Woodbury rubber dam holder. Advantages of the frame type: quickly and easily applied and does not interfere with the hair-do of the patient. Advantages of the strap type: permits good bracing, visibility, and access.

Advantages of the thinner rubber are its easy application and the comfort it provides the patient; advantages of the heavier rubber are its ability to retract soft tissue and its resistance to scuffing and tearing by the dental bur. Although individual preferences vary as to locations and use for each type, medium thickness is recommended for molar applications; heavy (or extra heavy) for anterior and bicuspid applications.

Clamps. Anchorage of the rubber at its distal end is accomplished by a clamp, which is available in a variety of sizes and shapes. The essential ingredients of any clamp are the two jaws, with the four prongs, the bow, the holes, and the wings (Fig. 9–6). Clamps vary primarily with respect to their mesial and distal prongs. Depending upon external circumference and tooth shape, the size of the clamp and location of its prongs are determined. The four prongs should engage the tooth precisely at its four corners. If the mesial and distal prongs are close together, they bite into only buccal and lingual tooth surfaces; if they are too far apart, they hang free in space, leaving the connecting metal to engage the tooth through tangential contact. Probably this kind of "fit" is notably worse than the former because the clamp tends to tip back and forth, eroding away soft cementum from the root and gouging the soft gingival tissue (Fig. 9–7). (Note how incorrect fit in Fig. 14–59 permits the tension of the rubber to tip the clamp forward.)

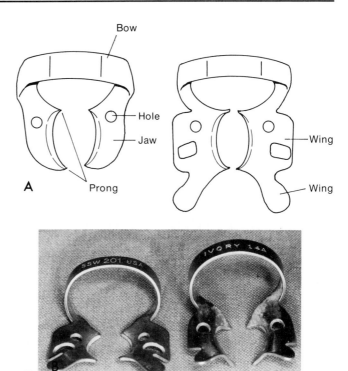

Figure 9–6. Clamp designs. *A,* Parts of rubber dam clamp labeled. The winged clamp holds the rubber out of the way, but it also restricts operating access. *B,* Inverted prongs of clamp on the right can more effectively engage partially erupted molars (Clamp No. 14A). Clamp on the left is typical.

Ratio and proportion are determined by the mind's eye of the operator as he selects a clamp for an anterior, a bicuspid, or a molar tooth. This is followed by experimentally fitting the clamp to the tooth. By trial and error the desired clamp is then chosen. An inordinately large variety of sizes and shapes of clamps have been designed. The bows of the clamps, being made of tempered spring steel, are heavier and more rugged for the molar clamps whereas bows of the clamps for smaller bicuspids and anteriors are more delicate. Although individual preferences differ, the wise operator can resolve most of his needs

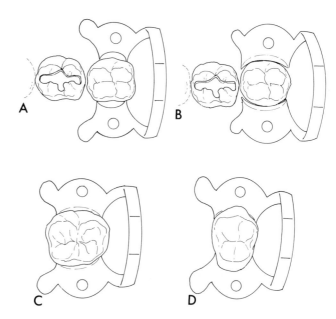

Figure 9–7. Method by which jaws of the retainer clamp grasp the tooth. The importance of proper fitting of the clamp cannot be overemphasized. *A,* Prongs are too close together for such a large tooth. *B,* The inner edge of the jaws engages the tooth, allowing the clamp to teeter back and forth. *C,* Correct prong and jaw alignment. The prongs securely grasp the tooth at its four corners. *D,* Proper fitting of premolar clamp.

Table 9–1. RUBBER DAM CLAMPS*

Teeth	Routine Use	Desirable Use	Occasional Use
Premolars	W2, Hygienic B-6	0, 1	00
Mandibular molars	7	SSW26, W3	14A (partially erupted teeth)
Maxillary molars	W22A, W23A	W8A	8AD
Primary second molars	W3, W2	W8A	
Anteriors	Hygienic B-6	0, 00 (wings removed)	9, Hygienic B-5

*All clamps are manufactured by J. W. Ivory Co. except those indicated as S. S. White and Hygienic. W: wingless.

with five or six clamps. (See Table 9–1 for suggested sizes of clamps that are frequently used.)

A partially erupted tooth is frequently difficult to grasp, requiring a clamp with inverted prongs (Fig. 9–6B).

The holes in a clamp must match the beaks of the clamp forceps. Frequently, holes are not matched by the beaks of the forceps. The beaks of many forceps may be small enough to fit into the holes of the clamp but are too large to release the clamp after it has been positioned on the tooth. Manufacturers of both clamp and clamps forceps are not careful with quality control in this regard, and modification by the dentist may be necessary to make them usable. Frequently, reducing the size of the forceps' beaks solves the problem more effectively than enlarging the holes of the clamp (Fig. 9–8).

A clamp may have as many as four projecting wings, two lateral and two anterior. Intended for restricting the rubber from the field of vision, these wings often obstruct the application of a matrix retainer and other instruments while operating. According to individual preferences, clamps can be purchased with or without* wings, or a winged clamp can be modified by cutting the wings off with a fissure bur (Fig. 9–9).

*Clamps prefaced by the letter "W" are usually devoid of projecting wings.

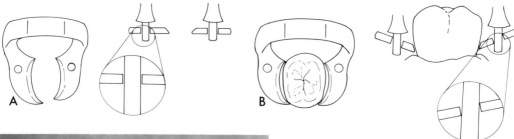

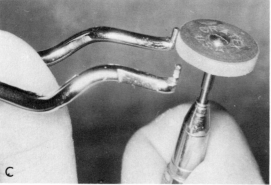

Figure 9–8. Mismatch of the holes in clamp and beaks of the forceps. A, In the closed position the beaks slide freely in and out of the holes of the clamp. B, While spread apart to engage a tooth in the open position, each of the beaks, now at an angle, is engaged by the metal edges, which will not release it. C, If predominant with most of the clamps, the beaks of the forcep should be carefully reduced in diameter with an abrasive wheel. If only an occasional clamp is involved the holes can be enlarged (see also Fig. 9–35).

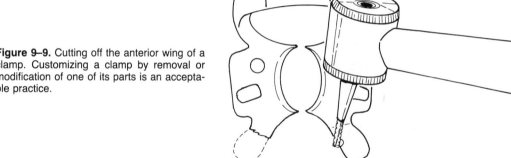

Figure 9–9. Cutting off the anterior wing of a clamp. Customizing a clamp by removal or modification of one of its parts is an acceptable practice.

At any rate, the student is encouraged to use the dam as often as possible. Each application presents its unique characteristics and only one with a thorough knowledge of its use can select clamps with impunity and apply the dam with skill and dispatch. Practice is necessary. The one who is skillful as an operative dentist first became skillful in rubber dam application.

Lubricant. A rubber dam is applied more easily when a lubricant is used. If the lubricant is oil soluble rather than water soluble, i.e., petroleum jelly, it penetrates and quickly rots the rubber. Shaving soap is first choice as a lubricant. Borofax,* an all-purpose lubricant, or ordinary bar soap make excellent lubricants. Rub the wet surface of the bar, pick up slurry on the finger, and rub it over the holes on the tissue side of the rubber (Fig. 9–10).

Napkins. Napkins† are worn for the comfort of the patient. Perspiration and saliva leakage are readily blocked by a napkin to separate the rubber from the skin (Fig. 9–11).

Rubber Dam Holders. The rubber must be stretched to provide wide access to the oral cavity. There are rubber dam holders of various types and designs. Essentially they involve (a) cervical traction,‡ with a strap going around the head or neck or (b) facial frames that provide circumferential stretching around the mouth itself.

The former is more advantageous from the point of view of the operator, since it reflects the rubber backward and keeps it flush with the face. Cervical traction provides greater access and improved finger bracing, because the

---

*Borofax is available from the pharmacy.

†Disposable cloth napkins manufactured by Hygienic Rubber Co. or Johnson & Johnson Company.

‡Woodbury-type rubber dam holder available from D.D.S. Industries, 1200 San Marcos Rd., Santa Barbara, California 93111.

Figure 9–10. Application of bar soap as a lubricant to the rubber dam. Lubricants are placed on the tissue side of the rubber to assist the teeth in slipping through their respective holes.

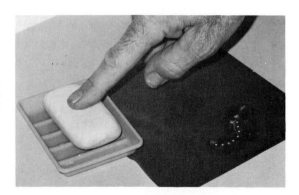

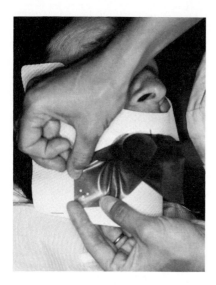

Figure 9–11. Rubber dam napkins are placed to absorb perspiration and saliva that might leak out the corners of the mouth. For short-time procedures a napkin is not necessary; for longer periods of time patient comfort requires its use. Note the identification holes for orienting the rubber on the lower right side.

operating hand can be brought closer to the working area. The strap sometimes annoys patients whose coiffure has been disturbed. It is also slightly more difficult to employ high-velocity suction and to control water flow during cutting procedures if strap fixation methods are used.

The facial frame (Fig. 9–5) is easier and faster to apply and more tolerable to patients. It does restrict the movement of the operator, however, and does not provide as much security and anchorage as the cervical type.

The use of either type may fulfill the needs of the operator, and both types should be on hand—the frame for the routine operation and the cervical type for the difficult or complex application (see Fig. 9–5).

Placement of the Holes

The holes are placed to conform to the curvature of the arch and spaced according to the distances between the teeth. Punching the holes in the rubber is not done until they are positioned and marked on the rubber. To assure the uniformity of rubber borders after application, two landmarks should be kept in mind. For maxillary applications, the incisors should lie one inch from the upper border; for mandibular applications, the most posterior hole is slightly right or left of the center of the rubber. Distances between the holes should be comparable to spaces between the centers of each tooth. The circumference of the arch is also reflected in the location of the holes, the object being to space the holes so the rubber will snugly engage each tooth without puckering. If the holes are placed too closely together or incorrectly aligned, they will fit over the teeth but will be stretched to the side, permitting saliva to leak by. If the holes are too far apart excess rubber stock remains and is puckered between the teeth (Figs. 9–12 to 9–14).

Although most punches can make five sizes of holes to match tooth size, it is suggested that only the three larger holes be used in order to avoid tearing the rubber during application. An extra large hole is suggested for the tooth that supports the clamp (Figs. 9–15 and 9–16).

A liberal number of teeth should always be included in a dam application for operative procedures. For example, an anterior application should include

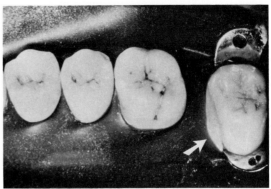

Figure 9–12. Holes in the rubber placed too close together. Leakage is likely to occur through open space mesial to the molar. (Courtesy of Dr. Dan Frederickson)

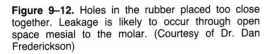

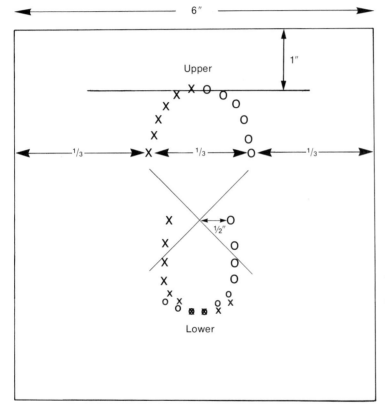

Figure 9–13. Positioning holes within the borders of the rubber. *Maxillary teeth:* Upper border should be one inch wide. The right and left borders in the molar region should be two inches wide (⅓ total width). The arch form is symmetrical. After application the rubber is folded to give a double thickness over the upper lip. *Mandibular teeth:* The borders must be larger for a mandibular application. It is important that sufficient rubber extend beyond the incisors to allow the dam to drape over the chin. The dead center of the dam—one-half inch either side—is the point of orientation for the most distal hole. Unlike the upper arch, the holes are punched in an asymmetrical pattern.

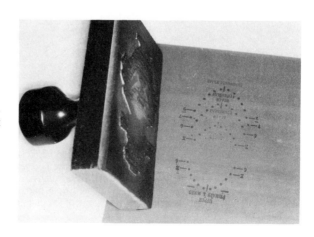

Figure 9–14. Hygiene rubber dam stamp. Although it is reasonably accurate, it does not always provide borders of equal width.

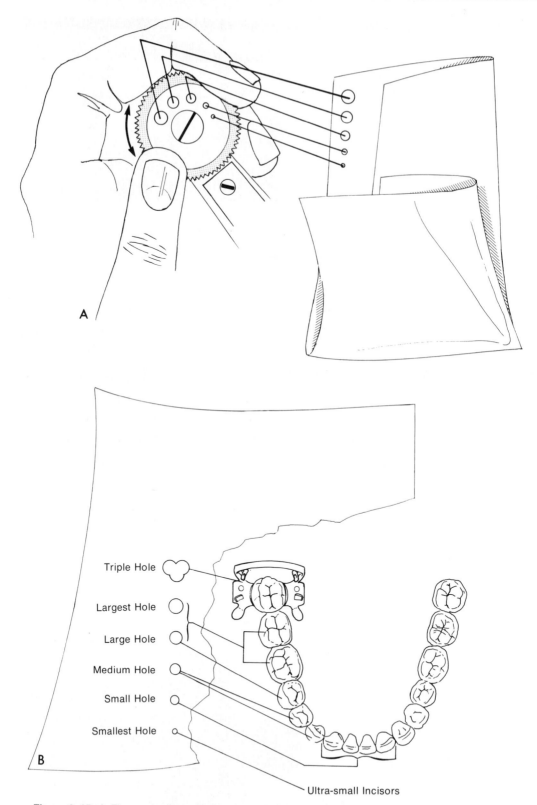

Triple Hole

Largest Hole

Large Hole

Medium Hole

Small Hole

Smallest Hole

Ultra-small Incisors

Figure 9–15. *A,* Five or six sizes of holes are available in most rubber dam punches. The punch is a delicate instrument and should be protected from damage. *B,* Seldom is the smallest hole used. To stretch the rubber over the bow and wings of the clamp a larger distal hole is needed.

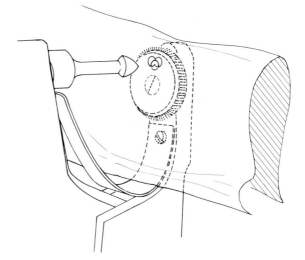

Figure 9–16. Position of rubber on anvil for punching an extra-large hole.

a minimum of seven teeth. A large number of teeth protruding through the rubber gives the operator access, reflects the lips, and provides an adequate number of dry anterior teeth to serve as finger rests. Posterior applications should usually reach from the first or second molar to the opposite cuspid. Ordinarily the clamp is attached one tooth distal to the tooth receiving treatment. Clasping third molars is usually possible and can be done if the need arises; however, patient comfort is greater if one can terminate the distal end of the application at the first or second molar.

Careful use and maintenance of the rubber dam punch cannot be overemphasized. It must be kept well oiled, it must never be autoclaved, and it should be stored in a dry place. *Above all else, the operator must be sure the punch cone is centered directly above a hole before it is depressed to punch the rubber.* If not, it is likely to shear off a fragment of metal around the edge of the hole and prevent it from cutting a clean perforation in the rubber. Carelessness in this regard virtually ruins this expensive instrument until a new cutting table is procured to replace the damaged one. Holes must be sharp and clean-cut. Holes with ragged edges will cause the rubber to tear when tightly stretched (Figs. 9–17 and 9–18).

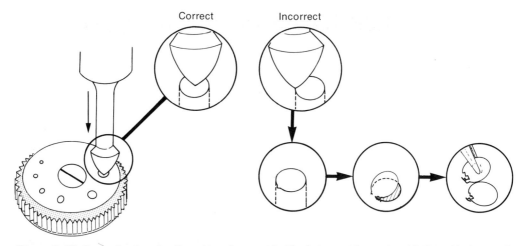

Figure 9–17. Precaution in using the rubber dam punch. The hole must be centered in line with the punch before closure. Any rubber cut from a hole with a chipped rim will have ragged edges and be subject to a rip or tear while slipping it over a tooth. Repair of the anvil requires resurfacing or purchase of a new anvil.

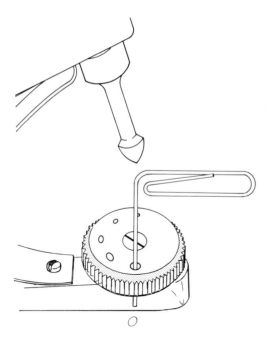

Figure 9–18. Removing rubber disks that have clogged a hole.

In applying the rubber dam, three steps should be taken: the preparation, the application, and the stabilization.

The Preparation

Procurement of the materials and the inspection of the teeth are of greatest importance.

Armamentarium

1. Basic four instruments: mirror, explorer, cotton pliers, plastic instrument
2. Rubber dam punch
3. Rubber dam clamp forceps
4. Rubber dam marked for punching
5. Rubber dam holder
6. Rubber dam napkin
7. Two pieces of dental tape 18 inches long
8. Rubber lubricant
9. Saliva ejector
10. Scissors
11. R-D clamp or clamps

Gross bits of calculus and other debris are removed, contact points are checked by the passage of dental tape, and sharp edges of enamel that might cut the rubber are removed. If the tooth to be prepared has an offending contact point (e.g., sharp enamel edge or rough amalgam surface), the wise operator frees the contact with a bur or instrument so that placement of the dam does not result in a torn rubber septum. The clamp to be used has been tried on the tooth and tested to be sure it will not be dislodged by the pull of the rubber against the bow. If a clamp can be readily dislodged by the mirror handle, another more secure clamp must be found. All clamps, particularly for second molar teeth, should be tested for stability before placing the rubber

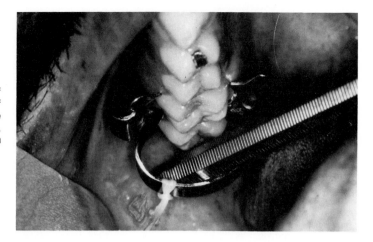

Figure 9–19. Testing stability of clamp before applying the rubber. If the clamp will be dislodged by the downward pull from a mirror handle, it will respond likewise to the tension of the rubber on the bow.

dam. Moreover, as a safety precaution dental tape should be tied in a bow as insurance against accidental dislodgement and aspiration of the clamp by the patient (Figs. 9–19 and 9–20).

Another preparatory act that lends comfort to the patient is the application of an emollient such as Borofax to the lips, especially at the corners of the mouth. It is also expected that the operator will have anesthetized the tooth and punched the holes in the rubber.

The Application

A variety of methods may be employed, but the following sequence is suggested:

1. Application of the clamp.
2. Lubrication of the rubber.
3. Placement of the rubber over the distal tooth and the clamp, including *all* of the wings. The large hole enables the operator, with his index fingers, to stretch and maneuver the rubber over the entire clamp so it can snugly encircle the tooth at its neck (Fig. 9–21).
4. Placement of the rubber dam napkin (Fig. 9–22).
5. Attachment of the holder. An identification mark in the form of a hole is placed at the lower right-hand corner of the rubber to serve as an aid in orienting the rubber prior to the attachment of the holder. Note that the

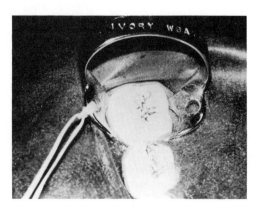

Figure 9–20. Dental tape attached to clamp as a security measure.

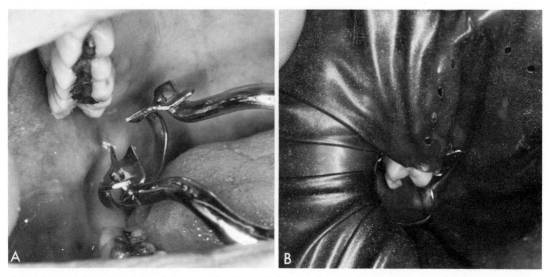

Figure 9–21. Initial placement of clamp and rubber. *A,* Clamp placement and testing for stability. *B,* Rubber stretched and passed over the bow and wings.

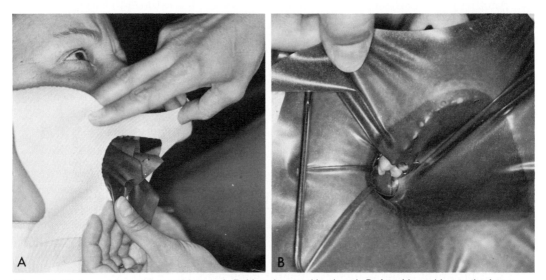

Figure 9–22. Assembling rubber and frame. *A,* Rubber dam napkin placed. *B,* Attaching rubber to the frame.

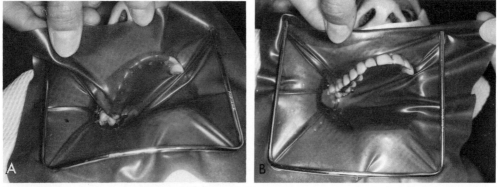

Figure 9–23. Teeth inserted through the rubber. *A,* The tooth at the opposite end of the holes is passed through first. *B,* Working back toward the clamp. Note the fold of the rubber, which makes a firm border under the lip.

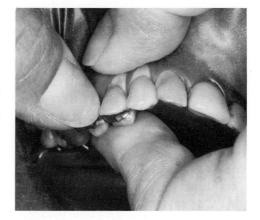

Figure 9–24. Stretching rubber with thumb and forefinger to make "elastic bands" above each contact point. The thumbnail of the other hand spreads the contact so the rubber can pass through.

clamped tooth is the only tooth protruding through the rubber at this stage of application. A fold at the upper border is desirable to enhance patient comfort (Fig. 9–22).

6. The rubber is then stretched over the opposite tooth, usually the opposite cuspid or first bicuspid (Fig. 9–23).

7. Working from this tooth back toward the clamp, the rubber is grossly stretched with the thumb on the labial and the index finger on the lingual to thin out the septal rubber so it can "pop" through the contact points. As an aid, the thumbnail of the opposite hand can wedge the teeth apart to allow passage of the rubber (Figs. 9–24 and 9–25).

8. Dental tape is now employed to pass the rubber through the remaining one or two contact points. If the rubber can be made to "knife" its way through the contact point as a single thickness of rubber, it is less likely to tear than if it is "folded" through in two or more thicknesses.

Waxed dental tape is preferred to dental floss or unwaxed dental tape. Often the passage of two to four strands of tape is needed to maneuver the rubber between tight contact points. To avoid tearing the rubber by removing the tape, additional strands are used, and removal of the tape from the gingival embrasure is postponed until all the rubber has passed through the contact point (Fig. 9–26).

It is not always possible to securely place a clamp on a tooth, and in these instances the rubber dam as an isolation modality must be abandoned. This usually occurs on incompletely erupted second or third molar teeth. In some patients the anatomy is such that the wings of the clamp placed on an

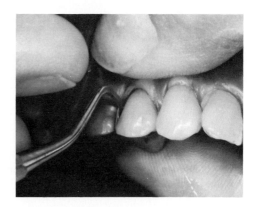

Figure 9–25. Opening the contact with an instrument to pry teeth apart.

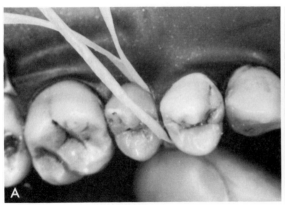
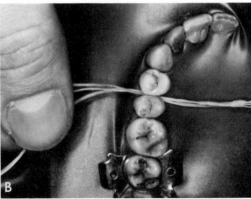

Figure 9–26. Passing rubber through contact with waxed dental tape. *A,* When multiple passes of the tape are necessary to manipulate the rubber between adjoining teeth, the pieces of tape accumulate in the gingival embrasure *(B)* until all the rubber has passed through. Then they are pulled out to the side.

upper second molar impinge upon the inner surface of the ramus of the mandible when the mouth is open. In such instances the rubber dam is not used.

Stabilization of the Rubber

To be sure the rubber remains intact to form a neat operating field the following should be inspected:

1. The rubber dam clamp is used, of course, to hold the distal end of the rubber around the most posterior tooth. Sometimes it is necessary to use another clamp to retain the rubber around the canine or first premolar on the opposite side of the arch. This may be prevented by cutting a wide piece of "rubber band" from the corner of the rubber dam, grasping and stretching it to simulate a piece of dental tape, and passing it through the contact point between canine and first premolar. Release of the tension permits the rubber to rebound and firmly engage itself in the gingival embrasure to prevent the rubber dam from slipping out from between the teeth (Fig. 9–27).

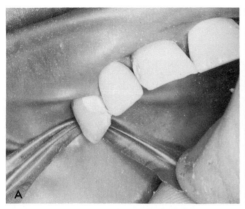
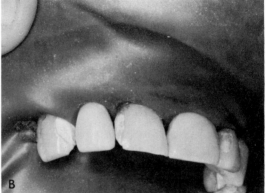

Figure 9–27. Clamp substitute. Where the tension is minimal and a clamp is not required, a piece of rubber 3 cm × 1 cm is stretched *(A)* and passed through the contact as one would a piece of dental tape. Release of the rubber and cutting off the ends *(B)* provides a neat rubber "wedge" to keep the dam in place.

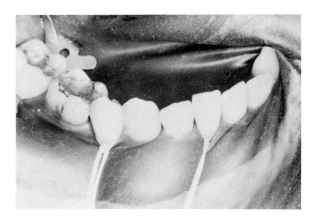

Figure 9–28. Invagination of rubber by using waxed dental tape; waxed dental floss is used for the smaller incisors.

2. Inspection of the rubber encompassing the clamped tooth may reveal a wing not encircled by the rubber or some distal gingival tissue included along with the tooth. Manipulation of the rubber with the fingers or a plastic instrument can readily position the rubber correctly to seal off oral fluids.

3. Invagination of the rubber around the necks of the teeth is necessary only in the area where operational activity occurs. However, tucking the rubber into the sulcus around all the teeth makes a most neat and tidy field of operation (Fig. 9–28).

4. The holder is checked for patient comfort and the rubber under the nose is inspected to insure free breathing.

5. By taking pleats in the rubber, excess wrinkles in the dam covering the chin can usually be eliminated.

6. Many patients do not need a saliva ejector but where required it should be comfortably positioned, preferably through a hole in the rubber dam (Fig. 9–29). The hole should be made opposite the operating area lest it obstruct use of the handpiece. As an option, the ejector may be passed underneath the rubber dam and face mask.

7. The area should be flushed, vacuumed, and dried.

Removal of the Dam

Removal of the rubber dam is relatively simple. The clamp is first removed and set aside. Stretching the rubber to either buccal or lingual, the operator cuts the rubber at each septum with scissors. The rubber mask is now removed,

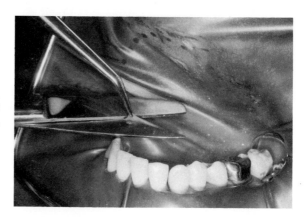

Figure 9–29. Cutting a hole for the saliva ejector. Using the cotton pliers to pick up the rubber, a disk is cut out. This method can also be used in lieu of a rubber dam punch to make an additional hole for another tooth after the dam has been applied.

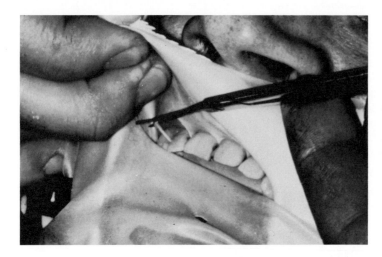

Figure 9–30. Removal of the dam involves cutting the interseptal rubber. The rubber is pulled to the side where the scissors can cut the interseptal portion.

followed by the application of a cool damp towel to wipe the lips and refresh the patient. Despite its ease of removal, careless cutting of the septal rubber can result in fragments of rubber being left behind unnoticed. Routinely the operator should hold the mask up to the light to examine it for missing fragments of rubber that might still remain in a gingival sulcus (Figs. 9–30 and 9–31.).

Customizing the Clamp

Selection of the proper rubber dam clamp is a matter of experience and common sense, tempered with some intuition. Some variations in clamp handling and placement are seen in Figure 9–32.

While its shape and size fit most teeth, alteration of its jaws, wings, and prongs should be done as a matter of routine. A husky fissure bur rapidly transforms a stock clamp into a customized one. Although a clamp has been modified, it need not be discarded; preserving it for future use proves to be worthwhile (Figs. 9–33 and 9–34).

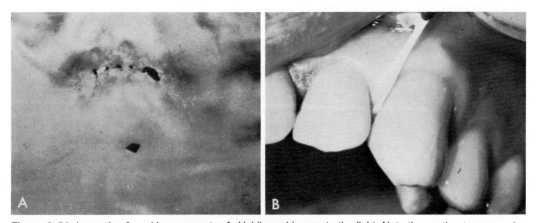

Figure 9–31. Inspection for rubber remnants. *A,* Holding rubber up to the light. Note the section torn away in the region of the cuspid. *B,* Torn fragment of rubber located under the contact point and removed. (Courtesy of Dr. Dan Frederickson)

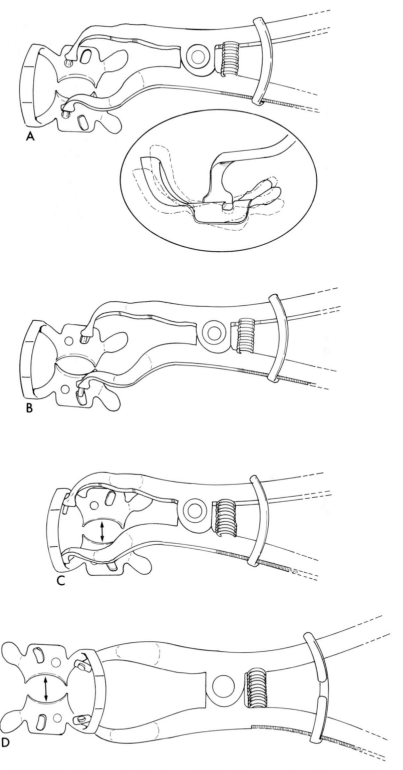

Figure 9–32. Methods for grasping the clamp. *A,* Clamp forceps under ordinary conditions fit into these holes. The clamp should be free to wobble, thereby assuring easy release of the forceps. *B,* These holes in the wings are not intended for the forceps and serve little purpose. *C,* A mesially tilted lower molar may require this position of the forceps to spread the jaws for placement. *D,* Grasp of clamp for reverse application.

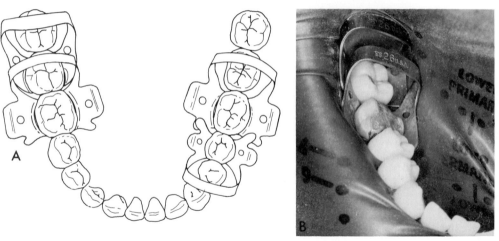

Figure 9–33. Double clamp application. *A,* Clamps may be mounted "piggy back" with bows in either direction. *B,* Extra security for operating on a lower first molar.

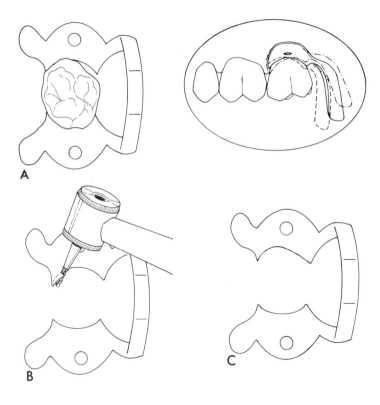

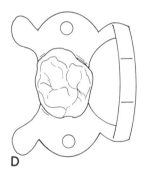

Figure 9–34. Customizing a clamp to fit a maxillary left 2nd molar. *A,* Disto-buccal prong does not engage the tooth, allowing the clamp to teeter from the tension of the rubber. *B,* Fissure bur is used to shape buccal jaw and mesio-buccal prong. Generous amounts of metal can be removed from the jaws without mutilating the clamp. *C,* Alternate grinding and fitting soon fashion the jaw so it fits the buccal surface. *D,* Clamp on the tooth.

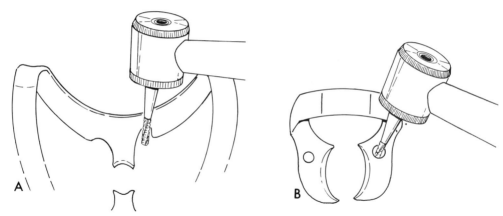

Figure 9–35. Modification of clamps with high-speed fissure bur. *A,* Deepening the lingual notch of the No. 212 clamp. *B,* Enlarging the holes.

A common necessary modification is to adapt the No. 212 clamp to the clamp forceps. More often than not, the notches for the clamp forceps are not sufficiently deep. Frequently the forceps slip out of the lingual notch when the operator attempts to maneuver the clamp in its "open" position. Deepening these two lingual notches is readily accomplished with a fissure bur (Fig. 9–35).

Other modifications can be made in the beaks so that the clamps fit flattened roots (Fig. 9–36) and narrow mandibular incisors. Overlapped and rotated teeth can frequently lend themselves to isolation by the use of a "half clamp" (Fig. 9–37). Although only minimal "spring" or grasping power is present, it is usually adequate to hold back the tissue and isolate the area.

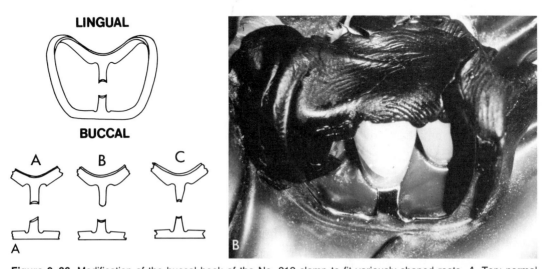

Figure 9–36. Modification of the buccal beak of the No. 212 clamp to fit variously shaped roots. *A,* Top: normal unmodified clamp. (A) Modified to fit sloped root surface; (B) modification of lingual beak to a rounded form for more versatile application (recommended by Dr. Lyle Ostlund); (C) buccal beak narrowed to fit the curvature of the labial surface of a lower incisor. Shaping the buccal beak is easily and rapidly accomplished with either a green stone or a carbide bur in the high-speed handpiece. *B,* Cohesive gold cavity prepared with a No. 212 clamp in position. Notice abundance of caulking compound to stabilize the clamp. Also note the modification of the buccal beak so it can seat firmly against the buccal surface.

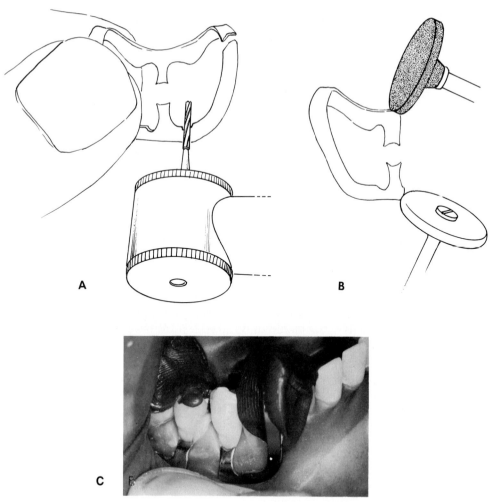

Figure 9–37. Half clamps applied for isolation of two adjacent lesions. *A,* Cutting off the fractured bow with a 557 bur. *B,* Rounding the corners. *C,* Two clamps in position securely stabilized with compound.

Class V Clamp Placement

The object of clamp placement is to stabilize the rubber and to isolate a working area on or near the root. Clamp placement is particularly crucial with the 212 type. Although other types of clamps for gingival retraction have been devised, none is as versatile as the 212 design. Perhaps its greatest value is its simplicity and its fragile bows, which permit access to the working area.

One requirement of this clamp that differs from all others is its passivity. All clamps, whether made from tempered stainless steel or chromium plated steel, do not lend themselves to bending. They will spring apart when stretched, and the application of forces that extend beyond their elastic limit results in fracture. This should not occur in the 212-type clamp. While a degree of strength and rigidity is present, this clamp permits itself to be bent and have its shape altered.

Once tempered, stainless steel clamps are difficult to anneal and make soft and pliable again. A high-carbon steel clamp, on the other hand, can be

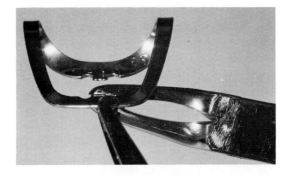

Figure 9–38. Bending beaks with two pliers.

annealed by heating it to redness and allowing it to bench cool. Soft untempered clamps of the 212 type are now available commercially.*

Naturally a passive untempered clamp does not hug the tooth as securely as a highly tempered one and must be handled with more care and discretion while it retracts the gingiva. If the beaks of the clamp have sprung too far apart, they can be squeezed back together again with the fingers and reapplied to the tooth. Customized fitting of the clamp to the tooth is done before rubber dam placement. It would be ideal if the location of the gingival border of the lesion on the buccal were at the same height as the marginal gingiva on the lingual. Unfortunately such is not the case. Pliers can bend the beaks upward or downward to achieve the desired fit (Figs. 9–38 and 9–39).

The actual effectiveness of a Class V No. 212 clamp is not provided by the metal itself but by the caulking material (impression compound) that fixes it rigidly to the teeth. Teeth may be scrubbed lightly with peroxide or coated with cavity varnish to assure better attachment of the compound.

Application of the compound is not difficult. The following hints are helpful in the application of the No. 212 clamp.

1. The fingers are coated lightly with lubricant (Borofax or petroleum jelly) to prevent compound from adhering to the fingers. (Some operators prefer water for this purpose as well as to temper the compound.)

*Soft untempered clamps designed by Dr. Hunter Brinker, B-6 and B-5 (narrow beak) are available from Hygienic Dental Mfg. Co, 1245 Holm Ave., Akron, Ohio 44310.

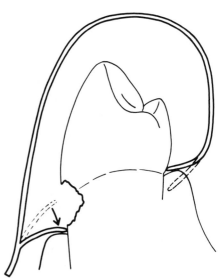

Figure 9–39. Versatility of the No. 212 clamp. Beaks can be bent upward or downward to conform to the lesion of a lower premolar.

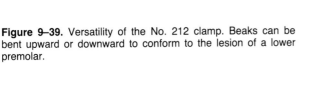

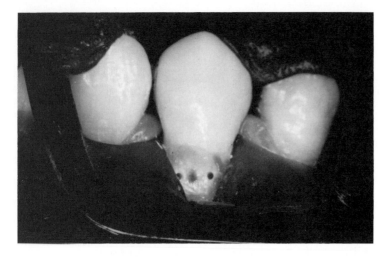

Figure 9–40. Strangulated tissue caused by punching the holes in the rubber dam too close together.

2. The clamp is stabilized by holding the buccal beak with the thumb until the compound has been completely applied, molded, and cooled.

3. First application of compound is under distal bow. After molding to form, it is repeated for the mesial bow.

4. After the compound has been applied and molded, cooling can be hastened by applying a moistened cotton roll to the compound. Evaporative action cools the compound as air is blown over the surface.

5. To prevent strangulation of the interseptal gingival tissue by the rubber (Fig. 9–40), the holes for the three teeth (the isolated tooth plus the two adjacent teeth) are spaced up to ½ inch apart, with the hole for the clamped tooth positioned well toward the buccal (Fig. 9–40).

Additional aids can be employed during a Class V clamp placement. Some operators will place an alum cord in the gingival sulcus prior to clamp placement. This provides an astringent action and aids in keeping the sulcus dry. Another practice commonly employed is the placement of a compound-cotton roll splint on the lingual (Figs. 9–41 and 9–42). The lingual beak of the clamp is directed into the cotton, where its force is disseminated over a broad lingual area, thereby protecting the lingual gingiva against trauma (Figs. 9–43 through 9–49).

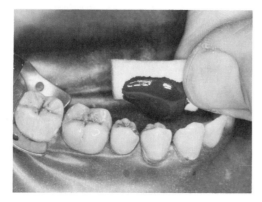

Figure 9–41. Half a length of cotton roll is coated with compound and pressed against the lingual side of the tooth to be clasped.

Figure 9–42. Immediately the lingual beak of the clamp is inserted into the side of the cotton roll while the buccal beak is positioned for caulking. The cushioning effect provided by the cotton compound support prevents the lingual beak from traumatizing the soft lingual tissue.

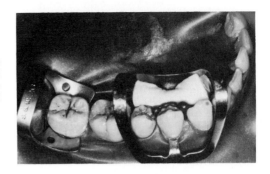

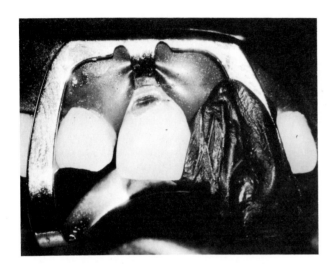

Figure 9–43. Maxillary central with gingival carious lesion. Cavity is prepared for composite resin. Notice excellent access and retraction provided by the clamp. Caulking with compound in this instance was accomplished by utilizing only one of the bows. (Courtesy of Dr. Dan Frederickson)

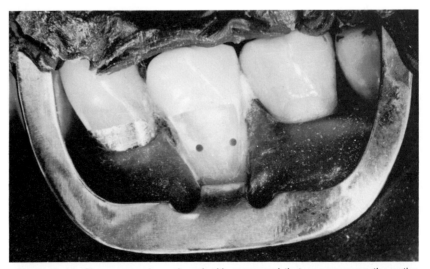

Figure 9–44. Clamp securely anchored with compound that encompasses the entire lingual surface. Following placement of two retentive pins, which straddled the pulp, direct gold was placed in this cavity.

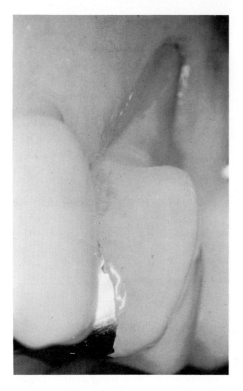

Figure 9–45. Repair of severe gingival erosion with direct gold. Two T.M.S. pins were placed for added retention. The disto-buccal root was unaffected by erosion.

Figure 9–46. Buccal beak of clamp bent inward and rootward to engage the mesio-buccal root. Bows were stretched to accommodate the thick molar. Note pencil line defining the outline of the preparation.

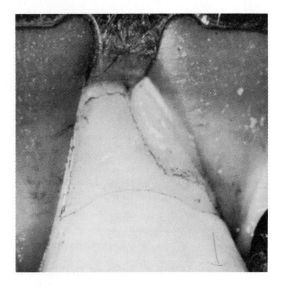

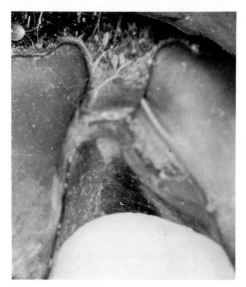

Figure 9–47. Finished restoration.

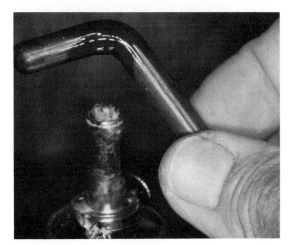

Figure 9–48. Heating red stick compound. Over an alcohol flame, 1 to 1½ inches of compound stick are gradually softened to chewing gum consistency.

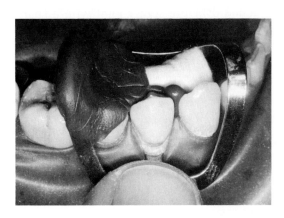

Figure 9–49. Applying the compound while the left thumb holds the buccal beak to prevent the clamp from moving.

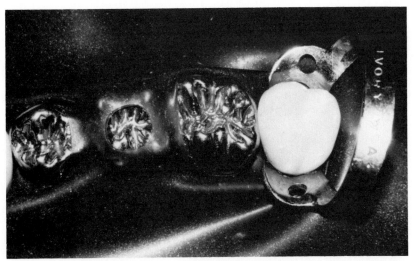

Figure 9–50. Rubber dam applied to fixed bridge. Lubricated dam applied over all teeth except the abutments and pontics. Larger holes are punched for these teeth. (Figures 9–50 through 9–53 courtesy of Dr. Dan Frederickson)

Isolation of a Fixed Bridge

Frequently it is necessary to isolate the tooth of a fixed bridge adjacent to a solder joint. In addition to standard materials, a No. 4 curved suture needle (dull point) and a needle holder are used. Holes are punched in a routine manner, including larger sized holes for each bridge unit. The rubber dam is applied over all teeth except for the fixed partial denture.

The suture needle is threaded with dental tape and passed through the buccal of the No. 1 hole (anterior abutment) under the anterior solder joint and out the lingual of *the same No. 1 hole.* Reversing direction, the needle is now threaded back through the lingual of hole No. 2 (pontic), but *still underneath the medial* solder joint, and out the facial side of hole No. 2. The two ends of the tape are drawn together and tied securely into a square knot and cut. In a similar fashion, the tape is then threaded underneath the *posterior* solder joint, through hole No. 3 (posterior abutment) in a lingual direction and back through hole No. 2 in a facial direction. The tape is drawn tight, tied, and cut (Figs. 9–50 to 9–54).

After completing the operation, removal of the dam is easily accomplished by cutting the interseptal rubber stretched over the solder joint with a sharp instrument. Small pieces of tape are removed and the mouth is examined for any residual fragments of rubber.

Isolation by Surgical Means

Despite the benefits derived from isolation by the rubber dam as well as the use of vacuum, cotton rolls, and so on, two other methods are available to the operative dentist as he seeks to obtain dryness and access in performing clinical service. Both of these methods involve surgical invasion of adjacent soft tissue. Both methods are used to gain access to root surfaces, which are substantially below gingival tissues.

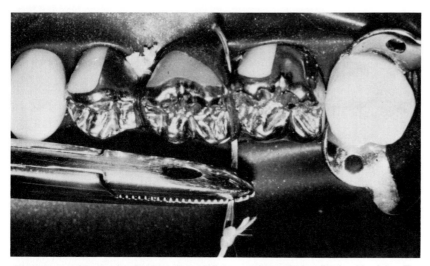

Figure 9–51. Blunted needle threads dental tape underneath the distal solder joint. The embrasures anterior to the pontic have already been sealed off.

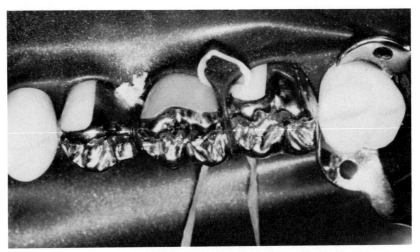

Figure 9–52. Tape looped around the rubber on the buccal and ready to be tied.

Surgical retraction is one way to provide this access. This is done by freeing the tissue from its attachment, often involving an incision, and reflecting the flap of tissue up (or down) out of the way. The rubber dam, with the clamp, is applied to control seepage and to hold back the gingiva while the operative procedure is taking place. When completed, the clamp and dam are removed and the tissue is re-positioned and held in place, usually with a suture or a periodontal pack.

The second method is the elimination of unwanted tissue by electro-surgery. Bleeding is not usually a problem with electro-surgery because the ends of the capillaries are cauterized by the cutting action. The major usage for electro-surgery is found in crown preparations; however, it is often used to expose facial surfaces of the teeth. This method therefore may or may not be used with the rubber dam, depending upon the task at hand.

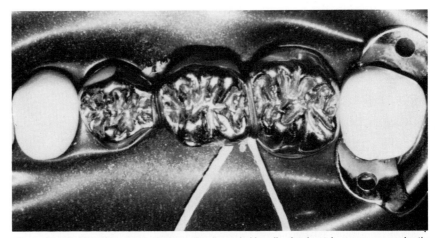

Figure 9–53. Knot has been tied on the lingual. Usually the knot is more conveniently placed on the buccal. If a class V clamp is to be placed, however, a buccal knot could obstruct the operating area.

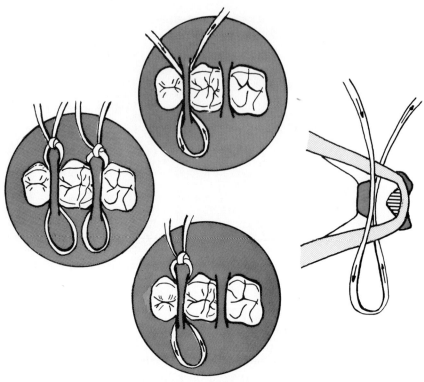

Figure 9–54. Diagrammatic illustration of threading dental tape around a solder joint. (Courtesy of Dr. Douglass D. Roberto)

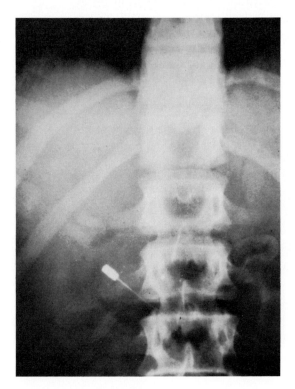

Figure 9–55. Root canal file swallowed during endodontic therapy. The use of the rubber dam would have prevented this accident. (From Christen, A. G.: Accidental swallowing of an endodontic instrument. Oral Surg. *24*:684, 1967)

In summary, all operative procedures are best done on dry and non-contaminated tooth surfaces so the materials can provide dentists with their optimal physical properties. On the other hand, the operator's eyes can see clearly and have non-distorted images when the area is dry and not cluttered with debris.

10

TOOTH-COLORED RESTORATIVES

A dentist in general practice will devote a significant amount of his time and energy restoring defects of the anterior teeth.

For reasons of personal esthetics, as discussed in Chapter 5, many patients are highly concerned about the appearance of their anterior teeth. Such patients will ignore the value of function and emphasize the importance of appearance. These people in particular need to understand the value of prevention, as suggested in Chapter 1.

The quest for a tooth-colored restorative material is one that parallels the history of dentistry. The utopian anterior restorative material is one that would be adhesive, permanently match the color of the remaining tooth, be biologically compatible with the tooth and soft tissue, be easily handled, and permanently maintain form and function of the tooth. Unfortunately, those requirements are not satisfied by any material available at this time. The dental profession has had to be satisfied with materials that only approach these requirements.

For many years silicate cement was the principal material used for this purpose. Its good and bad characteristics will be discussed later in the chapter. Currently, resin systems are used almost exclusively for anterior and other tooth-colored restorations.

Restorative Materials

Unfilled Resins

The first substitute for silicate cement was a chemically cured resin, supplied as a powder–liquid combination. These are referred to as Type I direct filling resins in the American Dental Association specifications. The powder is poly (methyl methacrylate) in the form of beads or grindings, while the liquid is methyl methacrylate, generally with some cross-linking agents. The color is incorporated into the powder beads. The energy source for completion of the hardening reaction is derived from the amine-peroxide reaction system. Although insoluble in oral fluid, the first resins had very poor color stability. Furthermore, the rate and completeness of polymerization was not dependable, which led to gross microleakage around the restoration. The leakage and improper pulp protection caused many teeth to lose vitality.

Table 10–1. DIRECT FILLING RESINS

	Units	Type I Acrylic	Type II (Composites)	
			Conventional	Microfilled
Working time	min	1.5	4	3
Compressive Strength (24 hr)	kg/cm²	703	2390	2812
	psi	10,000	34,000	40,000
Diametral Tensile Strength	kg/cm²	246	457	330
(24 hr)	psi	3,500	6,500	4,700
Modulus of Elasticity	kg/cm²	0.0239×10^6	0.15466×10^6	0.0457×10^6
	psi	0.34×10^6	2.2×10^6	0.65×10^6
Water Sorption	mg/cm²	1.7	0.6	1.4
Polymerization Shrinkage	%	7	1.4	1.7
Coefficient of Thermal Expansion*		7	3.1	5.3

*Ratios of linear thermal expansion coefficients of resins divided by that of tooth structure. (From Phillips, R. W.: Elements of Dental Materials, 4th Ed. Philadelphia, W. B. Saunders Co., 1984, p. 154.)

The physical properties of Type I resins are seen in Table 10–1. Unfilled resins have a volumetric shrinkage of 5 to 8 per cent on polymerization. However, the effects of this shrinkage are reduced by the care and methods by which the material is placed in the preparation and by the geometry of the contraction that occurs. Fortunately, the polymerization shrinkage is concentrated at the floor of the preparation rather than at the margins. Likewise, the use of techniques that will assure good adaptation to the tooth structure tends to inhibit any tendency of the resin to contract away from the preparation (e.g., acid etch techniques to be discussed later in this chapter).

Of all the restorative materials, acrylic has the highest coefficient of thermal expansion, in that it will shrink or expand almost seven times that of tooth structure for every degree change of temperature. The exact clinical significance of this property is not known. For example, the temperature changes that can be tolerated by the patient may not be as severe as those used in laboratory tests. Likewise, the low thermal conductivity of resin tends to reduce diffusion of heat and cold throughout the restoration. Nevertheless, this is not a beneficial property and may in time contribute to marginal leakage.

The early resins had poor color stability when exposed to ultraviolet light and would turn yellow or brown upon such exposure. However, by methods such as the addition of ultraviolet absorbers the color stability has been greatly improved. Unfilled resins are not adequately resistant to abrasive action and are subjected to rapid loss of contour as a result of masticatory or toothbrush abrasion.

A major advantage of the unfilled resin is that the technique of placement may be varied to include placement by a bulk method or by small increments using a brush. Also, the unfilled resins permit matching of the color of the teeth with relative ease.

Composite Resins

CONVENTIONAL COMPOSITES

The unfilled resins do not, however, provide the total answer as an anterior restorative material. Many of the physical properties of such a system are quite poor and this limits its usage and longevity. These acrylic resins

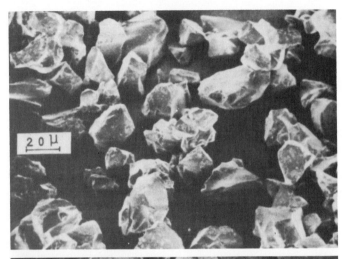

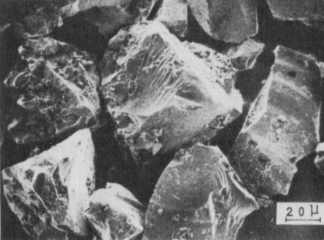

Figure 10–1. Scanning electron microscope picture of inorganic fillers employed in two commercial composite restorative materials. (From Phillips, R. W.: Skinner's Science of Dental Materials. Philadelphia, W. B. Saunders Co., 1982)

have now been replaced, to a major extent, by the composite resin, referred to as Type II direct filling resin in the American Dental Association specifications. This material is principally a result of the research conducted by R. Bowen.

The term composite material refers to a three-dimensional combination of at least two chemically different materials with a distinct interface separating the components. When properly constructed, such a combination of materials provides properties that could not be obtained with any one of the components acting alone. (Examples of composite structures are bone and tooth enamel.) A composite dental restorative material is one in which an inorganic filler has been added to a resin matrix in such a way that the properties of the matrix have been upgraded (Fig. 10–1).

It will be noted that the foregoing statement implies a discreteness in the formulation of the composite. A number of parameters have a marked influence upon the properties that will be obtained by the addition of macrofillers to a resin matrix. The geometry of the dispersed phase in terms of its shape, size, orientation, concentration, and distribution is very important, as will be discussed. Likewise, the composition of the continuous phase, i.e., the resin, is equally significant. Therefore, the term composite distinguishes this class of materials from unreinforced direct acrylic filling resins, including those materials to which small amounts of filler have been added.

Most of the present composite materials make use of the BIS–GMA molecule, which is the dimethacrylate monomer synthesized by the reaction between bisphenol-A and glycidyl methacrylate. This reaction is catalyzed by a peroxide-amine system. Recently other modifications of the BIS–GMA resin have been introduced, such as those based on urethane dimethacrylate. Among the materials used for macrofillers are ground particles of fused silica, crystalline quartz, or boron silicate glass. These particles, which make up 70 to 80 per cent of the material, tend to resist deformation of the soft resin matrix. The high filler content and the different chemistry of the resin matrix substantially reduce the coefficient of thermal expansion, as compared with the acrylic resin. The filler also reduces the polymerization shrinkage and increases the hardness. The refractive index and opacity of the filler particles are similar to that of tooth structure.

Properties. Naturally the properties of commercial composite resins vary to some degree from one product to another. These variations are due principally to the differences in the type and concentration of macrofillers employed.

Typical values for the mechanical and physical properties of composites, as compared with those of unreinforced resins, are shown in Table 10–1. Since the original source for this table included data from several reports and for different materials, these numbers represent values in the middle group.

It is obvious that the composite resins are superior to the unreinforced acrylic resins with respect to most mechanical and physical properties. This would be anticipated because of the strengthening effect of the filler and the differences in the properties of the resin matrix materials. The properties are compared in Table 10–1.

The composites are appreciably stronger than the direct acrylic filling resins when loaded in compression (2390 kg/cm^2, or 34,000 psi, and 703 kg/cm^2, or 10,000 psi, respectively), and the tensile strength is approximately twice as great. They have a much higher modulus of elasticity than the acrylic resins. This would suggest that the stiffer material should be less susceptible to elastic deformation when subjected to masticatory forces. They are considerably harder than the acrylic resins (49 KHN and 14 KHN, respectively) and are less vulnerable to abrasion, at least when abraded by slurries of abrasives such as silex, calcium carbonates, and pumice.

Because of the higher molecular weight and the effect of the filler, the polymerization shrinkage of the traditional or conventional composite resin restoratives (1.4 per cent) is markedly lower than that of acrylic resin restoratives.

The macrofiller and the resin matrix must be bonded together with a so-called coupling agent on the surface of the filler. If this is not done, the particles may be easily dislodged or may permit water sorption at the filler–matrix interface. Thus, the filler particles are coated with a reactive silane product.

In spite of this coupling system, the filler particles do become dislodged under abrasive action such as tooth brushing or by occlusal contact. This abrasive action likely affects the softer resin matrix, which becomes worn away and exposes the filler particles. When enough of the filler particle is exposed, it will break free of the resin. This process leaves a continual rough surface, and since the composites are 70 to 80 per cent filled, this surface roughness is clinically noticeable.

With the clinical experience of the passing years, there is a definite preference for use of smaller macrofiller particles. In the early materials it was

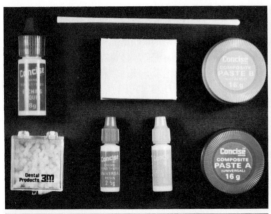
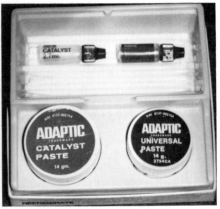
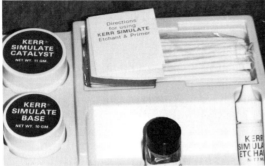

Figure 10–2. Examples of current commercially available composite materials.

common for the particle size to approach 100 μm, whereas now the coarsest particles would not exceed 50 μm. The average mean particle size of the fillers in many of the composites is in the 15 to 20 μm range. Now the trend is to reduce even further the filler size in these traditional composites. In some materials it may be as small as 1.5 μm and, in addition, the particles may be softer and rounded in shape.

Most of the conventional composite products are marketed in a paste form, which is convenient for the dentist or assistant to use (Fig. 10–2). The pastes are quickly measured volumetrically from the container according to the manufacturer's instructions. They are easy to handle and insert into the preparation. They take less time to polymerize as compared with unfilled resins. Because of the filler material, a composite resin is able to blend with its enamel surroundings, simplifying shade selection, which will be discussed later in the chapter. The major reason composite materials are popular is that the handling procedures are not difficult.

Although the use of composite resin is not technically complicated, it is still a demanding restorative material. The dentist must develop an appreciation of its good and bad characteristics and should cultivate a technique that will assure clinical success.

Microfilled Composites

A new series of restorative resin composites has now come on the scene. These are based upon the use of an extremely small filler particle and hence are called microfine, microfilled, or polishable resins (Fig. 10–3). The term microfilled will be used in the following discussion.

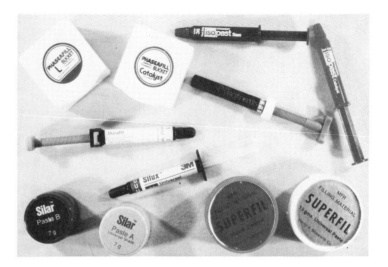

Figure 10–3. A variety of commercial microfilled products.

It will be recalled that the traditional dental composite resin makes use of filler particles, such as quartz or boron glass, imbedded in a BIS–GMA resin matrix. These particles are blends of varying sizes, usually ranging between 1 and 20 μm. A schematic drawing of the structure of such a system is shown in Figure 10–4.

In the microfilled resin the particle size of the filler—pyrogenic silica— is on the order of only 0.04 μm, which is below the wavelength of visible light. These particles of microfine silica may be dispensed directly into the paste but usually they are predispensed in a monomer. To achieve this the BIS–GMA resin monomer is thinned with a solvent such as chloroform and the filler particles, coated with the coupling agent, are dispersed in it. The solvent is evaporated and the resin polymerized. The polymerized resin, loaded with the micro-sized silica particles, is then pulverized into "splinter"- like particles of about the same size as the inorganic fillers in traditional composites. As a result of the process and filler content they are designated as "splintered prepolymerized particles." A small amount of pyrogenic silica may also be added to the matrix resin.

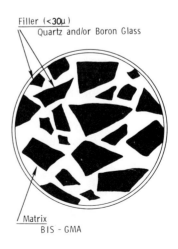

Filler (<30μ)
Quartz and/or Boron Glass

Matrix
BIS - GMA

Total Composition
80% Filler Particles - 20% Matrix

Figure 10–4. Schematic drawing of structure of a traditional composite, showing the filler particles dispersed in a BIS-GMA resin matrix.

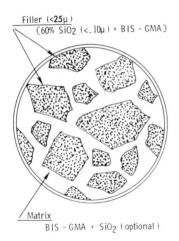

Filler (<25μ)
(60% SiO₂ (<.10μ) + BIS - GMA)

Matrix
BIS - GMA + SiO₂ (optional)

Total Composition
70% Filler Particles - 30% Matrix

Figure 10–5. Schematic drawing of structure of a microfilled composite. Very minute pyrogenic silica particles are dispersed in filler particles of a polymerized resin particle. These filler particles are then suspended in a typical resin matrix to form the paste supplied to the dentist.

The structure of such a resin is illustrated in Figure 10–5. This type of dispersion is often called an "organic filler," but obviously this is not strictly so, as inorganic pyrogenic silica is the filler used in the "organic" polymerized particle.

The interesting and appealing characteristic of the microfilled resins is their ability to be finished to an extremely smooth surface, which has always been a major problem of the traditional composites. During finishing of such a resin, one is cutting through filler particles that have an entirely different hardness and abrasion resistance as compared with that of the resin matrix. This leads to a rough surface, as seen in Figure 10–6, since particles are plucked out or are left standing up from the matrix.

In the case of the microfilled resins, during finishing the polymerized resin filler particles wear at the same rate as the matrix and a markedly smoother surface results, as is diagrammed in Figure 10–7. Even if some of the very small pyrogenic silica particles are dislodged, the surface irregularities cannot be detected by the eye. The difference in the surface of the two types of composites is seen in Figure 10–7B.

However, as with all dental materials, when formulations are changed to enhance one property, there is always the risk that certain other desirable characteristics may be altered or sacrificed. In this case, the problem centers on the fact that because of the small silica particle size and thus the very high surface area, the amount of filler that can be incorporated is reduced. It is generally only about 40 per cent as compared with a filler load of 75 to 80 per cent for the traditional composite. Thus, the microfilled composite is higher in its resin matrix content and certain properties are altered accordingly, as seen in Table 10–1. Such resins are softer, have a slightly higher coefficient of thermal expansion, and may have higher water absorption. Possibly more important is that color stability may not be as good.

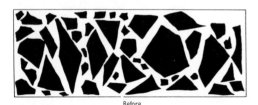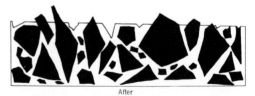

Before   After

Figure 10–6. Diagram of the surface before and after the finishing of a traditional composite resin restoration.

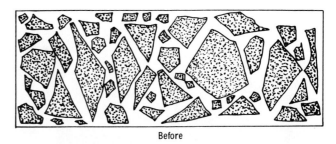

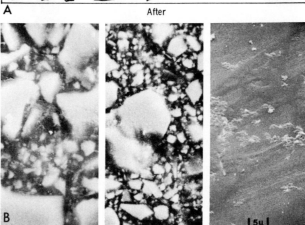

Figure 10–7. *A,* Diagram of the surface before and after the finishing of a microfilled composite resin restoration. *B,* SEM comparison of the surface of two conventional composites with a microfilled resin surface at right.

Whether this trade-off in such properties will lead to a less satisfactory clinical performance will be resolved only through well-controlled clinical studies. Although the microfilled resin system has been on the market for several years, a true clinical comparison with the traditional composite is difficult as there are distinct differences between them as related to appearance and physical behavior. These resins are more technique sensitive. For example, because of their translucency precise finishing of the margins is more difficult. However, the microfilled composite is an interesting one in that it does eliminate one of the real difficulties that every dentist faced with the previous type of composite, namely the inferior surface left after polishing.

The microfilled composites are mixed in the same manner as conventional composites, and the manufacturer's instructions are to be observed. The advisability of using a syringe will vary among the products, depending on viscosity of the material.

Hybrid Composites

The use of a pure traditional composite is no longer as popular. It has become common to admix some pyrogenic silica to the resin matrix in addition to the macrofillers in order to influence the viscosity and certain other characteristics. Since this combines two types of fillers the result is a "hybrid" composite. These are also referred to as "blends."

Thus the common type of hybrid currently used combines small traditional macrofillers with admixed pyrogenic silica as used in microfilled

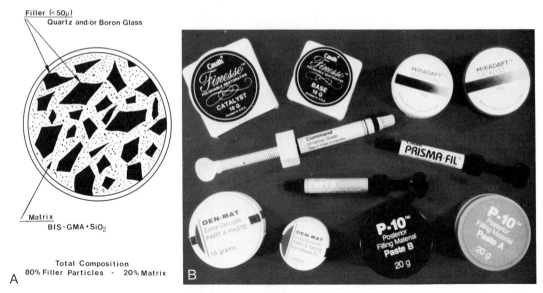

Filler (<50μ)
Quartz and/or Boron Glass

Matrix
BIS·GMA·SiO₂

Total Composition
80% Filler Particles - 20% Matrix

A

B

Figure 10–8. *A,* Schematic drawing of structure of a hybrid composite. The primary fillers are small macrofiller particles. The matrix contains pyrogenic silica as used in microfilled composite. *B,* Commercial examples of hybrid composite resins.

materials, both treated with a coupling agent and added to the resin matrix (Fig. 10–8). The in vivo tests demonstrate that the organic matrix of the traditional composites responded poorly to all kinds of wear. Thus to reduce the difference in properties between the macrofiller and matrix and for other reasons, the pyrogenic silica was added to help improve the performance and handling of traditional composite resin.

Since the surface characteristics of hybrid resins are not as smooth as those of microfilled resins they are not considered as ideal for certain types of anterior restorations where esthetics is a prime concern. While it is possible for a hybrid to be polished to an adequate smoothness, it will be of a temporary nature because of the wear patterns that accompany all macrofiller materials. In spite of this variance these resins find extensive anterior use if they are carefully polished. The acceptance level is greatly improved as compared with traditional composites.

Also one of the primary motivations in the development of these hybrid materials was to find a material that would compare favorably to dental amalgam in terms of wear resistance in Class II restorations. Furthermore, the use of heavy metal glass macrofillers offers the possibility of radiopacity, which is an essential factor when designing a posterior tooth composite. The use of composites in such situations will be discussed later.

Light-Cured Composites

Most composite resins are chemically activated by an amine-peroxide system. Currently there is an ever increasing interest in light-cured or light-activated composites. For all practical purposes these products do not differ in composition from the chemically activated resins, except for the curing mechanisms. However, light-curing provides an advantage in working time and other handling characteristics.

The first light-curing systems made use of ultraviolet light to initiate polymerization. These resins contain a photosensitive chemical, e.g., methyl benzoin ether. When this chemical is exposed to ultraviolet light, free radicals are formed that activate the benzoyl peroxide, which in turn initiates polymerization.

More recently visible light-cured resins have become available. The basic mechanism is the same as for the ultraviolet light system except that different chemicals are used (ketones), which are sensitized or activated by visible light of certain wavelengths (400 to 500 nm).

The visible light-cured resins have a number of advantages over the ultraviolet light-cured system and hence have largely replaced these original systems. The intensity of the ultraviolet light tends to gradually fall off with time, thus impairing the quality of the cure. For this reason it is necessary to test the ultraviolet light daily. The output of the visible light remains fairly constant throughout its life. Also, visible light is capable of polymerizing a greater thickness of resin than does ultraviolet light, and it will cure the resin through a layer of enamel (Fig. 10–9).

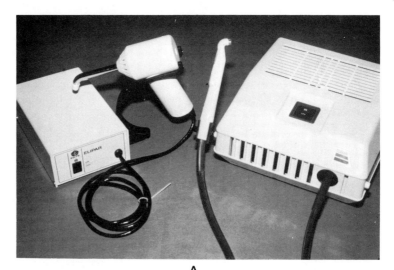

A

Figure 10–9. *A,* Two devices for polymerizing visible light curved resins. *B,* Examples of visible light activated composite resin materials.

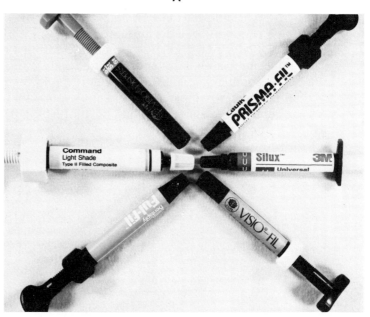

B

Treatment Selection

Indications for Resin Restorations

1. Interproximal (Class III) lesions of anterior teeth.
2. Facial (Class V) lesions of anterior teeth.
3. Facial (Class V) lesions of premolars.
4. Loss of incisal angles.
5. Fracture of anterior teeth.
6. Rebuilding of teeth to support castings.

These indications suggest an extensive range of lesions for which resins may be used successfully and, with the exception of rebuilding teeth to support castings, either filled or unfilled resins may be used. The unfilled resin provides a restoration with a smoother finish as compared with a composite, and this is particularly useful for facial restorations, which will be in contact with tissue.

The restoration of defective incisal angles or fractured anterior teeth is routinely done using resin. The choice of resin will be based on personal preference; however, if strength is a prime consideration the composite resin of macrofilled or hybrid type is recommended. On the other hand the hybrid type does not take a polish as well as a microfilled resin and certainly not as well as an unfilled resin.

Treatment of the results of trauma to anterior dentition is a continual problem for a general practitioner. This treatment is subject to the judgment and ability of the operator and the circumstances related to the problem. The age of the patient, amount of tooth loss, state of vitality of the tooth, and economics are among the variables that have a bearing on treatment. With extensive tooth loss a crown may be preferred, but if the patient is young or the expense a problem, it may not be feasible to place the crown. It is difficult to establish a fixed guide for the selection of a method of treatment.

The use of resin as a rebuilding material (indication 6) will be discussed in Chapter 15 in relation to preparations for castings.

Contraindications for Resin Restorations

1. Distal lesions of cuspids.
2. Routine posterior restorations.
3. Patients with high and poorly controlled caries activity.

Resin materials are not recommended for the distal lesions of canines, for when possible a metallic restoration should be placed. (See Fig. 11–82.) The normal forces in an arch tend to apply pressure toward the mesial, and a soft or abradable material will allow the distal contact to flatten, reducing the

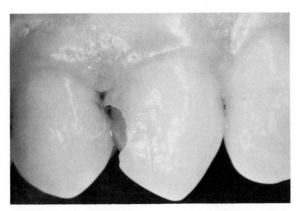

Figure 10–10. The inability of a resin system to maintain the canine mesial-distal width leads to gingival distress.

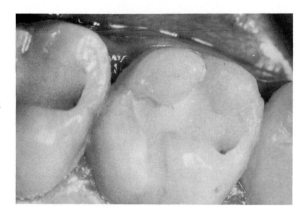

Figure 10–11. The loss of anatomic form of a posterior composite restoration is shown.

normal mesial-distal width of the canine, which in turn provides pressure on the interdental tissue, leading to constant gingival irritation (Fig. 10–10).

Resin Restorations for Posterior Teeth

The improved strength, hardness, and modulus of elasticity of composite resins, in conjunction with their low thermal conductivity and superior esthetics, suggest that they might serve as a suitable replacement for amalgam in the restoration of occlusal and proximal surfaces of posterior teeth. As a result of extensive clinical testing the performance of composite resins has proved to be inferior to that of amalgam. Fracture and marginal integrity do not appear to be problems but with time such restorations show a definite loss of material on the occlusal surface. This lack of wear resistance reflects in the loss of anatomic contour (Fig. 10–11).

There is great research effort currently in progress to develop an acceptable posterior resin system and a major breakthrough may occur soon. However, until composite resins have been developed that have better resistance to attrition than those being marketed for that purpose, they should not be used in posterior restorations, which are subjected to mastication. In addition to the physical problems, the difficulties of technique must be considered because careful attention is required to avoid gingival overhangs and to properly develop good anatomic form, while at the same time avoiding damage to existing enamel. Satisfaction in these points is much more easily achieved by the use of amalgam.

Nonetheless, it is valid to consider composite in posterior teeth where

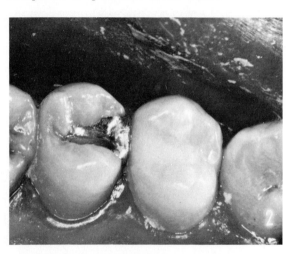

Figure 10–12. A disto-occlusal composite resin on an upper first premolar with good anatomy and margins.

esthetics is a compelling concern to the dentist and patients, such as the restoration of a premolar (Fig. 10–12). These restorations must then be routinely checked for signs of wear and replaced when loss of anatomic form is obvious.

Shade Selection

Before the rubber dam is positioned, the color of the replacement material must be determined (Fig. 10–13). After the teeth become dry, the color sensations are different, and very likely any color or shade selection made when the teeth are dry will not match as accurately as those made when the teeth are moist.

The powders for unfilled acrylic resins and silicate cements have several variations for color selection. A specific shade guide is available for each system, and from this guide a selection of the matching material is made. When selecting the color, the teeth as well as the shade tab should be moist. During selection avoid looking intently or staring at any tab and tooth; just look quickly and move the tab away. The process of shade selection will be discussed in greater detail in Chapter 20.

If it appears difficult to secure a direct match, select the shade on the light rather than the dark side. Also, it may be advantageous to mix two powders together in order to obtain a shade somewhere between the two colors. The objective is to have a perfect match, which may not always occur, but it must blend as closely as possible with the environment.

When the restoration calls for a composite resin, the color selection is simplified. The filler in the restorative material is the key to color success in that it is a glasslike material and thus is able to pick up color from its immediate surroundings. This composite guide is reliable to a certain degree but not to the extent that one might hope. The universal color system does very well for about 70 per cent of the situations but the remainder require modification, which is especially true if an incisal angle is involved.

When a precise color match is needed, most manufacturers provide color modifiers. For example, a pigmented paste may be added to the universal paste; the paste volumes are determined by trial and error to produce a matching color. Or, the universal paste may be substituted with a colored paste, which is matched to a shade guide to provide a predictable result.

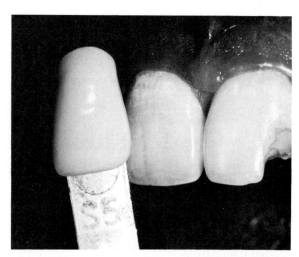

Figure 10–13. Shade selection must be done prior to rubber dam application.

Cavity Preparation

The cavity preparation designs for tooth-colored restorative materials are essentially the same, irrespective of which material will be placed.

First, the preparation must involve the surgical removal of the pathology caused by caries. The completed preparation should include the enamel, which demonstrates the effects of decalcification. It must permit ease in placement of the restorative material and finishing.

The rubber dam must be placed as part of the planned sequence of treatment. The resin systems, and most restorative materials, are not compatible with moisture and every effort should be taken to assure a dry field. For detailed information regarding the use and application of the rubber dam, refer to Chapter 9.

Class III Preparation

Armamentarium
1. Rubber dam, punch, clamp forceps, and clamps
2. Burs: Nos. 330, ½, 1, 2, 7901
3. Hand instruments: curved chisel, margin trimmer, Jeffery hatchets, hand excavator

Outline Form. Before proceeding with instrumentation, a decision must be made as to the proper direction of insertion for the restoring material. Whenever possible, it is preferable to make the opening from the lingual, as this will preserve the labial portion of the tooth. If the labial plate can be left reasonably intact, the esthetics will be superior (Fig. 10–14).

Many times the restoration will actually be a replacement for a defective existing restoration that has been inserted from the labial. With these conditions it is usually dictated that the new restoration will also be placed from the labial. There also will be situations in which caries has caused the greatest damage toward the labial. That type of situation will also dictate that the preparation will have a labial extension greater than preferred.

For example, in the case of a moderate interproximal lesion, the penetration will enter from the lingual surface. The high-speed handpiece, with a No. ½, 1, or 330 bur inserted, will accomplish most of the gross cutting of the preparation. The specific bur size will be related to the actual size of the teeth and the potential size of the preparation. The penetration from the lingual should occur so as to avoid cutting the adjacent tooth (Fig. 10–15).

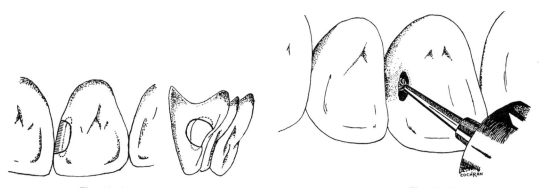

Fig. 10–14   **Fig. 10–15**

Figure 10–14. When feasible the preparation should be designed from the lingual. (See Fig. 2–21.) Note: The incisal part of the contact point is not removed.

Figure 10–15. Penetration is made to avoid injury to the contacting tooth.

The axial wall is located 0.5 mm beyond enamel into the dentin, and any variation from this will be dictated by the depth and the extent of caries. Where possible, the axial wall is placed at the ideal depth, and any carious penetration beyond this point is removed without involving the total axial wall. Usually there is no contact at the gingival with the adjacent tooth, which simplifies the restoring procedure.

The labial outline usually includes the labial part of the contact point, which places the labial margin in the labial embrasure. The gingival extension is restricted by the necessity to remove all defective enamel and dentin yet leave the remaining enamel properly supported by dentin. The enamel margin must be free of all decalcified material, otherwise the margin of the restoration will be faulty. The weakened enamel will be a source of continuing deterioration.

The finished Class III preparation outline does not require as precise a style as other types of preparations. It will usually have a rounded or curved form labially, incisally, and gingivally and will be made with the indicated rounded burs.

Resistance and Retention Form. The pulpal axial wall is placed into the dentin, as previously discussed under outline form. If caries extends beyond these limits it is removed, using either a slowly revolving bur or a hand excavator. The bur size will vary between a No. 1 and a No. 4, depending on the size of the lesion. The larger burs are used because they are effective in removing carious dentin and at the same time reduce the risk of accidentally involving the pulp.

When a hand excavator is used, it should be as large as convenient, although in the anterior teeth the smaller excavators are usually chosen. The carious material is removed until a firm non-yielding dentin wall is assured, as can be determined by appearance and surface texture.

Ideally, the enamel margins are supported by dentin. On occasion, a compromise may be advised to avoid a gross enlargement of the preparation wherein a segment of enamel may not have full dentin support. This is possible only if the enamel in question is free of any occlusal force.

The usual retention is a shallow groove placed across the gingival wall from labial to lingual. This will be made with a No. ½ or a No. 1 round bur, again using slow speed. The depth of this groove should not exceed the diameter of the bur. At times the retention may occur primarily toward the labial and lingual ends of the gingival wall, with the connecting groove being more shallow as compared with the primary sources of retention.

The same bur will be used to form a retentive area at the incisal (Fig. 10–16). If possible, the incisal retention is directed incisally, axially, and slightly toward the labial. The opening to the retentions should permit an

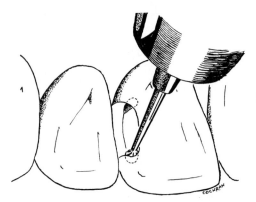

Figure 10–16. A round bur is used to place incisal retention.

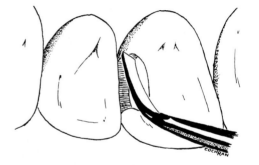

Figure 10–17. A sharp hand instrument is used to provide a smooth and beveled enamel margin.

easy flow of the restorative material into the retention areas; otherwise the restoration may not be adequately locked into position.

Hand Instrumentation. This type of preparation does not require unusual finesse with hand instruments.

When the labial surface is involved, a sharp No. 15 Wedelstaedt curved chisel is used to plane the enamel margin, helping to provide good support for the restoration. From the lingual, small enamel hatchets or marginal trimmers may be used to remove loose enamel at the margins and to help smooth the gingival and labial walls (Fig. 10–17; see also Fig. 8–1). Jeffery hatchets are also useful for the same purpose (see Fig. 6–26).

Bevels

Recent research indicates that preparations with bevels are more resistant to microleakage as compared with those without bevels when an acid etch technique is used. The bevel permits the acid to attack the enamel rods at the appropriate angle for maximum effect. Therefore, it is recommended that all preparations that will receive acid etching be beveled at the enamel margins. This improves the retentive capacity of the preparation and its resistance to marginal staining.

When possible an enamel bevel of 0.2 to 0.5 mm width is advocated as the final stage of preparation. This bevel is placed using a margin trimmer, Jeffery angle formers or, as convenience allows, a flame-shaped enamel finishing bur (No. 7901 or 242) at slow or moderate speed. The width of the bevel is restricted to avoid difficulties in finishing the resin restoration, because if the margin is indistinct it leads to either over- or underfinishing (Fig. 10–18).

Instrumentation Resumé for the Class III Preparation
1. No. ½, 1, or 330 used at high speed for penetration.
2. Same burs establish outline.
3. Axial wall located with the same burs.
4. Caries removed at slow speed using round burs as large as convenience allows.

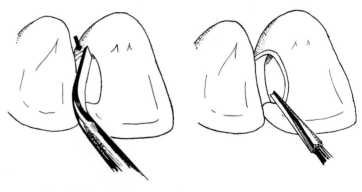

Figure 10–18. A definite bevel is placed on Class III composite preparations using either hand instruments or a bur.

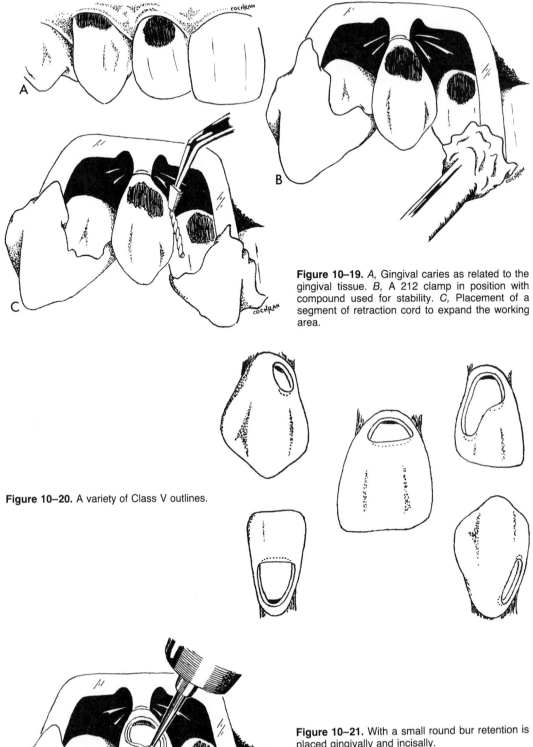

Figure 10–19. *A,* Gingival caries as related to the gingival tissue. *B,* A 212 clamp in position with compound used for stability. *C,* Placement of a segment of retraction cord to expand the working area.

Figure 10–20. A variety of Class V outlines.

Figure 10–21. With a small round bur retention is placed gingivally and incisally.

5. Hand excavator may also be used for caries removal.

6. Gingival and incisal retention is placed with No. ¼ or ½ bur.

7. Labial enamel is finished with a No. 15 Wedelstaedt chisel.

8. Gingival enamel is finished with small enamel hatchets, margin trimmer, or Jeffery instruments.

9. Bevels placed with margin trimmers, Jeffery angle formers, or 7901 or 242 finishing burs.

Class V Preparation

Armamentarium
1. Rubber dam, punch, clamp forceps and clamps, No. 212 clamp
2. Burs, Nos. 330, 256, ½, 1, 35
3. Hand instruments: curved chisel, mon-angle hoe, hand excavator

Outline Form. Isolation of the working area is the most significant item to be considered when dealing with any Class V lesion. Visibility and moisture control should have priority when placing a tooth-colored restorative. After placing the rubber dam, a No. 212 clamp is used to isolate the lesion for cavity preparation and placement of the restoration (Fig. 10–19). The details concerning rubber dam isolation are presented in Chapter 9.

The outline form of a Class V restoration is not uniform, as it will vary somewhat depending upon the caries or the degrees of decalcification (Fig. 10–20). When the diseased tissue has been removed and the margins are on reliable enamel, the outline will usually be rectangular with the corners round, ovoid, or kidney-shaped.

A No. 256 or 330 bur with high speed is suggested for establishing the outline. It is easy to overcut this preparation, as the tooth is quite small, so the No. 256 bur may be used with slow speed. Under most conditions the axial wall should be placed at a depth of 1.5 mm from the tooth surface.

The retention will be placed in the occlusal (or incisal) and gingival walls, at the junction with the axial wall, using a No. ¼ or ½ bur (Fig. 10–21). The mesial and distal walls should not be undercut. The depth of the retention will be governed by the diameter of the bur used, and it will not exceed the bur diameter and in some instances will be less. A mon-angle or Wedelstaedt chisel is useful for smoothing the walls and the enamel margins.

With the same reasoning as discussed with the Class III preparation, this preparation should also be beveled. The bevel is to be placed on all portions of the preparation that are surrounded by enamel and not where the preparation terminates in cementum. The bevel is placed by a hand instrument such as the No. 15 Wedelstaedt chisel or the enamel finishing burs Nos. 7901 or 242 (Fig. 10–22).

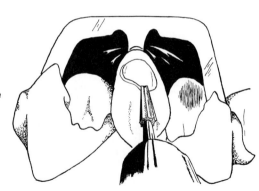

Figure 10–22. The enamel margins of a Class V composite preparation are beveled.

Instrumentation Resumé for the Class V Preparation

1. No. 256 or 330 bur for penetration and line.

2. Axial wall located with the same burs.

3. If required, caries is removed with a slow-speed round bur, as dictated by convenience.

4. Hand excavator may be advised.

5. Gingival and incisal retention placed with No. ¼ or ½ bur.

6. Enamel is finished and beveled with a No. 15 Wedelstaedt chisel and 7901 or 242 bur.

Class V Eroded Lesion

Improper use of the toothbrush and other causes frequently lead to abrasion or erosion of tooth structure at the gingiva. These so-called "eroded lesions" often become V-shaped, with large areas of exposed dentin and cementum. They are unsightly and usually sensitive to thermal or mechanical shock. Because they terminate on root surfaces, these lesions may be handled differently from the technique described previously, as will be discussed later in the chapter.

Class IV Preparation

Class IV restoration is required when an accident or extensive caries destroys or severely weakens the incisal angle. It is more difficult to provide the desired mechanical retention when the incisal portion of the tooth is lost. Also, the esthetics or color matching is more critical because of the size of the restoration. Because of its location, color change in a Class IV restoration is readily detected as time passes.

For many situations the Class IV is the most conservative approach for restorations that involve the incisal angle. This restoration does not require the great removal of normal tooth structure, as is required by a full crown preparation (Fig. 10–23). The youthful age of the patient may be a factor in the treatment plan, and the Class IV preparation may be a means of delaying a more complex restoration; if delayed, the eventual crown has a better chance for success. The pulp horns are very large in a young patient and interfere with good crown preparations. Also, as the patient proceeds through the adolescent and teenage years, the gingival tissue will continue to shift position, exposing more of the clinical crown. Furthermore, the Class IV is the most

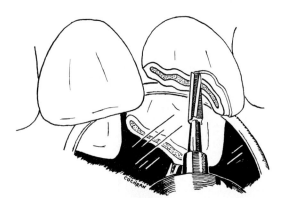

Figure 10–23. The enamel is prepared to increase the surface area for etching.

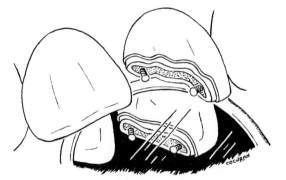

Figure 10–24. Pins are added to a fracture preparation for added stability.

economical option and so will frequently be chosen for that reason alone. However, the most predictable solution for the involved Class IV is the metal-ceramic crown, which will be discussed in Chapter 20.

If the incisal involvement is very slight, the same preparation as used for the Class III is satisfactory and the only variation would be to enlarge the incisal retention.

The success of many Class IV restorations will depend upon gaining retention other than that found within the cavity preparation itself. One is by the utilization of an acid etching technique, which will be discussed shortly, prior to placing the restoration. The other is by the use of threaded pins for support, which are to be discussed briefly here and in detail in Chapter 13. The use of pins for anterior resins has decreased markedly as the use of the acid etch technique has provided a high level of stability for these restorations. When the pins are used, they function as a supplement to the retention form available within the preparation (Fig. 10–24). The pin system recommended is the TMS threaded pin. The advantage of this system is that pins with diameters varying from 0.013 to 0.031 inch are available.

One or two pins are placed in the gingival wall, depending on need. If two are used, they are separated labial to lingual as far as possible. At times it would be an advantage to have a pin in the incisal area, but when the path of insertion creates a problem with preparation and pin placement, they should not be used.

Acid Etching and Bonding Procedures

A valuable adjunct for retention of resin systems is the technique of etching or demineralizing the enamel at the interface of the restoration. The technique has been especially helpful in the Class IV restoration. Sometimes the Class IV preparation is altered by preparing a minishoulder or chamfer in the enamel as far as possible around the preparation so as to make more enamel area available for the etching procedure. There are situations involving fractured incisal angles in which the total retention of the restorative material may be obtained by using the acid etch mechanism. There will be instances when this procedure, in addition to a conventional preparation, may be required for a successful restoration.

The determination to use acid etching exclusively or in combination with a preparation is based on:

1. The location and size of the pulp, as this may discourage the use of some preparation forms, with the exception of those limited to the enamel.

2. The incisal or occlusal involvement. Acid etching by itself will not be

able to support restorations that are subject to intense forces (see Figs. 2–22 to 2–24).

The acid etching of the enamel surface is very beneficial for retention of resin restorations for fractured anterior teeth. Likewise, it is beneficial in other types of restorations, e.g., the Class III and Class V, even though retention is adequate in those situations as a result of the preparation itself. However, the more intimate bond of the resin to the enamel at the margins reduces the tendency for marginal stain, regardless of the resin used.

INDICATIONS FOR ACID ETCHING

1. Class IV incisal angles of anterior teeth.
2. Enamel fractures, primarily upper centrals and laterals.
3. Class V, in occlusal or incisal enamel as added retention.
4. Class III, in addition to conventional retention.

Acid etching will not succeed if the amount of enamel is inadequate or if the restoration is subjected to heavy occlusal stress. Thus, many large restorations in the lower incisors will fail if acid etching is to be the primary support. In resin preparations with questionable retention, pins should be added as a means of support.

Dentin and Pulp Protection

Prior to application of acid for etching or the placement of the resin restoration the dentin must be protected by placing a liner. If a liner is not placed, either the acid used for etching or the resin will produce irritation to the pulp. This is true for either the composite or unfilled resin. As was noted earlier, zinc oxide–eugenol cement cannot be used under a resin, as eugenol interferes with the polymerization of most resin systems and tends to leave the resin soft at the interface between the resin and the cement. A varnish is generally not acceptable as a liner, as the monomer portion of the resin dissolves the varnish, which removes the protective barrier. Also the solvent in the varnish interferes with resin polymerization.

A calcium hydroxide base is recommended as the protective liner and, as detailed in Chapter 7, is applied as a thin layer under a resin (Fig. 10–25). In acid etch techniques, the phosphoric acid may dissolve some of the calcium hydroxide liner, necessitating addition of or reapplication of the liner material. The retention of the preparation should be checked and liner material that may have penetrated into those areas removed.

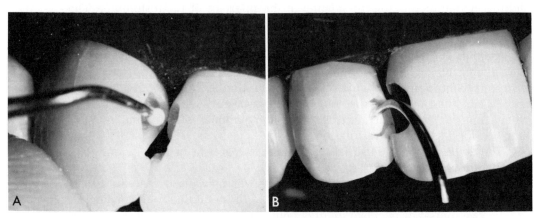

Figure 10–25. *A* and *B,* A calcium hydroxide liner is placed for pulp protection.

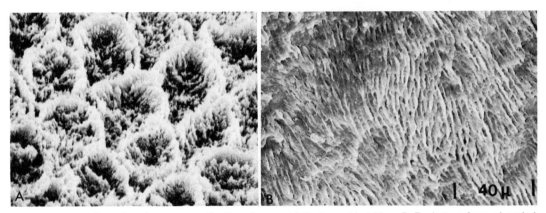

Figure 10–26. *A,* Scanning electron magnification of enamel following acid etching. *B,* Resin tags from a beveled enamel margin.

Etchant and Bonding Agent

The acid etchant applied to the enamel produces a markedly improved bond strength at the enamel–resin interface. One reason for this is that the acid leaves a clean enamel surface, which permits better wetting of the surface by the resin. More important, the acid attacks the enamel surface, leaving microscopic surface irregularities. The etchant thus creates peaks and valleys in the enamel, which allow for mechanical interlocking of the resin into the surface irregularities. The resin "tag" then produces a much improved bond of the resin to the tooth. The effective tag length as a result of etching on adult anterior teeth has been demonstrated to be approximately 7 to 25 μm (Fig. 10–26).

Phosphoric acid is the etchant employed. A concentration of 35 to 50 per cent is appropriate and most manufacturers supply these acid etch solutions or gels. The solution may also be obtained from a pharmacy. If the acid concentration is not in this range it will produce overetching, destruction of excessive tooth structure, and/or leave a tenacious debris on the surface that cannot be washed free.

In advance of placing the restorative material the dentin is protected with a liner and the acid solution is placed on the enamel using a small pellet of cotton or a fine camel's hair brush. Precaution is taken to limit application of the acid to keep it from running over unwanted peripheral areas of enamel. This illustrates again the virtue of having a well-placed rubber dam in position to help restrict the acid (Fig. 10–27). The acid is applied continuously and

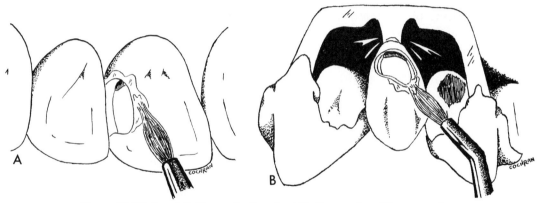

Figure 10–27. *A* and *B,* The application of acid to the margins of the preparation.

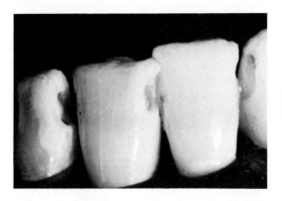

Figure 10–28. The frosty appearance of enamel following etching by acid.

left undisturbed in contact with the enamel for a minimum of 1 minute without any rubbing or smearing of the enamel surface. The acid and decalcified material are washed away thoroughly with water for a minimum of 30 seconds and evacuated and then gently air dried for 15 seconds. There must be assurance that there are no contaminants in the air line.

The etched enamel should have a frosty white decalcified appearance (Fig. 10–28). If that frostiness is not apparent, it suggests that the etching is not adequate and that the acid will have to be reapplied so as to produce an enamel surface appropriate to receive and hold the resin projections. Usually the single application is all that is needed, and the restorative procedure quickly follows. However, teeth of patients raised on a fluoride water supply possess enamel that is resistant to decalcification and often require reapplication of the acid etching procedure. In some situations, 3 or 4 minutes may be required to secure the necessary enamel decalcification. In contrast, immature enamel in a child is more rapidly etched than mature enamel in the adult patient.

Recently many manufacturers have introduced so-called enamel bond agents to be used in conjunction with acid etch techniques. The *bond agent* usually consists of the thinned BIS–GMA resin matrix material without filler or with only a very small amount of filler present. Bond agents are furnished in the form of either chemically activated resins or light-polymerized resins. After acid etching of the enamel the bond agent is applied. The theory is that the low viscosity resin will flow readily into the pores created by acid etching and assure maximum resin tag formation. The bonding agent thus achieves an intimate interlocking with the tooth. The composite resin is immediately inserted and in turn bonds to the intermediate layer of the resin bonding agent.

Probably the chief merit of such agents is that one is assured of good wetting of the tooth by the resin and formation of maximum resin tags. A relatively good resin–tooth bond strength can be attained with the use of an etchant and composite alone, but time is a more critical element. As polymerization proceeds, the fluidity of the composite decreases. With the decrease in fluidity the wetting capability of the resin diminishes. Although the decrease in fluidity does not, of course, occur with the light-cured systems, the use of a bonding agent is probably a good safety measure even with these resins. Also, it is advantageous for microfilled resins, which are somewhat more viscous.

The bond agent is a clear slightly viscous liquid that is easily applied with a small brush to the cavity walls and enamel margins. The bonding agent should form a thin and uniform layer throughout the preparation. The so-called adhesive dentin bonding agents will be discussed later.

Procedural Resumé

1. Local anesthesia.
2. Rubber dam isolation.
3. Preparation, outline, and internal form.
4. Caries removal.
5. Pin placement (optional).
6. Calcium hydroxide liner over dentin.
7. Acid etching (where indicated).
8. Recheck liner and remove from retention areas.
9. Place bonding agent.
10. Proceed to placing the restoration and finishing.

Placing the Restoration

The recommendation for all resin restorations, whether an unfilled acrylic or a composite, is that the acid etch technique be used prior to placing the restorative material. This is recommended even though acid etching is not used as a means of retention. In those situations, etching provides a more intimate marginal adaptation and thereby reduces marginal microleakage and thus stain, as noted by the marginal stain in Figure 5–15.

All tooth-colored restorative materials (silicate and resin) are pulpal irritants, as noted. Thus in cavity preparations where minimal dentin is present it is advised to place a calcium hydroxide liner over the dentin surface. This effectively protects the pulp against irritating components in the restorative material.

The technique for use of the unfilled and composite resins will be discussed since both are employed, although the composites are decidedly more popular, for reasons previously discussed.

When manipulating resins, the operator must carefully avoid including any impurities in the mixture. All instruments must be clean, and the material should not contact the operator's fingers before it has polymerized.

Brush Technique

Armamentarium
1. Dappen dishes
2. Sable brushes
3. Acrylic powder and liquid
4. Protective lubricant

Procedures. The so-called brush technique is used extensively with the traditional unfilled acrylic resins (Fig. 10–29). The selected powder is placed

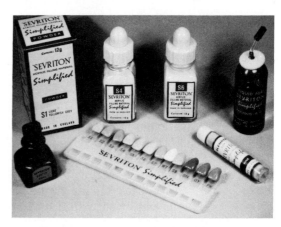

Figure 10–29. A conventional unfilled resin system.

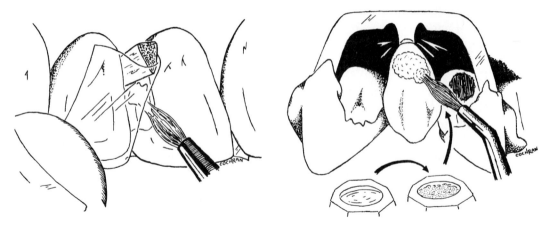

Figure 10–30. A brush is used to carry small increments of monomer and polymer to the preparation.

in one dappen dish and the monomer in another. A fine-tipped sable hair brush is used for placement into the cavity.

The preparation is first covered with a thin film of the monomer. Then the brush is dipped in the liquid. The wet brush is then used to pick up particles of powder, which in turn will turn into a fluid bead of resin that is then placed into the preparation. The fluid mix flows readily over the cavity wall already wetted by the monomer (Fig. 10–30). This process is repeated, and increments are added until the restoration is completed. The additions are made at a deliberate rate of about 10 to 15 seconds between increments, which will permit polymerization or hardening to begin in the previously placed beads of acrylic.

During this process precise care is taken to avoid dropping powder into the liquid or liquid into the powder, which would cause partial polymerization in both. To avoid this problem an additional dish of liquid can be provided and between each increment the brush is cleansed in the additional monomer. This type of assembly is commercially available.

Precaution must be taken not to allow an increment of resin to dry out before the next addition, as a laminating effect will possibly be visible. The restoration is filled to a slight overcontour and allowed to polymerize. The restoration should be coated with an inert material, such as cocoa butter, silicone lubricant, or vaseline, which prevents monomer evaporation and allows proper polymerization.

Before finishing can begin, the restoration must remain undisturbed until adequate hardening occurs. This will vary with different products, but a minimum of 8 minutes is a good general rule to follow.

Bulk or Pressure Packing of Composite Resin

Armamentarium
1. Mylar strips
2. Paper mixing pad
3. Disposable mixing spatulas
4. Composite materials
5. Syringe (optional)

Procedures. Owing to their viscosity and bulk, a bulk or pressure technique is employed with composite resins.

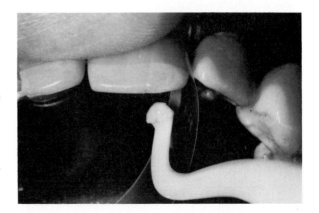

Figure 10–31. A clear plastic strip plus a wedge is used as a matrix.

A mylar strip is prepared to provide the desired contour (Fig. 10–31). The strip as usually supplied should be cut to one half the length, and the width should be reduced so as to provide a strip that will not protrude more than 1 to 2 mm beyond the incisal edge. The strip should then be placed in position between contacts, and the gingival margin should be enclosed.

Most current composites are supplied in a two-paste system and the manufacturer's instructions should be observed regarding storage and handling. One is a "universal" paste, and the other is the catalyst. A paper pad and disposable mixing spatulas are provided. The material can be mixed on a glass slab, but the composite is so abrasive that it will quickly etch a glass surface. The two pastes must not be cross-contaminated, so different ends of the spatula are used for the two pastes. Conventional metal spatulas are not used since the abrasiveness of the resin would lead to metal contamination of the mix, producing a color variance.

Equal amounts of the base and catalyst are placed on a mixing pad, which standardizes the polymerization and resultant color. The polymerization time is short, so with the disposable spatula the mass should be homogenously mixed and ready for placement in the preparation within 30 seconds (Fig. 10–32). A plastic-tipped instrument should be used to transport the material from the pad to the preparation. Increments as needed are wiped or placed into the cavity and this process is repeated until the cavity is filled with a slight overfill, helping to form a properly contoured restoration.

As the increments are being added, the trapping of air in the body of the restoration must be avoided (Fig. 10–33). The presence of voids in composite resin restorations is a greater problem than in unfilled acrylic resins. The material is relatively viscous and does not flow readily. It therefore tends to

Figure 10–32. The base and catalyst are mixed homogenously.

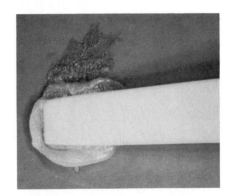

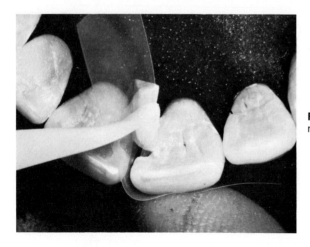

Figure 10–33. The material is inserted so as to minimize air entrapment.

"bridge over" and entrap air. Voids within the body of the restoration reduce the strength and impair the esthetics. A void at the margin is particularly serious, since such an area would be exceedingly vulnerable to caries attack. The technique of wiping the material into the cavity aids in reducing the possibility of trapping air. If a void is apparent, it may be necessary to remove the material and insert a new restoration. Again, speed is important, and the entire operation should be completed within 1 minute.

Immediately after the strip is adapted and in the desired position so as to provide contour, it is held tightly for approximately 4 minutes to allow polymerization to take place. Immediately after positioning the strip, a flat plastic instrument may be used to iron the margins, which tends to reduce the amount of excessive resin and ease the finishing process (Fig. 10–34). The strip protects the surface from oxygen, which would allow an oxygen-rich surface to develop and inhibit polymerization.

LIGHT-CURED COMPOSITES

The light-cured resins are generally furnished as a single paste since the chemicals that produce polymerization are activated only when exposed to light of the proper wavelength. Thus mixing of the components is eliminated. The resin paste is packed into the cavity and contoured by a matrix strip or by a premolded Class V matrix into proper contour and the restoration is polymerized by shining a small beam of light of the correct wavelength onto the restoration. If the restoration thickness exceeds 2.5 mm it should be developed by increments as there are limitations to the penetration by the light. The light tip is placed very close to, but not against, the surface of the restoration and activated (Fig. 10–35).

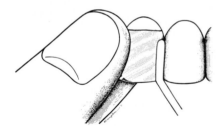

Figure 10–34. The matrix strip is held tightly against the tooth, and a plastic instrument is pressed over the margin to minimize flash.

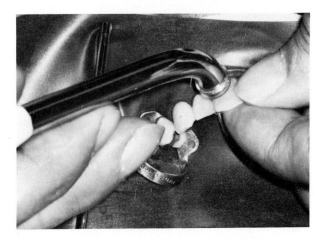

Figure 10–35. Employing visible light to polymerize a composite resin. The light source is held close to but not in contact with the restoring material.

The exposure time required to achieve polymerization varies to some degree with the shade of resin. Darker shades require longer exposure or cure time than do lighter shades. Forty to 60 seconds exposure per location of light is a good rule of thumb to obtain cure of a reasonable thickness with most shades of resin and to assure that the bottom of the restoration is completely polymerized. In the case of Class II and IV restorations, curing from both the facial and lingual surfaces is recommended.

There are some precautions to be observed with the light-cured resins. The resin should not be dispensed until the restoration is ready to be placed. If it is exposed for any extended period to the operatory lights, some polymerization may occur since they may emit a certain amount of light in the critical wavelength range. The curing lights are of high intensity, hence one should avoid looking directly at the light and care should be taken that the light is not directed into the patient's eyes. Some of the light sources employ glass fiber optics to transmit the light from the bulb to the handpiece. The cords containing the fiber optics should be carefully handled in order to avoid fracture of the fibers, which would reduce the amount of light emitted at the tip.

There are several advantages of light-cured resins over chemically activated ones. Since the mixing is eliminated there is less chance of incorporating air into the mix. Thus porosity in the restoration is minimized. The dentist can choose the working time since polymerization does not begin until the resin is exposed to the light. For this reason it is possible to mold and shape the restoration to the proper contour prior to polymerization. Therefore, the amount of finishing required is usually less than with chemically activated resins and it may occur immediately in the technique sequence. And, of course, polymerization is accomplished in a matter of seconds rather than minutes.

The light-cured systems allow for a generous versatility in providing treatment options in addition to conventional needs. The reader is referred to Chapter 5, where an esthetic spacing problem of anterior teeth is resolved using a light-cured resin.

Syringe Method

The restoration of a Class IV preparation poses more of a problem as compared with a Class III, as it is difficult to control the needed form for such a large segment of tooth.

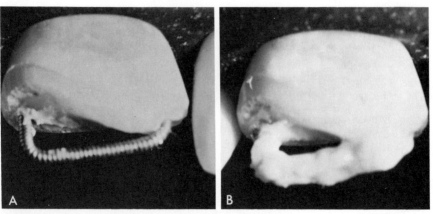

Figure 10–36. *A,* Threaded wire cemented across the incisal of the preparation. *B,* Wire covered with opaque resin material.

If pins have been used, there is a potential danger that the metal will shadow through the restoration, leaving an unsightly appearance. Thus, the pin needs to be masked or covered with a suitable material to prevent poor esthetics (Fig. 10–36). This may be done by coating the pin with a thin flowable mixture of cement or opaque liner material. A simple masking agent is a film of white liquid Nuba-Wax* or White Ace,† which is used for a shoe dressing (see Fig. 13–45).

---

*Nuba-Wax Division, Oil Kraft Inc., Cincinnati, Ohio 45223.
†White Ace, available from a variety store.

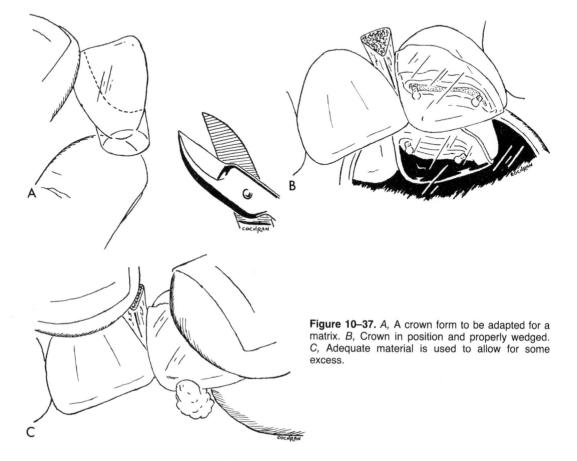

Figure 10–37. *A,* A crown form to be adapted for a matrix. *B,* Crown in position and properly wedged. *C,* Adequate material is used to allow for some excess.

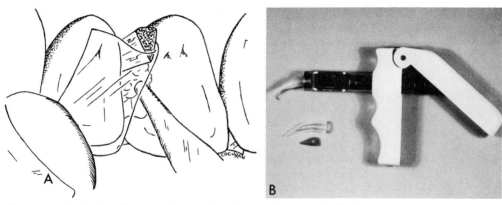

Figure 10–38. *A,* A syringe may be used to place resin materials. *B,* A syringe that is used to place composite restorative materials.

A matrix strip such as used for the Class III can be used, but it is difficult to control the intended shape and the excess resin. A plastic crown form, tailored to fit the preparation area (Fig. 10–37), is preferable. After the resin material is mixed, some of it is placed into the preparation and adapted to minimize amount of material.

A syringe that has disposable tips and plugs may be used to place the composite resins (Fig. 10–38). After mixing, the material is quickly picked up in the tip and a plunger inserted to permit extrusion of the resin into the preparation.* When the syringe method is used, it is important to work quickly, as the hardening may begin before the material is properly placed in a cavity. As an aid, the opening of the disposable tip may be enlarged by cutting it back a slight amount. The syringe method can be used with most types of preparations. Its primary advantage is that it tends to reduce the possibility of trapping air bubbles in the restoration. Also, it may simplify delivery of material because it is easier to determine the amount needed, although more material is needed to fill the syringe tip.

When employing a light-cured resin, it may be expressed from the ampule to the syringe tip and delivered to its precise location. If this provides a greater level of convenience for a given situation it is to be recommended.

When dealing with a Class IV restoration, a plastic crown form is tailored to fit and, if possible, is anchored into place by a wedge. Prior to this, a hole is cut in the incisal corner to accommodate the size of the syringe tip. With this method it is simple to fill the preparation, avoid air entrapment, and eject the needed amount of material. When injection is completed, it is simple to adapt the crown form tightly against the enamel margins, limiting the resin excess, which aids the finishing procedures.

Finishing of Resin Restoration

Armamentarium
1. Fine grit diamonds: designs vary from tapered cylindrical to round
2. 12- to 20-bladed carbide burs: designs may vary but include tapered flame-shaped and round
3. White tapered or round stones
4. Scalpel

---

*Clev-Dent, 3307 Scranton Road, Cleveland, Ohio 44109.

5. Finishing strips and Sof-Flex disks*
6. Fine cuttle paper disks†
7. White rubber cups
8. Glaze materials

UNFILLED RESINS

Procedures. The unfilled resin is the easiest of these materials to finish. Before finishing begins, polymerization must essentially be completed so as to avoid disturbing the adaptation at the resin–enamel interface. The contour is easily established with a conveniently designed finishing bur at slow speed. The bur may be either conventional steel or carbide. After the surface is contoured and smooth, moist flour of pumice and finely divided chalk is used in a white rubber cup to produce the final polish (Fig. 10–39). The white cup is preferred, as it decreases any possibility of the surface of the restoration being contaminated with the coloring in a grey cup. Also, when using a cup at the cervical edge of a Class V be extremely careful to avoid pressure on either the restoration or the cementum, as the cup will exert the greatest pressure at its periphery. Thus, it is possible to ditch or abrade the cementum, which may create a problem worse than that existing initially, for overpolished cementum may be very sensitive to temperature change or to touch.

CONVENTIONAL COMPOSITE, HYBRID, AND MICROFILLED RESINS

The smoothest and most desirable surface is that which remains after the properly adapted matrix is removed. However, it is difficult to adapt a matrix so accurately that additional adjustment to the margins or morphology is unnecessary.

A major problem with conventional composite resins is the rough surface produced during polishing, as has been discussed. During finishing, the filler particles are abraded less than the surface. Such a surface is more susceptible

---

*3M Company, Dental Products, St. Paul, Minnesota 55101.
†E. C. Moore & Son Co., Dearborn, Michigan 48126.

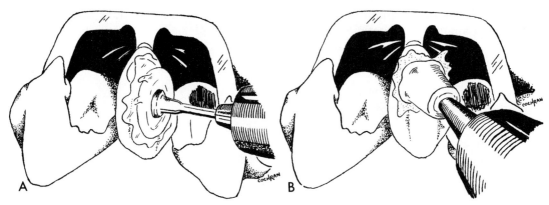

Figure 10–39. *A,* Paper disks used to provide a smooth surface. *B,* Polishing of a resin restoration with rubber cup and a polishing powder.

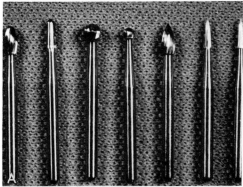

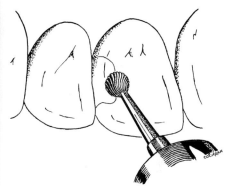

Figure 10–40. *A,* 12-bladed carbide finishing burs used to finish composite resin restorations. *B,* Carbide finishing burs used to provide desired contour.

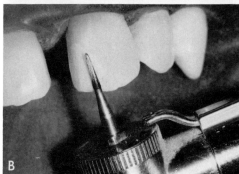

to staining and would be uncomfortable to the tongue. No polishing technique is perfect, but the following is satisfactory.

Procedures. The gross finishing or contouring is most easily done with fine grit diamonds* or carbide finishing burs,† usually at a moderate speed. The carbide bur is preferable, as it leaves a smoother surface than a conventional diamond (Fig. 10–40). Ordinary steel burs will discolor the surface. The smoothest surface is left if the bur has 12 or 20 blades. When the instrument is operated at high speed there is danger of cutting enamel, so slow speed is suggested for final segments of finishing.

The above sequence is used totally or in part, depending on the restoration size. If the restorations are small and located between the teeth, diamonds are not useful. The essential contour of larger restorations involving the facial or lingual surface, or both, is established with diamonds or burs, following which white stones may be used with water lubrication to improve smoothness (Fig. 10–41B).

The initial gingival or margin flash may be removed by using a scalpel or sharp gold knife, presuming that the amount of excess is not obviously bulky (Fig. 10–41A).

Traditional and hybrid composites are not polishable in the usual sense so the objective is to have them be as smooth as possible when finished. The variability between the hard inorganic macrofiller particles and the soft matrix resin makes a conventional and long lasting polished or smooth surface an impossibility. The traditional dental stones, disks, and diamond burs do not provide the best possible surface.

Plastic finishing strips that have an empty center gap are used for finishing

---

*Star Dental Manufacturing, Conshohocken, Pennsylvania 19428.
†Teledyne Densco, 3840 Forest St., Denver, Colorado 80207.

the interproximal surface. These strips are coated with aluminum oxide in the same manner as the disks (Fig. 10–41C).

Diamond instruments, which are very effective for contouring and finishing all resin systems, have become available (Fig. 10–42A).* These diamond instruments are supplied as fine, with diamond particles 40 μm in diameter, or superfine, wherein the diameter of the particle is 15 μm. These instruments are most effective when used at a low or moderate speed of 10,000 to 15,000 rpm in a constant whipping motion and with a generous water spray. These diamonds, when followed by the use of aluminum oxide disks, lead to the smoothest possible surface. They are particularly helpful in finishing of microfilled systems.

Whenever tooth contour and access permit, there are available highly flexible polyurethane-based finishing and polishing disks, which are coated with aluminum oxide particles. The sequence of grit size varies from a coarse cutting capability to a very fine finishing and polishing grit. These disks are compatible with water as a lubricant or with an intermittent air stream, and the selection at this point is related to personal preference. These disks are very effective whenever it is convenient to use them (Fig. 10–42B, C).

Again, as a reminder, damage to the enamel or cementum with any of the finishing procedures must be avoided. Examples of polished restorations are shown in Figure 10–43.

Unfilled resin "glazes" are also available from some manufacturers to coat the surface after polishing in the hope of eliminating the roughness. These glaze materials are the conventional BIS–GMA resin, with possibly a small

---

*Teledyne Densco, 3840 Forest St., Denver, Colorado 80207.

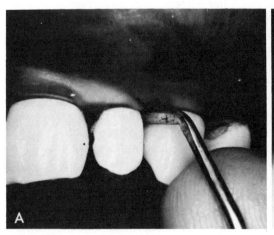
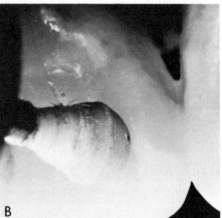

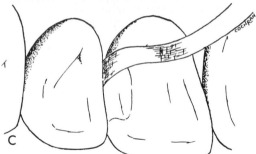

Figure 10–41. *A,* Gingival excess may be removed by a sharp gold knife. *B,* White stones are used to provide a smooth composite surface. *C,* Finishing strips are used for interproximal finish.

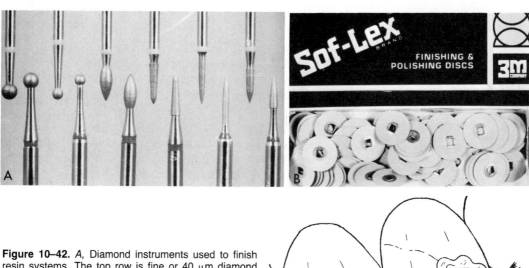

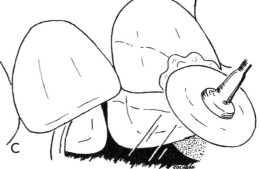

Figure 10–42. *A,* Diamond instruments used to finish resin systems. The top row is fine or 40 μm diamond particles and the lower row is superfine or 15 μm diamond particles. *B,* Flexible Sof-Lex polishing discs. *C,* Polishing disk in use.

amount of filler added. However, the resultant cured film is soft and thin and as a result is abraded away by the usual oral functions and hygiene procedures within a matter of months. In spite of the short duration, the surface veneer is worth placing if the patient is told that it will not last very long.

Resumé of Finishing
1. Remove gross flash with scalpel or diamond.
2. Contour with stones and/or finishing burs.
3. Finish interproximal with strips.
4. Polish facial and lingual with disks and polishing diamond instruments.
5. Polish unfilled resins with polishing powders.
6. Place resin glaze (optional).

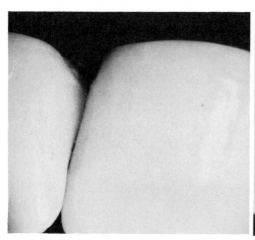

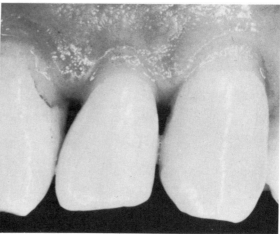

Figure 10–43. Clinical examples of conventional or microfilled composite restorations.

Eroded Lesions

The traditional method of restoring these lesions, in order to improve the esthetics and eliminate sensitivity, has been by means of a Class V restoration of amalgam, foil, or resins, as has been discussed. More recently, with the introduction of the acid etch technique for resin, it is possible to build these areas back to normal contour by etching the enamel at the margins. The mechanical bonding created thereby holds the resin without the use of a cavity preparation. The obvious advantages of such a procedure, as compared with the classic Class V restoration, are a saving of sound tooth structure by eliminating the instrumentation and also less chair time.

To restore these gingival lesions, rubber dam isolation is very important in order to prevent moisture contamination. Anesthesia can be used if gingival tissue comfort is a problem and at times a No. 212 clamp will be needed to reflect the tissue from the lesion (Fig. 10–44). A light application of pumice and water is used to remove plaque, and if the eroded area is deep, a calcium hydroxide base is placed.

The area is etched in the same manner as previously described, but in contrast to the enamel the dentin will not change color. The restoration is placed as specified by the manufacturer and the finishing will occur in the same manner as described for conventional composite resins.

Effective chemical bonding does not occur in dentin and cementum. As a result microleakage is prevalent in all areas of the margin not attached to enamel and when this occurs, it does not provide a satisfactory restoration. To minimize this leakage around the gingival margins and to improve its retention, it is recommended that mechanical retention be provided in the gingival segment in the manner described for the Class V restoration (Fig. 10–45).

A number of commercial "dentin bonding" agents have been marketed (Fig. 10–46). These involve phosphorus-containing agents or other mechanisms to provide adhesive bonding to dentin. Considerable research focuses on the effectiveness of such materials. More information is needed to determine their biocompatibility and especially their adhesive stability over a long period of time in the oral environment. Should such mechanisms prove to be effective in these matters then it would probably be possible to restore the eroded area without the necessity for any kind of mechanical retention. However, until this is resolved one is advised to instrument the lesion as described even when dentin bonding agents are used.

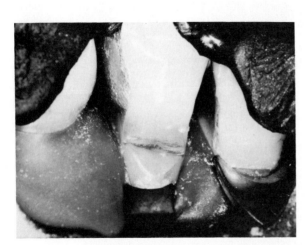

Figure 10–44. A clinical erosion lesion.

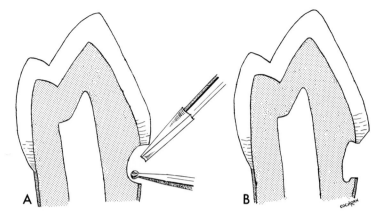

Figure 10–45. An eroded lesion (*A*) with beveled enamel for acid etching and mechanical gingival retention. *B*, Completed preparation.

Glass Ionomer Cement Restoration

There is still a third method that may be employed for restoration of the eroded lesion other than the conventional Class V restoration or the use of an acid etch resin technique without use of a cavity preparation. It involves the use of a glass ionomer cement (Fig. 10–47). Again, no cavity preparation is made, but bonding of the restorative material (the ionomer cement) to tooth structure is attained by chemical adhesion between the cement and one or more components of the enamel and/or dentin, rather than by mechanical bonding as for the acid etch resin method. The chemistry and characteristics of this type of cement were discussed in Chapter 7.

Following rubber dam isolation, the tooth surface is cleansed of plaque and debris with a non-fluoride prophylactic slurry. Pastes should be avoided, as they may have an oily film on the tooth that would deter bonding of the cement. The surface is cleansed further by scrubbing for 15 seconds with the solution supplied by the manufacturer for this purpose. That solution is 50 per cent citric acid, which would be contra-indicated for *cut* dentin owing to its irritational characteristics and its tendency to erode the odontoblastic process in the tubules. However, no harm occurs with a short treatment on these types of lesions because of the sclerosis of the dentin. Polyacrylic acid is better since it cleans the tooth surface effectively without etching or irritating

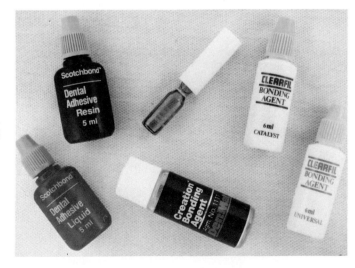

Figure 10–46. Examples of commercial products used as dentin bonding agents.

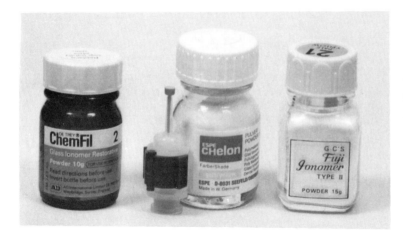

Figure 10–47. Representative commercial Type II glass ionomer cements. It can be seen that one of the products is also supplied in a pre-proportioned capsule and mixed in a mechanical amalgamator.

the odontoblastic process. A pumice wash may also be used for cleansing whenever sensitivity or pulpal irritation is a major consideration.

The surface is then thoroughly rinsed, dried, and maintained in a dry state. The powder and liquid are mixed to a thick creamy consistency (approximately a 3:1 powder to liquid ratio) (Fig. 10–48). The mix is completed rapidly and, as for the polycarboxylate cements, should have a gloss on the surface when carried to the tooth. This indicates that unreacted polyacrylic acid is still available to wet and bond to the tooth. The matrix is applied immediately and should be held in place for 6 to 15 minutes. That time is necessary in order to secure proper wetting of the cement to the underlying dentin and to protect the cement against moisture contamination during the initial set. Immediately after the matrix is removed the restoration should be coated with the varnish provided by the manufacturer. The excess cement is then carefully trimmed off. Only the gross excess is removed at that time, as the cement should not be disturbed unduly during its setting. Final polishing is delayed for at least 24 hours (Fig. 10–49).

A new generation of glass ionomer cement restoratives is now available. The main advantage of these new restorative materials is their ability to be finished immediately after matrix removal. These new materials are not sensitive to moisture contamination after initial set, but should be carefully finished using water owing to their increased sensitivity to dehydration.

Before the patient is dismissed, the surface of the restoration is revarnished. It is essential to provide protection during the continuing hardening of the cement. Chalky surfaces, accompanied by subsequent deterioration, can

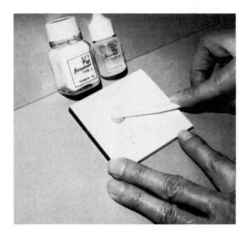

Figure 10–48. Glass ionomer powder and liquid are mixed thoroughly and quickly.

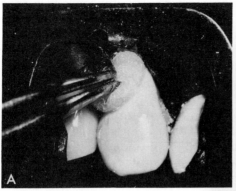

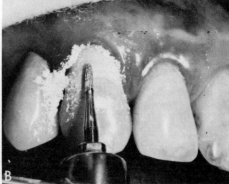

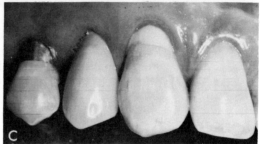

Figure 10–49. *A,* Following placement and initial contouring of a glass ionomer restoration, a film of varnish is placed over the surface. *B,* At the following appointment the finishing is completed and the use of a carbide finishing bur is illustrated. *C,* A finished clinical restoration with glass ionomer cement.

usually be associated with improper manipulation of the cement, premature removal of the matrix, or failure to use the surface protection agent.

Retention occurs in the majority of cases for at least up to 5 years following the use of the glass ionomer cement. However, owing to the low ductility of the material, it cannot be satisfactorily retained unless the lesion is quite definitely V-notched. Thus it is not suited for small, saucer-shaped lesions.

Yet another ionomer cement formulation has materialized. This makes use of a sintered ceramic–silver particle as a filler.* Certain properties, such as wear resistance, are enhanced. These "CERMETS" may in time extend the use of this type of cement to conservative Class I and even Class II restorations.

Silicate Cement

In selected patients with a high caries index, particularly in anterior teeth, resin is not the restorative material of choice. It is in the best interest of the patient to restore the teeth with well-placed silicate cement restorations. These restorations, reinforced by a good home care regimen, help reduce or control caries activity.

Silicate cements are supplied as a powder that is mixed with a phosphoric acid liquid. The mixture sets to a relatively hard, translucent substance resembling dental porcelain.

Silicate powders are finely ground ceramic materials, which are essentially acid soluble glasses. Most commercial silicate cement powders contain fluoride up to 15 per cent. The fluoride is present since a fluoride flux is added to permit proper sintering of the other ingredients.

The composition of the liquids for the silicate cements is not greatly different from that of the liquids used for zinc phosphate cements.

Ketac-Silver, BSPE, Germany

Clinical Significance of the Fluoride. The incidence of secondary caries is markedly less around the silicate cement restoration than around all other filling materials. This behavior is somewhat surprising when one examines the gross microleakage that occurs at the margins and through the restoration itself. Few, if any, dental restorative materials show greater leakage patterns.

This anticariogenic property is, obviously, associated with the fluoride present in the cement. Its action is actually twofold. One, it provides a source of fluoride uptake to the adjoining tooth structure during insertion and hardening of the cement. This results in a substantial reduction in enamel acid solubility, much as in a topical application of a fluoride solution. Also, the indefinite release of low concentrations of fluoride alters the chemical nature of the plaque, specifically by acting as an enzyme inhibitor and preventing microbial growth and acid production. As has been noted, the glass ionomer cements provide a comparable caries resistance since they are based on the silicate fluoride leach mechanism.

Although the silicate cement restorations exhibit good esthetic qualities for a short time after insertion, their greatest disadvantage is lack of stability in oral fluids with a loss of esthetic qualities. The rubber dam is essential for successful silicate restorations.

To anticipate maximum success with silicate restorations they must be mixed as thick as feasible to a maximum powder to liquid ratio. After insertion the surface must be protected with a film of cocoa butter or vaseline from premature moisture contact or dehydration.

The clinician will need to review the technical procedures concerning placement and finishing of silicate restorations stated by the manufacturer. The glass ionomer restoration is a superior one, however, as has been discussed.

Summary

The total process of placing successful tooth-colored restorations is based in part upon a scientific background. But it is also heavily based on subjective considerations on the part of the dentist. The dentist will make his selections with strong influence from such factors as ease of handling, time required for hardening, color results, and surface characteristics of the restoration. To obtain the best results each dentist will carefully blend scientific information with artistic ability, and this is the only way operative dentistry can bring satisfaction to patient treatment. Also, the reader will need to remain alert to the rapid transition taking place in this area and adjust his technology as progress occurs, as it most surely shall.

11

THE AMALGAM RESTORATION: TOOTH PREPARATION

Although amalgam has been used in the restoration of carious lesions since the 15th century or even earlier, it remains the one material most commonly employed. The most favorable qualities of dental amalgam are its relative durability and its ease of placement. Reasonably compatible with oral fluids, it is a relatively inexpensive restoration that can be placed in a single appointment. Without question, it can be said that at present amalgam may be the most important restorative material used by the dentist.

By definition, amalgam is an alloy of two or more metals, one of which is mercury. As will be seen, dental amalgam alloys are composed of three or more metals. The amalgam itself is prepared by combining the alloy with mercury through a process called amalgamation or trituration. The plastic mass is then packed or condensed into the prepared cavity where it hardens by crystalization.

It has been said that an amalgam restoration is "often much better than it looks." Obvious deficiencies are frequently noted on restorations that have been in service for a period of time, particularly deterioration of the margins, a so-called "ditching" of the material at the interface with the tooth. One would imagine that caries would almost routinely be present at such exposed margins owing to penetration of fluids, debris, and micro-organisms. However, this is usually not the case, even though the restoration may lose esthetics and be subjected to continued degradation. The explanation for this anomaly lies in a uniqueness of amalgam. As the restoration ages, corrosion products form along the restoration–tooth interface. These compounds then act as a mechanical block to the penetration of deleterious agents. This self-sealing mechanism thus accounts for the unusual durability of amalgam restorative material.

Nonetheless, daily observations in the dental office do reveal many amalgam failures. In addition to the marginal deterioration previously noted, failures may occur in the form of (1) secondary caries, (2) fracture, (3) dimensional change, and (4) excessive discoloration.

The American Dental Association specification for dental amalgam alloy has steadily decreased the number of inferior commercial products. Although certain types of alloys (e.g., the high copper system, to be discussed later) are superior, a high percentage of these failures are due to improper design of the preparation and/or faulty manipulation of the material or its contamination at the time of insertion. Each step in the procedure, from the time the alloy is selected until the restoration is polished, has a definite effect on the properties of the amalgam and, thereby, on the success or failure of the restoration.

The factors that govern the quality of the restoration can be divided into two groups: those controlled by the manufacturer, such as composition and manufacturing process, and those controlled by the dentist and his auxiliary. Matters such as trituration method and time, condensation technique, anatomical characteristics, and finishing procedures are governed by personnel within the dental office. Obtaining clinical success from amalgam is dependent upon meticulous attention to detail during manufacture of the material as well as during tooth preparation and insertion and finishing of the restoration.

Mercury Toxicity

The amalgam restoration is possible only because of the unique characteristics of mercury. It is this metal that provides the plastic mass that can be inserted and finished in the teeth and that then hardens to a structure that resists the rigors of the oral environment surprisingly well. However, it is also the element that so markedly influences the basic properties necessary to clinical success.

From the earliest use of amalgam, it has been asked whether mercury can produce local or systemic effects in the human. It is still conjectured that mercury toxicity from dental restorations is the cause for certain undiagnosed illnesses. It has been further suggested that a real hazard may exist for the dentist or dental assistant when mercury vapor is inhaled during mixing, thus producing an accumulative toxic effect.

Undoubtedly, mercury penetrates from the restoration into tooth structure. An analysis of dentin underlying amalgam restorations reveals the presence of mercury, which in part may account for a subsequent discoloration of the tooth.

However, the possibility of toxic reactions to the patient from these traces of mercury penetrating the tooth or sensitization from mercury salts dissolving from the surface of the amalgam is most remote. The danger has been evaluated in numerous studies. The patient's encounter with mercury vapor during insertion of the restoration is too brief and the total amount of mercury vapor too small to be injurious. Furthermore, any mercury leached from the amalgam is apparently not converted to the lethal form of methyl or ethyl mercury and is excreted rapidly by the body.

What about dental office personnel? Dentists and their auxiliaries are exposed daily to the risk of mercury intoxication. Although metallic mercury can be absorbed through the skin or by ingestion, the primary risk to dental personnel is from inhalation.

The maximum level of exposure considered safe for occupational exposure is 50 micrograms of mercury per cubic meter of air. This is actually an average value to be calculated by averaging instantaneous exposures over a standard work day. Mercury is volatile at room temperature and has a vapor pressure almost 400 times the maximum level considered acceptable. Mercury vapor has no color, odor, or taste and cannot be readily detected by simple means at levels near the maximum safe exposure. Since liquid mercury is almost 14 times more dense than water, in terms of volume a small spill can be significant. An eyedropper size drop of mercury contains enough mercury to saturate the air in a typical size operatory.

The American Dental Association has estimated that one dental office in

10 exceeds the maximum safe exposure level for mercury. However, only a few cases of serious mercury intoxication due to dental exposure have been reported, and the potential hazard can be greatly reduced, if not eliminated, by attention to a few precautionary measures.

Obviously the operatory should be well ventilated. All excess mercury, including waste and amalgam removed during condensation, should be collected and stored in well-sealed containers. If spilled, it must be cleaned up as soon as possible. It is extremely difficult to remove mercury from carpeting. Ordinary vacuum cleaners merely disperse the mercury further through the exhaust. Mercury suppressant powders are helpful but should be considered temporary measures. If mercury comes in contact with the skin, the skin should be washed with soap and water.

As noted earlier, the capsule used with a mechanical amalgamator should have a tightly fitting cap to avoid mercury leakage. When grinding amalgam, a water spray and suction should be used; eye protection and a disposable mask are recommended.

The use of an ultrasonic condenser with amalgam is not recommended. A spray of small mercury droplets has been observed surrounding the condenser point during condensation.

An important part of a hygiene program for handling toxic materials is periodic monitoring of actual exposure levels. Current recommendations suggest that this procedure can be conducted at least on an annual basis. Several techniques are available. Instruments can be brought in to actually sample the air in the operatory and yield a time-weighted average for mercury exposure. Film badges are also available that can be worn by office personnel in a manner similar to radiation exposure badges. Also, biological determinations can be performed on office staff to measure mercury levels in blood or urine.

The risk from mercury exposure to dental personnel cannot be ignored. However, close adherence to simple hygiene procedures will help insure a safe working environment.

One additional precaution related to handling mercury and mercury-containing materials should be noted. Mercury will rapidly amalgamate with most precious metals, especially gold (see Fig. 12–93). Watches, rings, and other jewelry should be removed before handling mercury or dental amalgam. Otherwise serious damage to the jewelry may result due to contact with mercury.

Principles of Tooth Preparation

Cavity preparations in teeth have been more or less designed to meet the needs of amalgam, with block-shaped cavities, edges with butt joints, and undercuts to lock it into the cavity. Because amalgam as a metal is an excellent thermal conductor, cavity preparations should be made shallow. A restoration that is too shallow, however, has a tendency to fracture because amalgam is a material that is quite brittle. Preparations therefore are made so the amalgam will be in the range of 2 mm thick. When carious dentin penetrates beyond this depth, a liner or cement base may be placed. (See Chapters 7 and 8.)

To compensate for the brittleness of the material, all cavities are more or less morticed into the tooth. Flat walls parallel with or perpendicular to the tooth surface compose the form of these box-like preparations. Anchorage of

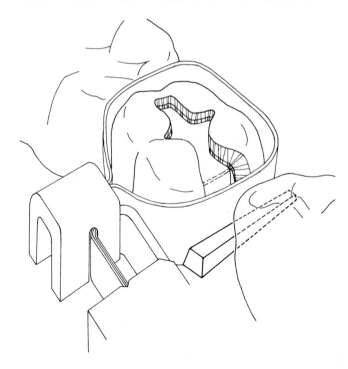

Figure 11–1. Tofflemire matrix band in position.

the material is achieved by parallelism of opposing walls or by slight undercuts in the dentin.

A putty-like, "crunchy" plastic material, the amalgam adapts itself to the internal shape of the cavity. Compound restorations, those involving two or more sides of the tooth, require a form or mold to confine the material so it can be packed into place under pressure. As a wooden form restricts concrete until it sets, the matrix band provides a secure wall against which amalgam can be packed (Fig. 11–1). After filling the cavity with the amalgam, the matrix is removed and the material carved to the original shape of the tooth. At a subsequent appointment it is polished (Fig. 11–2).

Class I Restoration

General Considerations. As was described in Chapter 2, the small Class I restoration is used to replace defective fissures and pits in the enamel. The

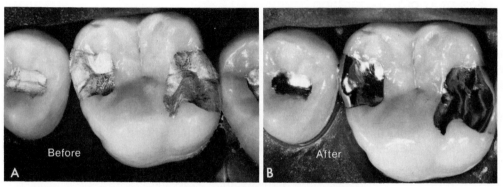

Figure 11–2. Amalgam before polishing and after polishing. (Courtesy of Dr. Loren V. Hickey)

Figure 11–3. Diagrammatic view of enamel removal in molar. *A*, Proper slopes on mesial and distal wall. *B*, Incorrect: mesial and distal marginal ridges have been weakened because of undercuts.

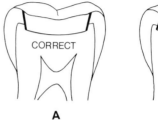

CORRECT

INCORRECT

A   **B**

large Class I amalgam restores occlusal enamel and dentin that has been lost or destroyed in the carious process. Amalgam is most effective, and adjacent enamel is best preserved when certain principles are followed in the design of the cavity.

1. Cavity depth is kept uniform within each tooth: "deeper" in teeth with thick enamel (molars) to "shallow" in teeth with thin enamel (premolars). Depth is usually carried just below the dento-enamel junction (Fig. 11–3).

2. The Class I cavity should be of sufficient width to include the defects but otherwise as narrow as possible, realizing, of course, that it must be wide enough to permit insertion of a small plugger (condenser) for placement of the amalgam into the preparation.

3. Cavity outline is a harmonious blend of definite curves or straight lines. (See Fig. 11–9 for cavity nomenclature.) Where a corner is formed in an outline its degree of angularity matches the circumference of a No. 700 or 55 bur (Fig. 11–4).

4. Mesial and distal margins are parallel with the marginal, transverse, and oblique ridges (Fig. 11–5).

5. Natural ridge contours in sound enamel usually separate pit and fissure cavities. Natural enamel ridges free from defective grooves (oblique ridges on maxillary molars and transverse ridges on lower first premolars) can usually be preserved and should not be included in the preparations (Fig. 11–5).

6. Mesial and distal walls adjacent to marginal ridges should taper outward slightly and should not undermine the enamel (Fig. 11–3).

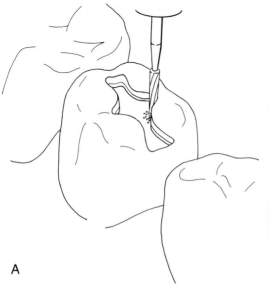

A

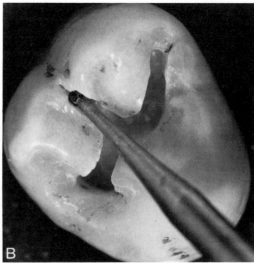

B

Figure 11–4. Diagrammatic extension of burs into grooves. *A*, Fissure bur, e.g., 55, 700; *B*, No. ½ round bur.

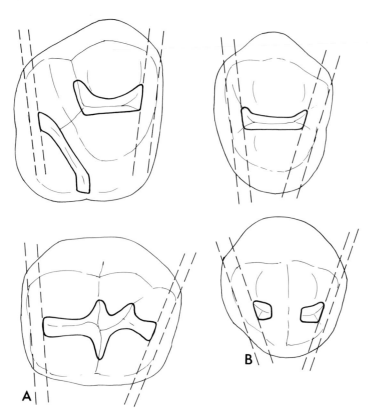

Figure 11–5. Occlusal outlines of two right molars (*A*) and two right premolars (*B*). Marginal ridges provide angulation and boundaries of the proximal borders of the preparations.

7. Ordinarily the pulpal floor is cut at right angles to the long axis of the tooth because most cusps are of comparable height. Where one cusp is shorter than another, e.g., the first premolars, the pulpal floor is sloped to parallel the cusp heights, and the shank of the bur is positioned to bisect the angle formed by adjacent slopes (Fig. 11–6).

8. Cavities on facial and lingual surfaces are prepared so their internal walls will parallel the outer tooth surface (Fig. 11–7). Unique features in the preparation of a Class I in a maxillary premolar and disto-lingual groove in a maxillary molar are shown and explained in Figure 11–8.

Armamentarium and Nomenclature

1. Burs
   FG Nos. 1/2, 330, 245
   RA, Nos. 35, 37, slow speed (steel preferred)

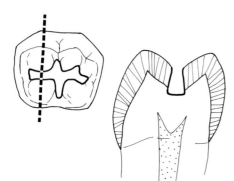

Figure 11–6. The shank of the bur (pear shaped bur) is positioned to bisect the angle formed by adjacent enamel slopes.

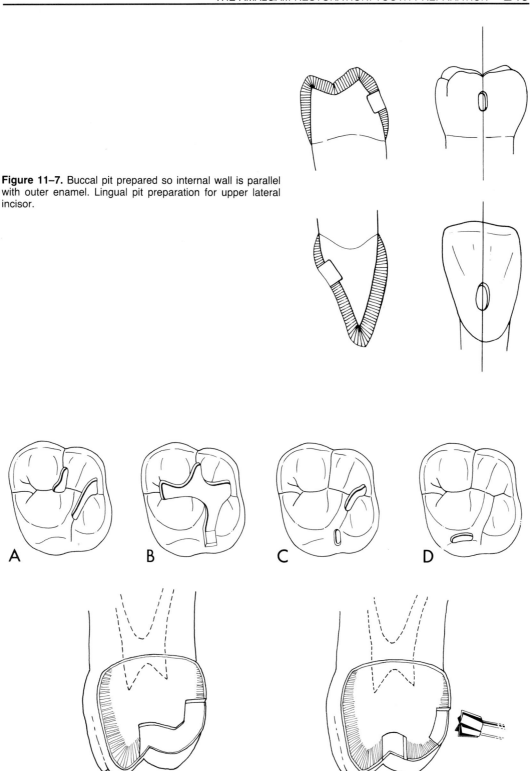

Figure 11–7. Buccal pit prepared so internal wall is parallel with outer enamel. Lingual pit preparation for upper lateral incisor.

Figure 11–8. Maxillary first molar: variations in design of distolingual groove preparations. *A,* Conservative design involving only central and distal pits; *B,* Caries-undermined oblique ridge (probably would need a cement base); *C,* Caries involving only distal and lingual pits; *D,* Preparation for defective groove alongside cusp of Carabelli; *E,* Sectional view through a typical DLG preparation; *F,* Angulation of bur for preparation of lingual groove (No. 35 or 37 bur).

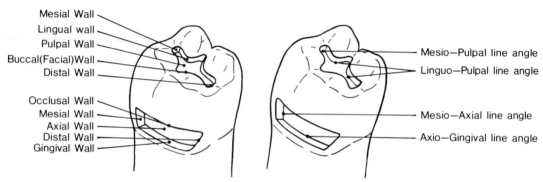

Figure 11–9. Nomenclature of major walls and line angles of Class I and Class V cavities of lower left second molar.

  2. Instruments
     Excavators
     Enamel hatchets (optional)
     Bin-angle chisels (optional)
     Curved Wedelstaedt chisels (optional)
  3. Identifying the parts of a Class I cavity is simple. Figure 11–9 labels the walls and the line angles of the Class I cavity.
  Sequence of Preparation. It is assumed that the dento-enamel junction has been penetrated but that no substantial amount of dentin has been

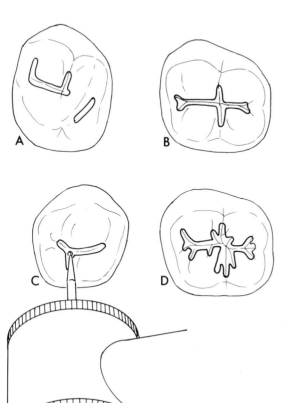

Figure 11–10. Initial pilot groove prepared in four teeth with a No. ½ round bur. Three of the teeth (*A, B, C*) have clearly circumscribed developmental groove patterns; *D,* molar is more diffuse with secondary groove involvement as well.

destroyed by caries. If caries penetration has been deep, attention is directed to optional step 4 below.

1. Enter the pit with a No. 1/2 round bur to a depth of 2 mm (1½ mm for small premolars; 3 mm depth for husky molars).*

2. Maintaining this depth, the cavity is extended out all grooves until evidence of defective fissures disappears. This includes supplemental as well as developmental grooves (Fig. 11–10). Proper depth of penetration is automatic with an experienced clinician; not so with a novice. Until such time as he is able to measure relative cavity depth with the naked eye, a measuring "tool" is indicated. This can be done by scoring the shank of a bur with a diamond disk and/or by painting the shank of the bur with a marking pen 2 or 3 mm from the end (Fig. 11–11). In use this can serve as a depth gauge as this small pilot bur mortices a guide groove for the cavity preparation. As mentioned earlier, this initial guide groove or slot is prepared with one major thought in mind—the elimination of potentially carious enamel fissures.

3. Use of the No. 330 bur is standard for this preparation although many clinicians also utilize other burs as well (Fig. 11–12; see also Fig. 3–11).

---

*Penetration of a lingual pit in a maxillary lateral may be only 1.0 mm.

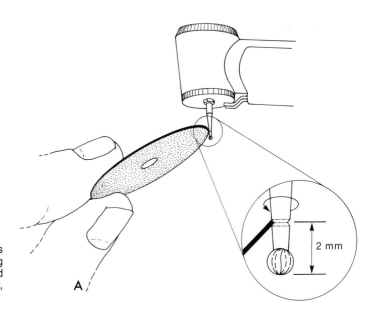

Figure 11–11. Use of a pilot bur as a depth gauge (no. ½ bur). A, Scoring the shank of the bur with a diamond disk at 2 mm or 3 mm length. B, Marking the shank with a felt pen.

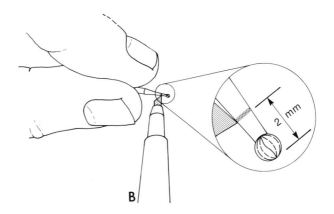

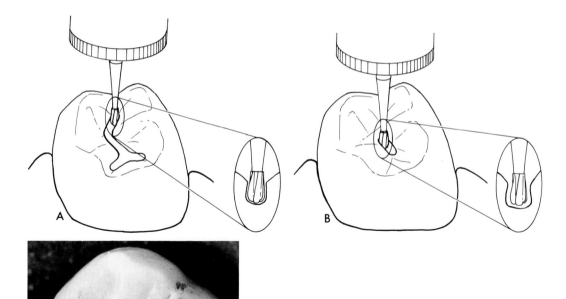

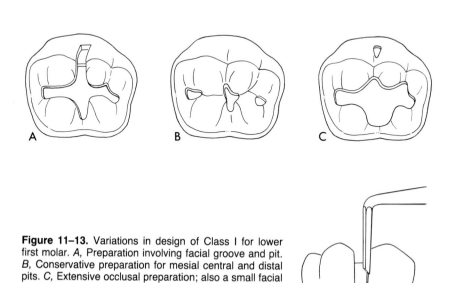

Figure 11–12. Effects from cutting with (A) and without (B) the pilot groove. The bur is less likely to "whip" and a more precise groove is possible if a pilot groove is first prepared with the No. ½ round bur. C, Opening created by the pear shaped bur restricts vertical withdrawal of the bur from the preparation.

Figure 11–13. Variations in design of Class I for lower first molar. A, Preparation involving facial groove and pit. B, Conservative preparation for mesial central and distal pits. C, Extensive occlusal preparation; also a small facial pit. D, Planing the wall with a posterior enamel hoe.

D

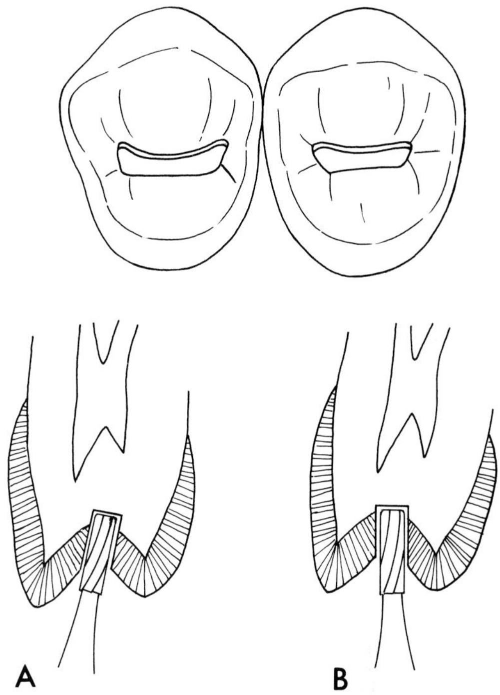

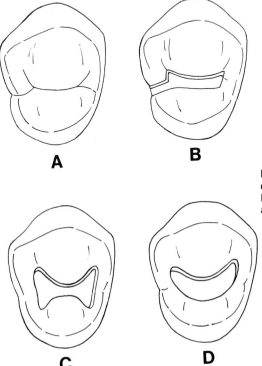

Figure 11–14. Conservative Class I cavity preparation for maxillary premolars (upper). Incorrect (*A*) and correct (*B*) bur angulation for preparation. *A,* A frequent mistake is made by tilting the head of the handpiece outwardly in order to enhance visibility. *B,* Correct angulation.

Figure 11–15. *A,* Maxillary left first premolar with mesial developmental groove crossing the marginal ridge. *B,* Preparation design for *A. C* and *D,* Incorrect "dog bone" and "crescent" designs.

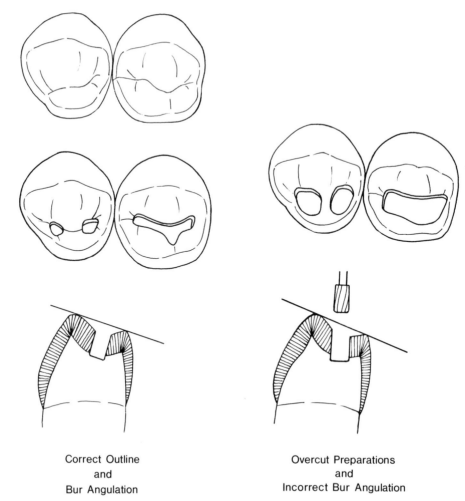

Correct Outline
and
Bur Angulation

Overcut Preparations
and
Incorrect Bur Angulation

Figure 11–16. Mandibular right premolars: *Left,* correct; *right,* common errors.

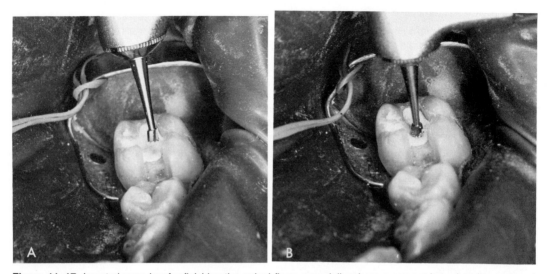

Figure 11–17. Inverted cone bur for finishing the pulpal floor, especially where a cement base has been placed. No. 35 and 37 steel burs are more effective than carbide burs. With light pressure and revolving at slow speeds they function like a floor polisher, eliminating irregularities and producing a smooth surface. *A,* No. 37 steel bur. *B,* Bur in use.

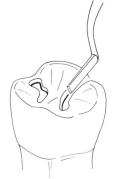

Figure 11–18. Planing the walls and margins of a disto-lingual groove with a bin-angle chisel. The instrument is reversed for planing the distal wall.

Endeavor to restrict the width of an isthmus so this pear-shaped bur cannot be withdrawn occlusally from the depth of the preparation because of the narrowed opening.

Variations in Class I outline and design for maxillary molars were shown in Figure 11–8. Similarly the variations in outline for the lower molars are found in Figure 11–13.

Because of their smaller size the premolars often fall prey to overcutting and overextension from the careless use of a bur. The proper outline for Class I cavities of maxillary premolars is shown in Figures 11–14 and 11–15, mandibular premolars in Figure 11–16. Another common error often made by the operator is to tilt the head of the handpiece toward the facial, presumably to obtain better vision. This makes a groove that is not properly aligned with the occlusal surface (Figs. 11–14 and 11–16).

4. (Optional step) Pulpal floors may now be rendered flat with a No. 35 or 37 slow-speed inverted cone bur. (Axial walls on lingual grooves of upper molars and facial grooves on lower molars may also be treated likewise (see Fig. 11–8F). Care should be taken not to unduly undermine the walls during this stage of the preparation.

5. If caries has extended below the optimal level of floor depth, the removal of carious dentin is postponed until the cavity has been essentially prepared. Carious dentin is then removed with an excavator or round bur (see Fig. 8–1).

6. When a cement base is placed to raise the pulpal floor to its proper height, it may be finished with a No. 35 or 37 bur so it will be smooth and flush with the adjacent dentin (Fig. 11–17).

7. Final finishing of the enamel margins is accomplished with hand instruments (Figs. 11–13 and 11–18) and with high-speed burs (No. 330 and 245) under light pressure.

Class II Restoration

General Considerations

By definition the Class II restoration is one involving a mesial or a distal surface of a posterior tooth. The reason why proximal surface lesions have their own special classification is because they occur on molars and bicuspids, which adjoin one anther, and it is difficult to keep them clean underneath their contact points.

Although the Class II lesion occurs on a proximal surface, it is generally considered a compound cavity, a cavity involving at least two surfaces, one of which is an occlusal surface. So frequently does this happen it is a common practice to allude to a Class II cavity as a mesio-occlusal (MO), a disto-occlusal (DO), or a mesio-occlusal-distal (MOD) (see Chapter 2). If the proximal lesion is so large that a cusp is destroyed, it might be called an "MOD with a mesio-buccal cusp replacement."

Access to the proximal lesion may be direct on rare occasions. The mesial surface of a first permanent molar of a child 12 or 13 years of age is a typical example. The second primary molar has exfoliated, leaving direct access to the mesial surface of the tooth distal to it. Before the premolar erupts into position, the tooth can be prepared and filled in a simple manner (Fig. 11–19).

However, inasmuch as the teeth are usually in contact, access to the cavity is obscured and one must approach it by cutting away tooth substance from the lingual, from the facial, or from the occlusal. The common method, of course, is to gain access from the occlusal; however, on occasion, when the lesion is near the cervical line, a facial or lingual approach is sometimes chosen (Fig. 11–20, see also Fig. 14–58).

Because the vast majority of Class II cavities are compound cavities, let us consider what design criteria might prevail if the entire crown were restored (the four axial surfaces plus the occlusal with all of its cusps). Such an amalgam crown would seldom be made, but if it were, it would contain five principles, which would prevail in all Class II restorations, be they small or large compound restorations.

1. Axial walls, pulpal and gingival floors* meet each other at right angles; in other words, all walls are essentially vertical or horizontal.

---

*Vertical planes in a tooth preparation are known as walls. Horizontal planes are identified as either walls or floors.

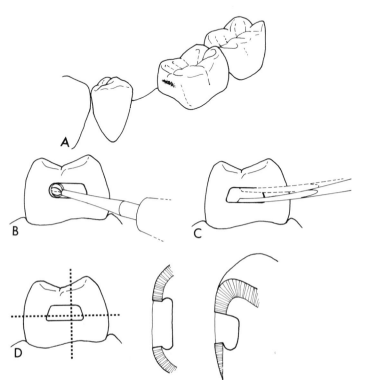

Figure 11–19. Incipient carious lesion on the proximal surface of a molar being restored by direct access. A, Lesion. B, Bur preparation (suggest No. 2, 4, and 6, which are sized for slow-speed, straight hand-piece). C, Marginal finishing (curved chisel). D, Internal design of preparation.

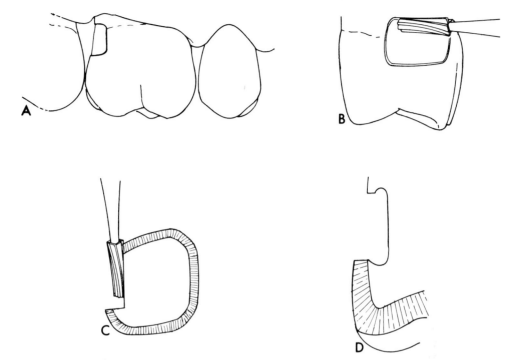

Figure 11–20. Lateral access to a Class II lesion on maxillary molar. Because of its gingival location and the massive amount of dentin and enamel between the lesion and the occlusal surface, access to the lesion from the buccal was chosen. *A*, Facial aspect of cavity outline. *B*, Proximal aspect. Tapered fissure burs and round burs (slow-speed) are used for this preparation. *C* and *D*, Cross-section and vertical section through the preparation.

2. Axial walls do not follow the bell-shaped contour of the crown but are parallel with the long axis of the tooth (Fig. 11–21).

3. Uniform peripheral thickness of tooth substance is removed so that the exterior shell of amalgam will not be too thin in some places and too thick in others. From both axial and occlusal directions, the tooth preparation has been kept somewhat shallow to limit the amount of metal used and to keep it at a reasonable distance from the pulp.

4. The pulpal and gingival floors are flat and parallel to the occlusal plane (right angles to the forces of mastication).

5. Cavosurface margins at the gingival floor are at right angles to the surface of the enamel or cementum.

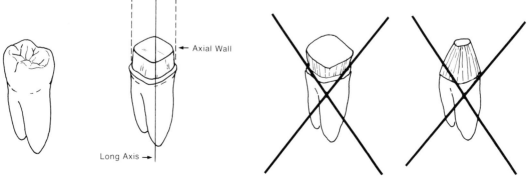

Figure 11–21. Proper preparation for an amalgam crown. Pulp protection, butt joints at the edges, and convenient access for preparing the tooth for condensing the amalgam and for carving and polishing. Note: any wall parallel to the long axis of the tooth is an axial wall.

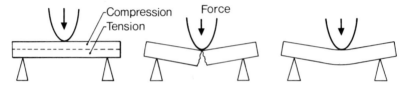

Figure 11–22. Any deflective force on a bar of metal will cause it to fracture if compressive strengths are greater than tensile strengths, e.g., dental amalgam (*center*).

Conversely, a metal with stronger tensile strengths, e.g., casting gold, will bend instead (*right*).

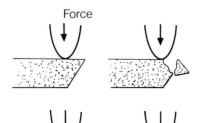

Figure 11–23. A brittle metal, e.g., dental amalgam, will be subject to more damage from trauma where it terminates as an acute rather than a right angle.

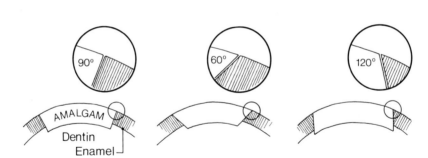

Figure 11–24. Diagrammatic interface of amalgam and enamel at the cavosurface margin. *Left,* Interface 90° angle best suits the enamel/amalgam interface. *Center,* An angular amalgam interface best suits the enamel, but is destructive to the amalgam. *Right,* An angular enamel interface is favorable to the amalgam, but is very destructive to the enamel because of the direction of its grain structure (enamel rods).

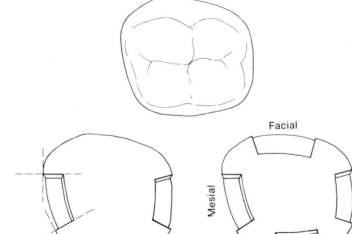

Figure 11–25. Occlusal view of uniform depth of axial walls.

Figure 11–26. Modified designs (diagrammatic) in which (A) no cusps are sacrificed in the tooth preparation; (B) one of the cusps is sacrificed; (C) diagonal cusps are sacrificed.

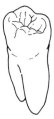
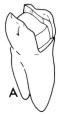
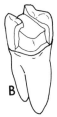
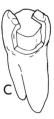

Amalgam is a brittle substance (Figs. 11–22 and 11–23). If only it could be bent or molded into another shape, tooth preparations might be substantially changed. However, amalgam is brittle and brittleness is a property that requires a cavity wall that will be at right angles to the surface of the enamel. When the amalgam is packed against it, the interface between the enamel and the amalgam will terminate as a butt joint. This adverse characteristic of amalgam is often called "edge strength" (Fig. 11–24). If these same lesions were to be prepared to receive a gold casting it would be quite permissible to prepare the tooth with a bevel or an obtuse angle because a gold alloy casting will not fracture and can retain its strength in thin sections.

Strength and marginal integrity are the two major criteria for deciding whether to retain a weakened cusp or whether to sacrifice it. If the latter is chosen—and this will be discussed later in the chapter—the entire cusp is cut away, removing approximately one third the total length of the crown so that a large enough mass of metal will remain to resist fracture during mastication.

Let us view a departure from the hypothetical full crown. Whether one or more boxes are used (Fig. 11–25) or whether cusps are replaced (Fig. 11–26) the same principles hold sway and the basic design remains unchanged. Furthermore, cavity nomenclature remains constant for all cavity types (Fig. 11–27).

Four types of anchorage can be used for retention of the restoration: (1) opposing undercuts in the occlusal or gingival area, (2) axial interlocks (facial and lingual grooves), (3) slots, and (4) dowels or pins.

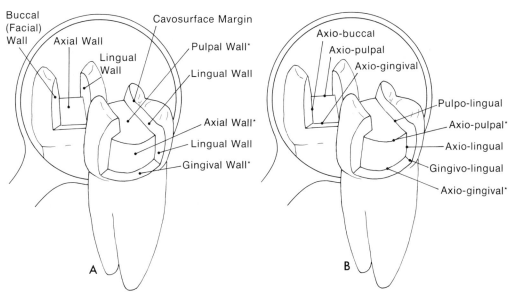

Figure 11–27. Diagrammatic tooth preparation, basic cavity nomenclature. Names with an asterisk are used more frequently. A, Walls and floors. B, Line angles. Pulpal and gingival "walls" may also be called "floors."

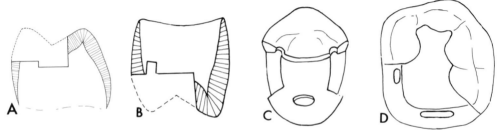

Figure 11–28. Resistance and retention form achieved by offsets and cleats. *A,* Occlusal offset prevents lingual displacement of the amalgam. *B* and *C,* Cleat placed in the bulbous part of the lingual of the crown of a premolar provides good anchorage. *D,* Slots placed in the gingival floor serve as cleats.

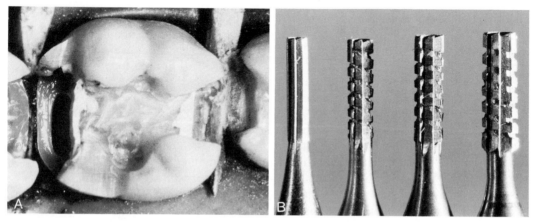

Figure 11–29. *A,* Illustration of a slot for an amalgam cleat. This 1½ mm deep slot must be prepared with precision. (Courtesy of Dr. Robert Birtcil and Masson Monographs in Dentistry). *B,* Fissure burs (left to right): 1. Straight fissure bur No. 55; 2. Straight cross-cut fissure bur No. 556; 3. Straight cross-cut fissure bur No. 557; 4. Straight cross-cut fissure bur No. 558. (The "5" preceding the size designates it as a cross-cut type.) No. 55 and 56 burs are best for preparing these slots.

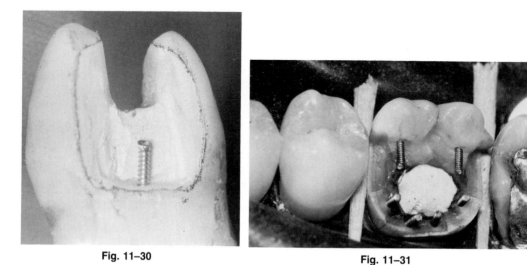

Fig. 11–30

Fig. 11–31

Figure 11–30. A wide (facio-lingual) preparation may receive auxiliary anchorage through a threaded pin placed midway in the gingival floor.

Figure 11–31. Pins used to fasten the amalgam to the tooth. Note the shallow offsets in the gingival floor to prevent lateral displacement. The use of the rubber dam should be routine in all cavity preparations. (Courtesy of Dr. Loren V. Hickey)

A slot is a clean-cut hole into which amalgam is packed. After hardening, it becomes an amalgam cleat with considerable anchorage value (Figs. 11–28 and 11–29). It varies in length from 2 to 4 mm and is approximately 1 mm wide. It is not placed too far toward the pulp, yet not too close to the surface lest the tooth substances peripheral to it fracture away. The opening to the slot must be large enough to receive a small condenser and its depth is 1 to 2 mm. The slot is first placed with a No. ½ round bur because it can make a pilot groove without skidding. This is then followed with a small straight fissure bur (e.g., No. 56) (Fig. 11–29B) to make the slot clean-cut and retentive. Because the need for tactile sense is most important this slotted retentive groove should be placed with the bur operating at slow speed.

On the other hand, pins are anchored to the dentin where they simulate concrete reinforcing steel for attachment of amalgam to the exposed ends (see Chapter 13). Where space permits, e.g., in the bulbous part of the crown, slots are probably preferred; in narrow cervical or root areas pins are recommended instead. Figures 11–30 and 11–31 illustrate application of these retentive modalities.

A fifth method for anchorage is the occlusal offset and the axial offset (Figs. 11–28A and 11–31). Either permits amalgam to be placed closer to the pulp, but an offset, if cleanly cut with sharp corners, can be quite effective at only 0.75 mm depth.

For purposes of understanding, Class II cavities can appropriately be divided into two categories; the incipient Class II amalgam is one that more or less plugs an entry site through which microbial activity can attack the tooth, and the extended Class II amalgam is one that replaces lost or destroyed tooth substance as well. Although a sharp line of distinction may not always exist between the two types, this concept of "plugging" versus "rebuilding" is important to understand as it may alter the execution of the treatment or even the type of the procedure itself.

The Incipient Class II Amalgam

Incipient lesions usually are small in area and, with teeth in normal alignment, lie immediately below the anatomical contact point of the tooth. In malpositioned teeth the *actual* point of contact may lie elsewhere, which in turn alters the location of the lesion. Figure 11–32 illustrates a second premolar that has become rotated and the lesions misplaced from where they would be if the teeth were aligned normally.

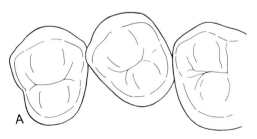

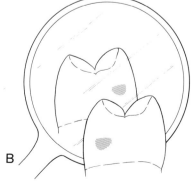

Figure 11–32. Rotated premolar. Potential caries may afflict the shaded areas because the contact points have shifted.

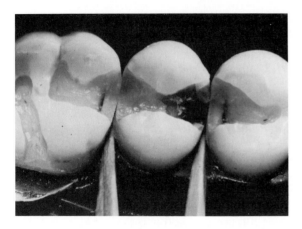

Figure 11–33. Mid-lesion cuts through the proximal surfaces of three teeth. Notice the incipient lesions on the distal of the first premolar and the mesial of the first molar. Soft and discolored dentin lies behind the apparently intact enamel. Such lesions must rely on the x-ray for detection.

Detection of an incipient Class II carious lesion is not readily accomplished. The bite wing x-ray is probably the best method for detection because adjacent teeth inhibit entering the site with an explorer (see Fig. 2–31C).* An additional complicating factor in cavity detection is graphically illustrated in Figure 11–33, mesial of the first molar and distal of the first bicuspid. The bur has exposed both incipient lesions, yet the enamel covering them appears to be intact. Obviously the enamel is not microscopically intact because it has allowed chemical dissolution and invasion of micro-organisms. Because the enamel retains sufficient strength to resist penetration by an explorer, in these two teeth at least, one cannot rely only on the probe (explorer) to ascertain the presence of a lesion. X-ray findings are more dependable for detecting this kind of Class II lesion.

When a lesion has been detected in a bite wing radiograph (Fig. 11–34) surgical intervention is indicated even though the lesion cannot be detected by probing. The tooth should be prepared to receive a Class II restoration. An incipient proximal lesion penetrates only approximately 1 mm into the dentin, and all carious material will automatically be removed in the natural sequence of preparing the cavity.

---

*Sometimes the lesion can be penetrated from the lingual embrasure with a No. 17 back action explorer.

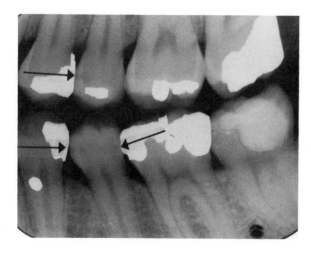

Figure 11–34. X-ray (bite wing) of interproximal carious lesions. Obvious lesions marked by arrows. Also notice the amalgam overhang on the distal of the maxillary bicuspid.

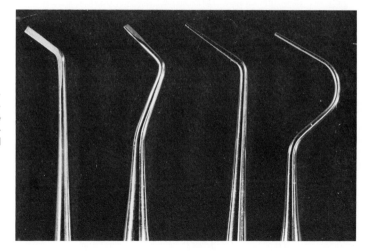

Figure 11–35. Small amalgam condensers (round and rectangular) designed by Dr. Miles Markley. These are essential for condensing amalgam into small restricted areas and around threaded retentive pins.

Outline of the Cavity Preparation

In general the outline should be small and conservative. An attempt is made to restrict the size of the cavity especially at its occlusal orifice. Unnecessary sacrifice of enamel is to be avoided, yet on the other hand keeping the orifice or "throat" of the cavity too small restricts operating access. However, use of small amalgam condensers (Markley design) can effectively condense amalgam into rather small occlusal openings (Fig. 11–35).

The cavity is sort of an inverted slot on the side of the tooth (Fig. 11–36). The gingival wall is parallel with the interseptal gingival border and extends below the lesion into sound enamel, usually 1 to 2 mm below the contact point. The total distance between the marginal ridge and the gingival floor is 3 to 4 mm, depending upon the size of the tooth and the location of the lesion.

The location of the facial and lingual margins is likewise determined by

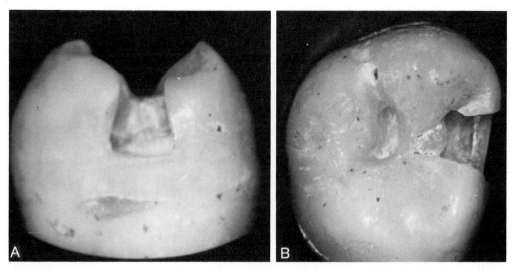

Figure 11–36. Mesial and occlusal views of the preparation of a tooth with an incipient carious lesion. Notice the enamoplasty, which reveals an immune fissure between the central pit and the proximal lesion. (Courtesy of Dr. Miles Markley)

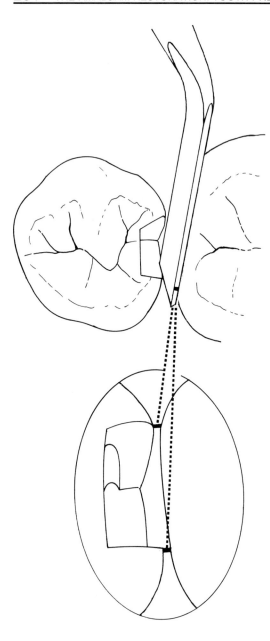

Figure 11–37. Use of a bin-angle chisel or enamel hatchet as a measuring tool to determine proper extension of buccal and lingual margins (space between the corner and the adjacent tooth). Where recurrence of caries is not anticipated, the thickness of the tine of an explorer (0.4 mm) is considered adequate.

Figure 11–38. Pear shaped bur (No. 330) is the classic bur for this preparation. No. 329 is a smaller bur that may be used for small bicuspids.

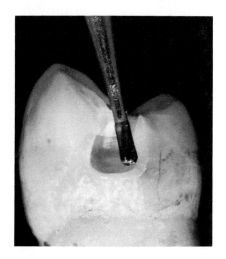

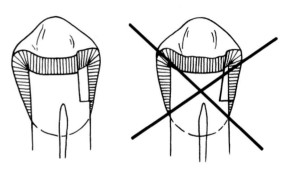

Figure 11–39. Proper direction of vertical or axial wall. *Left,* Parallel with long axis of tooth. *Right,* Parallel with the enamel surface.

the extent and character of the enamel. They should extend beyond the contact point and, of course, beyond the edges of the lesion. If pearly white enamel borders the lesion, these walls are not placed as far apart as they would be if the enamel is somewhat chalky in texture. The location of these walls is determined by the clearance between them and the proximal surface of the adjacent tooth (Fig. 11–37). In a relatively caries-free mouth, this clearance need be only the thickness of an explorer (0.4 mm). In caries-susceptible mouths this clearance may be 0.75 mm, which is approximately the thickness of a chisel or hatchet. The facial and lingual walls join the gingival in a rounded angle, an angle that approximates the contour of the end of a No. 330 bur (Fig. 11–38; see also Fig. 3–11).

Internal Form

Sharp, clean-cut walls form cavosurface margins throughout that are 90°. The cavity preparation is equally deep in all areas. The axial wall of the preparation is flat or convex in horizontal perspective; in vertical perspective it is flat and parallel with the long axis of the tooth (Fig. 11–39).

Facial and lingual walls are undercut to retain the amalgam restoration in place. These undercuts are not deep but they are uniform and extend from the gingival floor to where they fade away at the occlusal surface (Fig. 11–40).

Armamentarium
1. Burs: F.G. No. ½, 330
    R.A. Slow speed No. ½
2. Instruments: Gingival margin trimmers (small size: premolars; large size: molars)
    Enamel hatchets: mandibular teeth
    Bin-angle chisels: maxillary teeth

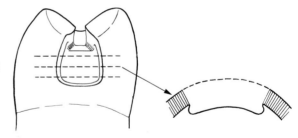

Figure 11–40. Diagrammatic view of preparation of tooth with a Class II incipient lesion.

Sequence of Preparation

The incipient Class II is essentially prepared with burs. Because it is incipient there will be no carious dentin to excavate with a hand instrument because the bur will automatically eliminate it during the course of the tooth preparation.

The first step in the preparation involves opening up the occlusal grooves and pits that need to be restored—the same as would be done for an occlusal Class I amalgam. This is done with a No. ½ round bur and refined with the 330 bur—the same as a Class I amalgam. As mentioned earlier, some pits and grooves will be considered immune to caries; in this case the operator moves directly to step two.

The second step is quite crucial because it requires the operator to decide how wide (facio-lingually) his "incision" will be for gaining access to the proximal lesion. Having made this judgment he then cuts a notch with a No. ½ round bur through the marginal ridge to expose the dento-enamel junction. Care should be exercised lest the adjacent tooth be nicked with the bur. It is also quite important that the operator has reached and identified the dentin (Fig. 11–41).

Step three is also accomplished with the No. ½ round bur. Having established the orifice of the "inverted slot," enter the dentin and cut a narrow groove facio-lingually underneath the proximal layer of enamel. Hold the bur lightly against the inside of the enamel plate, using it more or less as a guide to properly align the bur. The handpiece is held so the bur can be pendulated back and forth to gradually lengthen the groove as it extends downward toward the gingival. This pendulating movement to the facial and then to the lingual creates the inside (axial) wall of the preparation (Fig. 11–42). With careful intermittent inspections visually and with an explorer, one can detect when the carious dentin is gone and when the borders of the slot have been properly located, particularly the linguo-gingival and the facio-gingival corners.

Much of the cutting of the dentin is done without visual observation because the enamel and the handpiece are in the way. Tactile sense while using the bur is mandatory. Inasmuch as high-speed cutting reduces the tactile sense of the operator, slow speed is preferred for this step. Remember, the enamel plate is much harder than dentin and the bur tends to bounce off it

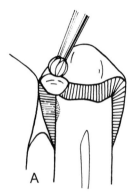
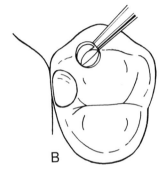
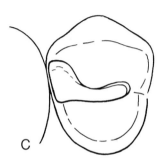

Figure 11–41. Illustration of step #2 in the sequence of preparation. *A* and *B,* Penetration through the marginal ridge until dentin is reached. *C,* Preparation that includes the occlusal fissure. Remember, the class II cavity preparation does not always include an occlusal groove component. "A" and "B" does not include the central groove; "C" includes the central groove.

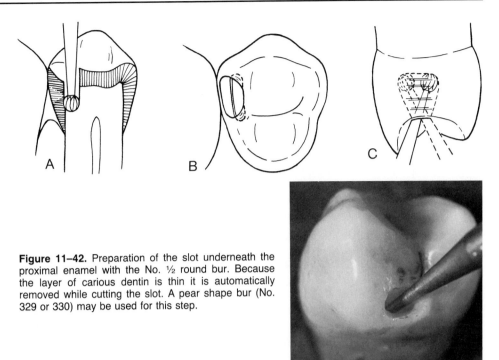

Figure 11–42. Preparation of the slot underneath the proximal enamel with the No. ½ round bur. Because the layer of carious dentin is thin it is automatically removed while cutting the slot. A pear shape bur (No. 329 or 330) may be used for this step.

and cut only dentin if the operator is atune to the feedback through the handpiece and into the fingers. Because of its uniform thickness the enamel can thereby guide a lightly held bur exactly where it is supposed to go.

When step three has been properly executed and completed, the enamel plate will still be intact; the internal part of the cavity preparation is now virtually completed; and all dentin has been removed from underneath the inside of the enamel.

Step number four is also done with a No. ½ round bur. Midway with a vertical groove, the enamel plate is penetrated (Fig. 11–43). Special care should be exercised to avoid defacing the enamel of the adjacent tooth.

In step five, with the enamel plate weakened by the groove the blade of an instrument (hatchet, chisel, or excavator), acting as a pry, can fracture off

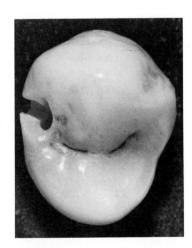

Figure 11–43. Penetration of the remaining enamel wall to permit cleavage of the undermined enamel.

the plate and eliminate it. If the undermining has been done properly the crystalline pattern of the enamel will fracture away neat and clean right up to the border left by the bur.

In step six, planing the margins is done with firm, well-directed forces applied through the correct instrument, which is sharp. (See cutting instrumentation for the extended Class II amalgam.)

In step seven, the No. 330 bur is now used to deepen the axial wall if needed, to redefine the axial grooves, and to accomplish necessary marginal refinements along the occlusal. It is too dangerous to use a rotating instrument along the margins of the box. Here use hand instruments only. Restricted access eliminates burs as an option for this location because they will invariably slip and cut into the adjacent tooth.

The cavity preparation is now complete.

The Extended Class II Amalgam

Attention is now directed to the larger Class II restoration. Extended amalgams are obviously larger because of cavitated areas (see second premolar in Fig. 11–33) or because of recurrent caries around existing restoration.

The size of the extended restoration depends on the needs of a given situation. If, for example, the caries undermines enamel along the gingival border, the gingival floor must be extended rootward to eliminate the unsupported enamel (Fig. 11–44). Also the facial and lingual extent of the caries determines the width of the cavity preparation. These three boundaries of the lesion are adjustable in almost every dimension to fit the needs (Fig. 11–45). These three walls are prepared more or less flat and straight, with their cavosurface angles at 90°. Unlike the incipient cavity preparation the facio-gingival and the linguo-gingival angles are preferably sharp rather than rounded.

The depth of the axial wall, or actually the width of the gingival floor, is not determined by the carious lesion or the old restoration. It is arbitrarily determined by the operator and is usually 1.0 mm wide for bicuspids and 1.5 mm for molars (Fig. 11–46). Factors that influence this width pertain to tooth anatomy, such as the location of the dento-enamel junction and the nearness of the gingival floor to the cervical line. The tooth is more constricted and the enamel becomes thinner as one approaches the cemento-enamel junction, and these anatomic features of the tooth itself are the determining factors of gingival floor width. But one thing that does *not* influence the width of the gingival floor is the depth of the "decay." One does not cut the cavity to bring the gingival floor width into conformity with the depth of the carious dentin.

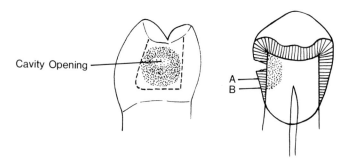

Cavity Opening

Figure 11–44. Diagrammatic views of the extended Class II carious lesion. *A,* Level at which an incipient lesion might have been terminated. *B,* Extended lesion from carious undermining requires the gingival floor to be dropped to this level.

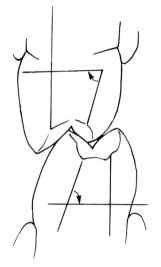

Figure 11–45. Diagrammatic outline of proximal surface. Site of entry or "throat" of the preparation should be as constricted as possible, usually at the expense of the supporting cusp. For esthetic reasons, in maxillary teeth some operators prefer to "curve" the facial wall inward at its gingival end.

If the carious dentin or the old restoration extends pulpward a base is added to bring the preparation back out to its optimal location or an application of calcium hydroxide is made to protect and insulate the pulp. In no instance, however, is the axio-gingival line angle brought inward to meet the depth established by the "decay."

The basic retentive component of the proximal box is the axial groove, one placed to the facial and the other to the lingual (Fig. 11–47). These grooves are deeper at their gingival ends and tend to fade out toward the occlusal. Most axial grooves are placed with a bur, but some prefer to have them angular for added retention of the amalgam. The wider the box, the larger the angle subtended by the facial and lingual walls and consequently the greater the depth of the groove required.

As this angle approaches 90°, an auxiliary retentive feature is required, namely a slot or a pin (see Fig. 11–30).

Reduction of 3.5 mm   Reduction of 2.5 mm

12.0 mm   9.0 mm

8.0 mm   6.0 mm

Figure 11–46. Comparative depths of axial walls. Dimensions are only approximate.

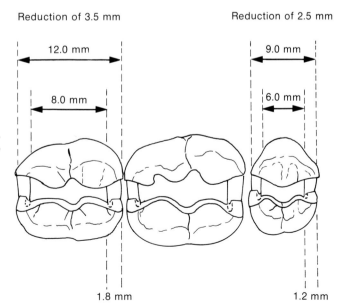

1.8 mm   1.2 mm

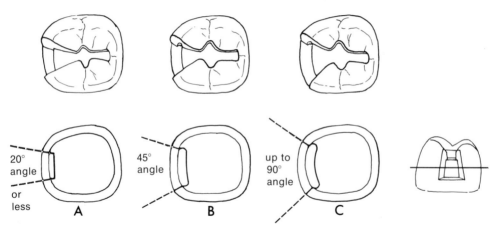

Figure 11–47. Axial groove depth as influenced by bucco-lingual exension. *A*, Small cavity with minimal extension (no axial groove required). *B*, Cavity begins to wrap around the tooth. Proximal retentive grooves indicated to lock the restoration into position to prevent lateral dislodgement. *C*, Large cavity extending around to cover a portion of the buccal and lingual surfaces. Note: Any further extension or increased bucco-lingual angle would justify placement of a pin or a trough (cleat) in the gingival floor (see Chapter 13).

Armamentarium
1. Burs: F.G. Nos. ½, 330, 55, 56 (556), 57 (557)
        R.A. (Slow speed) No. ½
             No. 700 (699) (tapered cross-cut fissure)
             Nos. 35, 37 (inverted cone)
2. Instruments: Gingival margin trimmers
                Bin-angle chisels
                Enamel hatchets
                Curved Wedelstaedt chisels
                Posterior enamel hoe

Sequence (Extended Class II Cavity)
With this particular type of cavity it is important to follow Dr. G. V. Black's steps in cavity preparation (see Chapter 8). It is particularly important that the final outline of the tooth preparation be fixed in the mind of the operator before any cutting is done. Having decided from x-ray study and so on what the final size and shape will be, the old restorations are removed and the occlusal portion of the cavity is prepared.

Rather than cut away the proximal enamel with a high-speed bur and risk cutting into the adjacent tooth, one should follow the same procedure as described for the incipient lesion. Using a bur, preferably the No. 700 tapered fissure bur at slow speed, the dentin directly underneath the proximal enamel is removed, followed by chipping it away and planing the margins. The successful execution of the box preparation is directly dependent upon the accuracy and exactness with which the undermining groove is made (Figs. 11–48 to 11–50).

This step, preparation of the slotted groove underneath the enamel, cannot be overemphasized. Carefully, one must judge whether the corners are sharp and clean cut, whether the slot has been sufficiently extended toward the facial and lingual, whether the gingival floor of the groove is flat and smooth, and also whether all the dentin has been removed from underneath the enamel—especially along the gingival floor. If the slotted groove is crudely

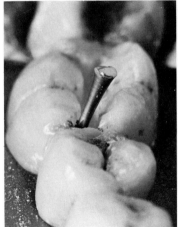
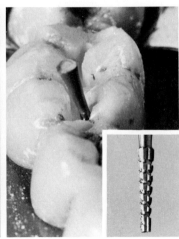

Figure 11–48. Undermining slot prepared with a No. 700 tapered cross-cut fissure bur. Steel burs operating at slow speed are best for this purpose. A pendulating action is most effective. Moreover, the No. 700 bur serves as a good depth gauge (length—4 mm).

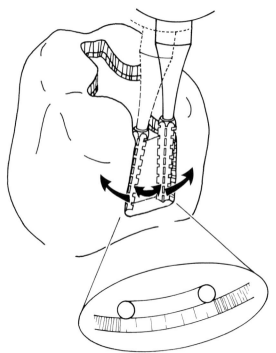

Figure 11–49. Slow-speed No. 700 bur cuts a slot. Special care must be given to prepare a clean-cut slot. The gingival corners, especially, should be sharp and well defined. All dentin must be removed so only the enamel plate remains.

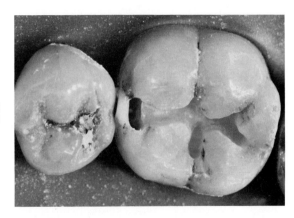

Figure 11–50. Prepared slot. Extension of the slot to the facial, lingual, and gingival is dictated by the size of the lesion.

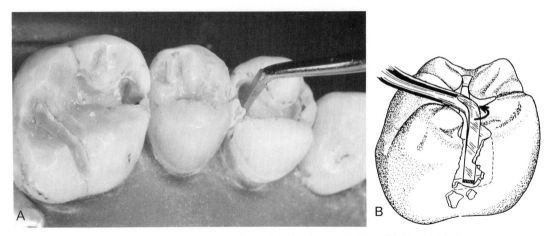

Figure 11–51. Fracturing away the undermined enamel with a chisel or hatchet.

prepared and some dentin remains inside the enamel, it will be most difficult to cleave with the hand instruments. In fact, the slot, if deftly and cleverly done, can actually become part of retentive grooves before the margins are planed.

When the operator has inspected the slot and examined it with an explorer, the enamel is chipped away (Fig. 11–51). If a restoration is being replaced, the procedure described above still prevails. The internal part of the box is cut to form in the dentin *before* the margins are planed with hand instruments.

The classic cutting instrument for a maxillary tooth is the bin-angle chisel. These come in 1.0 mm, 1.5 mm, and 2.0 mm widths and may be used wherever space permits. Ordinarily the largest size is chosen over the smaller sizes because it is more easily controlled. The classic cutting instrument for mandibular teeth is the enamel hatchet, which also comes in widths identified above. Preferred by some, the off-angle hatchet (see Fig. 3–49D) has the plane of its blade twisted at a 45° angle to the handle rather than parallel with it as is the standard enamel hatchet.

Gingival margin trimmers augment the chisel and the enamel hatchet because they have tapered rather than square cutting edges (see Fig. 3–42). The larger size is more easily controlled where space is available. The cutting edge, which is sloped away from the operator, is naturally inclined for planing the distal gingival margin; the slope toward the operator is for the mesial gingival margins.

Prior to usage the cutting edge should be tested, and if not perfectly sharp, should be sharpened (See Figs. 3–55 and 6–24). The primary function of cutting instruments is to plane and smooth margins in proximal box areas. They are also used to define internal retentive line and point angles (Figs. 11–52 to 11–54).

Another method to complete the instrumentation of the gingival floor, other than hand instruments, is to insert a wooden wedge firmly into the gingival space where it serves as a cutting guide to keep the bur in line so it will not slip off the edge or cut into the adjacent tooth (see Fig. 11–31). As an added precaution, one may place a matrix band protector around the adjacent tooth. The above step, in keeping with Dr. Black's rules, is the placement of the resistance-retention form.

Convenience form is usually accomplished automatically during the previous operation; however, access for removal of carious dentin, for matrix

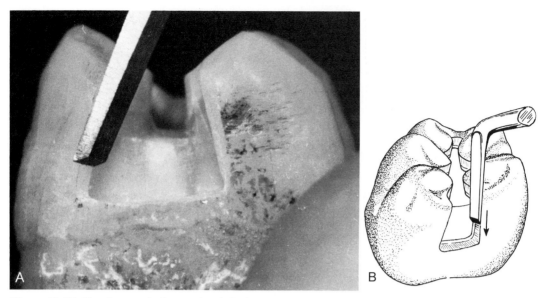

Figure 11–52. Cleaving marginal enamel and planing the walls with *A,* a chisel (maxillary molar) and *B,* a hatchet (mandibular molar). (Courtesy of Dr. Michael Cochran)

application, or for proper amalgam condensation may be restricted. In these instances one must remove offending enamel or dentin rather than jeopardize the placement of a faulty restoration because of inadequate access. The most classic area where access may be inadvertently overlooked is in the bucco-occlusal area called the *reverse curve.* During the preparation, on occasion, too little enamel is removed, which in turn results in insufficient access for the bin-angle chisel to plane the buccal wall to a 90° cavosurface margin (Figs. 11–55 and 11–56). The failure to square out the buccal part of the preparation causes the matrix band to restrict condensation because of an acute angle along the buccal margin. With inadequate space to receive the amalgam and with poor condensation, a faulty restoration with thin, friable edges will result. Such a restoration will be subject to failure at an early date.

Carious dentin is now investigated and removed as described in Chapter 8. Carious dentin removal is G. V. Black step No. 4.

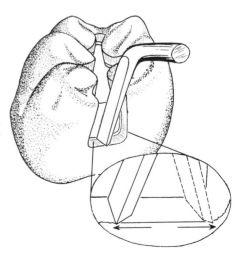

Figure 11–53. Instrumenting the gingival floor to render it smooth and free from irregularities; same instruments as used in Figure 11–52.

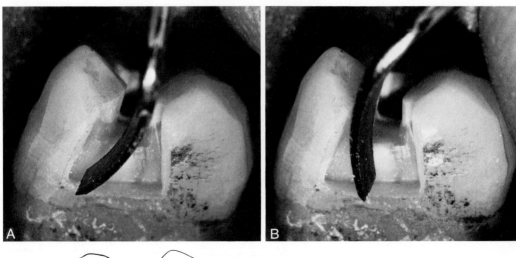

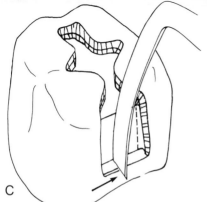

Figure 11–54. Use of a gingival margin trimmer to plane gingival floor and to eliminate loose enamel fragments. A, Cutting toward the facial. B, Cutting toward the lingual.

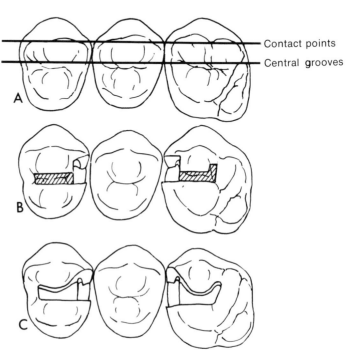

Contact points

Central grooves

Figure 11–55. Consolidation of the proximal Class II with the occlusal Class I. A, Class II lesions develop underneath contact points; Class I, in pits and central groove. B, Class I lesions (and preparations) are off-set to the lingual. C, Combined design into "reverse curve" in the outline. Seldom is it necessary to incorporate a "reverse curve" on the lingual. More often than not the lingual margin is straight or nearly straight.

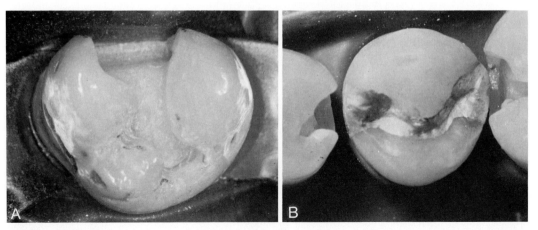

Figure 11–56. Typical reverse curve outlines. *A,* Mesiofacial margin of maxillary molar. *B,* Facial corners of mandibular premolar.

Internal refinement of the cavity is a matter of routine and involves inspection of areas that may have been overlooked such as deepening a cement base that might cause the amalgam (Fig. 11–57) to be high in occlusion or refining an occlusal wall or a line angle (Fig. 11–58). Proximal grooves may be altered at this time if one desires to deepen them (Fig. 11–59) or change a rounded axial groove into an angular one (Fig. 11–60). It is felt that an angular retentive groove enhances the retentive properties of the restoration. This can be accomplished with a sharp gingival margin trimmer. It is also a good suggestion to sharpen the axio-gingival line angle with the reverse end of the gingival margin trimmer (Fig. 11–61). This is G. V. Black step No. 5.

Marginal inspection is appropriately postponed until all else has been completed. Ripples along a facial wall can be re-planed with a re-sharpened instrument. Irregular bumps along the gingival floor can be made smooth with hand instruments and the reverse curve area of the occlusal can be planed with a sharp curved chisel (Fig. 11–62). Examine for debris, elimination of cement fragments adhering to the inner enamel, and dried blood. Three per

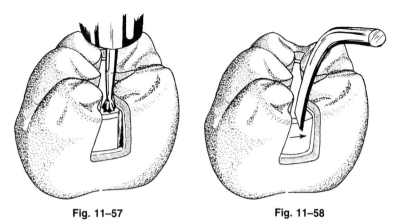

Fig. 11–57   Fig. 11–58

Figure 11–57. Use of a No. 37 inverted cone bur to refine the pulpal floor. (Courtesy of Dr. Michael Cochran)

Figure 11–58. Beveling the pulpo-axial angle with a gingival margin trimmer. (Courtesy of Dr. Michael Cochran)

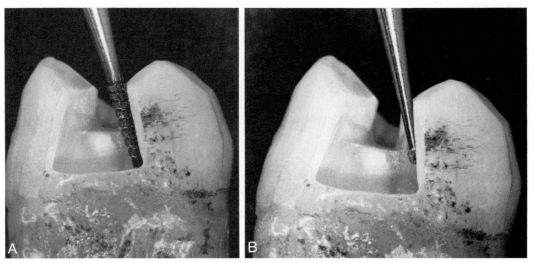

Figure 11–59. Refining retentive grooves with *A,* a No. 700 tapered cross-cut fissure bur and *B,* a No. ½ round bur.

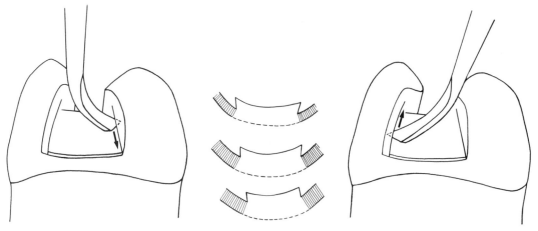

Figure 11–60. Transforming a rounded retentive groove into an angular one with gingival margin trimmers. *Left,* Cutting with a thrusting action. *Center,* Sectional view of three levels through the proximal box. *Right,* Cutting with a pulling or scraping stroke of the instrument.

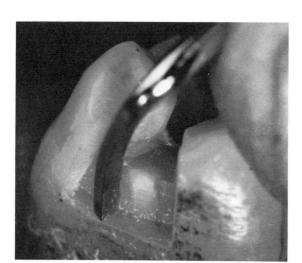

Figure 11–61. Refinement of the axio-gingival line angle with the reverse end of the gingival margin trimmer.

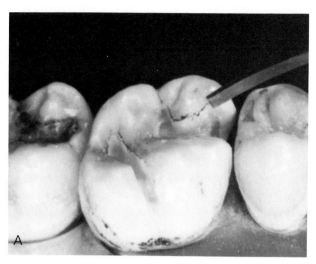 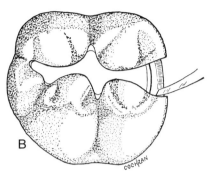

Figure 11–62. Planing the margin is the final step before placement of the matrix band and condensing the amalgam. *A* and *B*, Planning the reverse curve region.

cent hydrogen peroxide solution (see Fig. 8–6) is helpful in removing debris. This final refinement and cleansing is G. V. Black step No. 6.

Variation in Cavity Designs

Sloping Pulpal Floor

For all intents and purposes the posterior teeth are cuboidal in shape, a feature that makes the pulpal floor perpendicular to the long axis of the tooth. Two exceptions to this rule occur frequently enough to deserve attention; they both involve mandibular premolars.

Lower first bicuspids have small and short lingual cusps—much shorter than the facial cusps. On occasion a second bicuspid also develops similarly. A Class II compound cavity for this shape of tooth, e.g., a DO on a mandibular first premolar, should be prepared with a level gingival floor but a sloping pulpal floor (Fig. 11–63).

The mandibular second premolar, particularly a three-cusped premolar with "Y" type occlusal anatomy, develops with a mesial marginal ridge that is significantly higher than the distal marginal ridge. Probably this is to be expected because nature needed a lower distal marginal ridge here to provide space to accommodate a large cusp in centric occlusion. At any rate the pulpal floor should meet the axial wall at an obtuse angle so that the resultant

Figure 11–63. Disto-occlusal cavity of mandibular first premolar. Pulpal floor slopes to coincide with the height of the cusps, but the gingival floor is parallel with the soft tissue contours. Note: The preparation may extend beyond the transverse ridge if necessary, but ordinarily does not cross it.

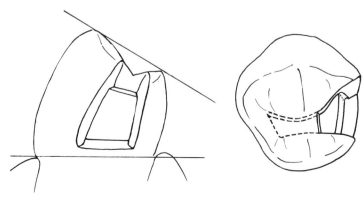

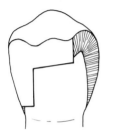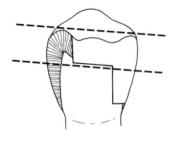

Figure 11–64. Right and left mandibular second premolars. Pulpal floor slopes to coincide with the occlusal morphology of the tooth (lingual aspect).

amalgam will be of equal thickness throughout (Fig. 11–64). If the natural tooth morphology presents a second premolar with a distal slope and the pulpal floor of the cavity is prepared without a similar slope, the operator risks traumatic occlusal forces from the occlusion of the lingual cusp of the upper second bicuspid and possibly a fractured restoration.

Cusp Capping

A classic rule among operative dentists as it pertains to the occlusal margins is "Extend the margins in all directions until full length enamel rods supported by sound dentin is reached" (Fig. 11–65). This is easily understood and interpreted where moderate sized lesions are concerned but may be confusing where large or extensive lesions are involved. If carious activity completely undermines a cusp on a molar, for instance, there is no way the enamel without its dentin support can be propped up and made functional again.

When a cusp is lost or must be sacrificed in the restorative process, it cannot be restored in a thin section. Because of the need to gain strength through bulk, one third the length of the crown must be removed (see Fig. 11–28). Restoring a cusp is quite properly accomplished with a thin gold casting but similar efforts to veneer a cusp with amalgam are destined to failure.

The primary reason for capping a cusp is loss of dentin support through caries. Caries can work its way from an occlusal opening (Fig. 11–66A to C) or it may work its way from the side of the tooth (Fig. 11–66E to G). In any event the treatment is still the same; the cusp must be removed in its entirety.

A common error in cusp replacement is to remove only the major portion affected by the caries and to preserve a small portion of the cusp that is not

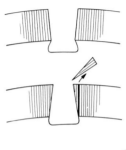
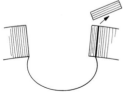

Figure 11–65. Diagrammatic illustrations for causes of enamel rod failure. *Upper,* Acceptable cavosurface margin. *Center,* Enamel rods adjacent to the orifice have been deprived of their inner dentin support. Outer portions can be easily damaged. *Lower,* Undermined enamel from caries is likely to weaken and be lost.

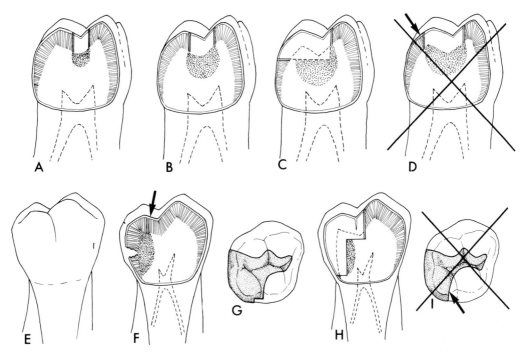

Figure 11–66. Cavity design (outline form) is determined by the size of the occlusal carious lesion. Small to moderate sized lesions can be restored by simply enlarging the access opening *(A and B)*. *C,* Proper location for terminating the margin on the lingual surface. *D,* Margin is terminated on the occlusal surface. This is unacceptable because the enamel will soon fragment. *E,* Lingual view of upper right molar. *F,* Cut-away view of distal caries that involves the tip of the disto-lingual cusp. *G,* Occlusal view of properly designed restoration for this tooth. *H,* Sectional view illustrating proper location of the mesial wall. *I,* Termination of the margin on the disto-lingual cusp. This is unacceptable because the enamel margin will tend to pulverize and fracture.

involved (Fig. 11–66*D* and *I*). Such restorations usually fail along the occlusal margin because the microstructure of enamel with rods perpendicular to the surface precludes terminating a margin on the downhill slope of a cusp (Fig. 11–67). It is quite acceptable to place the vertical wall of a preparation on an upward incline of a cusp because only the terminal ends of the enamel rods are lost in the process. The inward ends rest on dentin and still retain their "nourishment" and support from it. Terminating a wall through the cusp tip

Figure 11–67. Diagrammatic illustration of cusp replacement. *A,* Lesion that extends to the tip of the cusp and beyond. *B,* All carious dentin removed but the enamel rods are incorrectly aligned. *C,* All carious dentin removed plus all defective enamel. This is the proper location of a finish line.

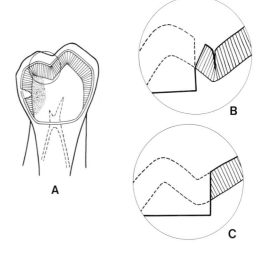

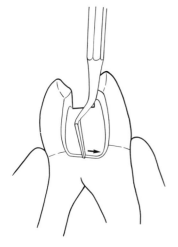

Figure 11–68. A deep carious lesion extending well into the root. A sharp chisel or hatchet is the most effective way to establish and execute a good gingival floor and margin.

or on a downward incline of a cusp results in the loss of the outer ends of the enamel rods. Without dentin support these enamel ends will soon disintegrate and will be lost, leaving a deep marginal defect and inviting new caries.

The following rule should prevail in such instances. If the carious process invades *beyond* the cusp tip the vertical wall and margin should be extended all the way out to the edge of the tooth (Fig. 11–66C) or it should be carried beyond the groove until it can be securely terminated on the upward incline of the cusp next to it (Fig. 11–66G).

Extended Margins

Cervical areas are susceptible to caries where careful cleansing by the patient is not possible, especially in areas gingival to old Class II amalgams. When the margin ends on the cementum, it may necessitate an alteration in cavity design.

Because the gingival floor is so deep it is very difficult to make it straight and flat. It is permissible in these instances to terminate the preparation as a rounded gingival outline as dictated by the lesion (Fig. 11–68). Lack of access in these places precludes the use of hand cutting instruments rather than burs.

Frequently in mouths where caries is quite active, proximal lesions are not restricted to areas underneath the contact point but extend to facial or lingual embrasures are well. Particularly does this tend to occur on lower molars. Naturally the margin cannot be terminated wthin decalcified enamel, yet on the other hand it is counterproductive to move the entire facial wall outward to include a small fingerlike extension of caries (Fig. 11–69). It is permissible to curve and indent the facial wall to include this portion,

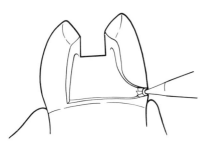

Figure 11–69. A Class II cavity afflicted with a facial extension. Marginal integrity, both in preparation and in condensation, is very difficult to achieve (also see Fig. 11–76).

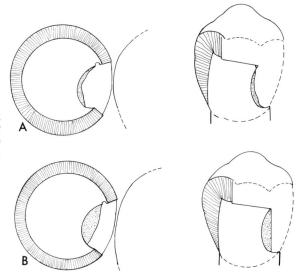

Figure 11–70. Two modalities of treatment for a deeper lesion. *A,* Calcium hydroxide liner to cover the deeper part of the cavity. *B,* Cement base placed to restore the axial wall to its optimum form.

remembering of course that this indentation must be readily accessible for condensation with amalgam after the matrix band has been placed. Moreover, inclusion of the defect must be cleanly cut to blend with adjacent enamel, and above all the cavosurface margin cannot be flared but must remain at a 90° angle.

Pulp Protection for the Moderately Deep Lesion. Frequently the pattern of caries involvement and its removal reveals some free standing enamel but no encroachment upon the pulp. After carious dentin has been removed and the peripheral walls have been planed smooth one of two methods is usually chosen to protect the pulp prior to placing the amalgam (Fig. 11–70).

The easiest method is the placement of an insulative and therapeutic liner, usually calcium hydroxide (see Chapters 7 and 8).

The second method is to restore the lost axial and pulpal walls to optimum form with cement: zinc phosphate, polycarboxylate, or reinforced zinc oxide–eugenol. A liner is indicated only with zinc phosphate cement.

Many operative dentists prefer to use only calcium hydroxide liner (Dycal) without building the axial wall back with cement (Fig. 11–70A). Others prefer to restore the cavity back to its ideal form before placing the amalgam (Fig. 11–70B). Arguments can be made for either method of treatment. A strong point in favor of the former is the additional strength provided by the additional bulk of amalgam. A point in favor of the latter is the added insurance and protection a thick insulative material provides the pulp.

Selection of one of the preceding methods involves some empiricism. Because practical treatment does not coincide with theoretical idealism, one clinician may suggest one method to treat a clinical situation while his colleague may choose another. Tolerance toward empiricism can justifiably be granted when one is faced day after day with the incongruities of clinical practice.

One glaring example of incongruity is the treatment of the shallow lesion in the gingival part of the crown of a lower molar. It is understood that if a barrier of dentin 2 mm or more remains, there is adequate thermal protection for the pulp. Clinicians are aware that post-operative sensitivity from thermal shock is probably most severe from an amalgam placed in a shallow lesion in the radicular half of the crown. When a lesion is deeper and a base is placed, post-operative sensitivity is markedly less. To make his patient more comfortable post-operatively, can one operator be criticized because he overcuts the depth of an otherwise shallow cavity so he will have room to place a calcium hydroxide liner in contrast to his colleague who attempts to reduce post-operative thermal shock by placing copal varnish in an ultra-shallow preparation?

The Class V Amalgam Preparation

General Considerations. This restoration, limited to the facial surfaces of bicuspids and molars (sometimes including the lingual surface of molars) is intended to replace carious and potentially carious tooth substance near the gingiva.

In general, the Class V cavity outline encompasses only the defective enamel and dentin. A common error is to restrict the length of the cavity and terminate the mesial and distal ends amid decalcified enamel. Several years following restoration this enamel breaks down, and recurrent caries develops at these locations (Fig. 11–71). While the Class V restoration is a single surface restoration, it may be a source of clinical frustration. Many are difficult to prepare, place, and finish. When observing existing Class V amalgam restorations, many are poorly finished and have irregular margins, which are a cause of irritation to the gingiva. In conformity to the convex outer surface, the axial wall is likewise prepared so the tooth will receive a convex plug of amalgam of equal thickness (Fig. 11–72). Ordinarily, the margins extend into the gingival sulcus, terminating occlusally at the height of contour of the facial surface.

The clinician's major task in tooth preparation is to maintain uniform cavity depth over the long expanse of a molar surface and to develop a butt joint throughout. Retention is expressed as undercuts occlusalward and gingivalward, and may be round or angular, depending upon the kind of bur that is used (Fig. 11–72). Because its flat end is not inclined to penetrate the axial wall and because its reverse tapered blades keep the bur centered in the cavity, a No. 37 (35) inverted cone bur is preferred by many clinicians over a straight fissure bur, especially when using slow speed.

Planing the margins of the cavity with a bin-angle or curved chisel eliminates cavosurface irregularities (Fig. 11–73). Cavitation from the carious process is handled with an excavator and by alteration in outline to eliminate unsupported enamel (Fig. 11–74).

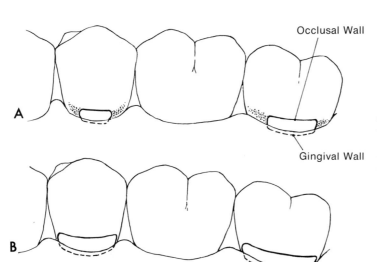

Figure 11–71. Tooth preparations for gingival lesions. *A,* Underextended. Decalcified enamel at the ends of the cavities could break down and caries recur at a future date. *B,* Cavities extended to include the decalcified enamel.

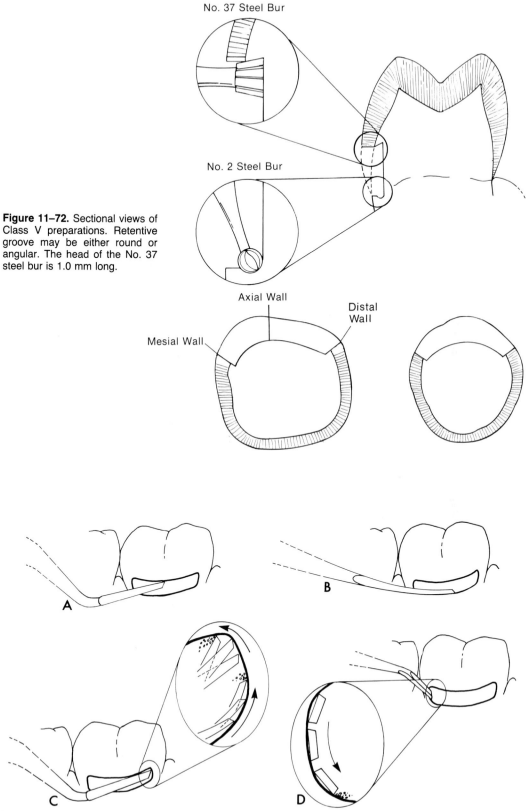

No. 37 Steel Bur

No. 2 Steel Bur

Figure 11–72. Sectional views of Class V preparations. Retentive groove may be either round or angular. The head of the No. 37 steel bur is 1.0 mm long.

Axial Wall

Distal Wall

Mesial Wall

Figure 11–73. Use of hand instruments to plane the margins *(A, B, C)*. The curved and bin-angle chisels are effective in eliminating marginal irregularities. The mon-angle hoe (10–4–8 and 10–4–14) is shown in two views. The mesial margin is best planed (or scraped) with the side of the blade as its corners rub back and forth against the mesial wall.

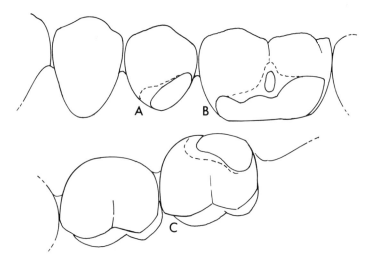

Figure 11–74. Variations in Class V cavity designs. Solid lines indicate the lesion, dotted lines the probable outline of the finished preparation. *A,* Lower premolar. *B,* Union of a gingival lesion with a buccal pit into one single cavity. *C,* Disto-buccal corner of maxillary second molar frequently found in the mouths of teenagers. This is caused by poor diet and poor plaque control.

Armamentarium

1. Burs
   FG Nos. 245, 330
   Slow-speed CA Nos. 37, 35, 56, 57; HP No. 2, 4, 6
2. Hand Instruments
   Bin-angle chisel
   Curved chisel
   Excavator
   Mon-angle hoe 10-4-8 (10-4-14)

Because of many non-specific conditions, this smooth surface cavity preparation lacks a definitive armamentarium, which may vary considerably from one operator to another.

Sequence of Preparation. If visibility is good and if finger bracing is ideal, high-speed instead of slow-speed cutting can be used. If not, however, tactile sense mandates the use of slow-speed burs. The rubber dam should be applied and the area isolated as well as possible. (See Chapter 9.) Uniform cavity

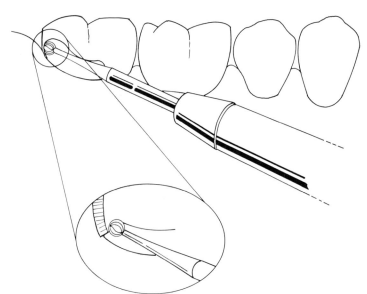

Figure 11–75. Access for disto-buccal corner of lower molar with straight handpiece and large round bur.

Figure 11–76. Restoration of a gingival carious lesion extending across the buccal surface of a molar. *A,* Restoration of proximal surface in amalgam adjoining decalcified gingival enamel. *B,* Buccal aspect of partially prepared Class V cavity. When fully prepared both ends will terminate in previously placed amalgam.

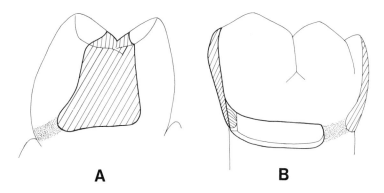

A   **B**

depth is not easily controlled as the operator moves the bur and handpiece over the convex buccal surface. For this reason, it is desirable to use a large inverted cone bur (No. 37CA slow speed) for bulk cutting. Its shape prevents it from slipping out of the cavity, while the length of its blades serves as a depth gauge to the operator. Because of additional retentive demands for the Class V cavity, the internal line angles may be sharp and angular instead of rounded.

After the cavity form is prepared, the bin-angle chisel and/or the curved chisel is used to plane the irregular and jagged enamel surfaces to render them straight or in definite curves. One should bear in mind that the occlusal margin should meet the surface at right angles, thereby paralleling the direction of the enamel rods. Gingival and occlusal undercuts need not be excessive but should be definite, with sharp internal line angles where possible.

The ramus of the mandible obstructs access in disto-buccal areas of second molars, thereby obstructing the space required for the head of the handpiece. Often the distal ends of these Class V cavities (second molars) can only be reached by direct vision with a round bur in a straight handpiece (Fig. 11–75). Although the operator may compromise the internal form of the preparation in the "difficult to reach" disto-buccal areas, he should always prepare 90° cavosurface margins and adequate retentive features.

In some instances the defective enamel extends beyond the corners of the tooth into the proximal of a previously placed amalgam restoration. In such cases it is perfectly proper to extend the cavity into the adjacent restoration, terminating the cavity as though it were ending in enamel (Fig. 11–76).

Figure 11–77. Gingival restorations that are breaking down near the margins. Note recurrence of caries toward the distal surface of the canine. (Courtesy of Dr. Daniel Frederickson)

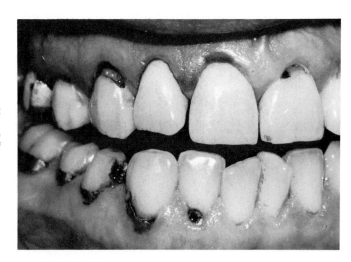

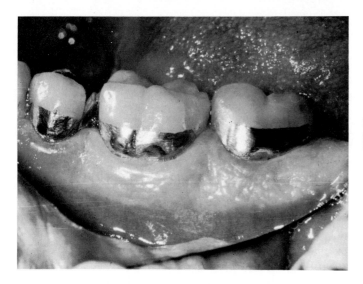

Figure 11–78. Restorations placed and completed. (Courtesy of Dr. Daniel Frederickson)

Special care should be taken to maintain dryness during amalgam condensation. Lest tissue fluids leak into the cavity where they wet the dentin and contaminate the amalgam, a rubber dam and an appropriate clamp should be used wherever possible (also see Chapter 16, for tissue management). With special consideration, lesions as shown in Figure 11–77 can be restored as shown in Figure 11–78.

Miscellaneous Considerations

Frequently a tooth develops a lesion on the opposite proximal side from which it was previously restored. It is customary to remove it and place a combined mesio-occlusal-distal restoration (MOD). If, instead, the restoration is sound, a typical proximal restoration encompassing the new lesion can be placed in a typical fashion, with one exception. The occlusal portion penetrates to only half its usual depth where it interlocks into the existing amalgam (Fig. 11–79).

Frequently, old amalgams must be removed. Unless anchored by pins, they can usually be sectioned and split away from the tooth structure with an enamel hatchet or bin-angle chisel. Sectioning is done with a round-ended bur of approximately No. 4 size. Penetrating through the occlusal amalgam

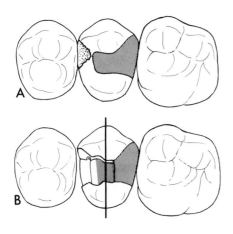

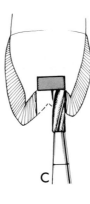

Figure 11–79. Repair of the opposite side of a tooth that has already been restored with amalgam. *A,* Before. *B,* After preparation with secondary occlusal locks and pulpal floor that does not disturb the inner half of the existing restoration. *C,* Sectional view of the prepared occlusal.

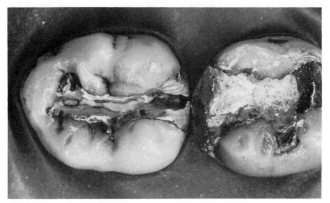

Figure 11–80. Method for removing old amalgam. A No. 4 *round* bur is used to section the restoration into buccal and lingual halves. It is necessary, especially at the gingival, that the restoration be completely separated into two parts. The existence of a white cement base improves visibility while the amalgam is being separated.

until underlying dentin, or cement, is seen, the bur is moved in a mesial and distal direction until the proximal boxes are reached. Penetrating gingivalward into the box with an increased orifice to the slot, careful inspection is made to ensure *complete* severance of the amalgam into two separate facial and lingual halves. The amalgam sections then can usually be deflected inward, leaving a cavity devoid of amalgam fragments (Figs. 11–80 and 11–81).

If occlusal portions resist dislodgment, additional sectioning to the ends of the buccal and lingual grooves usually releases any remaining frictional lock and permits easy removal of the fragments.

Prophylactically, the wise operator views the structural components of the tooth after it has been prepared to see if it is sufficiently strong to resist fracture. If structural integrity is questionable, prophylactic cusp capping is indicated. This is particularly true in the maxillary bicuspid, for after excavating deep proximal lesions the dentin that connects the facial and lingual cusps may be lost or badly weakened. Replacement as a simple MOD is an invitation to fracture, particularly of the lingual cusp. In instances such as this, the lingual cusp should be cut away and replaced in amalgam along with the MOD.

The maxillary canine is a unique tooth fitted into a unique location in the mouth, contacting the lateral on its mesial and the first premolar on its distal. Whereas a mesial lesion is treated as an "anterior" restoration, a distal is treated as a "posterior" cavity and is filled with amalgam.

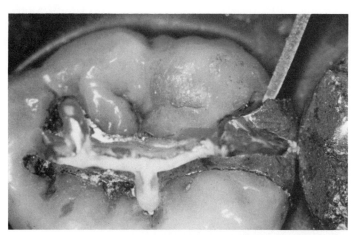

Figure 11–81. Hand instrument separating the amalgam from the tooth.

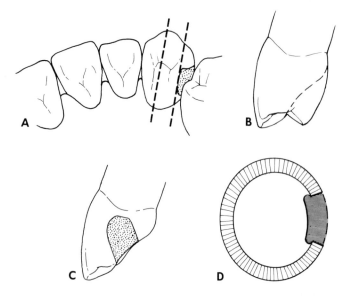

Figure 11–82. Preparation for an amalgan on the distal surface of a maxillary canine. *A,* Lingual aspect. *B,* Distal view of maxillary premolar; with dotted lines it becomes a canine. *C,* Distal aspect of preparation. *D,* Sectional view of facial and lingual retentive grooves.

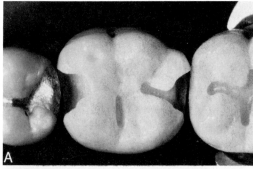

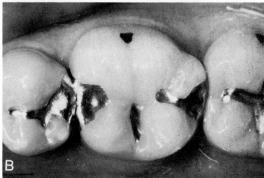

Figure 11–83. Conservative amalgam preparation and restoration, which did not weaken the supportive tooth structure any more than necessary. (Courtesy of Dr. Michael Hanst)

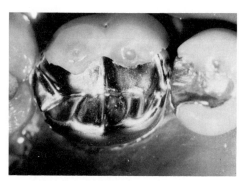

Figure 11–84. Large amalgam restoration restoring proximal surfaces and lingual cusps. (Courtesy of Dr. Loren V. Hickey)

The distal of the canine is best not restored with composite because of the occlusal forces that are brought to bear upon it from the mandibular first premolar. Because its cingulum tends to simulate a lingual cusp of a premolar, a modified slot is suitable as a preparation. It is instrumented in the same way as a typical Class II preparation (Fig. 11–82).

Larger lesions require additional anchorage in the form of a dovetail, which involves the lingual surface. In these instances the pulpal floor parallels the lingual surface of the enamel.

Amalgam, although a brittle material, can adequately serve the needs of many teeth. However, common sense and judgment in cavity design are vital factors controlling its use. The wise operator who views each preparation with a discerning eye can render the patient an excellent service (Figs 11–83 and 11–84).

12

THE AMALGAM RESTORATION: INSERTION AND FINISH

Although the restoration of a tooth is a relatively simple matter, the procedure requires care and an appreciation of certain fundamental principles. The clinical success possible with amalgam restorative material is dependent upon meticulous attention to detail. Thus, the method of inserting and finishing the restoration will have a marked effect upon the properties of the amalgam and the anatomy of the restoration.

If the prepared tooth represents a circumscribed cavity, e.g., Class I or small Class V, it is readily filled with amalgam and carved to shape. If, on the other hand, a side of the tooth is missing, a false wall must be placed to confine the material as it is packed in under pressure. This false wall, a matrix, is usually a piece of thin metal held securely in place while the material is condensed. It may vary, however, from a tag of metal blocking out the space to a complete collar encircling a root so an entire crown can be built (Figs. 12–1 and 12–2; see also Fig. 11–1).

At least a dozen different kinds of matrix retainers have been developed by inventive dentists, each allegedly with certain advantages over the others. Others have used spot-welded bands customized to fit the tooth and adjusted in height so that the patient can close the teeth with it in position. Three types of retaining devices will be described: (1) the Tofflemire matrix band and retainer (Fig. 12–1); (2) the non-yielding customized retainer (Fig. 12–3); and (3) the Automatrix (Fig. 12–4).

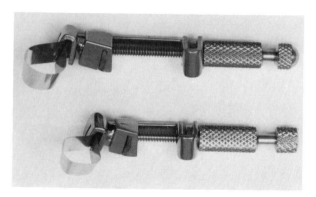

Figure 12–1. Tofflemire matrix retainers. *Top,* Universal. *Bottom,* Junior type, suitable for lingual application and for tipped molars.

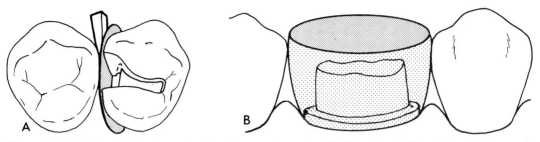

Figure 12–2. Matrices. *A,* Simple metal strip with a wooden wedge. *B,* Circumferential band of copper to encase the entire crown.

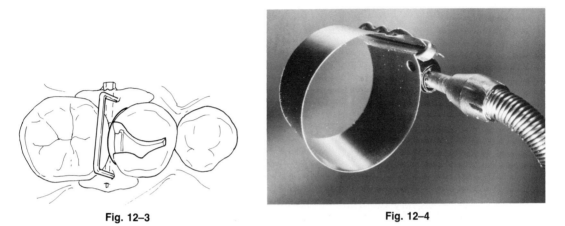

Fig. 12–3   **Fig. 12–4**

Figure 12–3. Rigid nonyielding matrix. Band material is supported by a wooden wedge and acrylic.
Figure 12–4. Automatrix is very useful for cusp restorations. The tightening ratchet is released after it is in position.

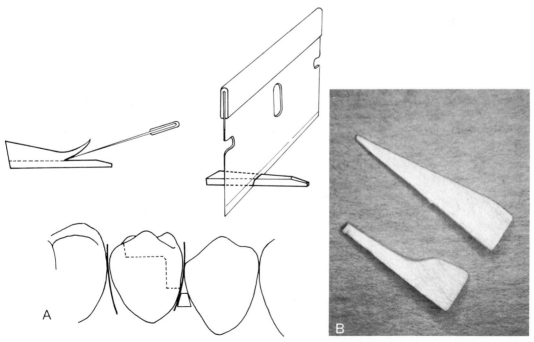

Figure 12–5. Wooden wedge cut with razor blade. Finished wedge in position. Photo: Optional shape wedge trimmed with a handle.

To prevent the band from springing open under pressure and to prevent the extrusion of amalgam out the gingival border, a wedge is placed against the next tooth to hold the band intact. The wedge is a short piece of wood cut from tapered triangular wedge stock or cut to proper form from a toothpick or a tongue blade (Fig. 12–5).

Specifications of a Matrix

To achieve optimal results, the matrix must meet the following requirements:

1. EASE OF APPLICATION. From the standpoints of both usage and instructing auxiliaries, the band and its retainer should be simplistic in design, easily applied, and readily sterilized.

2. NOT BE CUMBERSOME. The retainer or its handle should not interfere with amalgam condensation or patient comfort.

3. REMOVABILITY. Subsequent to condensation, the band should be easily removed without disturbance of the soft amalgam.

4. RIGIDITY. Within limits, the band need be rigid enough to confine the material under pressure, especially for large restorations to prevent the band from bulging outward with excessive unwanted amalgam. Deflection toward the facial and lingual pulls the band away from the proximal contact areas and may leave them deficient.

5. VERSATILITY. Cavities being confined for amalgam condensation present a large variety of problems. Some teeth are bell shaped with narrow necks and wide contact points; others are rotated with adjoining teeth overlapping the cavity; other teeth have gingival contours that restrict matrix placement. Insofar as possible, a matrix, to be effective, should have sufficient versatility to provide the desired proximal contour for condensation.

6. HEIGHT. The retainer and band should be small enough and short enough so that they extend only a short distance beyond the length of the tooth. Hardware projecting above the occlusal plane of the teeth in the operating area can greatly restrict visibility and necessary condensing movements.

7. PROXIMAL CONTOURS. While it is not expected that a band can reproduce a tooth surface, it is more important with proximal surfaces than with facial and lingual surfaces, which are readily accessible to carving. A good matrix will provide sufficient bulk of material for carving a physiologic contact point while preventing excessive amalgam from being pushed beyond the gingival margin.

The Tofflemire type of matrix is the most popular because of its versatility and its ease of usage. Encompassing the tooth at the gingival border more tightly than at the occlusal, tooth form can be readily reproduced for either two or three surface cavities. On the other hand, the Automatrix is more rigid and adaptable than the Tofflemire for cusp restorations.

Tofflemire Matrix Application

Armamentarium
1. College pliers
2. Wooden wedge (see Fig. 12–5)

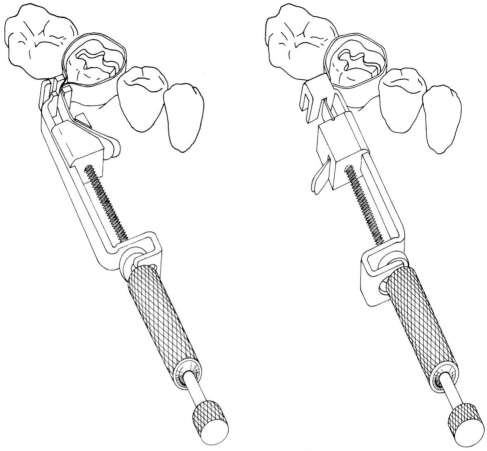

Figure 12–6. Retainer placed upside down.

Figure 12–7. Retainer placed correctly.

3. Razor blade or scalpel
4. Scissors (curved crown shears)
5. Lubricant (Borofax or soap)
6. Matrix retainer (Tofflemire type)*
7. Matrix band (regular and convoluted)

Sequence of Application

1. The regular band† is fitted into the retainer so the handle will preferably be in the buccal vestibule. The slot openings in the retainer always open toward the gingival to permit easy removal of the retainer (Figs. 12–6, 12–7, and 12–14).

2. After the band has been placed into the retainer and fixed with the retaining screw, it is placed loosely over the tooth. Inspection of the gingival border is then made to be sure the band extends below the prepared cavity. If it does not cover the gingival border, it is removed and replaced with a convoluted band and trimmed so the bulge will match the areas of the cavity (Fig. 12–8). A pre-contoured† band designed by Eames rather than a flat band

---

*Tofflemire retainer and bands, available from Teledyne-Getz Corp., Elk Grove Village, Illinois 60007.

†"Dixie-land Bands," available from Teledyne-Getz Corp.

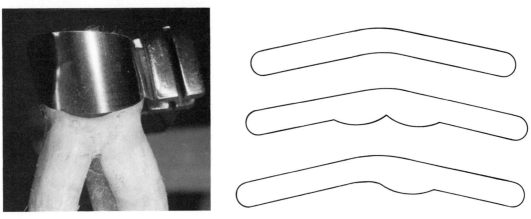

Figure 12–8. Convoluted band covering deep gingival area on extracted tooth.

has been popular among many clinicians to reproduce convex proximal surfaces (Fig. 12–9).

3. The band is then checked for height. If it extends more than 2 to 3 mm beyond the occlusal edge of the cavity, it is trimmed back with crown shears (Fig. 12–10). Trimming of a band in any location is encouraged in order to customize its fit and improve its ease of application.

4. The band is then tightened and prepared for insertion of the wedge.

5. The wedge, 5 to 6 mm long and trimmed for proper taper, thickness, and width (see Fig. 12–5), is inserted from the buccal, the widest side of the opening to the gingival embrasure.

6. Access for insertion of the wedge for a mesial cavity may be obscured by the handle of the retainer. In such a case, it is temporarily loosened about two turns, the handle reflected outward, and wedge inserted (Fig. 12–11). Lubricating the wedge with Borofax* is helpful during insertion so it will slip into place without sticking to the rubber dam. The wedge should engage the band at, or slightly gingival to, the cavity floor. Serving as a snug prop, it prevents excess extrusion of amalgam as it is condensed into the proximal box.

7. Inside the cavity, the gingival border covered by the band is inspected

---

*Borofax, a common therapeutic lubricant found at most pharmacies.

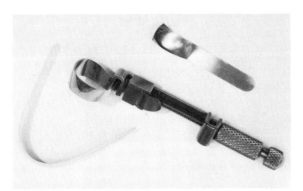

Figure 12–9. Pre-contoured band for developing a convex proximal surface. Band cut through the center illustrates its curvature. (Designed by Dr. Wilmer Eames)

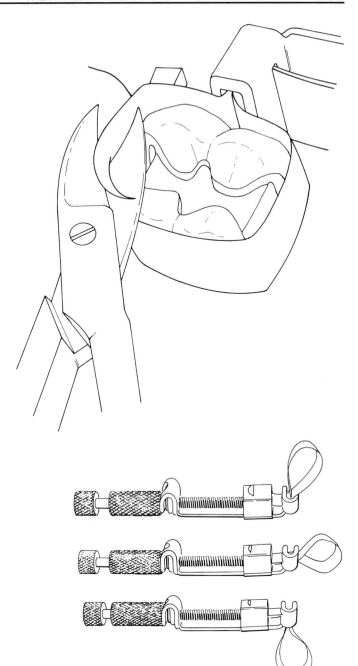

Figure 12–10. Trimming occlusal height of the matrix band. At the convenience of the operator the handle of the retainer may lay parallel with the teeth in the vestibule, alongside the tongue, or it may project outward.

to be sure no rubber from the dam or any gingival tissue is impinged between the tooth and the band (Figs. 12–12 and 12–13).

    8. Fragments of debris or bits of blood can be washed out with water or hydrogen peroxide.

    9. Inspect for copal varnish application (varnish should have been applied before the matrix was placed).

    10. After condensation, the handle of the retainer is first removed, followed by removal of the band (Figs. 12–14 and 12–15). The band is slipped out sideways from between the teeth; removal in an occlusal direction invites fracture of the newly placed amalgam.

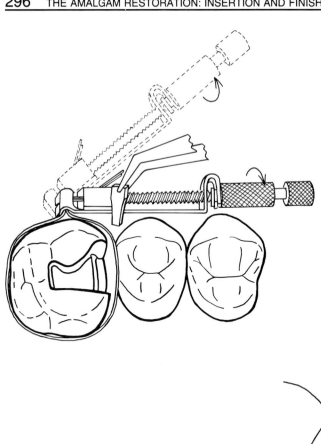

Figure 12–11. Reflecting the handle to permit insertion of mesial wedge. (Courtesy of the Journal of the Southern Calif. Dental Association)

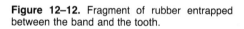

Figure 12–12. Fragment of rubber entrapped between the band and the tooth.

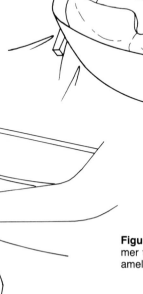

Figure 12–13. Gingival margin trimmer to remove debris and fragile enamel next to the matrix band.

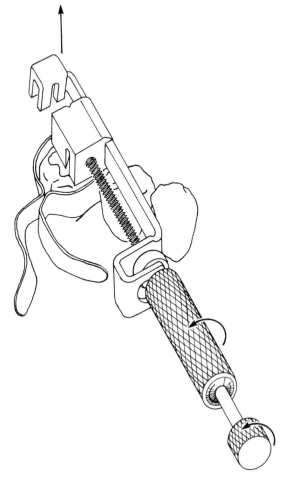

Figure 12–14. Removal of the handle; stabilizing the band with the fingers while releasing the knob insures against fracture of the soft amalgam.

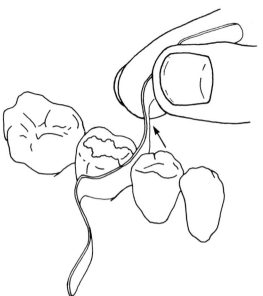

Figure 12–15. Removal of the band in an angular direction.

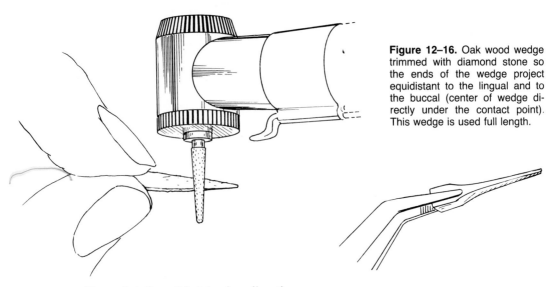

Figure 12–16. Oak wood wedge trimmed with diamond stone so the ends of the wedge project equidistant to the lingual and to the buccal (center of wedge directly under the contact point). This wedge is used full length.

Non-yielding Matrix Application

The custom-made matrix utilizes only a short strip of metal and no matrix retainer. Although more time is required for its placement, it is more rigid and more versatile for relatively small cavities that do not extend far below the adjoining gingivae. Moreover, it has the advantage of freedom and access for condensation because there is no handle to get in the way. Although this matix is used for condensing direct gold, the reader should realize that it is also acceptable for amalgam, with impression compound being substituted for acrylic.

Armamentarium
1. Long wooden wedge
2. Quick curing acrylic and dappen dish
3. Scissors, pliers, wire cutter
4. Matrix band, standard thickness
5. Paper clip, large size

Sequence of Application (Figs. 12–16 through 12–29)
1. Cut elliptical piece of matrix band and curl it to encircle the tooth.
2. *Carefully* trim wedge to pass through the gingival space so both ends extend equally to the facial and lingual.

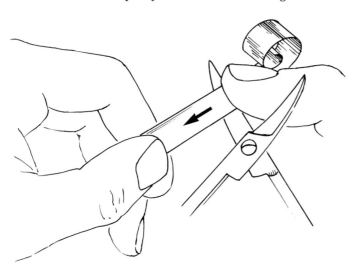

Figure 12–17. Curling the band like a decorative ribbon. Pulling the band over a sharp corner produces a natural curl to fit through the contact and hug the lingual and buccal surfaces.

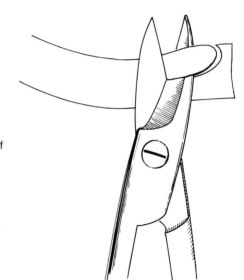

Figure 12–18. Cutting an elliptical matrix band from the strip of material.

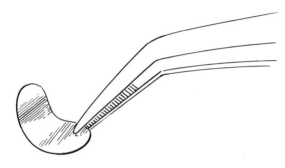

Figure 12–19. Correct height and length of band are quite important.

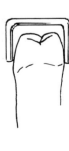

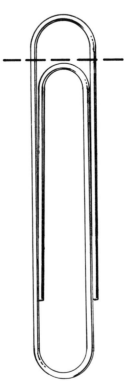

Figure 12–20. Cutting and shaping the staple to proper height and width are also important.

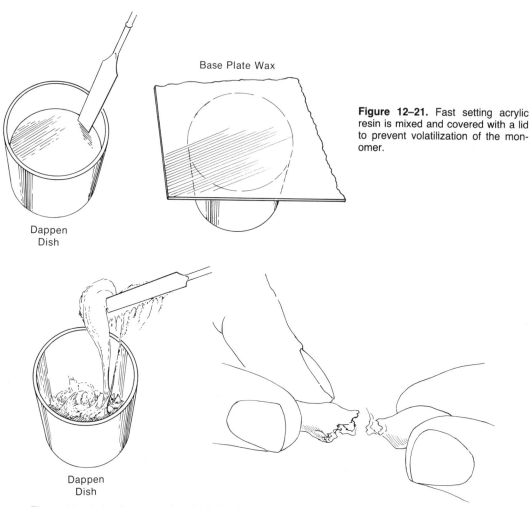

Base Plate Wax

Dappen
Dish

Figure 12–21. Fast setting acrylic resin is mixed and covered with a lid to prevent volatilization of the monomer.

Dappen
Dish

Figure 12–22. Acrylic not used until it is hard enough to be pulled apart with a snap. At its optimum texture, acrylic has only 30 seconds working time.

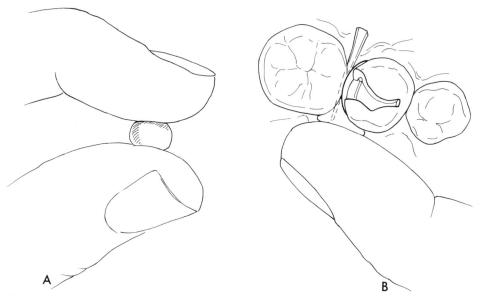

A

B

Figure 12–23. Acrylic ball rolled in the fingers (A) is pressed over the wedge (B) and squeezed toward the wedge and gingival embrasure.

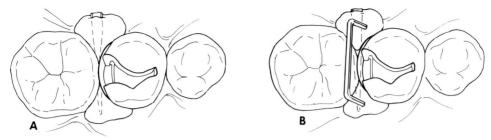

Figure 12–24. Application is identical for buccal acrylic *(A)*. *B*, Staple is quickly inserted and seated to its premeasured fitting.

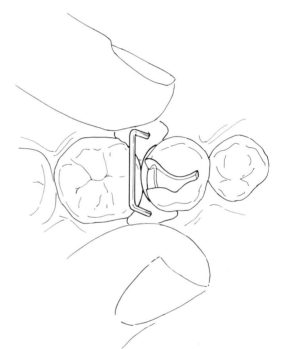

Figure 12–25. Buccal and lingual acrylic supports are held with thumb and forefinger while hardening.

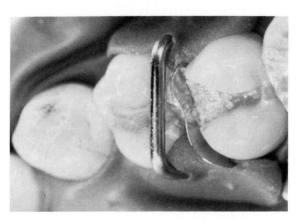

Figure 12–26. Finished application with cavity partly filled. Inspection should reveal ready access for condensation, acrylic that has not squeezed into the area of the contact point, and acrylic that does not lock into the holes of the rubber dam clamp. The staple should lie close to the tooth and not obstruct access to the cavity.

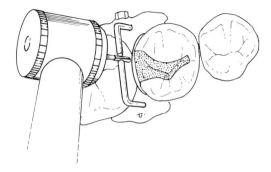

Figure 12–27. Cutting paper clip for removal.

Figure 12–28. Grasping band and pulling it out toward the buccal.

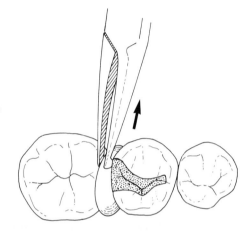

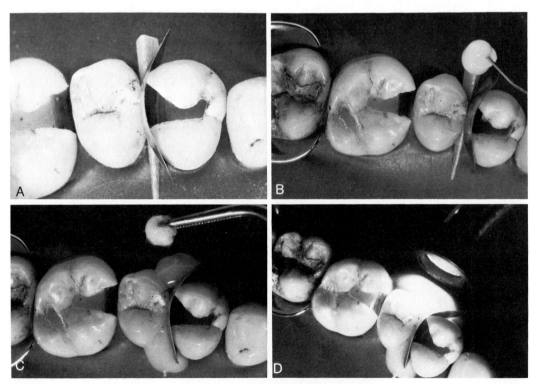

Figure 12–29. Customized matrix using light-cured resin (recommended by Dr. Adalbert Vlazny). *A,* Matrix metal and wedge in position. *B,* Clear resin being applied to facial embrasure. *C,* Molding resin into the embrasure with cotton pellet dampened with alcohol. *D,* Resin being polymerized with visible light.

3. Cut, band, and fit a section of the paper clip staple so its arch *does not obstruct access* to the cavity preparation.

4. Mix acrylic and cover the dappen dish so monomer cannot escape by evaporation.

5. Lightly coat fingers with vaseline or other lubricant.

6. When acrylic has reached texture of heavy chewing gum, select and roll a piece the shape of a large pea in the fingers. Compress this firmly into the lingual embrasure and around the wooden wedge.

7. Repeat procedure for buccal embrasure.

8. Insert staple into the acrylic to previously fitted position.

9. With thumb and forefinger, maintain the position of the acrylic tabs until heat of polymerization indicates that hardening has taken place. The cavity is now filled with amalgam (or gold).

10. The paper clip is cut with a fissure bur to release facial and lingual halves so the matrix can be removed.

11. After removal of the wedge and the acrylic, the metal strip is grasped with pliers and pulled toward the facial.

Light-cured microfilled resin can be substituted for the acrylic. Because it is very passive and does not have an elastic memory as does acrylic, it is readily forced underneath the contact point and around the wedge. Moreover a reinforcing wire staple is usually not required (see Fig. 12–29). A cotton pledget dampened with alcohol serves as a plunger to force the material where it is wanted.

A translucent, non-opaque resin facilitates the transmission of the light from the activator, which is applied from both facial and lingual sides. Because the resin is clear, deep penetration of the light rays is possible. If a large mass of material is used, better results are obtained with a second application of resin and light to insure polymerization in the interproximal region (Fig. 12–29).

Automatrix Matrix Application

Armamentarium
1. Kit of assorted bands (4 sizes)
2. Ratchet to tighten band
3. Cutting pliers
4. Wedges
5. Razor blade or sharp knife

Sequence of Application (Figs. 12–30 to 12–32)
The automatrix system uses pre-formed disposable bands. These bands are not convoluted, and seldom is the band trimmed to fit the tooth or the cavity. The band is wound tightly, simulating a clock spring, where its tension is maintained by a retainer clip.

1. Select the most likely fitting band and place over the tooth. The clip is usually on the buccal side.

2. The ratchet is used to cinch the band securely to the tooth.

3. Wedging is not usually required but may be used to depress the band against a concave area of the root.

4. After condensation the clip is released by cutting it in two.

5. Sliding the band sideways, it is removed from the tooth in an angular direction.

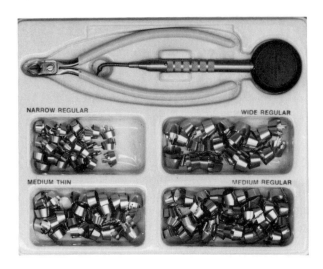

Figure 12–30. Automatrix bands, ratchet for tightening, and cutter for removing the band. Four sizes of bands are available.

Miscellaneous Matrices

Copper bands of assorted sizes make excellent matrices, but they are cylindrical and do not flare outward to engage distant contact points. They are susceptible to stretching and shaping with contouring pliers after the band has been rendered soft (Figs. 12–33 and 12–34). Bands are softened by heating to redness in a flame and quenching in water.

After selecting the proper size for fit, the band is cut to length and the fitting process begun. Fitting consists of flaring the mesial and distal while

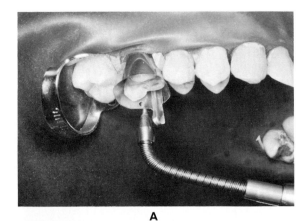

A

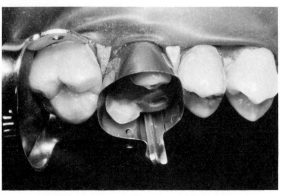

B

Figure 12–31. *A,* Band on tooth being tightened with ratchet. The band can be tightened or loosened at will by turning the sleeve in a clockwise or counterclockwise direction. *B,* Band in position and ready for condensation.

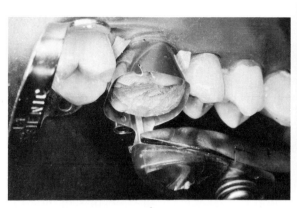
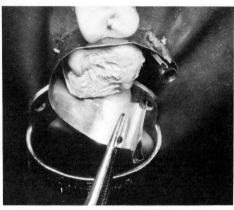

A   **B**

Figure 12–32. *A,* Cutting the retainer clip to release the assembly. *B,* Removal of the band.

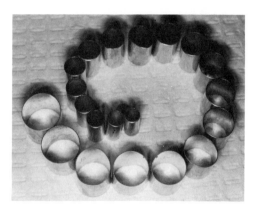

Figure 12–33. Assorted copper bands, sizes 1 to 20. The size of a No. 1 band is 4 mm in diameter, and the size of a No. 20 band is 12 mm in diameter, with a wall thickness of 0.15 mm.

Figure 12–34. Heating and then quenching in water.

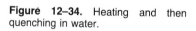
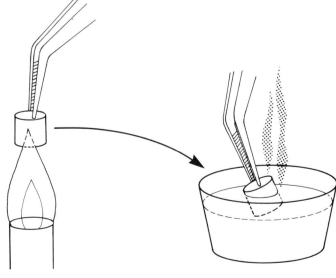

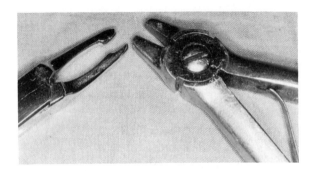

Figure 12–35. Pliers for shaping copper band. *Left,* Contouring pliers to bend the edges of the band. *Right,* Stretching pliers. By pinching the metal the band becomes thinner and spreads apart.

constricting the buccal and lingual. Because it is necessary for the finished amalgam to engage its neighbor in proximal contact, the thickness of the band should be reduced with a green stone at the contact point. Concurrently with this occlusal shaping, the gingival border is crimped inward to seal off the gingival margins. To complete the customization, the band is trimmed free of occlusion.

Stabilized in position with wooden wedges, the amalgam is condensed, the occlusion checked, and the edges of the band inspected for roughness. Wedges are removed and the patient is then dismissed while the amalgam hardens. At the next appointment, the band is sectioned with a bur and removed. Carving and shaping that could not be accomplished with the band in place must then be done with burs and stones (Figs. 12–35 through 12–38).

As can be envisioned, the copper band matrix, while yielding excellent results, is quite time consuming. Stainless steel strips can be fitted and spot-welded to produce comparable results. The wall thickness of the stainless steel (less than the copper band) is an added advantage; however, the ability of the copper to be shaped and contoured as well as its rigidity must not be overlooked.

In the absence of the spot welder, another type of matrix is used that is not encumbered with a handle. The "T" band, available in narrow and wide widths, curved or straight, is made of brass instead of steel. The tags fold outward to the facial, creating a channel for cinching the band tightly around the tooth. Quite flimsy in structure, it is inferior to most other bands, but it is very easily and rapidly applied (Fig. 12–39).

The Class V cavity on a sharply convex surface defies confinement during the condensation process. While condensing the mesial-buccal portion, the disto-buccal portion pushes out; while condensing the distal end of the cavity, the amalgam in the mesial end is dislodged. The use of a stainless steel strip wrapped around the lingual surface serves as an acceptable matrix for these

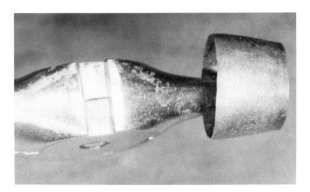

Figure 12–36. Stretching pliers in use to enlarge and contour the sides of the copper band.

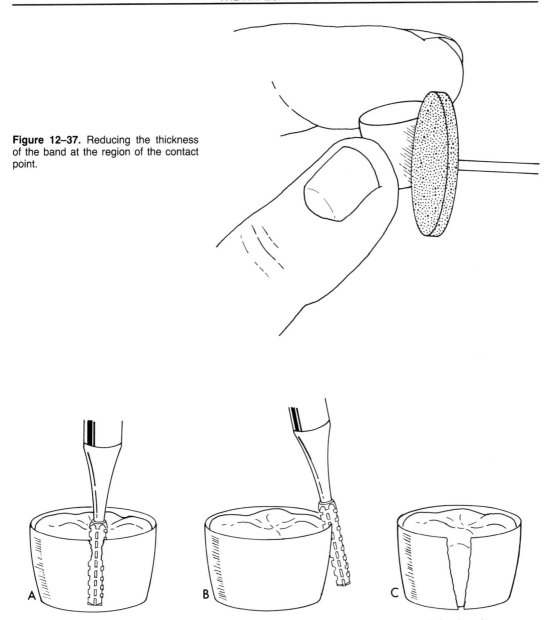

Figure 12–37. Reducing the thickness of the band at the region of the contact point.

Figure 12–38. Cutting the band off the tooth after the amalgam has sufficiently hardened.

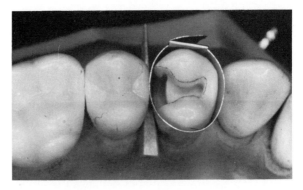

Figure 12–39. "T" band (available from Pulpdent Corp.).

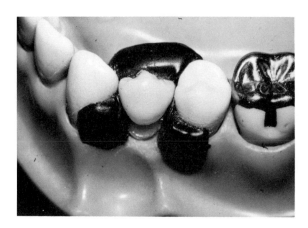

Figure 12–40. Matrix for large Class V restoration extending into interproximal spaces. Standard stainless steel band material 0.002 inch × 1 inch long is festooned around the lingual side of the tooth and secured mesially and distally with wooden wedges whose ends have been coated with soft compound. (Courtesy of Dr. Daniel Frederickson)

long cavities. Stabilized with wedges and compound the two protruding ends of the band provide walls so the material can be suitably compressed (Fig. 12–40).

Dental amalgam is particularly indicated for restoring gingival lesions in the posterior part of the mouth. The customized kind of matrix described above is not always possible to apply. A second method for condensation during its final stage is the mechanized vibrator with concave points for molars and bicuspids (Fig. 12–41).

Confinement of the cavity to restrict the amount of excess material can invariably become a problem when restoring cusps. The band continues to flare, whereas the contour of the natural tooth presents more closely aligned cusps and ridges. This unnecessary waste of material and effort can be controlled by the use of an occlusal "prop." After inserting one or two short strips of metal inside the fitted band, one or two wedges are inserted between it and its outer support. The band then tips inward and a restricted occlusal table will then be formed automatically as condensation is completed (Fig. 12–42).

Wedges

Unfortunately, many dentists and dental students see the insertion of a gingival wedge as a gesture rather than an important segment of the wall (matrix) that is built to confine the amalgam. Arbitrarily stuffed between the band and the adjoining tooth, it often does more harm than good (see Fig. 14–43).

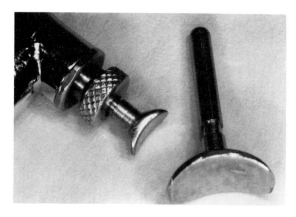

Figure 12–41. Mechanical condenser with molar and bicuspid points for condensing large gingival amalgam restorations, especially when spherical amalgam is used. (Amalpac condenser and points available from Midwest Sybron)

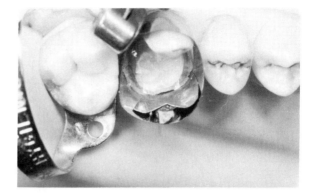

Figure 12–42. Matrix insert to confine the occlusal space. Compound may be needed to stabilize the inner band.

Wedges can be long or short, hard and rigid, or soft and compressible (Fig. 12–43). Whether made from wood or from plastic, the following rules must prevail when using them:

1. *Not all cavities need to be wedged.* Collectively, more wedges are probably used than needed. A gingival floor placed on a convex proximal surface, e.g., mesial of a lower 2nd bicuspid, does not need a wedge. A milder or flatter convexity, such as might be found on a mesial or distal surface of a maxillary 2nd bicuspid, should be braced with a wedge. Flat and concave surfaces naturally require wedging.

Unlike other restorative materials, amalgam has a strange property similar to crushed ice. When packed into a crevice or semi-flexible mold (proximal box of a Class II cavity), it wedges itself into the space and retains its position even after the condenser has been removed. Repeated tamping with more material spreads the space and pushes the band even farther from the axial wall. With regard to the contact point, this accumulative spreading is a desirable property because it creates tension on the periodontal membrane so that positive contact will prevail even after the tension has been partially released by the removal of the metal band.

2. *Wedges must not restrict the band from bulging outward to develop a good contact point.* A wedge that is so high it produces too large a gingival embrasure is definitely contraindicated (Figs. 12–44 and 12–45).

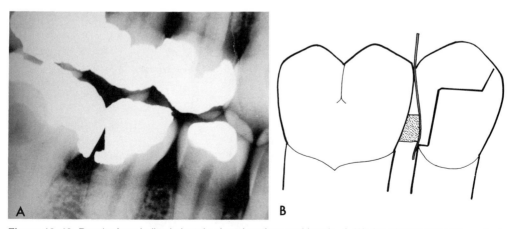

Figure 12–43. Results from indiscriminately placed wedges and bands. *A,* Wedge placed alongside a short band, forcing it to bulge inside the cavity. *B,* Gingival wedge inserted at the wrong level. The band bends inward and creates a concavity in the gingival third of the restoration. (Courtesy of the Journal of the Southern Calif. Dental Association)

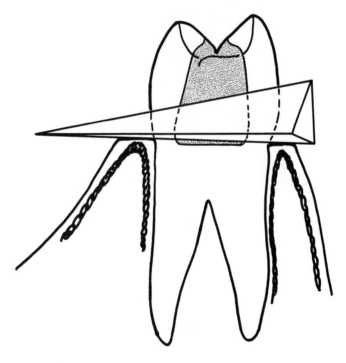

Figure 12–44. A high wedge can interfere with the development of a physiologic contact point.

3. Gingival margins that terminate above the gingival crest may be routinely braced with any wedge that fits the space and props the band against the tooth (Fig. 12–46). It is those cavities whose gingival floors terminate on the root that present the real challenge. To prop the band against tooth structure in these regions precludes the use of a long wedge.

Anatomically and clinically, the interseptal gingivae seem to be more depressible than the adjoining buccal cortical plate. A short wedge of compressed soft wood* functions most effectively here (Fig. 12–47). Although it induces some trauma and bleeding, it remains in position less than 20 minutes and no permanent damage is induced by its presence. Inasmuch as the wedge

---

*"No-Hem" wedges, The Doctor's Company, Hayward, California 94500.

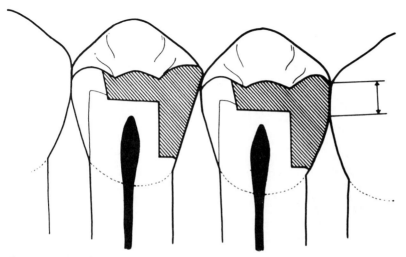

Figure 12–45. Correct *(right)* and incorrect *(left)* proximal contour for Class II amalgams. (Courtesy of the Journal of the Southern Calif. Dental Association)

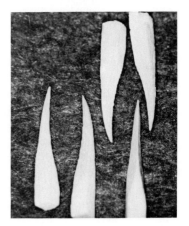

Figure 12–46. Well-designed long wooden wedges. Note curvature near the tip and triangular shape to not restrict the proximal contour.

has no handle for its removal, it must be pushed outward from the lingual with a small condenser.

4. *Wedges should usually be inserted from the facial.* Although one finds it more convenient to insert the wedge into the lingual rather than the buccal embrasure because the handle of the matrix retainer is in the way a wedge is more effective when its taper matches that created by the sides of the adjacent teeth. Because teeth tend to be closer together at their linguals the natural taper of the wedge adapts itself more appropriately to close the space if inserted from the facial side.

5. *Wedges must be fitted and customized.* There is no "Universal" wedge, and each one must be fitted for its individually intended space. Trimming can best be accomplished by a scalpel, a gold knife, or a diamond stone (Fig. 12–16).

Amalgam: Physical Properties and General Considerations

The Alloy

SILVER. Conventional modern amalgam alloys contain 67 to 70 per cent silver. The general effect of silver is to form metallic compounds with mercury, which largely determine the dimensional change that occurs during the hardening. It tends to increase the expansion at that time. It also increases the strength.

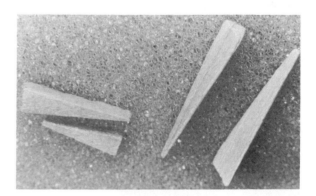

Figure 12–47. Wedges made from soft pine *(left)* and hard oak *(right).* The pine (No-Hem) wedge is compressible on insertion; the oak (Wizard) wedge is not. A customized wedge may be only 4 to 6 mm in length.

TIN. Tin, present in concentrations between 25 and 27 per cent, influences the amalgam in an opposite manner to silver in that it tends to reduce expansion during setting. Because of its affinity for mercury, tin improves the amalgamation of the alloy. Unfortunately, when tin combines with mercury in the amalgamation process, a tin-mercury compound forms that reduces the strength and increases corrosion, as will be seen.

COPPER. Copper, traditionally 6.0 per cent or less, is added to amalgam to increase the strength and hardness. It also tends to increase the expansion during hardening. In the past few years, several new alloys that contain markedly higher concentrations of copper have been introduced. For the sake of convenience, these products will be referred to as "high copper" alloys, in order to distinguish them from the classic silver-tin system. It is more appropriate to delay a discussion of the rationale for the added copper and its effect upon the alloy until we have described the setting reactions that occur during hardening.

ZINC. Zinc may or may not be present (a maximum of 2.0 per cent is pemitted in the American Dental Association specification for amalgam alloy). It is generally used as an aid in minimizing the oxidation of the other metals present in the alloy. When the metals are melted together during the manufacture of the alloy, there is always danger of oxygen contamination. The zinc readily reacts with any oxygen and prevents the combining of the oxygen with the silver, tin, or copper. Oxides of these metals would weaken the amalgam.

LATHE-CUT ALLOY. The manufacturer carefully melts the proper concentrations of these various metals and then casts them into an ingot or rod, which is heat-treated to produce a uniform composition throughout. It is then ready to be cut into small particles so that it can be mixed readily with mercury by the dentist. This is done by means of a milling machine or lathe, producing small particles or grains that can then be sifted and graded as desired. This is the classic method of preparing the alloy and the resulting filings are referred to as lathe-cut alloy (Fig. 12–48).

SPHERICAL ALLOYS. The alloy particles may also be made in the form of small spheres. One method of preparing such an alloy is by an atomizing procedure. A fine mist of the molten metal is sprayed into a cold, inert gas atmosphere. Upon solidification the particles form small spheres, as illustrated

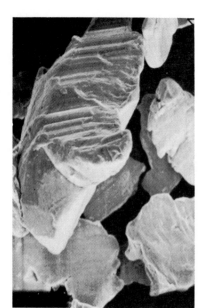

Figure 12–48. Particles of a lathe-cut alloy showing small filings (× 2000). (Courtesy of G. Wing)

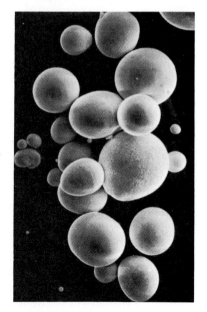

Figure 12–49. Particles of a spherical alloy (×2000). (Courtesy of G. Wing)

in Figure 12–49. Such alloys are referred to as "spherical alloys." Some products may be a mixture of both lathe-cut and spherical particles.

Spherical alloys amalgamate very readily. Therefore, amalgamation can be accomplished with smaller amounts of mercury than is generally required for many filing-type alloys. Spherical amalgam alloys have a somewhat different feel during manipulation as compared with lathe-cut alloys. The condensation pressures are less, and spherical alloys tend to "flow" into and adapt themselves more readily to internal cavity detail. On the other hand they do not have the "body" and "holding ability" (crushed ice property) that is present with the lathe-cut alloys (see Fig. 12–48). Forcing the band against the opposing tooth to develop a positive contact becomes more of a problem with spherical alloys.

Condenser and plugger section therefore becomes important with the type of alloy used. Lathe-cut alloy that does not flow ahead of the condenser will resist adapting itself to the angles and corners within the confines of the matrix. Very small condensers with deliberate thrusts (see Fig. 12–65B) must be applied in a patient, thorough manner to ensure a solid mass and to eliminate entrapment of voids, especially in acute angles alongside the matrix.

Spherical type alloys require attention to detail during initial stages of condensation in the deeper parts of the cavity as well. However, the major concern with this type of alloy centers around its inability to "stay put" once the condensing force has been removed. The prudent operator therefore will be sure that his matrix band rests passively and firmly against the adjacent tooth and that larger condensers are used as he packs and settles the particles as firmly as possible against the band in the region of the contact point.

Therefore, the dentist should familiarize himself with the particular alloy selected before placing clinical restorations. In this manner, the desired alloy-mercury ratios may be established and the necessary experience gained with the varied condensation and carving characteristics presented by different alloys. Over 100 commercial amalgam alloys are certified by the American Dental Association. The brands vary somewhat in terms of ease of amalgamation, rate of hardening, character of the carved surface, and similar factors that influence the selection.

PROPORTIONING THE ALLOY AND MERCURY. The amount of alloy and mercury to be used is defined as the *alloy-mercury* ratio, i.e., the parts by weight of alloy to be combined with the proper amount of mercury. For example, an alloy-mercury ratio of 5:8 indicates that 5 parts of alloy are to be used with 8 parts of mercury by weight. It may also be stated as the *mercury-alloy* ratio, in which the relative percentage of the mercury is given first. The manufacturer's directions should be consulted in regard to the correct ratio to be used with any particular brand of alloy.

The ratio will vary for different alloys and for the particular technique and handling characteristics desired by the dentist. With the modern, small-grained alloys, the mercury-alloy ratio has steadily decreased. Use of ratios equivalent to 50 to 51 per cent mercury is now common, and with some alloys as little as 46 or even 45 per cent mercury may be employed. The use of these low mercury-alloy ratios is referred to as the *Eames* or the *minimal mercury technique*.

As the consistency of the amalgam will be influenced by the amount of mercury in the original mix, trial mixes should be made at different ratios. The appropriate one can then be selected for the technique preferred for placement of the restoration.

A wide variety of alloy and mercury dispensers, or proportioners, are available, and most are satisfactory if properly adjusted. The dispenser may not be set accurately by the manufacturer; thus, it should be adjusted for the brand of alloy being used. This can be done by dispensing the alloy and mercury and checking the weights of the spills on a simple pharmaceutical balance.

Accuracy is particularly important when the minimal mercury technique is employed. At these very low alloy-mercury ratios, a variation of as little as 0.5 per cent mercury may have a marked effect upon the handling characteristics and properties of the amalgam.

PRE-WEIGHED ALLOY. In addition to the powder form, the alloy may also be dispensed in the form of a pre-weighed tablet or pellet (Fig. 12–50). In this case, the alloy particles are subjected to enough pressure that they adhere, but not so much that they cannot be readily separated during amalgamation. The process is much like making a pill. A small amount of mercury may also be added to assist in holding the particles together. Either the powder or pellet form of the alloy is acceptable, although the pellet has the advantage of convenience.

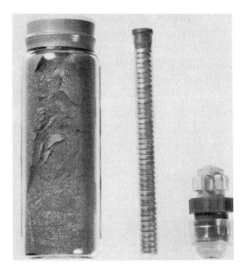

Figure 12–50. Various forms in which dental amalgam alloy may be supplied. *Left,* powder; *center,* pellets; *right,* disposable pre-weighed capsules.

Probably the best method for measurement of the alloy and mercury is to use pre-weighed pellets of the alloy and to dispense the mercury from a volumetric dispenser, which has been properly regulated to deliver the correct amount of mercury. If the amalgam alloy and the mercury dispenser are from different manufacturers, it will be necessary to weigh the pellet on a pharmaceutical balance. The manufacturer of the dispenser does not usually supply the proper setting for an alloy of a competitor. Having obtained the weight of the pellet, the amount of mercury required for the desired ratio can be calculated. Increments of mercury may then be dispensed and weighed on the balance until the desired setting to provide the proper alloy-mercury ratio has been attained.

Disposable capsules are now available. They contain pre-weighed alloy and mercury in separate compartments. There are disadvantages to the disposable, pre-proportioned mercury-alloy capsule other than the higher cost per mix of amalgam. Obviously, there is a restriction to a given size mix, as well as to the mercury-alloy ratio established by the manufacturer for that capsule. In other words, there is no opportunity to make minor adjustments for wetter or dryer mixes if desired.

However, the advantages are considerable. Their use standardizes the amalgam technique, as most products provide acceptable accuracy in the weights of alloy and mercury from one capsule to another. They are convenient to use and save time by eliminating the need for proportioning. Also, the chance for loss of mercury from the capsule during amalgamation is minimal, thereby reducing the possibility of mercury contamination of the office environment.

In any event, the correct amount of alloy and mercury must be measured before the start of trituration. Excess mercury at the start, or addition of mercury after the trituration has started, results in a restoration that is high in mercury content. The influence of the final mercury content upon the properties of the restoration is extremely important.

Setting Reactions

The reactions that take place during the hardening of amalgam are complex and not as yet completely understood. Thus only the principal one will be summarized. This information is essential in order to appreciate the roles that the various compounds (phases) play in regulating the properties of the final structure.

The main component in the original alloy particle that reacts with mercury during trituration is the *gamma* phase, Ag_3Sn. Initially some absorption of mercury into the particles occurs, which is then followed by the crystallization of a silver-mercury compound (Ag_2Hg_3), the *gamma-one* phase, and a tin-mercury phase (Sn_8Hg), the *gamma-two* phase. These crystals produce a hardening of the amalgam, much as in the setting of plaster.

The reaction that occurs between the alloy particles and the mercury can then be summarized as follows:

Silver-tin alloy + Mercury		Silver-tin alloy + Silver-mercury + Tin-mercury		
Ag_3Sn	Hg	Ag_3Sn	Ag_2Hg_3	Sn_8Hg
(gamma)		(gamma)	(gamma-one)	(gamma-two)

Thus, the hardened amalgam is a multi-phase structure composed of unreacted particles of the original alloy that remain, surrounded by a matrix of silver-mercury and tin-mercury compounds, the gamma-one and gamma-two phases, respectively.

This reaction has been reasonably well understood for many years. What is relatively recent, though, is an appreciation of the contribution that each of the three phases makes in regulating the properties of the amalgam and thereby the clinical behavior of the restoration. The strongest component is that with which one starts, the original silver-tin phase. The weakest is the tin-mercury, gamma-two phase. Likewise, the gamma-two is decidedly more susceptible to corrosion than are the other two phases. Thus, to an extent, the strength and corrosion resistance of the restoration are dependent upon the relative percentages of each component. More specifically, it follows that the bad actor is the tin-mercury phase. This knowledge has led to a marked transition in alloy formulation based upon the use of mechanisms whereby the amount of the gamma-two phase that forms during the setting reactions may be markedly reduced or eliminated.

Acquaintance with the basic reaction between the alloy and mercury and the significance of the end products that form makes it possible to discuss more intelligently the newer commercial amalgam alloys that deviate from the classic silver-tin systems described so far.

High Copper Alloys. Many new alloys have recently appeared on the market, and all are based upon the concept that the properties and performance of the material can be enhanced by altering the formulation in some manner so that the weak, corrodible gamma-two phase is virtually eliminated during the hardening of the amalgam. The most popular method has been to increase the copper content of the alloy above the traditional maximum of 6 per cent. The terminology for such alloys remains somewhat nebulous. An acceptable term to differentiate them from the conventional silver-tin alloys is *high copper alloys*. A number of such products can be seen in Figure 12–51.

The copper content of commercial high copper alloys varies considerably

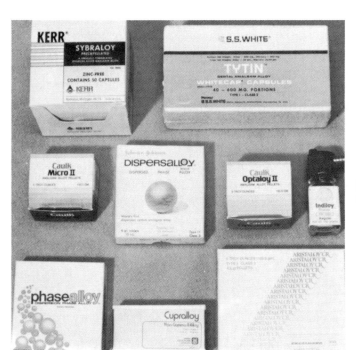

Figure 12–51. A number of the commercial "high copper" amalgam alloys.

from one brand to another. In a few instances they may contain less than 10 per cent copper while in others the copper content is as high as 30 per cent. There are two basic types of high copper alloys, admixed and single composition.

Admixed Alloys. The oldest type or form of the high copper alloy is the *admixed* alloy (Fig. 12–51, center). In the admixed alloy system the alloy powder purchased from the manufacturer is composed of a mixture of powders of two alloys, each of a different composition. One of the alloys is the traditional low copper alloy, containing silver, tin, and less than 6 per cent copper. The increase in the overall copper content of the product is achieved by adding a second powder prepared from a copper-rich alloy, i.e., a silver-copper eutectic. Thus the rationale for the term *admixed alloy* is obvious. (Alloys of this type are sometimes referred to as a *dispersion* alloy, but from a scientific standpoint this terminology is incorrect.)

The total copper content of commercial admixed alloys ranges from about 9 to 20 per cent. The alloy particles can be either spherical or filings. A common, although not universal, approach with these alloys is for the particles of one alloy to be filings while the particles of the second are spherical. The result is a mixture of filings and spheres.

Single Composition. The other approach to increasing the total copper content of amalgam alloys is to increase the amount of copper in the silver-tin-copper alloy particles. Since such an amalgam alloy contains powder particles of only one composition, this type is referred to as a *single composition* high copper alloy (Fig. 12–51, top). Again the copper content varies considerably from one manufacturer to another. The copper content of different brands of alloy of this type ranges from about 13 per cent to as much as 30 per cent. Some of the single composition alloys marketed today also contain small amounts of indium or palladium.

Physical Properties

The clinical behavior of the restoration is based upon the physical properties of the amalgam. Therefore, a proper understanding of these properties and their control is necessary in order to appreciate the importance of the various manipulative factors that are to be discussed.

Dimensional Change. Most metals shrink when they freeze. Since the hardening of amalgam is actually a freezing process, dimensional changes are to be expected. As explained, amalgam can expand or contract, depending upon its manipulation. After the restoration is inserted, dimensional change should, of course, be at a minimum.

The current American Dental Association specification for amalgam alloy states that at the end of 24 hours, the dimensional change should be zero plus or minus 20 microns (micrometers) per centimeter. When one considers that 1 micron is only 0.00004 inch, it is apparent that in general these changes during the setting of amalgam are very small, and *minor* deviations from these recommended limits are apparently not clinically significant. However, since manipulation does influence the magnitude of the dimensional changes that occur, every care must be taken to prevent undue expansion or contraction.

Strength. Sufficient strength to resist fracture is a prime requisite for any restorative material. Fracture, even on a small area, or fraying of the exposed margins will hasten recurrence of caries and subsequent clinical failure. For this reason, the material must be handled in a manner that will assure maximum strength.

The strength of amalgam is usually measured by subjecting a specimen to compressive stress. Although the principal stress involved during mastication is compressive, other types of stress are also involved. Whenever those forces tend to induce a tensile stress, fracture may be more likely to occur. The tensile strength of amalgam may be only approximately one-eighth of the compressive strength. However, compressive strength provides a convenient yardstick by which the general strength characteristics of the material may be assessed. The manipulative variables that alter the compressive strength invariably seem to influence the other strength properties. Undertrituration results in low strength and, when within reasonable limits, longer trituration increases the strength.

The rate of hardening is of considerable interest. A patient may be dismissed from the chair within 20 minutes after trituration of the amalgam, and thus the question of whether the restoration is strong enough to support biting forces is a vital one. Amalgam does not gain its strength as rapidly as might be expected, or desired. The strength during the first few hours is low, and it is probable that most of the amalgam restorations that fracture do so at that time, even though the break may not be evident for several months. For that reason, it is advisable for the dentist and/or his auxilliary to suggest that the patient avoid biting on the restoration for the first few hours after leaving the dental office. He should pay special attention to the occlusion before dismissing the patient to be sure a cusp or ridge is not occluding heavily. One of the advantages of some of the new high copper alloys is that they tend to gain their strength very rapidly, thus making the restoration less susceptible to early fracture.

The strength of amalgam is governed by two factors other than the influence played by the composition of the alloy. One is the effect of the amount of residual mercury that remains after condensation. Whenever the residual mercury exceeds approximately 54 per cent, a marked loss in strength results. Second is porosity. There are always internal voids in the amalgam mass and, as their number increases, the strength decreases. Thus, for attaining maximum strength the manipulative procedure must be designed to control the mercury content in the final restoration and to minimize porosity (Fig. 12–52).

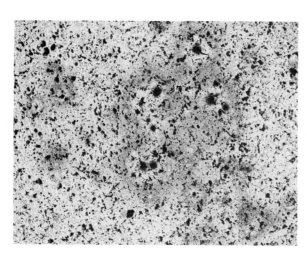

Figure 12–52. Voids and open spaces in condensed amalgam. (Courtesy of Dr. Y. Katoh)

Flow and Creep. When a metal is placed under stress, it will undergo plastic deformation. This characteristic is referred to as flow or creep. The flow test has long been used in evaluating amalgam alloys. Generally it is considered that if the flow is high, the restoration will be more likely to result in failures, such as flattened contact points or even protrusion of the proximal surface in a stress-bearing restoration.

Possibly of greater pertinence is the characteristic of creep, which measures the deformation after the material has completely hardened, as is the case in the continual application of masticatory stress to the restoration day after day. The creep values of commercial alloys vary widely, from as high as approximately 4 per cent to as low as 0.10 per cent. The high copper alloys, as compared with conventional silver-tin alloys, usually tend to have lower creep values. As with all properties, creep is influenced by manipulative variables. However, alloys that inherently possess low creep values seem to be less sensitive to manipulation than those that are high in their normal creep values.

Amalgam restorations have been placed with alloys having different creep values and their clinical behavior evaluated. Generally, it has been noted that the lower the creep value of the amalgam, the better is the marginal integrity of the restoration, at least with the traditional alloy.

Certainly factors other than creep may be involved in the complex mechanism of marginal breakdown of the amalgam restoration, such as corrosion (as influenced by the amount of gamma-two phase present), variation in strength, or a combination of all of these. At the moment though, the creep test is a useful screening device for determining the clinical performance characteristics of amalgam alloys.

If routinely satisfactory restorative dentistry is to be achieved, an appreciation of these properties is obvious. Failure to control them can only result in a clinical failure.

Amalgamation

Recognition* of properly mixed alloy is quite important because there is no magic formula or method whereby one can expect to always produce ideal mixes. Variations in operation of the equipment frequently prevent this from happening. In speed alone, amalgamators differ markedly from each other and produce mixes that may be quite dissimilar.

Probably more amalgams in dental offices are undermixed than overmixed. A grainy amalgam is undermixed; smooth plastic amalgam may be properly mixed or it may be somewhat overmixed* (Fig. 12–53).

Mulling. Most pre-weighed capsules include a metallic pestle, which helps rub the particles together during oscillation to remove their oxide surfaces so mercury can attack the bare metal—namely the silver, tin, and copper components. If after initial trituration the mass appears too grainy, additional trituration is done in a more gentle fashion without the metallic pestle. This process is known as "mulling." Another means of mulling is to twist the amalgam into a fold of a rubber dam where it is kneaded and massaged with the fingers. A rubber finger cot serves the need equally well, but it must be turned inside out lest talcum powder contaminate it. After 15 to 20 seconds of mulling, a grainy material will become more plastic and permit itself to be more readily manipulated (Fig. 12–54).

---

*Advice and assistance from an experienced operative dentist can be helpful in identifying material that has been properly triturated.

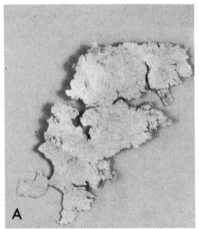

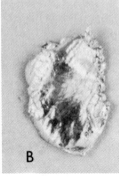

Figure 12–53. Undertriturated *(A)* and properly triturated *(B)* amalgam. The mass on the left *(A)* has low strength and poor resistance to corrosion.

Figure 12–54. Amalgam inside a piece of rubber dam. Massaging vigorously with the fingers or against the heel of the hand serves to mull the amalgam and make it more plastic.

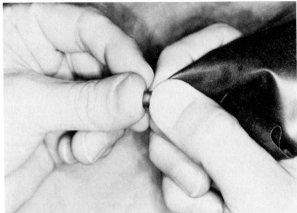

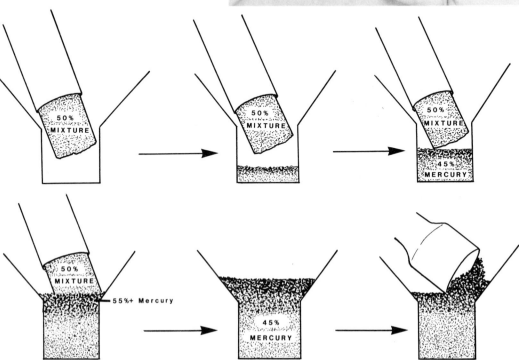

Figure 12–55. Sequential condensation of amalgam within a cavity. Thorough condensation brings mercury toward the surface. When the cavity has been overfilled the excess mercury-rich amalgam is scraped away and discarded. Care should also be exercised in the final stages lest mercury-rich material be allowed to accumulate along the margins.

Condensation

The recognition of properly mixed amalgam cannot be overemphasized. If it is undertriturated it will seem "grainy"; if it is overtriturated it will be crumbly as though it were beginning to set. The desired plastic texture lies between these two extremes and it is essential for obtaining a solid metallic restoration.

The basic purpose during condensation is to eliminate the void spaces inside the cavity or, more tersely put, to squeeze all the air out of the material and to fill the nooks and crannies with amalgam. Deliberate condensation of all parts of the cavity is necessary as it is built from the bottom to the top. Lack of concentration may result in air spaces that could be left unnoticed in one of the underlying layers. Generally speaking small condensers are used in corner areas and along the deeper portion of the cavity, changing to larger condensers as the filling nears completion.

Another objective in filling a cavity is to draw off as much mercury as possible in the process. When ready to condense, the material contains slightly more mercury than will appear in the final product. Figure 12–55 graphically illustrates a hypothetical amalgam, which has a 50/50 blend of mercury and alloy. As the first increment is placed in the cavity and condensed, some of the mercury is drawn to the surface. After placement and thorough condensation of the second increment, the lower portion of our hypothetical amalgam contains, e.g., only 45 per cent whereas the surface material may contain 55 per cent. As additional increments are added and as packing continues, the mercury underneath is drawn up to the surface where it is subsequently scraped away. The remaining mass is then carved and shaped to its desired form as setting begins to take place.

Selection of the Alloy

A number of factors enter into the selection of an alloy, and the weight given to each will vary with the individual. Certainly, the first criterion is to make sure that it meets the requirements of the American Dental Association Specification No. 1 or a similar specification.

The manipulative characteristics, such as ease of amalgamation (see Fig. 12–53), rate of hardening, and smoothness of the finished surface, are extremely important and a matter of subjective preference. Coincident with this is the delivery system provided by the manufacturer, its convenience, expediency, and capability to reduce human variables. The physical properties discussed earlier in this chapter should be reviewed in light of claims made for superiority over competing products. Lastly, documentation as to performance, in the form of well-controlled clinical studies, must be requested. This is especially necessary for alloy formulations that may depart from traditional compositions.

Condensation and Carving of Occlusal Forms

Armamentarium
1. Condensing instruments
   Large round condenser DE
   Small round condenser DE
   Other designs of choice (optional)

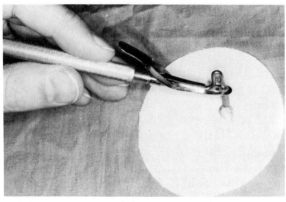

A

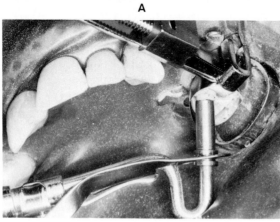

B

Figure 12–56. *A,* Loading the amalgam carrier (gun). Amalgam may be placed on a squeeze cloth or in an amalgam well. *B,* Injecting the amalgam into the cavity.

2. Amalgam carrier
3. Amalgam well (optional)
4. Squeeze cloth
5. Carving instruments
   Cleoid-discoid (No. 4–5)
   Hollenback or Ward carver (No. 3 or ½–3)
   Other carvers (optional)

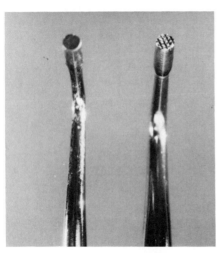

Figure 12–57. Smooth vs. serrated condensers. Serrated condensers "bite" into the material better, whereas smooth-faced condensers skid over the surface.

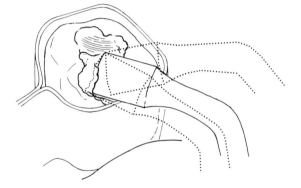

Figure 12–58. Excess amalgam scraped off the surface with a large amalgam condenser.

6. Burnishers (suggested types):
   PKT wax carver, No. 3 (blunted ends)
   Small ball burnisher
7. Pumice slurry and rubber cup (optional)
8. Articulating paper

Procedure

1. After the amalgam is mixed as previously described, it is placed in an amalgam well or on a squeeze cloth so the barrel of the carrier (amalgam gun) can be loaded (Fig. 12–56).

2. After ejecting the load into the cavity it is pressed into position with positive firm pressure (Fig. 12–56). Careful condensation must include "stepping" the condenser over all parts of the cavity.

3. Additional increments are added where they are successively condensed, first with small condensers, then with large sizes.

4. Excess material is built over the edges of the cavity where it is scraped off with the large condenser.

Some clinicians prefer condensers with faces that are smooth, whereas others prefer serrated (Fig. 12–57). A smooth faced condenser tends to slip around over the surface without effectively engaging the amalgam, whereas one with serrations can more effectively hold the amalgam and maneuver it into position. On the other hand the serrated face tends to clog up with amalgam and must be cleaned immediately after use. Once amalgam has hardened within the serrations cleaning becomes quite difficult.

5. After scraping off the excess amalgam with a large condenser, a damp pledget of cotton is rubbed over the surface to eliminate gross excess of material (Figs. 12–58 and 12–59).

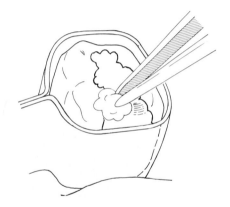

Figure 12–59. Surface rendered smooth and free of gross excess material with a tightly twisted cotton pledget.

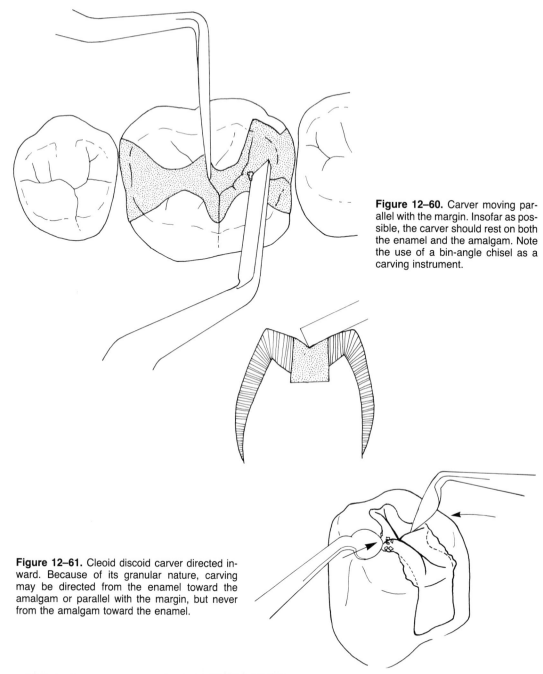

Figure 12–60. Carver moving parallel with the margin. Insofar as possible, the carver should rest on both the enamel and the amalgam. Note the use of a bin-angle chisel as a carving instrument.

Figure 12–61. Cleoid discoid carver directed inward. Because of its granular nature, carving may be directed from the enamel toward the amalgam or parallel with the margin, but never from the amalgam toward the enamel.

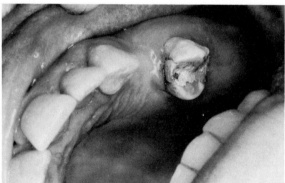

Figure 12–62. Articulating paper (carbon paper) marking the spots that are "high" in occlusion. The patient must close his teeth together gently lest the amalgam fracture, especially if the restoration is a Class II.

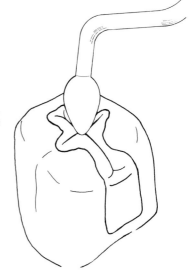

Figure 12–63. The surface is ironed smooth with a burnishing instrument. This is done after the carving has been completed and the amalgam has begun to harden.

6. Carving is then done. Strokes with the carver are parallel with the margin, with the carver resting on the outer enamel surface to prevent it from digging into the material (Fig. 12–60). With a delicate touch carving can most effectively be accomplished by directing the strokes from the tooth toward the amalgam (Figs 12–60 and 12–61).

7. The patient is instructed to close the teeth together lightly with the carbon marking paper inserted between them. High spots on the amalgam, if present, will be readily marked and can then be carved away (Fig. 12–62).

8. With a thin pumice slurry in a flexible rubber cup the surface is smoothed to eliminate the scratches from the carver (this step is optional).

9. The surface is then ironed to a shiny finish with the appropriate size burnishing instrument (Figs. 12–63 and 12–64).

It should be understood that burnishing is not a substitute for polishing. Burnishing is done immediately after carving, but not before the amalgam gives evidence of firm clinical hardness.

Condensation and Carving of Proximal Forms

Armamentarium
1. Condensing instruments
   Large round condenser DE
   Small round condenser DE
   Other designs of choice (optional)

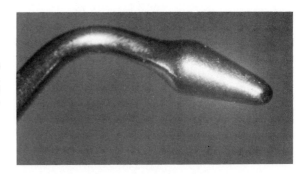

Figure 12–64. Burnisher, highly polished with no sharp corners. This particular instrument is a P.K.T. No. 3 with a blunted end. A round ball-shaped burnisher, as well as the reverse side of an excavator, is also very useful.

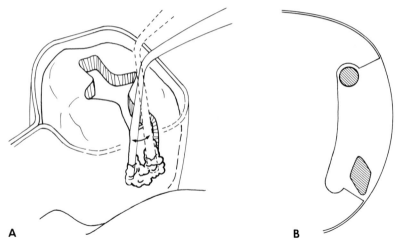

Figure 12–65. *A,* Condensation with the side rather than the face of the plugger is helpful in filling the corners alongside the matrix band. *B,* Properly shaped condensers should match the corners they are intended to pack.

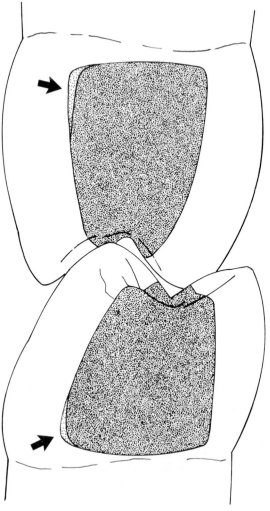

Figure 12–66. Common site for careless condensation. More vigorous lateral movements with the side of the condenser, especially "pulling" movement, would have forced the material into the bucco-gingival corners.

2. Amalgam carrier
3. Amalgam well or dappen dish (optional)
4. Squeeze cloth
5. Carving instruments
   Cleoid-discoid (No. 4–5)
   Hollenback or Ward carver (No. 3 or ½–3)
   Inter-proximal carver DE
   Other carvers (optional)
6. Burnishers (suggested designs)
   PKT wax carver No. 3 (blunted ends)
   Small ball burnisher
   Back side of an excavator
   Beavertail or egg burnisher (optional)
7. Pumice slurry and rubber cup (optional)
8. Articulating paper

Procedure

1. Apply one carrier of amalgam to the gingival floor and thoroughly condense it to place. The first increment of amalgam is the most crucial and should require more attention than subsequent ones. If poor condensation is to occur, it will most likely be found along the buccal margin near the gingival floor. For that reason a buccolingual action, with amalgam being forced ahead of the shaft of the condenser, is more effective in filling this crucial area than condensation with a vertical thrust (Figs. 12–65 and 12–66).

2. In condensing subsequent increments the band can be pressed against the contact point of the adjacent tooth to insure positive contact with the material after the band has been removed.

3. Increments of amalgam are condensed at will into the cavity, thoroughly "stepping" it to eliminate all voids (Fig. 12–67) and to fill carefully and consistently all of the retentive and undercut areas. When pins are used, amalgam should carefully and meticulously be adapted around them and into their serrations.

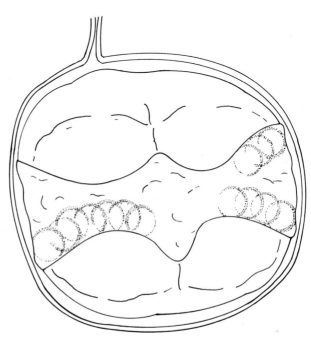

Figure 12–67. "Stepping" the amalgam. The condenser is moved systematically forward and sideways to cover the previous location with half the face of the condenser. Each particle is thereby insured of being condensed at least twice.

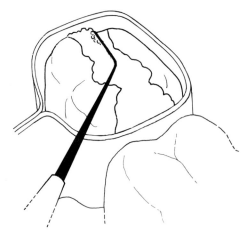

Figure 12–68. Explorer tine serving as a scraper to level the marginal ridge to its proper height. The tip also provides relief alongside the band so the amalgam will not be as likely to fracture during band removal.

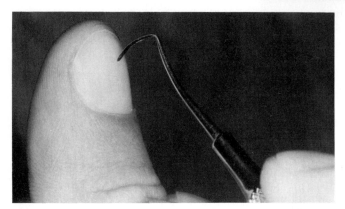

Figure 12–69. Proximal amalgam carver in position for carving lingual embrasure.

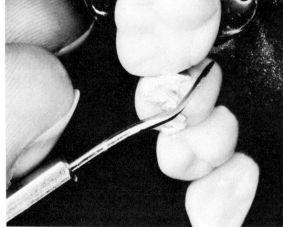

Figure 12–70. Proximal carver blade is flexible, thin (0.2 mm), and sharp. It is slipped into the space occupied by the matrix band, and the amalgam is carved with a slicing action.

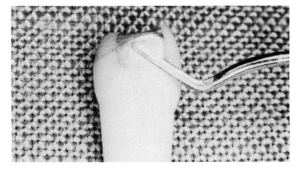

Figure 12–71. Comparative size of carver and proximal amalgam surface. (Courtesy of Connecticut State Dental Association Journal)

4. The occlusal portion of the cavity is filled to completion and excess material removed with the condenser.

5. Using the end of the explorer as a scraper, the form and height of the marginal ridge is established as the excess amalgam is scraped away (Fig. 12–68).

6. With the index finger holding the band secure the screw is released to permit removal of the handle (see Fig. 12–14).

7. The band is carefully unwrapped from around the tooth so that the restored contact point remains undisturbed. With the band free in all other areas it is grasped at either end and slipped out in a tangential direction (see Fig. 12–15).

8. Using the appropriate end of the thin proximal amalgam carver, the blade is slipped into the proximo-gingival sulcus and excess amalgam sliced away (Figs. 12–69 and 12–70). Utilizing this knife-like carver, the "overhangs" of amalgam are removed and the proximal surface carved to contour to reveal normal buccal, lingual, and gingival embrasures (Fig. 12–71).

9. Following the technique outlined for the Class I amalgam, the occlusal surface is carved to form. As the occlusal contour involves the marginal ridge, it is wise to use a proximal carver to establish the occlusal embrasure as well.

10. Interference in occlusion is best checked after the rubber dam has been removed. A thin piece of carbon paper is inserted between the teeth as the patient closes together lightly. Abrupt or forceful closure can likely result in fracture of the marginal ridge or a cusp. After "high" spots have been carved away the patient can be dismissed with reasonable assurance that the amalgam will not fracture. Notwithstanding this, however, the patient should be advised to eat with caution for the first 2 or 3 hours. It is not necessary that occlusal contact be made between the amalgam and the opposing tooth, yet deep over-carved surfaces are not desirable.

11. Some clinicians prefer to remove the rubber dam and check the occlusal heights before occlusal carving. At this stage the amalgam is softer and is not as likely to fracture as after the carving has been completed. The wise clinician, prior to his cavity preparation, will place carbon paper between the teeth to mark occluding areas. This provides him with a visual image of preliminary occluding patterns, an image that he can reproduce in his finished amalgam carving, thereby decreasing the amount of occlusal adjustment that may be necessary. To protect the marks from being rubbed off during cavity preparation the area is covered with cavity varnish (Fig. 12–72).

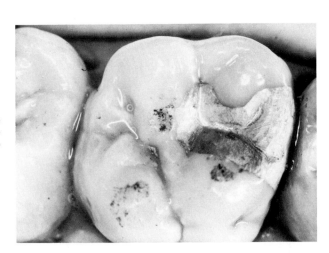

Figure 12–72. Carbon paper markings on the surface of the enamel. Prior to preparing the cavity, occluding areas should be identified to guide the operator in the occlusal carving.

12. Large restorations, to be condensed thoroughly, require more time than smaller ones. Several separate successive mixes of amalgam can provide the operator with fresh material to condense. After removing the band, however, the operator may discover the earlier mix may have already started to harden and be resistant to carving instruments, so much so that he must resort to burs and sharp chisels. Where multi mixes will be required it behooves the operator to work rapidly and to remove excess material as soon as possible.

13. Burnishing is accomplished best after the amalgam has begun to harden. The convex side of a spoon excavator (large and small) may be used in proximal areas and marginal ridges, whereas the blunt wax carver (PKT No. 3) is very effective in occlusal regions.

Condensing and Carving the Class V Amalgam

Armamentarium
1. Amalgam condensers
   Large round DE
   Small round DE
   Back action (optional)
2. Amalgam carrier
3. Squeeze cloth
4. Amalgam well (optional)
5. Carvers
   Hollenback or Ward type (No. 3 or ½–3)
   No. 6 explorer
   Other carvers (optional)
6. Burnishers: PKT wax carver No. 3 (blunted ends)
7. Pumice slurry and rubber cup (optional)

Following the technique already described, the Class V cavity is filled and condensed. Unlike the others, the Class V wraps around the buccal surface, making confinement of the material quite difficult, with material squeezing out at one end as pressure is applied at the other. As mentioned earlier, a custom-made matrix should be applied to confine the amalgam (see Fig. 12–40) or a mechanical condenser may be used (see Fig. 12–41).

It should be pointed out that with the Class V restoration a back action condenser is helpful in "hard to reach" areas, e.g., the distal buccal surface of a 2nd molar (Fig. 12–73; see also Fig. 3–52).

Carving is best accomplished with the No. 6 explorer, with its tip gliding

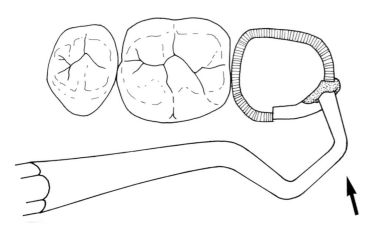

Figure 12–73. Back action condenser in use.

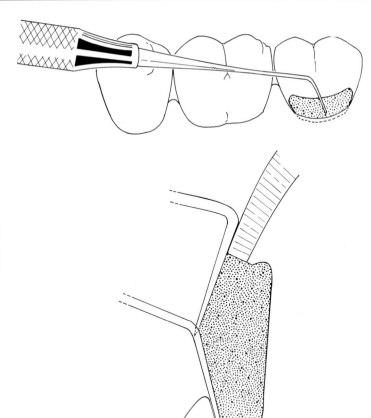

Figure 12–74. No. 6 explorer serving as an amalgam carver and burnisher. With the tip riding low in the sulcus and resting against uncut tooth, the tine can be used to scrape off excess amalgam and carve the surface while the material is still soft.

along the root surface as its side wipes away the unwanted material (Fig. 12–74). An effort is made to retain a convex surface that can be reduced to its desired form as the amalgam begins to harden. On occasion a pledget of damp cotton makes an effective "carver" for gingival restorations.

With a rubber dam and gingival clamp isolation, the cavity vision is good and carving is easy. If one must rely on the "feel" of the carver inside the gingival sulcus, it is very easy to misinterpret the location of the gingival margin and inadvertently carve a ditch inside the gingival margin. On the other hand it is easy to procrastinate and delay carving until the amalgam has become so hard that an unwieldy gingival overhang results. It behooves the operator, therefore, to remove excess material as soon as possible and to use a delicate carver (e.g., a pointed explorer), which will give the operator maximal tactile sense in establishing a smooth and accurate gingival finish.

As with other amalgams, surface smoothness is imparted with a pumice slurry inside a rubber cup followed by burnishing of the surface.

Finishing the Amalgam Restoration

Studies in progress will determine the necessity of polishing the new alloy systems, but until results indicate otherwise it is best to polish the hardened amalgam. Polishing naturally must come at a subsequent appointment when the completely hardened surface has greater resistance to corrosion.

Aside from making the surface attractive, polishing eliminates surface scratches and blemishes following carving. These imperfections, if not elimi-

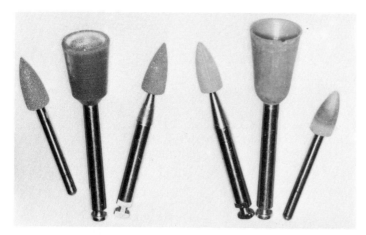

Figure 12–75. SHOFU rubber polishing system. "Brownies" on the left and "Greenies" on the right are, respectively, coarse and fine abrasive polishing points and cups.

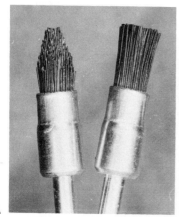

A

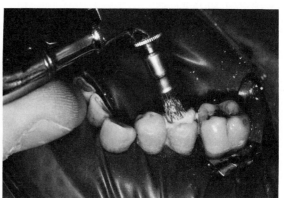

B

Figure 12–76. *A,* Polishing brush cut to a point with scissors. *B,* Tufted brush in use.

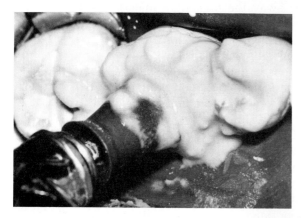

Figure 12–77. Pumice slurry in a rubber cup polishing amalgam restorations. Isolation of the area with a rubber dam is highly desirable.

Figure 12–78. Polished Class I amalgam restorations. (Courtesy of Dr. Loren V. Hickey)

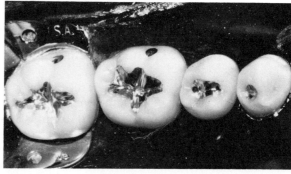

nated, tend to act as centers for corrosion. Polishing can be accomplished in a variety of ways, the selection of which way being a matter of personal choice and preference. Basically, however, the hardened surface is abraded smooth with a stone or finishing bur. This action eliminates irregularities and makes the surface flush with the enamel.

Having accomplished this, the scratches are reduced in magnitude so that a smooth, relatively shiny surface results. As noted, a smooth surface is desirable because it is more compatible with gingival tissue and is less likely to retain microbial plaques.

Occlusal and gingival surfaces are relieved of irregularities with a green stone, either SHP or RA. Stones for this purpose are tapered (pointed) or in the shape of an inverted cone (see Figs. 3–17, 3–19, and 14–20). Tapered stones function most effectively when dressed to a point. Inasmuch as the point wears down first, it should frequently be re-dressed against a diamond stone to provide it with a new tip (see Fig. 3–20).

Additional finishing of occlusal surfaces is then accomplished with finishing burs (see Fig. 14–23) of appropriate sizes and shapes (e.g., Nos. 4 pear, 2 round, and 242 flame) or the Shofu abrasive polishing system (Fig. 12–75). Another method employs pumice slurry (coarse grit denture pumice followed by fine flour of pumice). A final shine is obtained by using tin oxide, powdered chalk, or Amalgloss. This pumice slurry is used wet and is applied by tufted bristle brushes or by a rubber polishing cup. The powdered chalk, tin oxide, or Amalgloss is applied as dry powder. A final shine can be obtained as shown in Figures 12–76 to 12–78).

Proximal surfaces are very difficult to polish because of their inaccessibility. From routine bite wing radiographs during a routine dental examination it is quite apparent that it is difficult to even carve away the excess amalgam that overlaps the tooth, much less be able to polish the proximal surface (see Figs. 11–32 and 12–43). In fact many practitioners routinely take post-operative bite wing radiographs to be sure an inadvertent "overhang" has not been left undetected.

Using files, spoon excavators, and gold knives the operator can remove excess material and render the surface reasonably smooth. A sharp spoon excavator is especially helpful in trimming and shaping proximal surfaces (Fig. 12–79). A sharp discoid carver, for example, may be used to cut away unwanted amalgam in the mesial concavity of maxillary first bicuspids (Fig. 12–80).

After finishing the proximal surface as much as possible with hand instruments efforts can be made to impart a polish with finishing strips. A narrow finishing strip* can be threaded underneath the contact point (Fig.

---

*Extra-long linen finishing strips (fine grit, extra narrow width) available from Moyco Co., 21st and Clearfield St., Philadelphia, Pennsylvania 19132.

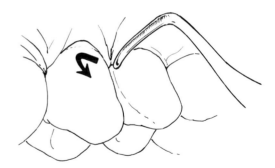

Figure 12–79. Spoon excavator with cutting side against the tooth. It can serve as a proximal carver when the amalgam begins to harden and is even effective at times in removal of overhangs from old restorations.

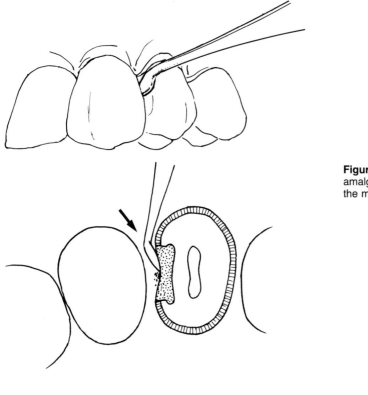

Figure 12–80. Discoid carver removing amalgam from the mesial concavity of the maxillary first premolar.

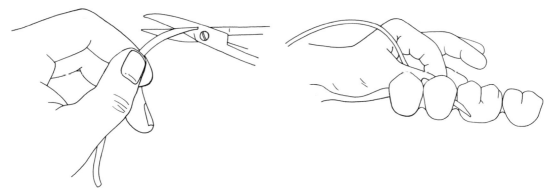

Figure 12–81. Polishing beneath the contact point with an abrasive strip.

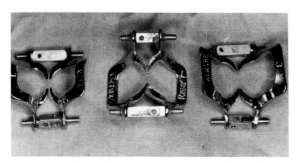

Figure 12–82. Ferrier separators, sizes No. 1, 2, 3 (Almore International). Size No. 2 is intended for cuspids or large incisors. Size No. 3 (right) is for premolars.

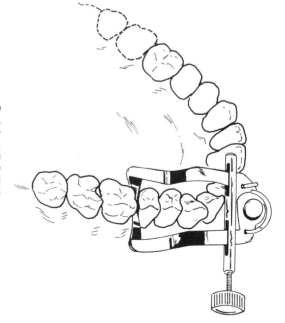

Figure 12–83. Elliott separator (often known as the crab-claw separator). Less forceful than the Ferrier type, it often requires compound for stabilization while polishing the proximal surface. It is rapidly and quickly applied. The tightening screw can be removed and inserted from the other side if one chooses to separate teeth on the right side of the arch. This separator is available with straight or curved jaws; also anterior and posterior types are available.

12–81), where it can be passed back and forth to impart a degree of polish to the gingival half of the restoration.

Unfortunately there is no ideal method for polishing a contact point. Although somewhat cumbersome, a separator can be applied to jack the teeth apart enough to gain space for an abrasive finishing strip. Two kinds of separators, the Ferrier type (Fig. 12–82) and the Elliott type (Fig. 12–83) can be used for this purpose. Because mesial distal separation is usually achieved only with great force, the Ferrier separator* is more effective. The bows can be braced with compound on the occlusal surfaces of the teeth to prevent the separator from sliding up the roots as force from the turnbuckles is applied (Fig. 12–84). If on the other hand the teeth are somewhat mobile the Elliott† separator is more conveniently and quickly applied.

---

*Ferrier separators available from Almore International, P.O. Box 25214, Portland, Oregon 97225.

†Elliott separators available from J. W. Ivory Co., 6019 Keystone St., Philadelphia, Pennsylvania 19135.

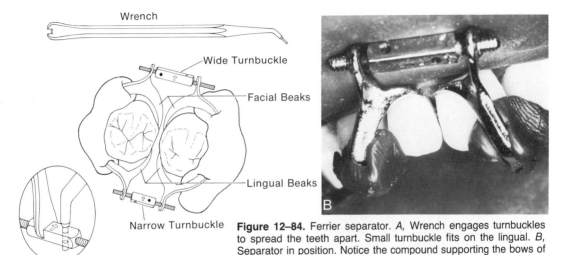

Figure 12–84. Ferrier separator. *A,* Wrench engages turnbuckles to spread the teeth apart. Small turnbuckle fits on the lingual. *B,* Separator in position. Notice the compound supporting the bows of the instrument so it will not slip gingivalward.

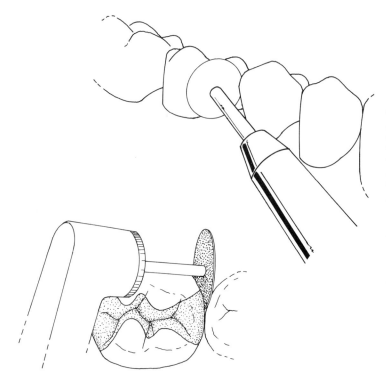

Figure 12–85. Finishing margins with tiny abrasive disks. The use of the straight handpiece for accessible amalgam surfaces is obvious (above). The technique for finishing the mesial surface of an amalgam below the height of contour is not so obvious. These mesiobuccal and lingual surfaces can be polished with an "inside mounting" of the disk in a contra-angle mandrel (below). "Inside mounting" versus "outside mounting" refers to whether or not the abrasive surface faces the head of the handpiece.

Accessible proximal margins and occlusal embrasures are best finished with small garnet and cuttlefish disks (Fig. 12–85; see also Fig. 3–33A). Lack of access caused by the adjacent tooth restricts their use to only the embrasure areas; however, many contact points and proximal surfaces can be polished completely with disks if the operator plans ahead. Figure 12–86 illustrates a mesial surface of a mandibular molar being polished before applying the matrix to condense a disto-occlusal restoration in the second bicuspid.

Final polishing of the Class II amalgam is accomplished similarly to the Class I or the Class V restoration. When shaped to a point, tufted bristle brushes are good for concave surfaces, especially occlusal pits. Flexible rubber cups are suitable for convex surfaces. One should revolve them slowly and avoid the production of frictional heat (Fig. 12–87).

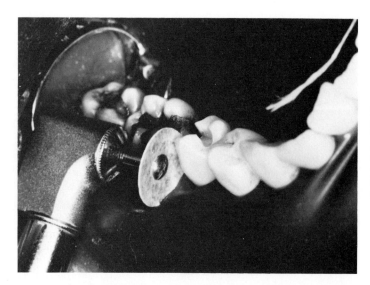

Figure 12–86. Polishing a proximal surface adjacent to a prepared cavity. This added service to a patient takes only a few moments and it can assist the patient in flossing the contact point. Note thin-headed mandrel and ⅜-inch diameter disks (see Fig. 3–33).

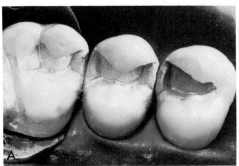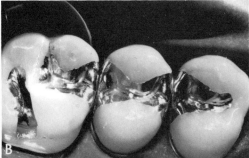

Figure 12–87. Amalgam restorations after carving *(A)* and after polishing *(B)*. Notice the polish extending into the proximal areas.

Miscellaneous Considerations

Marginal Ridges and Occlusal Embrasures. In the process of carving Class II amalgams the operator is inclined to carve the occlusal surface before the proximal. In so doing he will establish an occlusal groove pattern with mesial and distal pits placed too far apart. This results in a marginal ridge without occlusal embrasures (Fig. 12–88). Had the proximal surfaces of the first bicuspid (Fig. 12–88) been carved before placing the pits this optical illusion of distance would not have taken place and this error would have been averted. The thin interproximal carver is an effective instrument for carving the facial, lingual, and gingival embrasures and it will serve equally as well for placing the occlusal embrasure. When they are placed before attempting the occlusal anatomy, the carvings are more proportional and the marginal ridges are correctly located.

Another method for forming this embrasure and a good contact point is to use the Palodent sectional matrices with BiTine rings* (Fig. 12–89). These matrices are swaged to simulate the proximal form of a posterior tooth, including the occlusal embrasure. After the tooth has been prepared a sectional matrix band is gently pinched together so it will conform to the radius of the tooth at contact level as well as fit closely to the facial and lingual enamel surfaces. High gingivae may require trimming off some of the metal from the

*Sectional matrices and BiTine rings available from Palodent Co., 75 Bear Gulch Drive, Portola, California 94025.

Figure 12–88. Maxillary bicuspid carved without occlusal embrasures. Mesial and distal pits placed too far apart to provide space for proper marginal ridge contour.

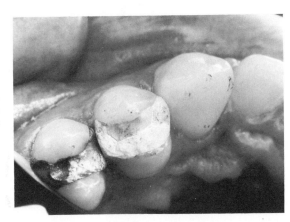

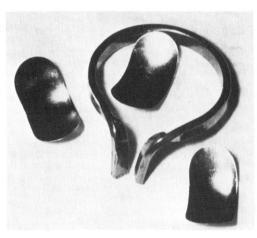
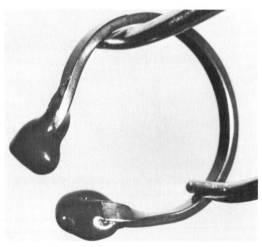

Fig. 12–89 Fig. 12–90

Figure 12–89. Sectional matrices with preformed contours and BiTine ring. (Courtesy of Dr. Alvin Meyer)

Figure 12–90. BiTine ring held in spread position with rubber dam clamp forceps. Note red compound over the tines. (Courtesy of Dr. Alvin Meyer)

matrix in order for it to fit into position. When it is seated a wedge is placed in a conventional manner.

The BiTine ring (Fig. 12–90) is shown with a 3 mm globule of compound applied to each of its tine tips. Grasping the ring with rubber dam forceps, it is quickly stabbed into an alcohol flame to plasticize the outer layer of compound without melting the inner layer. The ring is carried to the mouth, placed into the embrasures, and allowed to collapse. The spring action firmly and rigidly seals the band around the cavity as well as imparts a supplemental separating action.

The gingival seal is checked. The matrix is massaged with a ball burnisher to perfect the contour before condensing the amalgam (Fig. 12–91). After condensation is complete the ring is spread apart and removed, followed by a lateral removal of the matrix. The teeth will tend to return to their original positions and dimple the amalgam at the contact point, leaving good proximal contour and a pre-carved occlusal embrasure (Fig. 12–92).

Mercury Contamination of Gold. As mentioned previously, mercury has an affinity for tin and silver. This attraction is only casual compared with the

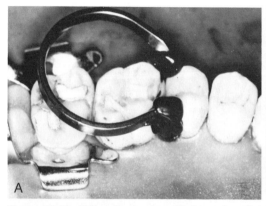
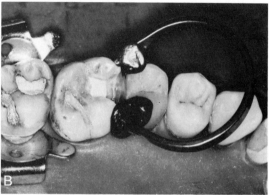

Figure 12–91. BiTine ring in place (*A,* forward or *B,* backward) to stabilize the sectional matrix and to provide some separation.

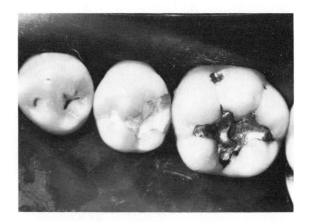

Figure 12–92. Finished Class II amalgam with proper embrasure form and contact area. (Courtesy Lori Harner)

aggressive manner in which mercury attacks a fresh surface of gold. Nothing is quite as frustrating as to see a nicely polished gold casting become "silvery and white" from untoward contact with fresh amalgam (mercury).

Prevention is the best advice that can be given when fresh amalgam is used on or near gold. Prevention consists of the following measures:

1. Coat the gold surface with a copal varnish insulator.

2. Isolate potential areas with a rubber dam barrier.

3. Impart no rubbing action to the gold that would disturb an oxide layer and permit the mercury and gold to make contact.

4. Never use on gold a polishing cup that has recently encountered fresh amalgam.

If contamination does occur and is discovered before the patient is dismissed, it can be abraded away before it "sinks in" and crystallization occurs. Copious amounts of pumice in a rapidly revolving rubber cup will usually render the crown surface yellow again and the mercury will be gone.

If a period of time elapses and in-depth contamination has occurred, the scars of the amalgamated gold will reveal themselves as dark gray blotches. These will be permanently embedded in the surface, and efforts to grind them out are usually impractical.

If a gold casting becomes contaminated with mercury outside the mouth, it is simply held in an alcohol (or gas) flame at 500° F, whereupon the mercury evaporates. Needless to say, mercury bound up in crystals with silver, tin, or copper poses no problem whatever; only freshly mixed amalgam is of any concern in this regard (Fig. 12–93).

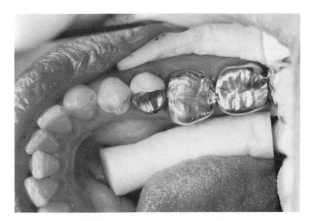

Figure 12–93. Molar crown contaminated with mercury. An access entry for endodontic therapy was closed with amalgam without care being exercised to protect the surrounding gold with varnish.

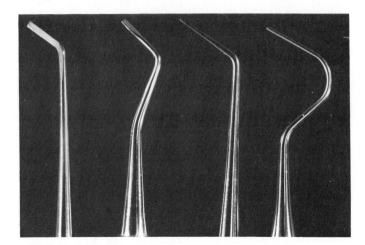

Figure 12–94. Amalgam condensers designed by Dr. Miles Markley are excellent for condensing amalgam around pins. Round condenser on the right measures 0.5 mm in diameter, rectangular on the left, 0.5 × 0.9 mm.

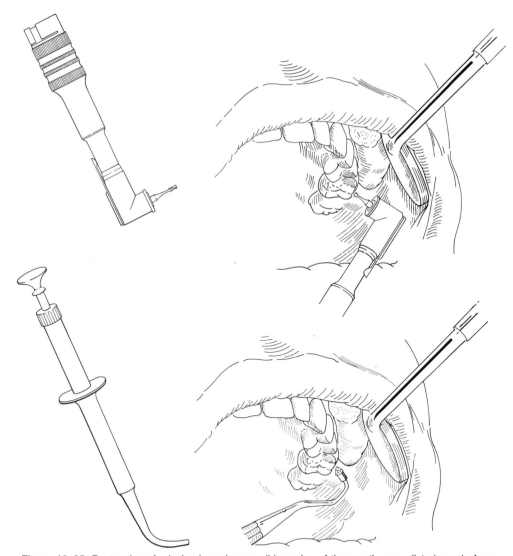

Figure 12–95. Restoration of a lesion in an inaccessible region of the mouth, e.g., disto-buccal of an upper second molar. Miniature head right angle handpiece with short neck burs (see Fig. 3–6) is used to prepare the cavity. Tactile sense is very important here; hence the need for slow-speed cutting. Amalgam is deposited with a right angle amalgam carrier and packed with a back action condenser.

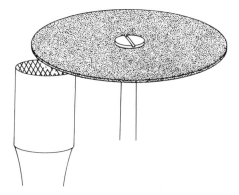

Figure 12–96. Reduction of a serrated surface to a smooth one.

Condensation Around Pins. Amalgam may be fast setting or slow setting, depending upon factors controlled by the manufacturer. In most restorations it is to the advantage of the experienced operator to work with a fast setting material so carving need not be delayed and the patient can be dismissed without danger of amalgam fracture. On the other hand, a slower setting amalgam could sometimes be preferred.

Particularly does this become important in a large restoration with pins present. The first capsule is mixed and placed into the base of the cavity in a traditional fashion. To maximize the benefits from this plastic property the amalgam in the base of the cavity is condensed one carrier load at a time. Intricate adaptation around crevices, slots, pins, and so on is thereby permitted, especially when small properly shaped condensers are used (Fig. 12–94).

As mentioned earlier, lathe-cut alloy does not adapt itself to surface irregularities as well as spherical alloy. The spherical particles allow the material to be more readily molded and adapted against threaded pins. The concerned operator therefore would do well to use spherical alloy—at least for the first capsule—for large restorations involving threaded pins or other intricate internal details.

If use of the amalgam carrier delays insertion, it may be laid aside and increments placed into the band with cotton pliers. A large condenser is used to settle the material into position, followed by one of medium size to pack it securely in place. In this manner the bulk of the restoration is rapidly built to size.

Figure 12–97. Cross-hatching a smooth-faced condenser to transform it into a serrated surface (see Fig. 3–66). Note the shape of the knife edge disk in Figure 3–65.

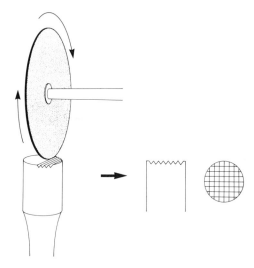

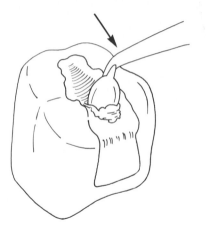

Figure 12–98. Carving without an enamel guide frequently leads to a scooped-out occlusal surface.

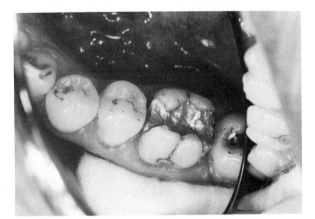

Figure 12–99. A common mistake in occlusal carving. Too much amalgam has been removed from the occlusal area.

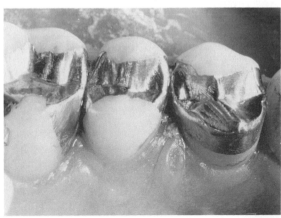

Figure 12–100. Maxillary amalgam restorations. Note replacement of lingual cusp of first premolar. (Courtesy of Dr. Robert Birtcil, Masson Monographs in Dentistry)

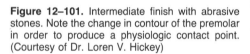

Figure 12–101. Intermediate finish with abrasive stones. Note the change in contour of the premolar in order to produce a physiologic contact point. (Courtesy of Dr. Loren V. Hickey)

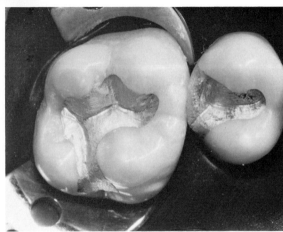

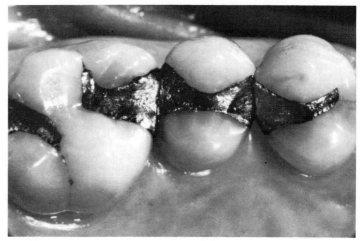

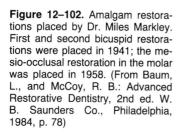

Figure 12–102. Amalgam restorations placed by Dr. Miles Markley. First and second bicuspid restorations were placed in 1941; the mesio-occlusal restoration in the molar was placed in 1958. (From Baum, L., and McCoy, R. B.: Advanced Restorative Dentistry, 2nd ed. W. B. Saunders Co., Philadelphia, 1984, p. 78)

Difficult-to-Reach Areas. Disto-facial corners of maxillary second molars, for example, can pose a challenge in condensation. Because the angle of the barrel must be at 90° to the tip, most carriers are unsuited for placing amalgam into these cavities. Moreover, the use of a back action condenser is also helpful in directing condensation forces properly (Fig. 12–95).

Serrated condensers are not always available. Although not as nicely cut as those produced by the manufacturer, a smooth-faced condenser can be rapidly transformed into a serrated one and a serrated surface reduced rapidly to a smooth one. A carborundum disk sharpened to a wedge (see Fig. 3–65) can crosshatch a smooth surface and make it serrated (Figs. 12–96 and 12–97).

Occlusal Considerations. The strength of the amalgam depends upon its bulk. While no restoration should be "high" in occlusion, it is not necessary to reduce the occlusal surface beyond physiologic occlusion. A common error is to overcarve (undercontour) occlusal surfaces. Causes for occlusal "bathtubs" may be conceptual or manipulative, but the end result leaves insufficient material inside the occlusal surface. Carving parallel with the margins with a cleoid or discoid carver will invariably result in too much amalgam being scooped out of the occlusal area (Figs. 12–98 and 12–99).

Where cusps must be restored it is usually wise to build them back slightly short of their original height. Particularly is this true of buccal cusps of maxillary molars and lingual cusps of mandibular molars. Supporting cusps, however, cannot be arbitrarily shortened. When they are depended upon to provide the vertical stability of the tooth, the restored cusp should make centric contact during closure. Delicate controlled closure on articulating paper by the patient is necessary so that equal loading between the restored cusp and the enamel supporting cusp of an adjacent tooth is achieved.

Restoring teeth with amalgam can be an enjoyable experience, both in the performance of the procedure and in the sense of satisfaction derived from providing a superior restorative service for a patient (Figs. 12–100 through 12–102).

13

RETENTIVE PINS IN OPERATIVE DENTISTRY

Restorations, as observed in Chapters 10 and 11, are customarily anchored by small undercuts in dentin. When a large portion of the crown is missing because of caries or for other reasons, it is difficult to obtain this anchorage. Pins anchored in the dentin serve this need quite nicely, as the restorative material is packed around them (Fig. 13–1).

Pins are made of gold-plated stainless steel; however, titanium pins have recently become popular. Pins vary in diameter from 0.35 to 0.8 mm and are approximately 5 mm long, one end fastened into dentin, the other surrounded by amalgam or composite resin. Knurled or serrated threads extend their full length to provide better anchorage into the dentin and filling material surrounding them.

Pins fall within one of two categories: those whose diameters are slightly larger than the drills that prepared their channels and those whose diameters are slightly smaller than the corresponding drill. The latter require a cementing medium to attach them to the tooth;* the former rely upon the elasticity of the dentin to secure their retention. The most popular pin, the TMS self-threading pin,† falls in the former category and is screwed into position with a kind of miniature wrench. Its popularity is based primarily upon its anchorage value, which may be 10 times that of the pin that is cemented. Needless to say, a self-threading pin must have a precise fit lest the threads strip the inner lining of the hole; if the hole is too small, the pin will fit too tightly and fail to reach full depth of the pin channel. Another danger of a tight-fitting pin is the risk of splitting off a piece of the tooth while inserting it, especially if the tooth has received endodontic treatment.

The Twist Drill

Success with a pin technique requires a working knowledge of three things: the drill, the pin, and the dentin. Foremost in developing a precision technique is the use of the twist drill. As one compares its shape to that of a dental bur, a marked difference is apparent. It cuts only on the end; a dental bur, which is a router, cuts on all sides. The two cutting blades of the drill

---

*Because of limited usage, this chapter will not deal with the cemented pin.
†Whaledent, Inc., 236 Fifth Ave., New York, New York 10001.

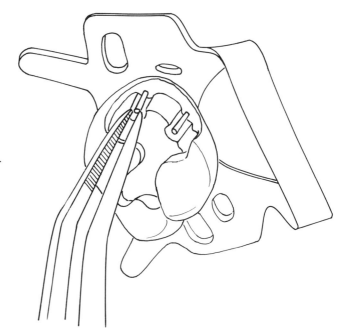

Figure 13–1. Pins are used to fasten amalgam to the tooth.

tip are sloped so that they will cut only when the drill is turning in a clockwise direction (Fig. 13–2) (also see Figure 3–1). A masonry drill (Fig. 13–3) has a bi-bevel end, which pulverizes the material and carries it away with the spiral edges of the shaft.

Figure 13–4 shows two twist drills with different helix patterns. For cutting dentin, the one on the right is preferred because its flutes are less likely to become clogged with dentin; the one on the left is designed for cutting metal and to withstand strong torquing forces, which are not encountered when cutting dentin.

Four things should be kept in mind when using the twist drill: (1) run the drill at a slow speed, (2) be sure the drill is sharp, (3) withdraw the drill frequently to allow the flutes to be cleared of pulverized dentin (Fig. 13–4), and (4) maintain good hand bracing lest uncontrolled movements result in a hole with an enlarged orifice.

Conquering fear is a major factor in drilling pinholes. The student would

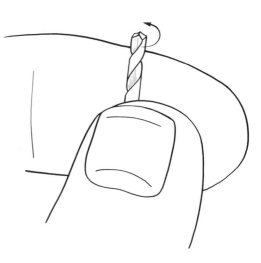

Figure 13–2. Proper rotation of the drill is necessary for effective cutting.

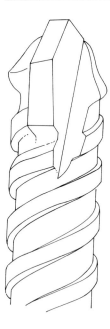

Figure 13–3. Masonry drill with cutting blade on the end. When sharpening a dull drill, identical slopes and bevels are reproduced.

do well to drill holes at random in an extracted tooth to gain familarity with the drill and its actions. Particularly important in this regard is the recognition of a dull drill from a sharp drill. With some experience a dentist can recognize a dull drill by its "feel" while cutting dentin and he need not resort to a microscope to determine whether the drill is dull or sharp (Fig. 13–5).

Insofar as possible, drilling should be done against a flat surface. Drilling against a sloping surface makes calculation of pinhole depth difficult (Fig. 13–6). It is the general consensus among operative dentists that pinholes should be approximately 2 mm in depth. Accordingly, manufacturers are inclined to place a depth-limiting shoulder on the drills, which of course,

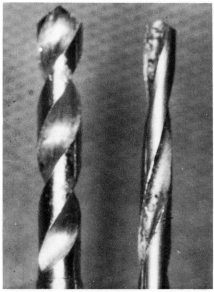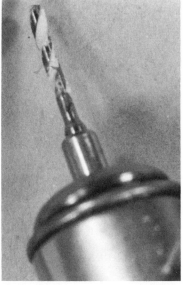

Figure 13–4. Two twist drills with different helix patterns. Because of their spiral pattern, the flutes on the left drill are more likely to become clogged with dentin chips. Clogged flutes can cause enlarged holes or crazed lines in the dentin.

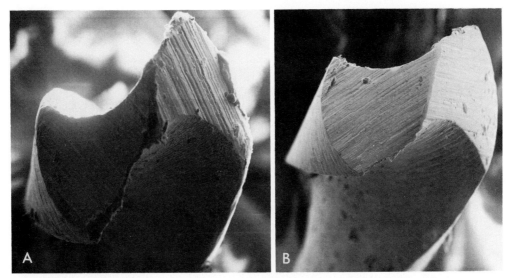

Figure 13–5. Under a microscope a dull drill can be quickly recognized. Note the rounded corner of the leading edge of the dull drill in *A*.

restricts the placement of a deeper hole. Furthermore, it restricts sharpening of the drill because sharpening even further reduces its length (Figs. 13–7 and 13–8; see also Fig. 3–62).

Ultra-slow speed is not required in drilling a pinhole, but high speed is definitely contraindicated. Operating at a relatively slow speed in the regular contra-angle handpiece, the twist drill is a very efficient cutting instrument.

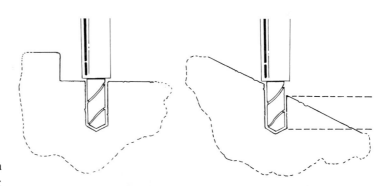

Figure 13–6. Drilling against a sloping surface and a flat surface. Effective pinhole depth is reduced by nearly 50% when the pinhole is placed in a sloping surface and a self-limiting drill is used. The "stop" of the self-limiting drill also tends to impair the vision of the operator.

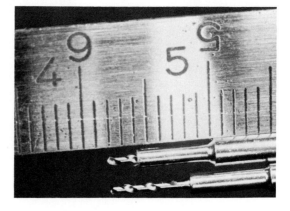

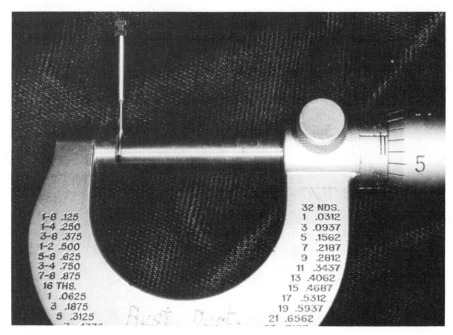

Figure 13–7. Machinist's micrometer measuring drill diameter. Each revolution of the rod measures .025 in.; each mark on the dial measures .001 in. Such an instrument is a valuable aid in pin procedures and may be purchased at a hardware store.

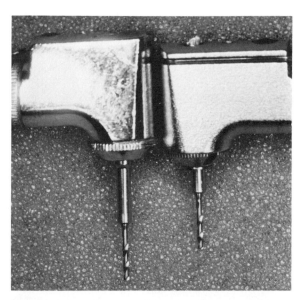

Figure 13–8. Drills of unequal overall length, but with the ability to drill holes of equal depth. The drill on the left is preferred because the handpiece head is less likely to restrict vision; the drill on the right is more suitable for work on molars, because of restricted space when the mouth is open.

The Retentive Pin

As mentioned earlier, many pins are made of gold-plated stainless steel and correspond in size to the diameter of the matching drill. Composite and microfil resins are translucent. A steel-colored pin is less desirable than a gold-plated pin for use in anterior teeth because the gold plating helps mask out the discoloration of the darker metal.

Occasionally pins require bending, which is best done with a special tool (miniature pickle fork) (see Fig. 13–32). Following placement, pins must frequently be cut to provide proper length. Perhaps this would best be accomplished with miniature wire cutters; however, most clinicians use a bur with sharp corners to cut through the pins, as shown in Figure 13–9. Because they are made from stainless steel, pins cannot be cut readily with a bur, especially a dull bur. Tending to work-harden, the metal becomes tough and generates considerable heat from friction of the bur. So inclined are they to temperature rise that they should be cooled when they are being cut. Water coolant is not necessary if a generous stream of air is employed and the nozzle of the air syringe is held close to the bur. Figure 13–9 illustrates the most effective position for holding the bur to cut the pin. Figure 13–10 illustrates the incorrect angle for cutting off a pin.

Pins are prepared with deep threads (Fig. 13–11) to suitably engage the dentin at one end and the restorative material at the other. The pitch of the threads is right-handed, the same as a wood or metal screw, and is turned clockwise to advance the pin into the channel. In the process of using a dental bur to cut off a pin, the bur also has a clockwise direction of rotation. The surface friction from the bur engages the side of the pin and tends to unscrew it out of its pinhole. This tendency can be offset if the pin is grasped by a hemostat or with cotton pliers as a second choice. This also helps stabilize the pin and keeps it from chattering during the cutting process (Fig. 13–12). Vibration can also cause a loosely anchored pin to fall out of the pinhole.

Total pin length is approximately 4 to 5 mm. Half of its length (2.5 mm) is anchored in the dentin, half in the composite or amalgam. Longer lengths are not especially advantageous. Length has some bearing with regard to pin diameter, however. Pins with smaller diameter naturally have reduced holding power and are shorter in length. Sizes of pins, measured in diameter at the crest of their threads, are shown in Table 13–1.

Despite the intriguing delicacy with which the smaller pins are made, it must be recognized that the larger pins, sizes 0.6 mm and 0.75 mm diameter, are more useful in ordinary operating procedures; the former for premolars,

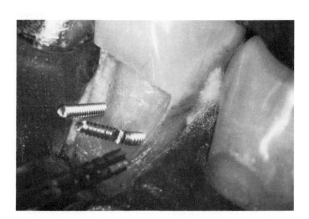

Figure 13–9. Correct angulation for cutting off a pin. The bur cannot have a rounded end, and its blades must be very sharp to restrict heat generation.

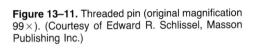

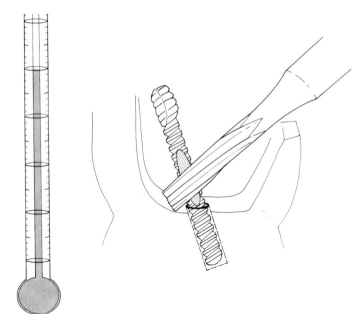

Figure 13–10. Incorrect angulation of a bur for cutting a pin. Air coolant, with the syringe tip close to the pin, is mandatory whenever any pin is cut.

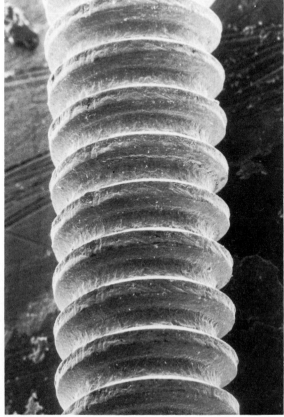

Figure 13–11. Threaded pin (original magnification 99×). (Courtesy of Edward R. Schlissel, Masson Publishing Inc.)

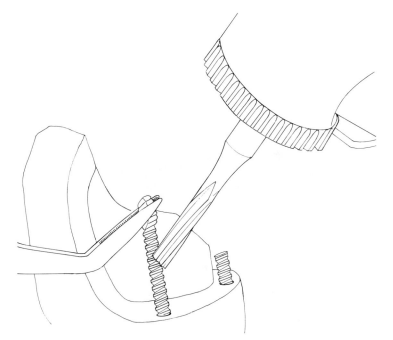

Figure 13–12. Stabilization of the pin while cutting. A mosquito hemostat is preferred over cotton pliers.

the latter for molars. Although no hard and fast rule can be applied, one should lean toward using the larger pins. As a carpenter selects the size of nail to be used in a given location, so the operative dentist will select the size of pin to match the amount of available dentin. Figure 13–13 shows two stiff regular-size pins being employed to add length to a mandibular lateral incisor for a geriatric patient.

For purposes of insertion, pins are flattened on the end to enable the wrench to engage the pin. The regular type of pin has only a flattened end; the self-shearing type is necked (Fig. 13–14) to a smaller diameter so it will break free and not require cutting to the proper length. This feature is advantageous from one point of view but disadvantageous from another. A self-shearing pin might encounter unusual resistance during its insertion and break free from its handle after only 5 or 6 threads have become engaged, leaving the terminal end of the channel unused (Fig. 13–15). Once broken free from its shank, it cannot be engaged by a wrench for removal but must be used as it is.

With the universal acceptance of retentive pins by the profession, other manufacturers have developed innovative designs. One of the most interesting has been the incorporation of the chuck wrench and the pin into one single piece of metal*, which fits into the latch-type right-angle handpiece (Fig. 13–

---

*Stabiloc pins, Pulpdent Corporation of America, Brookline, Massachusetts 02146; PHILPINS, available from Filhol Dental Mfg. Co. Ltd., High St., Chipping Campden, Glas. GL 55 6AT England.

Table 13–1. TMS PIN/DRILL SIZES

Size	Pin Diameter at Crest of Threads	Pin Diameter at Depth of Threads	Drill Diameter
Regular	0.76 mm (.030 in.)	0.60 mm	0.68 mm (.027 in.)
Minim	0.60 mm (.024 in.)	0.46 mm	0.52 mm (.021 in.)
Minikin	0.48 mm (.019 in.)	0.38 mm	0.42 mm (.017 in.)
Minuta	0.37 mm (.015 in.)	0.31 mm	0.34 mm (.0135 in.)

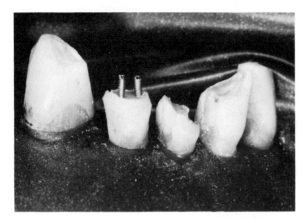

Figure 13–13. Two regular size TMS pins inserted in a lateral incisor for a geriatric patient. (Composite resin will be added to restore the incisal third of the crown.) Alteration of the pins to make them self-tapping permits the placement of such large pins in a small space.

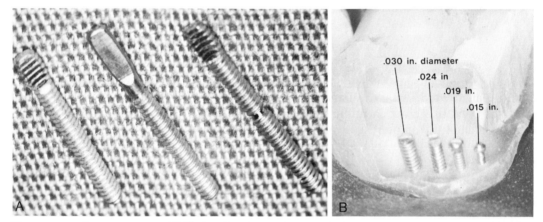

.030 in. diameter

.024 in

.019 in.

.015 in.

Figure 13–14. Styles and sizes of TMS pins. *A, Left*: standard basic type; *center*: self-shearing; *right*: two-in-one. *B,* Comparative sizes, left to right: regular, minim, minikin, minuta.

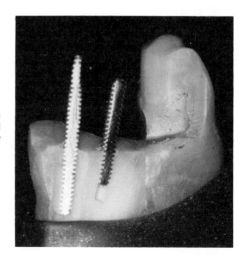

Figure 13–15. Sectional view of basic pin seated full depth in its channel *(left)*, and two-in-one pin with 1 mm of its channel unused *(right)*. The pin sheared before it had been completely seated.

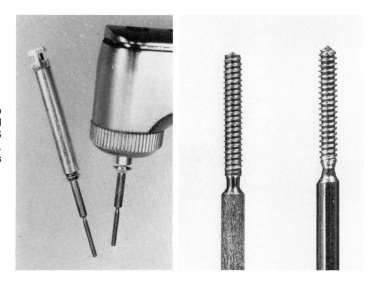

Figure 13–16. *Left,* Pin attached to metal chuck. *Right,* Titanium and stainless steel pins. (PHILPINS available from Filhol Dental Mfg. Co. Ltd., Chipping Campden, Glas GL55 6AT, England)

16). After insertion of the pin into its hole, the wrench becomes disengaged and is thrown away. The major advantages are the elimination of a separate chuck wrench and less effort during insertion of the pin (Figs. 13–17 and 13–18).

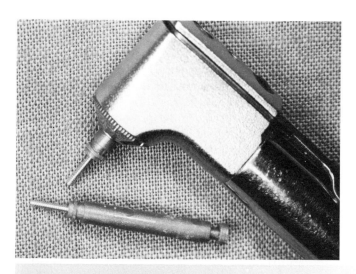

Figure 13–17. Link pins with plastic chuck to fit into the handpiece. When seated the pins strip free from the plastic chuck. (Distributed by Whaledent)

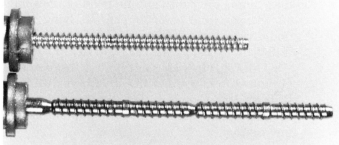

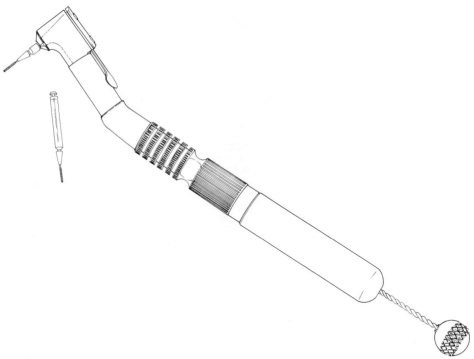

Figure 13–18. Stabiloc pin in pin setter. Like the Link pins, the Stabiloc pin shears off the disposable metal chuck. (Cable-drive pin setter available from Golden West Dental, Inc.)

Dentin as an Anchorage Medium

Simulating ivory or a kind of plastic, dentin can be cut, abraded, or drilled with comparative ease. Its inherent elasticity,* unlike wood or metal, produces a medium that requires different treatment when it is being instrumented. Wood fibers crush under pressure and automatically create a pathway for the crest of the thread of a wood screw. Metal screws permanently deform sheet metal as pathways are prepared for their insertion. Unlike wood or metal screws, dentin screws (pins) are effective to only a limited degree in crushing or deforming dentin to provide grooves for the edges of the threads. Despite sharp edges (Fig. 13–19), the threads of a pin do not produce the desirable grooves in the surface of the pin channel. Instead, they seem to stretch the dentin as they worm their way into position.

It is axiomatic, therefore, that the use of a precision pin technique confine all drilling and pin insertion within the elastic limit of the dentin. Exceeding these limits can cause minute fracture lines internally around the dentin (Fig. 13–19) or crazed enamel. The overlying enamel is not as forgiving as the underlying dentin and responds by developing vertical cracks, the result of a dull drill, clogged flutes, or oversized pin, or all of these (Fig. 13–20).

Drilling pinholes can stretch the dentin if the flutes of the drill are permitted to clog up with pulverized dentin or if the leading corners of the drill blades become dulled. Pin insertion is probably more likely to cause internal trauma than drilling the pinhole, especially when the larger size pins are used.

*Teeth that have lost pulpal vitality are not as elastic as teeth that have normal vital pulps.

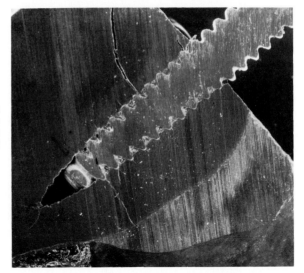

Figure 13–19. Cracks developed from inserting a tightly fitting, self-threading pin. Notice how they tend to develop and radiate where the crest of the thread presses against the dentin. (Courtesy of Schlissel et al., J. Dent. Res.)

All pin insertion is attended by friction and resistance to screwing the pin into place. For a given hole, a larger pin is more resistant (fits more tightly) than a smaller pin. Because of human factors in preparing the holes and the need for the unstressed anchorage of the pins in dentin, tactile sense plays an important role in ascertaining the degree of friction encountered during pin insertion.

Only the hand wrench and the cable-driven pin setter provide the operator with tactile sense for insertion (Fig. 13–21). The hand wrench is suitable when access is possible, e.g., in the premolars and anteriors; the pin setter is more suitable for molars where access is difficult. The pin setter is a latch-type contra-angle handpiece, modified with an extension to provide a handle and flexible shaft with finger knob to transmit rotational forces through the gears to the chuck holding the pin (see Fig. 13–28).*

---

*Available from Golden West Dental Inc., P.O. Box 777, Garden Grove, California 92642.

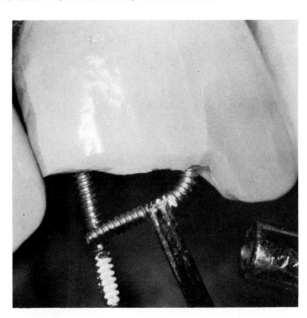

Figure 13–20. Crazed lines in enamel caused by a non-precise technique for pin insertion. Had the self-tapping concept been employed, this crazing would probably have not occurred. Note the incorrect angulation of the bur for cutting off the pins.

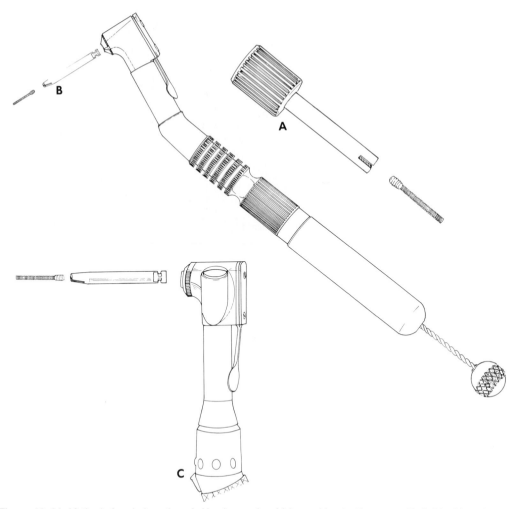

Figure 13–21. Methods for pin insertion. *A,* Hand wrench, which provides tactile sense. *B,* Cable-drive pin setter, which provides tactile sense. *C,* Auto clutch with reduction gear is motor driven and does not provide tactile sense.

If, during insertion, only minimal resistance is encountered, the operator continues turning the wrench until he feels the bottom of the hole, whereupon he *stops* turning.

If, during insertion, strong resistance is encountered, the operator knows that the pin is too large for the hole. Resistance increases with each turn until the self-shearing link breaks loose from the handle. Perhaps it does not reach the bottom of the pinhole; perhaps it is engaged by only several threads (see Fig. 13–15).

If, on the other hand, he has used a standard (not a self-shearing) type, the resistance will reach a magnitude at which he cannot determine whether or not the pin has reached the end of its hole. Because the pin is still intact it can readily be removed and modified to fit properly.

So frequently does the operator encounter a tight fit that he becomes highly suspect of the self-threading procedure for 0.75 mm diameter pins and frequently for the 0.6 mm pins as well. Smaller size pins do not encounter the strong frictional resistance found in the larger sizes, and a mismatch in drill and pin sizes is not as easily detected.

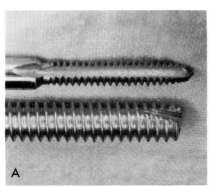
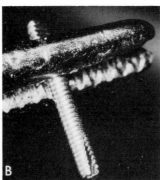
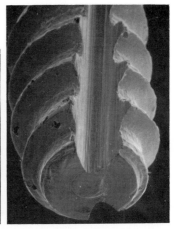

Figure 13–22. *A,* Machinist tap and self-tapping screw. Longitudinal channels in a threaded rod expose sharp corners to cut pathways for the threads. *B,* Makeshift tap prepared from TMS pin. *Left,* Prepared pin held in mosquito hemostat forcep. *Right,* Scanning electron microscopic picture of prepared grooves. This procedure, namely the cutting of two opposing grooves, can be used for regular and minim size TMS pins.

This does not mean that larger size threaded pins should not be used; indeed, they can be most effective in even delicate locations (see Fig. 13–13), but they must be precisely inserted, first by a tap to *cut* the threads rather than by an attempt to mash or crush them into the smooth intact suface of the pin channel.

A separate instrument or tap is not required to place threads in the pinhole. After an attempt is made to insert a pin and tactile sense reveals that the fit is too tight, the pin is removed, grasped by a hemostat, and two V-shaped grooves cut into it to form a self-tapping pin. The self-tapping pin is then inserted into the pinhole by intermittent forward, then backward, turns to enable the exposed sharp corners of the threads to cut grooves into the wall. A well-tapped pinhole provides only modest resistance to the pin, which seats precisely to the full depth of the hole (Figs. 13–22 to 13–25).

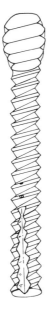

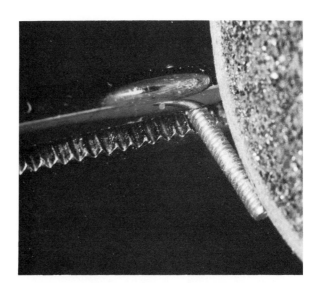

Figure 13–23. Self-tapping pins (preferred method). Cutting grove with altered carborundum disk. Only the terminal 4 to 5 threads need be involved. It is important that the carborundum disk be dressed down with the diamond stone to an ultra-sharp edge (see Fig. 3–65). Binocular loupes or some form of magnification may be necessary when executing these cuts.

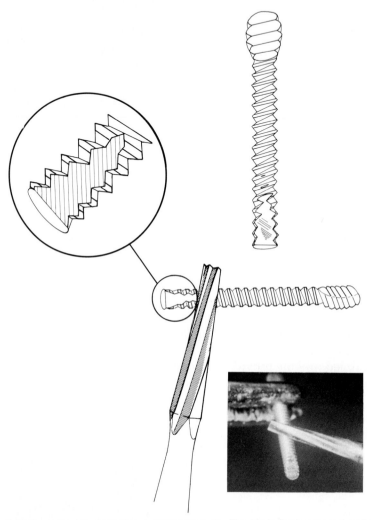

Figure 13–24. Substitute method for preparing a self-tapping pin. The pin is firmly grasped and a high-speed bur is drawn across the edge of the terminal 4 to 5 threads (one side only). Usually one pass with a sharp bur is sufficient to expose sharp corners suitable for cutting threads. Examination of the cut threads should not reveal any round corners.

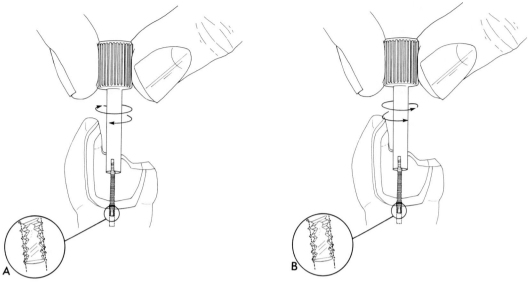

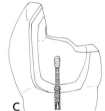

Figure 13–25. Tapping procedure. The prepared pin is easier to start in the hole than an unprepared pin (*A* and *B*). After about three turns to the right, it is reversed for ½ turn. The pin is advanced forward for 1½ to 2 turns, then reversed for ½ turn. The process is continued back and forth until the pin seats firmly against the end of its channel. *C,* The pin should turn freely with back and forth movements before it is advanced farther into its channel. It is not necessary to remove the pin to clear away pulverized dentin.

Drilling and Pin Insertion

Armamentarium

Successful pin placement does not require a large number of specialty items. The procedure might be compared to hanging a picture on the wall. One simply needs matching drills and screws (drill and pin) and a screwdriver (wrench). Depending upon the brand of pin system used and upon the variety of sizes selected, a most simple armamentarium may suffice. The use of specialized handpieces, depth gauges, self-limiting drills, and so on may be helpful to some degree but not actually necessary most of the time. Two lists of instruments and materials have been provided, a basic list and an optional list (Figs. 13–26 and 13–27).

Basic List	*Optional List*
Contra-angle handpiece (latch type)	Auto clutch handpiece (including chucks)
Drill	
Pin	Altered carborundum disk
Hand wrench	Sharp fissure bur
Bur with sharp corners	No. ½ round bur
Bending tool	Hemostat forceps (needle holder)
Cable-driven pin setter (including chucks)	Magnifying glasses

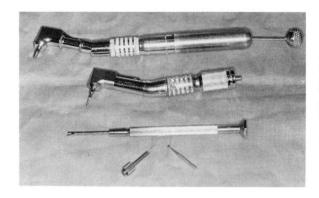

Figure 13–26. Basic setup for pin placement. Contra-angle handpiece (latch type) for drilling pinholes; drill (in handpiece); pin (in hand wrench); hand wrench for accessible pin insertion; cable-drive pin setter for inaccessible pin insertion; bending tool (see Figs. 13–35 and 13–36); bur with *sharp* corners for cutting pin to length.

Use of items in the optional list varies primarily with the accessibility of the site for placement and the individual preferences of the operator. The use of a gear-reduction handpiece (auto clutch handpiece) to insert a pin deprives the operator of the valuable tactile sense. Until a thorough working knowledge is gained, it behooves the student to use a finger-driven rather than a motor-driven wrench (Figs. 13–28 and 13–29).

Trouble Shooting

Of all hazards in pin placement, pulp penetration probably looms greatest in the mind of the beginning student. The experienced clinician on the other hand is more concerned about perforation out the side of the root into the periodontal space. Avoidance of either is possible if the operator exercises reasonable care and planning. Greater perceptibility in tooth alignment, root contours, and pulp morphology will prevent a majority of errors in pulpal penetration or periodontal perforation. Bite wing x-rays, obviously, are of help in this regard.

Pulpal Penetration. Only rarely should pins be placed without rubber dam isolation. If, when drilling in a dry field, a pulp exposure occurs, it is not necessarily a total disaster. Several factors shed some optimistic light on the outcome of such an accidental exposure (Fig. 13–30).

If the rubber dam has been placed and the area is relatively free from microbial contaminants, a sterile pin can produce a hermetic seal to occlude the space and provide a kind of pulp capping. The pinhole that caused the

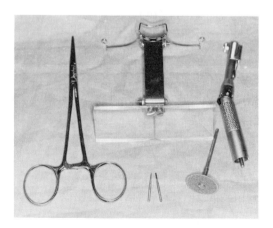

Figure 13–27. Optional setup for pin placement. Auto clutch handpiece for pin insertion without tactile sense; altered carborundum disk with V-shaped edge to prepare self-tapping pin; sharp fissure bur for preparing self-tapping pin; No. ½ round bur as a center spot locator for the pinhole. Hemostat forcep to grasp pin while cutting; magnifying glasses for attaching to eyeglasses. (See Fig. 6–33.)

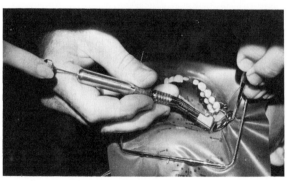

Figure 13–28. Starting the pin. Utilizing the mouth mirror, the operator positions the pin at the orifice of the hole. The dental assistant then turns the knob about two or three revolutions to engage the threads.

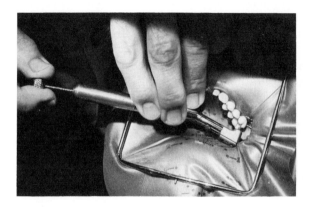

Figure 13–29. Continuing the insertion. The mirror is put aside. The left hand grasps the handpiece for stability while the operator's right hand turns the knob. Tactile sense is achieved as the pin threads its way to the end of the channel.

Figure 13–30. Secondary dentin formation following an experimental pulp exposure of the buccal pulp horn of a maxillary 1st premolar. This pinhole exposure was capped with a TMS pin 4 months prior to this picture. (Courtesy of Dr. Raymond Dolph, D. Clin. N. Amer.)

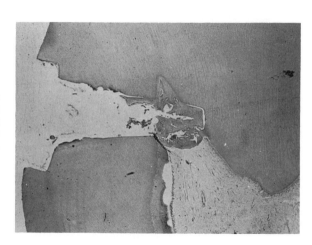

exposure penetrates healthy, not carious, dentin. A seal against leakage and pressure is one of the major clinical requirements for successful direct pulp capping procedures. As with any direct pulp capping there is some risk involved. When one considers the options, namely endodontic therapy, followed possibly by the placement of a ceramo-metal crown, the patient will likely decide to take the risk.

In light of preceding considerations, the operator, following an inadvertent pulp exposure, may choose to insert a sterile pin and continue with the intended restorative procedure. Follow-up examinations with pulp testing at 3 to 6 month intervals should reveal whether or not endodontic therapy might be necessary. If so, access for endodontic treatment can usually be obtained through the occlusal surface without dislodging the restoration.

Periodontal Perforation. Perforation into the periodontal membrane cannot be viewed with the same optimism as a pulp exposure. If penetration is occlusal to the gingival attachment, the floor of the cavity is lowered to eliminate the pinhole. If the perforation is apical to the attachment, there is no ideal method of treatment that can be followed. Some would suggest that the hole be left open and that no treatment be done at all, leaving the opening as a permanent defect in the root. Others would suggest the discreet placement of a pin whose end terminates flush with the surface of the root. Others would suggest the laying of a gingival flap and repairing the hole from the external surface of the root.

Regardless of which option might be chosen, the best results prevail when there is no perforation to repair. A thorough working knowledge of the equipment and self-confidence are great deterrents to pulpal or periodontal involvement. Practice drilling of pinholes in extracted teeth, especially in the cervical regions, is very helpful in this regard.

Broken Drills and Pins. Because of inaccessibility of certain oral locations and because of their delicate nature, broken drills and pins are potential hazards. The primary cause for fracture of a drill is static usage. One cardinal rule should prevail: never insert a drill into a pinhole unless it is turning (revolving). Whether it is inserted when mounted in the handpiece or whether it is inserted digitally (Fig. 13–31), a slight lateral movement by the patient or operator can easily snap the drill.

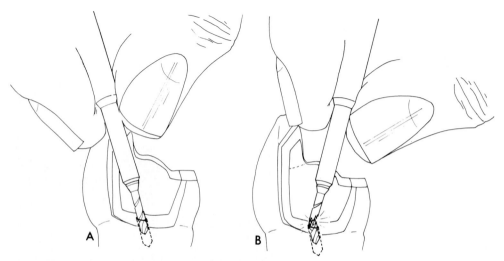

Figure 13–31. *A,* Probing a pinhole with a drill held in the fingers. *B,* A misdirected movement can cause the drill to break.

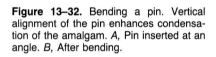
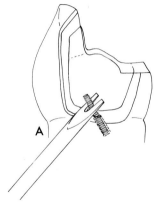
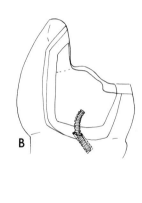

Figure 13–32. Bending a pin. Vertical alignment of the pin enhances condensation of the amalgam. *A*, Pin inserted at an angle. *B*, After bending.

Bending Pins. A most common use of pins is for an amalgam or composite build-up (Fig. 13–33). Insertion of the pin frequently leaves its end extending out beyond the confines of the final preparation, thereby necessitating a change in its direction. Bending a pin, especially if it is made from stiff rigid metal (T.M.S. pins), can be done either correctly with a gradual curve or incorrectly with a sharp bend (see Figs. 13–32 and 13–34). Avoiding pin fracture during bending requires a special bending tool; never use an amalgam condenser to push it to the side.

Customized bending tools are sometimes necessary and should be kept on hand so they can be used for inaccessible locations. Easily fabricated from the end of a bin-angle chisel, discoid carver, or even the end of a large excavator, such tools can be prepared chairside with a carborundum separating disk (Fig. 13–36).

Fracture of a pin can also occur while cutting it to length. Stabilization with a curved mosquito hemostat eliminates the risk of the pin snapping off from the vibration induced by the bur.

The response to a fractured pin or drill is rather simple. Do not attempt removal; simply leave it entombed in the dentin and make another pinhole.

Enlarged Pinholes. If as a result of one or more causes, as discussed earlier in the chapter, the pin fails to engage itself and the threads do not hold the pin in place (Fig. 13–37), the hole obviously has become too large for the pin. One of three things can be done to make the pin more secure: (1) drill the hole deeper and re-insert a fresh pin, (2) redrill a larger hole and use a larger pin, or (3) cement the existing pin in place. Clinical judgment should prevail as to which option should be chosen.

Drill Will Not Cut. A most frustrating experience is to operate the drill

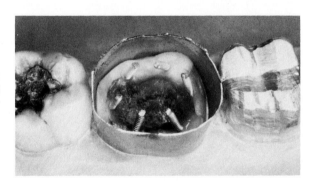

Figure 13–33. Pins, especially for amalgam and composite cores, are bent inward so they will not be exposed by axial reduction of the crown preparation.

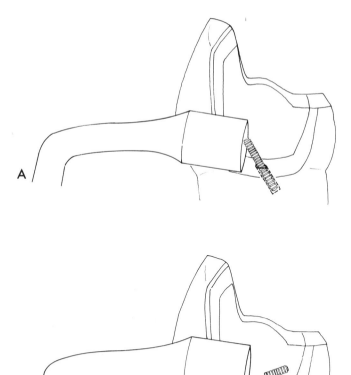

Figure 13–34. How not to bend a pin. *A*, Pins are very rigid and will not tolerate an abrupt bend. *B*, Notice the contrast between the gradual convex bend in Figure 13–32 and the abrupt angle induced by a direct lateral thrust.

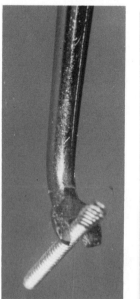
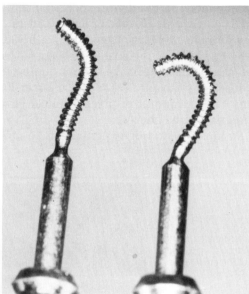

Figure 13–35. Bending tool fabricated from a discoid carver to fit a minim size pin (regular size pin requires a No. 3 discoid carver). The bent instrument permits access to pins placed interproximally. Not all pins are equally susceptible to bending as shown by the PHILPINS on the right.

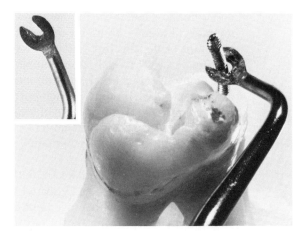

Figure 13–36. Fabricating a bending tool from an enamel hatchet. An excavator serves as a bending tool. (Courtesy of Dr. David Newitter)

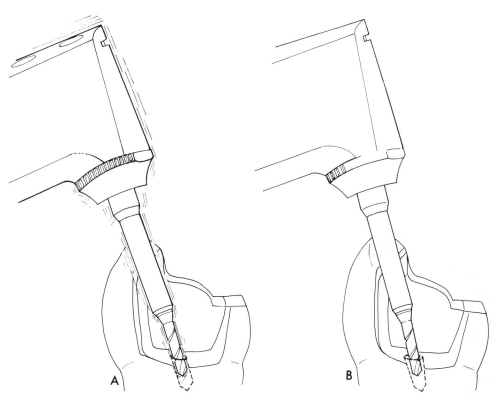

Figure 13–37. Movement of the handpiece during drilling. *A,* Lack of proper bracing and direction during drilling. *B,* Funnel-shaped hole resulting from uncontrolled movement. Salvage of the pinhole can probably be accomplished by cementing a pin in place (see Fig. 13–42).

and discover that it is neither cutting nor making a hole. Inspection should reveal one of the following as the cause: (a) the drill is revolving in the wrong direction, (b) the drill is dull, or (c) the end of the drill is resting on enamel or composite material. In placing a horizontal pin into a buccal cusp, the enamel plate may be much thicker than anticipated. After drilling through 1 to 2 mm of dentin, the drill encounters the inner surface of the enamel and cutting ceases. Enamel is not subject to the cutting action of a twist drill. If, for some reason or other, enamel must be involved in the placement of a pin, a No. ½ round bur in the high-speed handpiece is recommended to assure proper penetration through to the dentin. It also might be mentioned at this point that drilling against enamel or composite is the primary cause for a drill becoming dull. When this happens, always resharpen the drill before using it again.

In developing competence with a pin technique, nothing is quite as important as practice and repeated usage. This will develop skill in the use of the drill and in the management of the pins, and a better knowledge of the internal anatomy of the tooth, particularly in the region of the cervix of the tooth. Last but not least is the psychological boost that practice gives the operator. Fear and apprehension, for some reason or other, cause a student to hold back and not use pins when they are clearly indicated. Repeated practice tends to remove this apprehension and twist drills will become as commonplace in his hands as dental burs.

Sizes, Numbers, and Locations of Pins

When called upon to provide additional anchorage for a restoration the operative dentist must decide what size pins to use, how many are needed, and where they should be placed. Because so many factors are involved, the decision must necessarily be an empirical one.

Pin Size. The approach to pin size is quite simple. Because of its threads, the pin provides retention against vertical withdrawal. This may be thought of as *retention form*. As a rigid prong in the dentin, the pin prevents lateral shifting of the amalgam superstructure because its stiffness resists skidding, torquing, and shifting movements under the forces of mastication. This may

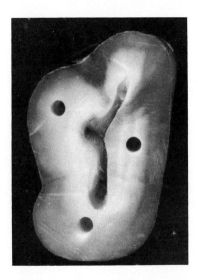

Figure 13–38. Section through the trunk of a maxillary right molar exposing pulp chamber and pin holes from a regular size drill (.030 in. diameter). A thorough knowledge of tooth morphology coupled with a working knowledge of the materials can make pin retention a most common modality in everyday operative procedures.

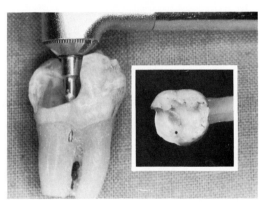

Figure 13–39. Drilling over a bifurcation. Especially on the lingual side of a lower molar the drill is likely to perforate the side of the root.

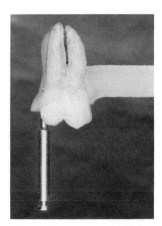

Figure 13–40. Common optical illusion created by angulation of a molar root surface. Disto-buccal perforations out the side of the root are common occurrences.

Figure 13–41. Pin placed in gingival floor. A large proximal preparation, because of its extension to the buccal and lingual, may require additional anchorage to supplement its axial grooves. A single pin placed in the gingival floor fulfills this need nicely. Notice the space behind the pin for easy condensation of amalgam around it. Inset: tooth before removal of carious dentin.

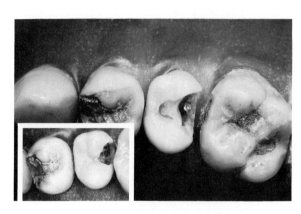

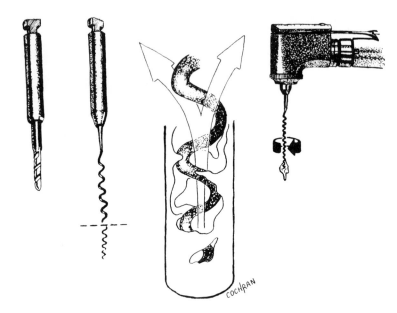

Figure 13–42. A twist drill and lentulo spiral with terminal half removed. The configuration of the spiral permits air to escape through its center while the cement is being spun against the walls of the pinhole. (Courtesy of Dr. Michael Cochran)

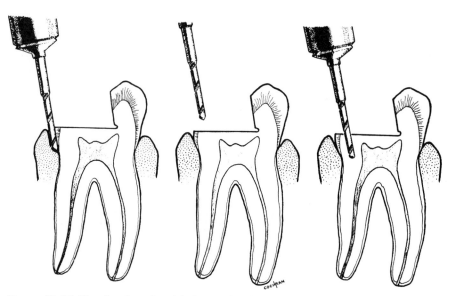

Figure 13–43. The direction of a pinhole may be determined by holding the twist drill parallel to the adjacent external tooth surface. (Courtesy of Dr. Michael Cochran)

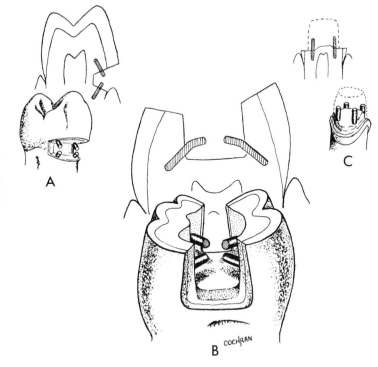

Figure 13–44. Pin-retained amalgam. *A,* Splinting crown to root in badly eroded Class V lesion. *B,* Splinting buccal and lingual cusps together. *C,* Building an amalgam core for anterior crown. (Courtesy of Dr. Michael Cochran)

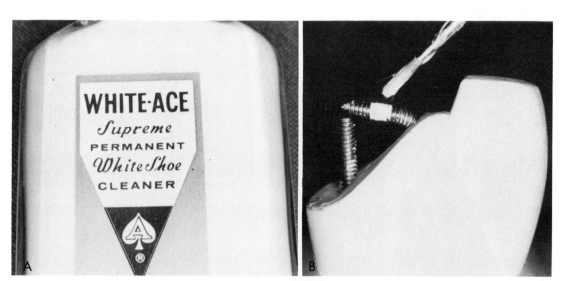

Figure 13–45. Masking pins prevents a metallic cast from showing through the resin. *A,* Shoe polish is thin and dries rapidly. *B,* Painting the labial side of the labial pins to mask the metal.

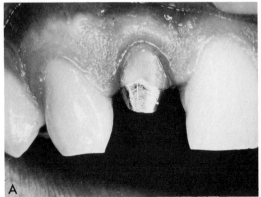

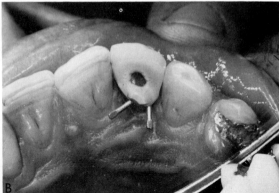

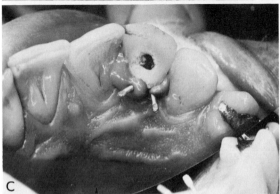

Figure 13–46. Use of pins in an emergency situation to temporarily salvage a poorly fitting crown. *A,* Preparation with severely tapered walls. *B,* Holes drilled through the lingual apron and 2 mm into the tooth. Crown and pins are assembled together. Note: when drilling through a cast gold alloy, the drill should be freely coated with Vaseline as a lubricant to prevent the drill from binding in the metal. *C,* The pins and crown are removed, the cement is mixed, the crown is recemented, and the pins are replaced in their channels. After hardening, the pins are severed flush with the surface of the gold and polished with a disk.

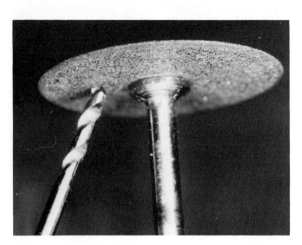

Figure 13–47. Sharpening a twist drill. Simulating the slopes and bevels of a masonry drill (see Fig. 13–3), comparable slopes on the twist drill are redefined with the safe side of a carborundum disk.

be thought of as *resistance form*. Resistance form exceeds retention form by a factor of at least 10 to 1 and must be given major concern in the design of any restoration. Large diameter pins are stiffer than smaller diameter pins and will provide greater resistance form. Categorically, therefore, the operator should use the largest size pins possible. Regular (large) size pins are generally intended for molars; minim size pins for premolars, canines, and some incisors. The smaller sizes, minikin and minuta, are reserved for thin sections of dentin and other areas of restricted space.

Common sense and judgment should prevail when selecting pin size. It is quite reasonable to choose a regular pin for anchoring a restoration into a husky cuspid or even a central incisor. On the other hand, from esthetic considerations, the choice of two small pins in lieu of a single large one might be made in a composite restoration because of proximity of the metal to the surface.

Number of Pins. Because pins provide anchorage and anchorage values are quite relative, pins can vary in number according to the needs of the case at hand. When cusps are lost and axial surfaces of teeth are replaced, a good rule of thumb is to use one pin for each missing cusp and one pin for each missing proximal surface. An MO amalgam with one cusp missing would require two pins; an MOD with both lingual cusps missing would require four. A pin build-up for a premolar could require four if the entire crown was missing.

An excessive number of pins makes amalgam condensation difficult and much of the time the tooth could be restored safely with one or two fewer pins than are actually placed.

Location. Dentin bulk is naturally greater in the coronal part of the tooth because of the location of the pulp cavity. Any pin below the cemento-enamel junction is placed, more or less, in a wall of dentin bordered inside by the pulp and outside by the periodontium. Tendencies are to drill holes closer to the outer border of the wall than toward the inner (pulpal side). More than adequate space is available to place pinholes and the operator should not be reticent to place them in the gingival wall. Only lower anterior teeth and small maxillary lateral incisors provide limited bulk of dentin for pin placement in cervical regions. (Fig. 13–38).

Where this wall of dentin is flat or of uniform contour, pin placement can be routine. Where there are bifurcations or other aberrations, e.g., mesial concavity of maxillary first premolar, pinholes should be avoided. Generally speaking, however, there is a wide range of space available for pin placement, and distribution of these pins to provide suitable anchorage is the goal (Figs. 13–39 to 13–41).

The reader is also directed to Figures 13–42 through 13–47 for miscellaneous hints in using drills and pins. Examples of tooth preparations involving their use can be seen in Chapter 11.

14

DIRECT GOLD AS A RESTORATIVE MATERIAL

General Considerations

Since antiquity, pure gold has been a metal of special intrinsic and practical value. It would be redundant to review the importance that has been placed on this material by individuals and cultures of all ages. From the dawn of civilization until the present time, man has utilized gold in some form or other in the practice of dentistry.

In its pure form, gold has the unusual ability to cohere to itself at room temperature. This is true with certain other metals, but the presence of oxygen in the atmosphere produces an oxide film on the surface of most metals, preventing this welding from taking place. Gold is also quite soft and in a compressible form increments can be welded by pressure into a solid metal mass inside a prepared tooth cavity. The metallic bonding between the overlapped increments produces the "direct gold" restoration.

Another unique feature about gold that has made it an unusual restorative material is its inertness. Under most conditions it does not tarnish, corrode, or stain. The long history of the excellence and permanence of the material prompted the establishment of a special academy* in organized dentistry. As gold has captured the fancy of civilized man throughout history, so has direct gold as a restorative material generated the respect and admiration of sophisticated and exacting operative dentists.

Nevertheless the direct gold restoration is a demanding one. Because of the care and cleanliness required in handling the metal and the organization and skill necessary in its use, cohesive gold has acquired a reputation as a material that embodies perfection in the hands of a skillful, well-trained operative dentist. It is impossible to achieve acceptable results using careless or sloppy techniques.

Lest direct gold be envisioned as the ideal material for all restorative purposes, attention should be first directed toward its limitations, to give the student a proper perspective of its applications.

The lesion to be restored must not be subject to heavy chewing or biting forces. The use of gold is contraindicated for corners of teeth subjected to heavy masticatory stresses. The cavity must not be excessively large because

---

*American Academy of Gold Foil Operators: co-sponsor of *Journal of Operative Dentistry.*

more time and effort is required to place gold than composite or amalgam restorations. Large restorations therefore can be tiring to both operator and patient.

Chalky or mottled enamel could contraindicate the use of gold. Finishing the gold at the marginal area requires forces on the enamel, which could pulverize the surface if it is not of a glassy or "pearly" white texture. The lesion and site of operation must be accessible, as good visibility and operational access are important with this material. Last but not least, a display of gold in a smile could be a deterring factor when used in certain locations in the anterior teeth and maxillary premolars.

Notwithstanding these contraindications, direct gold has its value in all kinds of cavities and in many places within the mouth. It can be used to restore Class I, II, III, IV, and V lesions as well as to repair holes in crowns. Common sense and judgment, tempered by experience, will guide the conscientious operator in the proper use of this material.

Types of Direct Gold

As a raw material for use by a dentist, gold is supplied in three different forms: (1) gold foil, (2) electrolytic precipitate (commonly called mat gold), and (3) powdered gold (Fig. 14–1).

Gold Foil. The oldest form is foil, in which pure gold, being readily malleable, is rolled into extremely thin sheets. Beating these with a mallet produces a leaf of gold with a thickness on the order of 1.5 micrometers. During this process the gold crystals become elongated and under the microscope have a fibrous appearance. Sheets of commonly used dental gold (No. 4 gold foil) cover 16 square inches (4″ × 4″), are approximately 1.5 micrometers thick, and weigh about 250 mg. To render it usable, gold foil is crumpled up into small pellets. The best pellets are made by hand from varying sizes of

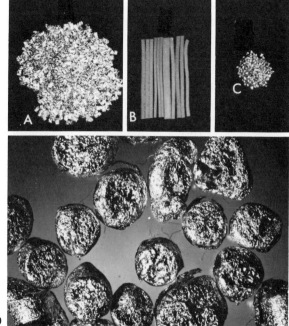

Figure 14–1. Direct gold in common usage. *A,* Gold foil; *B,* mat gold; *C,* powdered gold. The increments of gold are ready to be heat treated and packed into the prepared cavity. *D,* Enlarged pellets of powdered gold (Goldent).

foil (usually ½″ × ½″ square). Gold foil "cylinders," mechanically prepared pellets, are also available.

Mat Gold. Mat gold is prepared by electrolytic deposition, which is similar to an electroplating process, albeit at an accelerated rate of deposition, so the resultant material has a spongy structure of loosely aligned crystals. During a subsequent heating process the branch ends are rounded and tend to weld themselves together (see Fig. 14–13). During condensation these crystals are compacted into a solid mass within the prepared cavity. This mat material is supplied in conveniently sized strips or loaves that can be cut to fit the size of the cavity when they are ready to be used.

Worthy of note is a popular crystalline gold, Electralloy R.V.,* which contains small amounts of calcium as an alloying agent, which produces a harder surface to the restoration.

Powdered Gold. Powdered gold is a blend of atomized and precipitated powder embedded in an organic matrix. From this material variously sized pellets are cut, encased in gold foil wrappers, and packaged for use (Fig. 14–1).

Other direct golds in various forms and modifications could be described, but they can be classified as one of these three types: foil, mat, or powdered. Another material, platinized gold foil,† imparts a white color to the material and increases its hardness.

Heat Treatment of Gold

Gold should be kept in a closed container when not in use and never exposed to contaminants. It is axiomatic that instruments, fingers, and environment be ultra-clean and that gold be used only in a dry field. All three types of gold must receive heat treatment just prior to condensation. This is done to de-gas the surface of the gold and render it cohesive. Some of these gases may be driven off by heat; others are irreversibly attached. Gases composed of sulfur and phosphorus compounds fall in this latter category and are readily produced by matches. These gases to some degree are inherently present in a smoggy environment.

Reversible contaminant gases, i.e., oxygen, can be readily removed by treatment with heat in the range of 900° to 1300°F. Heat treatment (annealing) may also alter the crystalline formation of the metal, making it more cohesive. For whatever reason, de-gassing or change of grain structure, heat treatment renders the material cohesive and workable, although too much heat in time and temperature causes gold to become brittle.

Heat treatment may be accomplished in an open flame or on a hot plate (Fig. 14–2). With gold foil or mat gold, either method is acceptable; with powdered gold and its volatile matrix, only flame annealing is acceptable (Figs. 14–3 and 14–4).

Flame Annealing. For flame annealing the pellet is skewered with a non-corrosive wire over an alcohol flame. Either ethyl or methyl alcohol produces a clean flame and is available at most pharmacies or hardware stores. The pellet is brought to a dull red glow, removed from the flame, and carried to the cavity. Heating of powdered gold‡ is essentially no different from flame

---

*Electralloy: Williams Gold Refining Co., 2978 Main St., Buffalo, New York 14214.
†Platinized foil: sheet of foil consisting of gold with 15 per cent platinum.
‡Goldent: Williams Gold Refining Co., 2978 Main St., Buffalo, New York 14214.

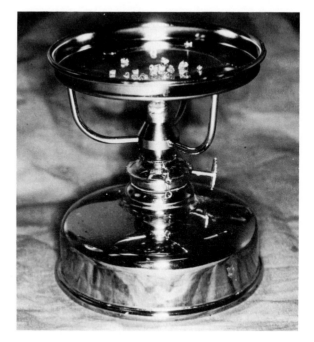

Figure 14–2. Pellets of gold foil being heated on a tray.

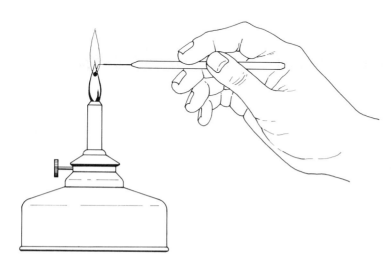

Figure 14–3. Flame annealing of Goldent. Held near the top of the flame, the Goldent pellet "catches fire" and burns until volatile substance is eliminated. Continued heating elevates the temperature to redness. It is then removed from the flame.

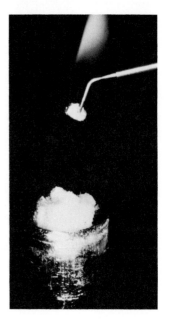

Figure 14–4. The alcohol flame is transparent; the flame from the pellet is visible. (Courtesy of Dr. Adalbert L. Vlazny)

treatment of mat gold. Because of its organic filler the pellet catches fire and burns until all volatile ingredients are eliminated. After the flame burns out the pellet then reaches a dull red glow, whereupon it is removed from the alcohol flame and carried to the cavity for condensation. Insufficient heating of the pellet causes it to be "powdery."

Hot Plate Annealing. Hot plate pre-heating is more prolonged and at a lower temperature than flame annealing, but equally as effective for gold foil or mat gold. It is unacceptable for powdered gold. Several pellets at a time are placed on the surface of the plate. After 15 to 60 seconds, depending upon the temperature of the plate, they are ready for use. As mentioned earlier, brittleness and "stiffness" identify gold that has been overheated. An underheated gold pellet is not cohesive and does not stick to the prior condensed surface. Obtaining a working knowledge of annealing procedures is one of the first requirements in mastering the use of direct gold.

Properties of Direct Gold

The Brinell hardness number (BHN) of pure gold is approximately 25. During condensation the hardness rises to as high as 75. Likewise, the tensile strength rises from 19,000 psi to 32,000 psi, while a yield strength of essentially 0 increases to 30,000 psi. The exact mechanism whereby these properties of pure gold are so enhanced by condensation is not completely understood. In addition to strain hardening, it is possible that a certain amount of recrystallization may occur, even at oral temperatures.

A measurement of the density of restoration indicates that the ideal of 19.3 grams per cubic centimeter is never realized in practice. At best one can expect a maximum of approximately 18.0 grams per cubic centimeter. The difference is due to the presence of porosity and voids.

A comparison of these properties with those of dental gold alloys indicates that direct gold is inferior. Thus the use of direct gold should be restricted to situations where the material is employed to "fill" rather than to "recontour." Because direct gold is not strong enough to resist deformation, it cannot be used as a crown or to restore a cusp.

The process of condensation is a critical one. Even the best restoration, while appearing dense, will contain some few void spaces between the individual layers of particles of the gold. The greater the void space, the lower the strength and hardness. Air spaces at the gold–tooth interface enhance microleakage and thereby the possibility of sensitivity and secondary caries. Thus it can be seen that although the theoretical density of pure gold cannot be truly attained, only by proper condensation can it be approached.

Condensation

General Considerations

As mentioned earlier, to become a solid mass, gold must be deprived of its air or porosity. This involves work (energy) for the operator as he (1) manipulates the gold fragments into position and (2) imparts a compacting force to drive out the air and to condense the gold into a solid mass. Too frequently little care or attention is given to the former, resulting in a lumpy surface and open spaces, which invite microleakage. The best condensation is achieved when the gold is delicately maneuvered and spread out into position before applying compacting forces.

Successful condensation is dependent upon the ability of the operator to

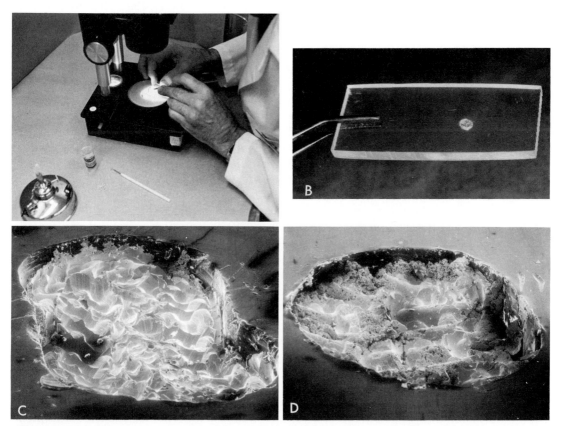

Figure 14–5. Experimental condensation of powdered gold in the laboratory. *A,* Plexiglass block with a simulated cavity is being filled under a binocular microscope (20×). *B,* Plexiglass block permits direct and reverse side observation. *C,* Complete condensation of gold in a cavity (75×). *D,* Incomplete condensation; note fragments of uncondensed powder.

recognize properly condensed gold. It is very easy for an operator to be fooled into thinking the gold is condensed when actually it is quite porous. To some extent this is also true with mechanical condensation, but it is particularly true with hand condensation because of the wide variation between individuals in manipulating hand instruments. One operator must exert himself to produce two pounds of operating force whereas another operator will apply eight pounds with ease (see Fig. 6–5). A low-power binocular microscope (approximately 20×) is helpful in understanding and in developing a working knowledge of direct gold. A simulated cavity in a plexiglass block (Fig. 14–5) can be filled under the microscope where the student can observe condensation internally as well as externally.

Hand (Static) vs. Mechanical (Malleting) Condensation

Hand condensation is accomplished simply by pressing the gold into the cavity. Not so simple, however, is the application of force in the right direction and the proper magnitude to accomplish compaction of the gold at the bottom of the cavity. Instrument size and shape must be equated or balanced out with the force being applied. For example, a rectangle-shaped condenser (parallelogram) will require three times the force of a small round condenser (Fig. 14–6). More time is naturally required to condense with small pluggers than with larger ones. Hand condensation therefore requires the operator to be thorough in his condensation, using instruments compatible with his ability.

Malleting forces can be produced by two methods, the hand malleting method and the mechanical condenser. The former relies upon the team effort of dentist and assistant who work together, the dentist placing the instrument in the proper position while the assistant taps it with a mallet weighing about 50 grams (Fig. 14–7).

The mechanical condenser,* which accommodates various shapes of condenser points, has a small mallet in the handle of the instrument. Through an ingenious design the mallet in the handle remains dormant until the operator wishes it to function (Fig. 14–8A, Hollenback, and Fig. 14–8B, McShirley). Condenser points are similar in size and shape to the hand condensers, with adaptors for usage in either the straight handpiece or the angle handpiece.

It matters little whether one uses hand or mechanical condensation as long as the end product is non-porous. Reliance upon a piece of equipment (mallet) to achieve this result may create a false sense of security with the thicker materials such as mat or powdered gold. An average pellet of gold foil when condensed has a thickness of only 50 micrometers, whereas a condensed pellet of powdered gold is 5 times as thick (250 micrometers). A loaf of mat gold when condensed has a thickness of 175 micrometers.

There is no evidence that the mechanical properties of direct gold restorations are influenced to any significant extent by the type of gold employed or by the method of condensation, i.e, mechanical or hand. The properties are more likely determined by the competence of the operator. Some operators prefer to use one type of gold to fill a cavity; others prefer to mix their golds, e.g., mat gold as a base, powdered gold for the bulk of the restoration, and gold foil as a veneer. Gold is gold. Whether one uses crumpled

*Hollenback Condenser, Clev-Dent Corp., 3307 Scranton Rd., Cleveland, Ohio 44109; McShirley Condenser, McShirley Dental Products, 653 San Fernando Rd., Glendale, California 91201.

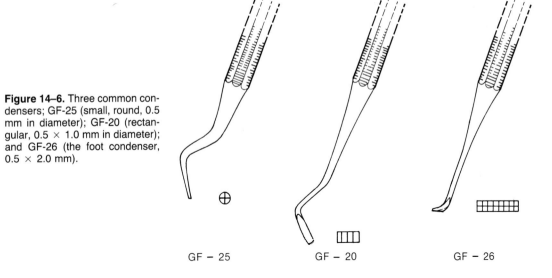

Figure 14–6. Three common condensers; GF-25 (small, round, 0.5 mm in diameter); GF-20 (rectangular, 0.5 × 1.0 mm in diameter); and GF-26 (the foot condenser, 0.5 × 2.0 mm).

GF – 25   GF – 20   GF – 26

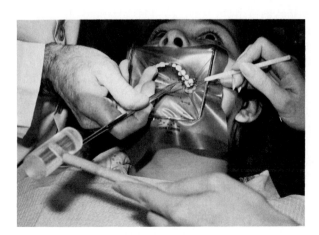

Figure 14–7. Condensation by hand malleting. With rhythmic blows from a small mallet, the dental assistant imparts the condensing and welding force, while the operator directs the angle of the instrument and moves it over the surface.

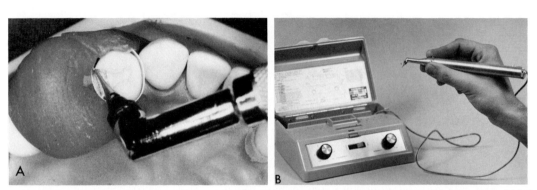

Figure 14–8. Mechanical condensers: *A,* Hollenback condenser filling the box of a Class II cavity with gold foil. (Courtesy of the Annals of Dentistry *23*:14–23, March 1964). *B,* McShirley condenser with the angle attachment for the posterior part of the mouth. A variety of condenser points are available for either HP or RA handpieces.

miniaturized "sheet metal" (gold foil), a loosely bound structure of crystals (mat), or miniaturized sand and gravel (powdered gold), it becomes a homogeneous metallic restoration if it is condensed properly.

Condensation in its best form requires proper direction of forces and an absence of "bridging." Bridging is the covering up of small crevices and pits that were present in the deeper portions of the cavity, especially adjacent to cavity walls. This can be avoided by maneuvering the raw gold into a smooth concave surface before condensing it. Forces, insofar as possible, should be angled outward toward the walls of the cavity so the surface will be "dished out" rather than "humped up" in the center of the cavity. Enamel walls should be covered with gold as soon as possible, leaving the central portion to be filled last (Fig. 14–9).

Crushing the enamel on the cavosurface margin is a frequent mishap that occurs with the novice operator. He becomes so intent in condensing the gold he does not notice the trauma being caused by the shank of the instrument (Fig. 14–10). If such an injury is recognized in time, deft planing by a curved chisel can re-establish another clean-cut margin and condensation can continue toward completion.

Recognition of an improperly condensed gold surface can be made clinically with a stiff explorer or in the laboratory with a microscope.* The explorer is thrust firmly into the gold, especially adjacent to a corner area. If it penetrates the surface and leaves a hole (Fig. 14–11), air pockets are yet present; if only a surface dent is made, condensation has been acceptable. The beginning conscientious operator is constantly searching for "soft spots" in his restoration as he builds it to completion.

Cohesion, naturally, is a key factor in successful condensation. Clean instruments and a dry field virtually mandate the use of a rubber dam. Exhaust fumes from the air-rotor handpiece will also contaminate the gold, as will fumes from the patient's breath. Contaminants afflict a condensed gold surface

---

*To establish a knowledge of his ability to condense gold properly, each student should fill a simulated cavity under the magnification of a low-power binocular microscope. Pits and uncondensed gold particles, which would normally escape attention, are brought out in bold relief when observed under magnification. To "fill the cavity," i.e., eliminate voids, the operator will logically select condenser points of the proper size and shape and push the gold into the open spaces. Once having gained a working knowledge by microscopic condensation the operator can, with reasonable confidence, relate this knowledge to condensing gold in a clinical situation.

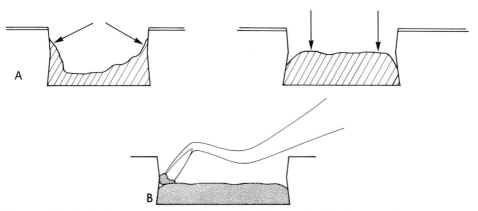

Figure 14–9. Application of condensation forces. *A, Left,* correct; *right,* incorrect. Improper positioning of gold causes incomplete condensation along the walls. *B,* Attempting to condense gold into a tight crevice results in bridging. Part of the gold must be cut away to provide access so small fragments can be condensed and the surface brought up to the desired level and concave contour.

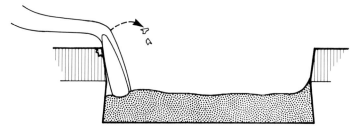

Figure 14–10. Condenser inadvertently damaging the corner of the enamel with its shank.

so that subsequent pellets will not adhere. When this occurs and succeeding pellets fail to "stick," the surface gold must be cut away to expose clean non-contaminated material beneath before new pellets will attach.

Condensation of Gold Foil

Unlike the other golds, gold foil does not tend to fragment under the pressure of a condenser. This is advantageous because its "toughness" permits the condensation of bevels and less access to the cavity is needed. This same feature, however, impedes initial placement of the material because condensation forces tend to "pull" the material out of the undercuts in the tooth preparation. To lock a foundation or base layer of gold foil in a cavity is often difficult and requires precisely and sharply cut line angles to provide secure locks for the material.

A holding instrument is also required to stabilize already condensed gold to prevent it from shifting out of position while additional pellets are added to build the gold, one pellet at a time, to the opposing undercut (Fig. 14–12). Once this has been done and a secure base of condensed gold lines the floor of the cavity, additional pellets, one pellet at a time, can be heat treated and added to build the contour to its desired form. As mentioned earlier, gold foil can be heat treated in an open flame or atop an annealing tray.

Because of its toughness and its smaller mass per unit volume, a pellet of gold foil can be maneuvered into a smaller space. The cavity designed for gold foil therefore can have a smaller orifice than one designed for mat or

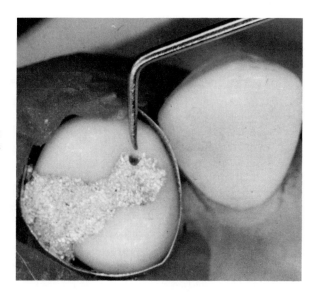

Figure 14–11. Clinical inspection of a condensed surface with a sharp explorer readily discloses the soft porous areas (voids).

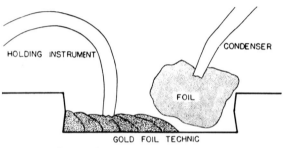

GOLD FOIL TECHNIC

"TYING-IN" BETWEEN OPPOSING RETENTIONS

Figure 14–12. Starting gold foil with a holding instrument. Each pellet is built onto the previous one and must be stabilized until the mass can be wedged between opposing cavity walls. Otherwise the mass of condensed gold will tend to shift around within the cavity.

powdered gold, which tend to fragment when first manipulated within the cavity. Gold foil, moreover, can be condensed effectively over beveled edges. Generally speaking, gold foil is condensed with a malleting force because of its relatively small mass, and stepping the condenser over the surface is recommended (see Figure 12–67). The skill required to condense gold foil, except for veneering purposes, and to prepare cavities to receive it is substantially greater than the skill required for powdered gold or mat gold.

Condensation of Mat Gold

The internal portion of the tooth preparation is the same as that for gold foil, e.g., precisely cut line angles and point angles to retain the gold. Two or three pieces, the size and shape of the cavity, are cut from a loaf of mat gold (Fig. 14–13). Following heat treatment (flame or hot plate), a section of mat gold is fitted into the cavity and deftly condensed as a gold blanket over the floor or axial wall of the preparation (Fig. 14–14). This frequently requires two condensers, one in each hand, to stabilize the material and prevent it from shifting. A second layer is applied in a similar manner, care being taken to fold the excess gold neatly into the retentive and corner areas. Two blankets of gold usually provide a metal base of sufficient thickness to resist buckling and dislodgment during subsequent condensation. Mat gold can be cut into any size and shape desired. Condensation can be by hand pressure or by

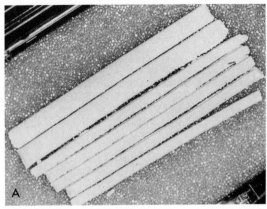
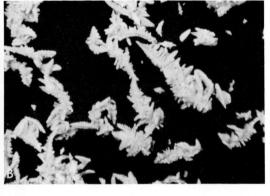

Figure 14–13. Mat gold. *A,* Strips of mat gold ready for use. With a razor blade or a scalpel several pieces of gold are cut to the proper size and shape for the cavity. *B,* Microscopic view of mat gold crystals. (Courtesy of Williams Gold Co.)

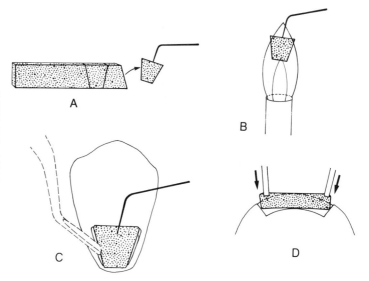

Figure 14–14. Mat gold for the base of a Class V cavity. *A,* Pieces to fit the cavity are cut from strips. *B,* Heat treat in the flame or on annealing plate. *C,* Position the piece within the cavity. *D,* Press the piece into place. Sufficient excess should be present to wedge the gold between occlusal and gingival walls.

malleting. The best results seem to be achieved by hand pressure followed by malleting. Mat gold can be used to fill the entire cavity; however, most clinicians prefer to substitute gold foil for the surface layer.

Condensation of Powdered Gold

Of the three types, powdered gold appears to be the easiest material to condense, often creating a false sense of security in the mind of the operator unfamiliar with its use (Figs. 14–15 and 14–16). Precisely cut line and point angles are not necessary with powdered gold, rounded retentive grooves (No. ½ to No. 1 round bur sizes) being adequate to retain the gold. Because of its tendency to fragment and spread out when initial pressure is applied, cavity preparations should be box-like, with sides, ends, and a floor. Flares and

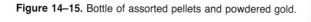

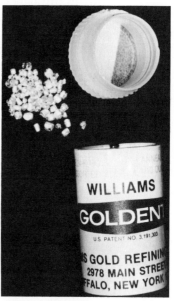

Figure 14–15. Bottle of assorted pellets and powdered gold.

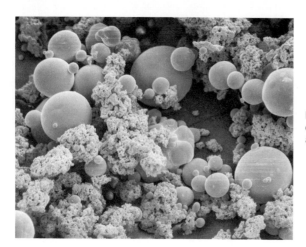

Figure 14–16. Powder consists of spherical particles, ranging up to 75 micrometers in diameter,
amid a matrix of finely precipitated gold powder.

bevels are minimized because powdered gold finishes more easily against a
butt joint.

After heat treatment of a large pellet, it is placed in the cavity and pressed
into position with a large amalgam condenser. If the cavity is so large that
one pellet will not spread out enough to engage opposing walls, two or three
pellets are added to fill up the space. It is best to place a generous amount of
raw gold into the cavity at this stage, so the condensed layer of gold should
be at least one pellet thick (0.25 mm or 0.010 inches) (Fig. 14–17).

Condensation of these initial pellets does not occur until the mass has
been firmly wedged between opposing walls. Having accomplished this, heavy
pressure with small-faced condensers is directed toward retentive areas first,
to create a solid peripheral ring of condensed gold before condensing the
center areas (Fig. 14–17).

Once the initial mass has been condensed, one pellet at a time is annealed
to build the contour, care being taken to direct forces outward against the
vertical walls of the cavity (Fig. 14–18). Condensers with a small face
presenting a convex surface are ideal. Condensation with a rocking motion
utilizes full benefit from the convex face of the condenser.

Small inaccessible areas within the cavity require attention to detail. To
reduce the mass of material being packed into a specific spot, the pellet may
be broken apart and small fragments packed into corners and crevices or a
small pellet of gold foil may be used instead.

As with mat gold, powdered gold can be used to achieve final contour of
the restoration or, as some clinicians prefer, a veneer of gold foil can be
applied.

Finishing of Direct Gold: Indirect Condensation

Cohesive gold in general and powdered gold in particular are subject to
two forms of condensation, direct and indirect. Pressure from pluggers or
condensers provides the former; finishing procedures provide the latter.

Indirect condensation is necessary because of the inability of the operator
to achieve absolute and complete condensation by direct thrusts with the
condenser. Although appearing dense, small voids or air spaces exist throughout the mass of gold and make themselves apparent when the gold is polished.

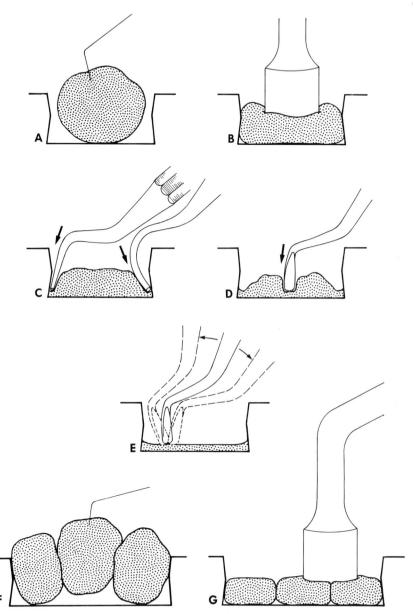

Figure 14–17. Starting procedure for powdered gold. *A,* A large pellet is placed in the cavity. *B,* It is compressed with an amalgam condenser to engage the vertical walls. *C,* The internal corners are condensed first. *D,* The central area is condensed last. *E,* A rocking motion aids condensation. *F,* A cluster of pellets fills a large space. Do not attempt to condense until enough pellets are present. If there is any doubt, add another pellet. *G,* Pellets are fixed firmly in place with a large faced condenser. Follow through as in *C, D,* or *E.* If the condensed gold slides around in the cavity, more pellets should have been placed prior to condensing.

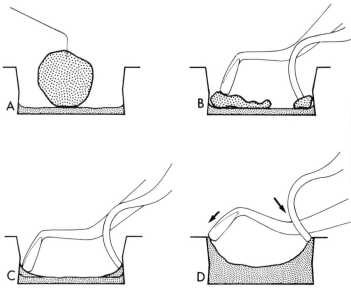

Figure 14–18. Building the contour after the base is placed. *A,* One pellet at a time is added. *B,* The pellet is fragmented. *C,* The corners are filled in first. *D,* The edges of the cavity are covered as soon as possible to protect the enamel.

When condensation is complete, the surface must receive special treatment to eliminate all surface porosity. This is accomplished by creating a surface "crust" of perhaps 0.1 to 0.2 mm thick. A dense crust is produced by rubbing the surface with hand instruments.

Rubbing or ironing the surface to develop a dense crust is best accomplished with an instrument with a blunt edge. If the edge is too sharp, i.e., gold knife, it tends to cut or tear the surface; if it is too rounded, i.e., ball burnisher, the force is disseminated over a large area and its action is ineffective.

"Ironing" the surface with heavy hand pressure cannot be overemphasized, particularly with respect to mat and powdered gold. Direction of force follows from the gold toward the enamel.* Instruments of choice for this purpose are the Spratley finishing instrument, discoid and cleoid carvers, and gold files whose serrated edges impart this "ironing action." A beavertail burnisher is also preferred by some. To impart the force required, the use of the palm grasp or modified palm grasp is expected. Gold files are excellent for this purpose when huskier instruments are inaccessible. Because gold files are made to function with a "push" or a "pull" action, the manufacturer designates the end for pushing with two rings around the shank (Fig. 14–19).

Concave surfaces (occlusal pits and grooves) can be similarly treated by the use of coarse grit finishing stones. When rotated under pressure and at a relatively slow speed, the surface of the stone imparts an "ironing" effect. Along with its ability to remove excess gold, it can function quite effectively in both contouring and finishing the surface. A small inverted cone stone with a dulled corner is recommended for this purpose (Fig. 14–20).

Gold, unlike amalgam, has a tendency to lap over the edge of the cavity as a "flag" or "tag." Whereas thin amalgam fragments flake away during the carving stage, gold that has overfilled and overlapped the edge of the cavity tends to remain firmly attached, making it difficult to tell where the cavity ends and the tooth begins (see Figs. 14–23 and 14–26). Precautionary measures

---

*This heavy force adjacent to enamel with decalcified or soft texture is contraindicated, as it will tend to pulverize the enamel.

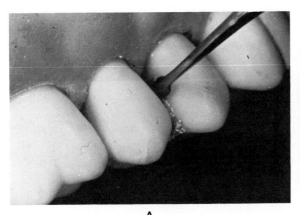
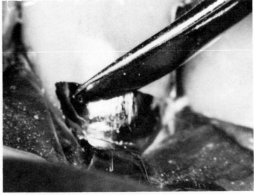

Figure 14–19. Burnishing ("ironing" or rubbing) the gold surface. *A,* Gold files, GF-30 DE and GF-31 DE. Each file has a "push" end and a "pull" end. *B,* Beaver tail burnisher.

during tooth preparation (e.g., straight walls and sharp angles in the cavity outline) can greatly assist the operator in detecting and removing excess gold over the margins as the original form takes shape.

Once the contour has been established, marginal excess has been removed, and a reasonably thick crust of gold has been formed, polishing procedures may continue. Polishing is most effectively accomplished with medium (fine) garnet disks followed in order by cuttle disks, damp flour of pumice, and Amalgloss.* Round finishing burs in groove and pit regions leave an acceptable polish. It should be borne in mind that indirect condensation with heavy hand pressure is one thing and polishing is quite another. If the pressure is minimal and it produces only a thin crust, which will be worn away by disking and polishing, a pitted surface is the inevitable result.

Indirect condensation in finishing prevails in all cohesive gold restorations regardless of type or location. References hereafter to specific instruments will be made in light of the preceding techniques and the ability of the dentist to use them in their respective locations.

---

*Tin oxide, whiting, and other polishing agents are also effective.

Figure 14–20. Use of an inverted cone stone for initial finishing of distal groove. Stone should revolve from the gold toward the enamel at slow speed and with firm pressure.

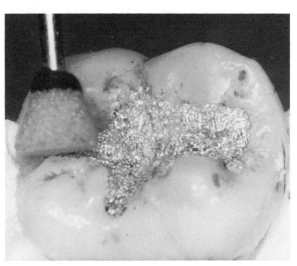

Specific Applications of Direct Gold

The Class I Cavity

A tooth with minimal facets of wear and one that will not likely be susceptible to subsequent caries invasion is a candidate for direct gold. Moreover, the tooth should be free from extensive supplemental grooves.

The preparation is more or less identical to that for an amalgam restoration (see Chapter 11). The cavity preparation for cohesive gold should have all cavosurface enamel margins very carefully honed to a sharp edge. Moreover, the margins should be in straight lines or definite curves.

After a base of gold has been built over the pulpal wall, individual pellets are heated and condensed as described earlier, forces being directed laterally with appropriate condensers to build up the edges before the central part of the cavity (Figs. 14–21 and 14–22). Condensation is completed after all margins are covered, but with a minimum of overfilling.

Essentially two rotating instruments, a coarse grit inverted cone stone (SHP) and multi-bladed round burs (Nos. 2, 4, 6), are used in contouring. The former trims excess gold from the recesses of occlusal grooves; the latter contours the surface and removes excess gold from the margins (Fig. 14–23). Direction of rotation of the stone should be from the gold to the enamel. Whenever rotating instruments (burs or stones) are used, additional air cooling should be used to prevent the friction from overheating the tooth. Some operators prefer the use of Vaseline on the cutting surface. Hand instruments are used to increase surface density and improve surface hardness (Fig. 14–24).

Small garnet and cuttle disks (Fig. 14–25) can be used along with pumice powder to impart a smoother surface. If all excess gold flags have been removed from the periphery of the cavity, the surface left by finishing burs is acceptable; however, polishing with pumice and Amalgloss is preferred (Figs. 14–26 and 14–27).

The Accessible Smooth Surface Proximal Cavity

When direct access can be obtained because of a missing tooth or portion thereof, the direct gold Class II or Class III provides the patient with an excellent service.

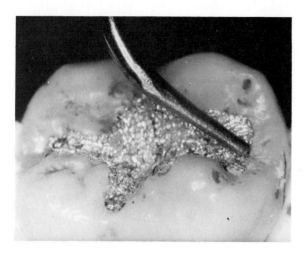

Figure 14–21. Direction of condensation forces for a left molar (mesial is to the right) with a GF-21 condenser directed against the mesial wall. Forces that pull the gold against an enamel wall are more likely to be overlooked than thrusting forces.

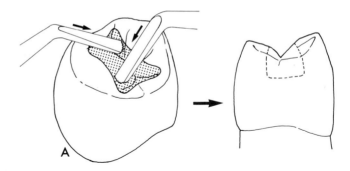

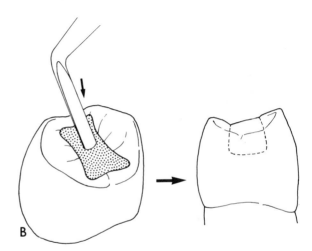

Figure 14–22. Overfilling in central areas should be avoided. Proper condensation follows the contour of the occlusal anatomy. *A*, Correct. *B*, Incorrect.

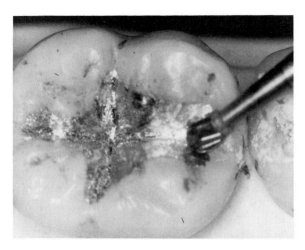

Figure 14–23. Finishing bur on the occlusal. Direction of rotation is toward the enamel. Note the "tag" of gold with its ragged edge in front of the bur awaiting removal.

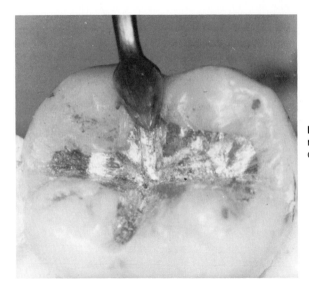

Figure 14–24. Instruments with heavy force burnishing the surface. Direction of movement of cleoid carver is toward the enamel.

Figure 14–25. One-quarter inch diameter pinhole disk for polishing the occlusal surface. These disks are available in garnet and cuttle, ⅜" diameter and ¼" diameter. These disks can only be used with small-headed mandrels.

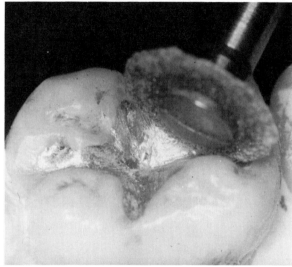

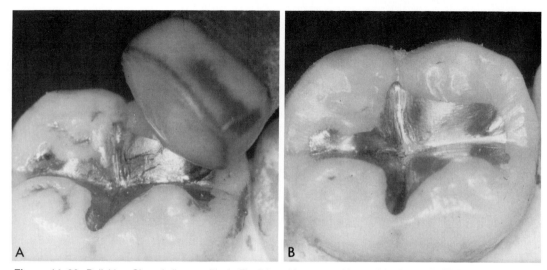
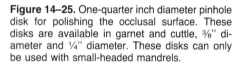

Figure 14–26. Polishing Class I direct gold. *A,* Flexible rubber cup with pumice slurry. *B,* Finished restoration. Notice the marginal adaptation of the gold at the enamel interface. Also note the small "tag" of gold over the mesial marginal ridge that was inadvertently left in the finishing process.

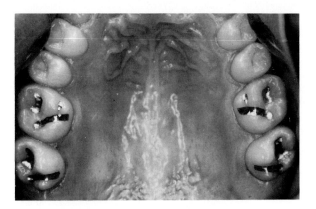

Figure 14–27. Defective pits and fissures restored with direct gold.

Figure 14–28 illustrates the mesial surface of a lateral incisor. The central incisors are being restored with crowns, and the proximal lesion is clearly exposed for access. Restoration of the lesion would naturally be accomplished before the crown is cemented.

The preparation is established with a No. 4 or 6 round bur; retention with a No. 1 or 2 round bur (Fig. 14–28). Diagrammatic sections of prepared cavity are shown in Figure 14–29.

Condensation is routine, comparable in manner to that employed in a Class I cavity. Special care should be directed to "pull" the gold toward the labial and incisal to insure adaptation of the gold to these margins. Only condenser points that fit into the cavity should be used.

Finishing of the smooth surface cavity is best done with gold files, which in turn are followed by ⅝″ diameter disks of garnet and cuttle. Extra-long finishing strips (18″ long) prove quite effective in polishing these surfaces.

The Gingival Restoration

Teeth that are *not* good candidates for Class V direct gold restorations are most molars, because of inaccessibility, and many maxillary anteriors, because of esthetic concerns with the display of gold.

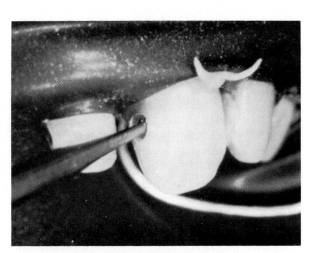

Figure 14–28. Restoration of proximal lesion with unlimited access. The adjacent tooth has been prepared for a crown that will be cemented after the lesion has been restored. Retention is established with a round bur. Only the straight handpiece is used; the contra-angle handpiece would obscure access.

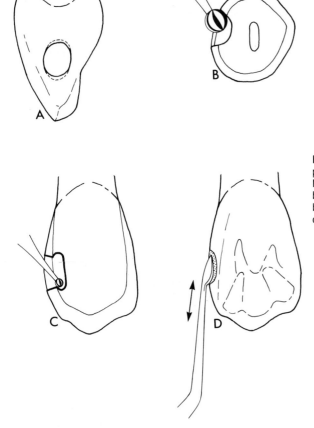

Figure 14–29. Diagrammatic restoration of a proximal lesion (cuspid). *A,* Proximal view. *B,* Margins bevelled with a No. 4 or No. 6 round bur. *C,* Retention established with a No. 2 round bur. *D,* Gold file (GF-30 or -31) contouring the condensed surface.

With respect to molars, the issue is one of isolation with the rubber dam and retraction of the tissue with the No. 212 clamp.* If this can be achieved, tooth preparation and placement of the gold are usually possible.

With respect to maxillary anteriors, the height of the lip line and the wishes of the patient are the prevailing factors. Naturally, the central and lateral incisors would be of greater concern than the canines and, except for small inconspicuous restorations, direct gold is contraindicated in the maxillary anterior region (Fig. 14–31B). All other areas are acceptable locations, with special indications in the mandibular canines and premolars.

Restoration involves four steps: (1) isolation of the lesion with the rubber dam and the retainer clamp, (2) preparation of the cavity, (3) filling and condensing the cavity with gold, and (4) finishing and polishing the restoration. Each of the four phases requires a comparable amount of time and will be discussed in order. When restored with direct gold, the Class V incites more trauma to the tooth than does the Class II or III. For this reason the procedure should never take more than three hours. The trauma produced by condensation of the gold and the prolonged application of the No. 212 clamp can restrict blood supply to the periodontium and pulp, with possible irreversible damage. For this restoration, therefore, it is essential that the student be well prepared and organized so he can apply the No. 212 clamp and move on rapidly to completion of the restoration.

---

*The B-6 clamp (Hygienic Dental Mfg. Co.) is an excellent substitute for the No. 212 clamp.

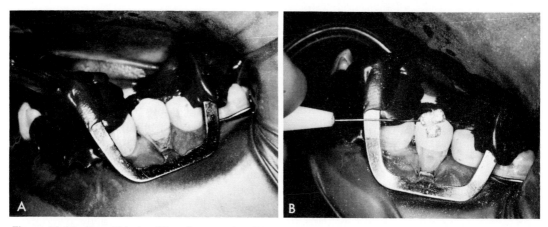

Figure 14–30. Class V lesion *(A)* and preparation *(B)*. Notice the pencil line, which marks the extension of the cavity outline before any preparation is made. *B* also shows a cluster of Goldent pellets ready to be placed in the cavity to form the base.

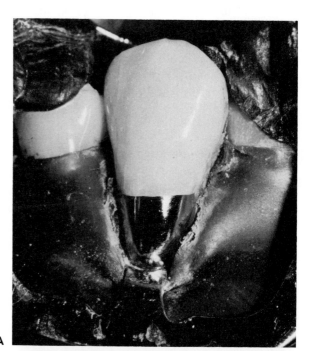

Figure 14–31. *A,* Class V restoration completed and ready for clamp removal. It is not wise to remove the clamp and the rubber dam until the final polish. *B,* Conservative direct gold restoration on maxillary central incisors. Heavy musculature of the upper lip identifies a patient with a low lip line who rarely shows his teeth when smiling.

A

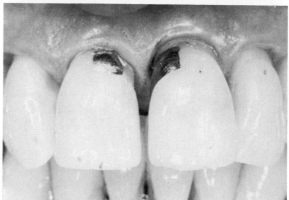

B

Design of the Preparation. The placement of the clamp (see Chapter 9) permits an accurate outline for the cavity. The tissue that has now been stretched by the buccal beak determines most of the cavity margins, gingival, mesial, and distal. The length of the gingival margin is determined by the buccal beak of the clamp and it lies 0.5 mm from it (Fig. 14–30). The mesial and distal walls are tucked under the edge of the reflected rubber. This retraction of the tissue by the rubber allows the cavity edges to terminate in areas of the root that will be covered by gingiva after the tension is released. In essence these three margins (mesial, distal, and gingival) form the new "cervical line" after the restoration is finished (Fig. 14–31A).

Occlusal and incisal margins are determined not by the position of the clamp and rubber dam but by the location of the lesion and the height of contour of the tooth. Foremost, the occlusal (incisal) wall should be flat or convex—never concave. It should also be extended to the height of contour (Figs. 14–32 and 14–33). Termination of an incisal margin gingival to the height of contour is done only on maxillary anteriors and occasionally on a maxillary first premolar. Finesse and contour are sacrificed in preference to display of gold (Fig. 14–31B). Insofar as possible angular patterns and internal line angles and point angles should be placed with angle formers or other hand instruments (Fig. 14–34).

It is a wise practice, for even the experienced operator, to draw the outline on the tooth with a lead pencil prior to actual tooth preparation. Mesial and distal walls flare out to produce a 90° cavosurface margin (Figs. 14–35 and 14–36). Retentive areas are predominantly at the gingival with some minimal undercuts at the occlusal corners. It is quite acceptable for a direct gold restoration to terminate against a previously placed amalgam or gold restoration.

Preparation of the Cavity. Two burs and three hand instruments provide the necessary provisions for cavity preparation.

Armamentarium
1. No. 35 inverted cone bur, SHP (HP)
2. No. ½ round bur, SHP (HP)
3. Curved chisel (large, medium, or small)
4. Angle former (large, medium, or small)
5. Mon-angle hoe 10-4-8 or 6½-2½-9

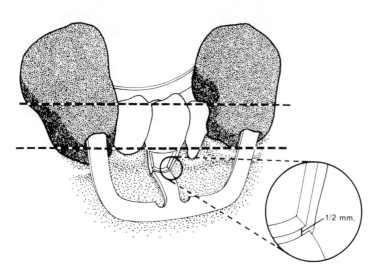

Figure 14–32. No. 212 type clamp application. The beak of the clamp locates the gingival margin; the folds of the rubber dam into the sulcus locate the mesial and distal margins (see Figure 14–31A). The occlusal margin is parallel with the occlusal plane and terminates at the height of contour of the tooth.

1/2 mm.

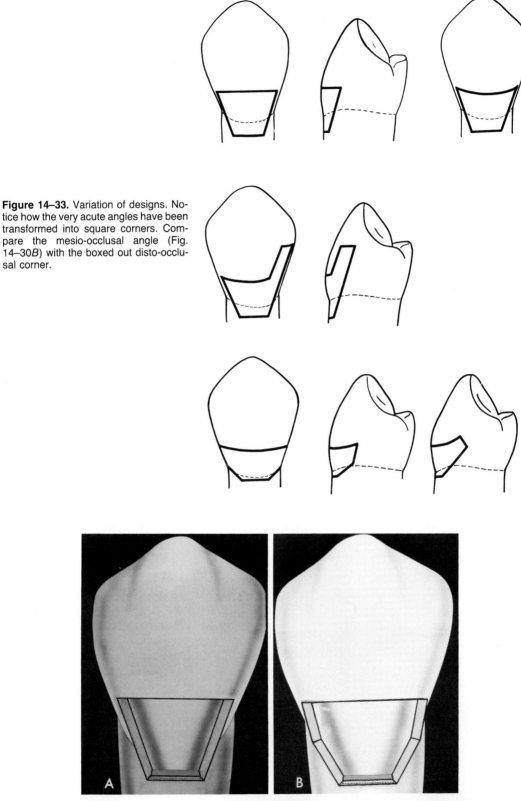

Figure 14–33. Variation of designs. Notice how the very acute angles have been transformed into square corners. Compare the mesio-occlusal angle (Fig. 14–30*B*) with the boxed out disto-occlusal corner.

Figure 14–34. Two basic forms of Class V design. Retention is predominantly along the gingival border but also in the occlusal corners. *A* is more likely indicated for maxillary premolars. *B* is more commonly used for lower bicuspids. Slightly rounded corners in the outline are acceptable.

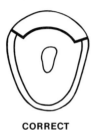 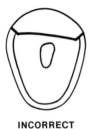 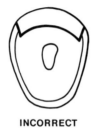

CORRECT   INCORRECT   INCORRECT

Figure 14–35. Cross-section of correct convex axial wall with proximal walls that flare outward to provide a 90° cavosurface margin.

Prior to the use of the first bur (No. 35), a thin coat of shaving soap or other lubricant is placed over the rubber to prevent the bur from becoming entangled in the rubber dam if it slips out of the cavity. The bur is inserted only part way into the handpiece to provide greater shank length, and in turn, greater visibility (Figs. 14–37 and 14–39).

With the bur extending radially from the surface, the four corners are connected by an X-shaped slot across the surface. Corners are then connected with the same bur as the crudely shaped trapezoid is roughed out. The No. 35 bur (SHP) operating at slow speed in its several positions removes the bulk of the material for the preparation (Figs. 14–37 and 14–38). A curved chisel forms the internal walls and angles of the cavity. The No. ½ round bur provides the retentive features, which are later sharpened and refined with the medium or large angle former. Final gingival bevel and margins are finished with an ultra-sharp curved chisel. A bevel is placed on the outer ¼ of the gingival floor only. No cavosurface bevel is used along any other part of the cavity (Fig. 14–40). Retentive features occur primarily at the gingival floor but also to a slight degree at incisal (occlusal) corners (see Fig. 3–40B). The 10-4-8 mon-angle hoe (or 6½-2½-9) as well as the curved chisel can be used with a sideways scraping action. The sides rather than the end of the blade do the cutting (see Figs. 3–40 and 11–61).

The angle former with its sharp point often breaks off unnoticed during use. The end should be inspected frequently, as it may reveal a missing tip (Fig. 14–41, magnified). When this occurs, it must be re-sharpened before further use.

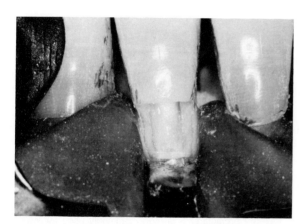

Figure 14–36. Class V preparation for a narrow lateral incisor.

Figure 14–37. Preparation made primarily with a No. 35 inverted cone bur in the straight handpiece. Contra-angle handpieces would restrict visibility and access. Notice that a soap slurry or Borofax is used as lubricant so the shank of the bur will not catch in the rubber dam.

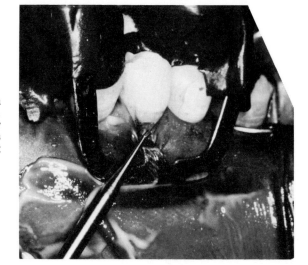

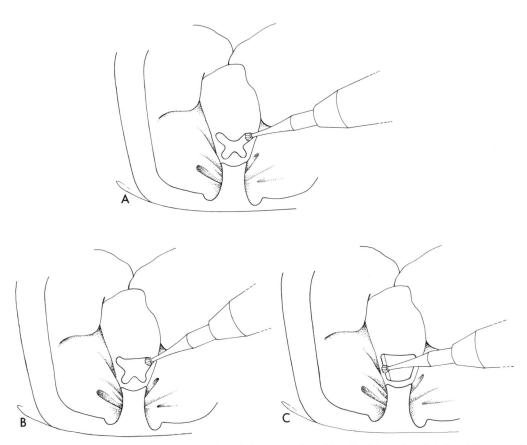

Figure 14–38. Establishing the size and location of the preparation with a No. 35 steel straight handpiece bur. *A*, "Butterfly" outline carries the preparation to its trapezoidal corners. *B*, Extensions are connected to form straight walls. *C*, End of the bur planes mesial and distal walls. Notice close proximity of the bur to the rubber dam. Apply a generous amount of rubber dam lubricant to the rubber to prevent snagging with the bur if it slips out of the cavity.

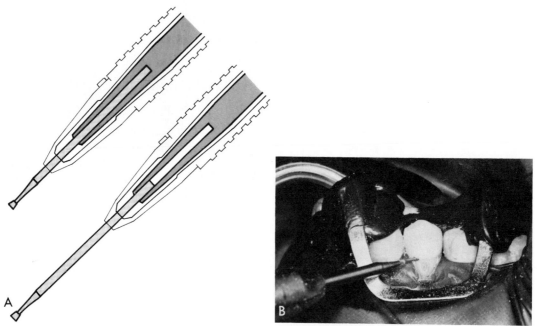

Figure 14–39. Better visibility and access using a SHP bur. *A,* Bur partly ejected from the handpiece to produce greater length. *B,* Straight handpiece bur can approach cavity at all angles within the constraints of the bow of the clamp.

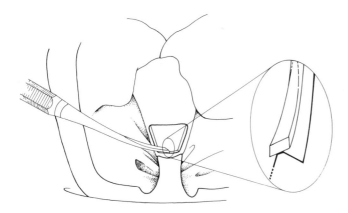

Figure 14–40. Refining the basic preparation (also see Fig. 3–40). Curved chisel (or bin-angle chisel) is the basic instrument to plane the gingival and other margins. Minimum distance of ½ mm, maximum of 1.0 mm, between gingival margin and the beak of the clamp (see Fig. 14–32). It is desirable to terminate the margin as close to the clamp as possible, yet if it is too close, the clamp may slip over the edge and its beak may drop into the cavity.

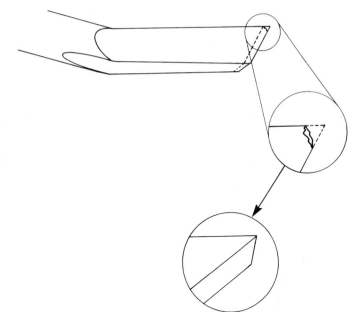

Figure 14–41. Repair of a fractured angle former. If the tip fractures, the entire length of the blade must be shortened to establish a new angle. A broken tip can easily escape notice and is caused from prying with the instrument rather than cutting away the unwanted dentin.

Cavity varnish is now applied (Fig. 14–42). Aside from serving to restrict microleakage, it helps stabilize the gold to the dentin surface during initial condensation.

Filling the Cavity. Condensed gold of at least 250 micrometers (.010 inch) thick should cover the axial wall and be locked into the retentive angles of the cavity as a solid base upon which to begin building the contours.

With Goldent this is accomplished with a cluster of pellets heated over the alcohol flame (Fig. 14–43) and then positioned and pressed into the cavity. When the pellets are lodged securely between gingival and occlusal walls, the parallelogram (No. 20) and the small round condenser (No. 25) are used to depress the gold into the retentive spaces and into all the internal line angles. This is followed by overall condensation of the axial.

If one uses mat gold as a base, the properly sized section of mat gold (usually a trapezoid shape) is packed into the cavity to form a base as described earlier. If the axial surface of the preparation is quite convex, the gold, when being pressed into the distal, will bend and be dislodged at the mesial. Pressure applied at the mesial will cause it to pull loose at the distal. If it appears as though the base is too thin (less than .010 inch), another section

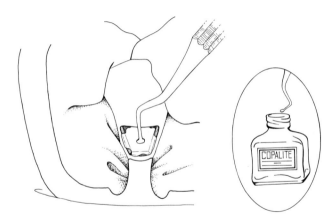

Figure 14–42. Cavity varnish being applied with a hand instrument (e.g., excavator). Gravity permitting, copal varnish can be applied more easily and with more control with a hand instrument than with a cotton pellet.

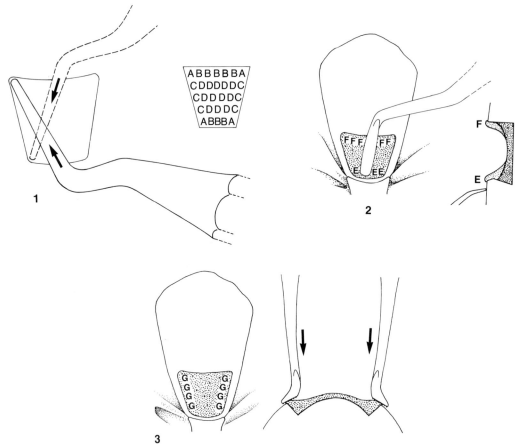

Figure 14–43. Condensation procedures. A cluster of Goldent pellets that will generously fill the cavity is annealed and packed loosely into the cavity with a large amalgam condenser (see Fig. 14–30B). If the gold is not well wedged between the occlusal and gingival walls, add another pellet before condensation. *1,* The four internal point angles are condensed first with a GF-25 condenser (**A**). The sequence of condensation is diagrammed. **A, B,** and **C** are condensed first; the central portion, **D,** is condensed last. *2,* Additional pellets are added and condensed with a GF-20 condenser (**E** and **F**). *3,* As soon as the mesial and distal margins are covered, a switch to the GF-26 (foot condenser) is desirable (**G**).

of mat should be added before attempting condensation (see Figs. 14–13 and 14–14).

Additional increments of gold are added to bank the walls of the cavity and create a "dished-out" contour, with a special effort to complete the gingival and distal walls first. The distal wall is completed because it is the least accessible; the gingival wall, as insurance against clamp dislodgment. Nothing is quite as devastating during the condensation as having the clamp beak slip into the cavity. If the gingival portion of the cavity has been filled and accidental dislodgment of the clamp occurs, the beak will be restricted from slipping occlusalward.

Mesial and occlusal walls are covered and the contour of the restoration is completed with only a slight excess of gold. Viewing the surface from two or three perspectives is helpful in determining proper contour. The surface should be as smooth as possible and free from bumps and irregularities.

The use of the GF-26 foot condenser is most valuable in packing the bulk of the restoration. With a "rocking" motion and by "walking" the condenser across the surface, efficient condensation with a smooth contour is achieved.

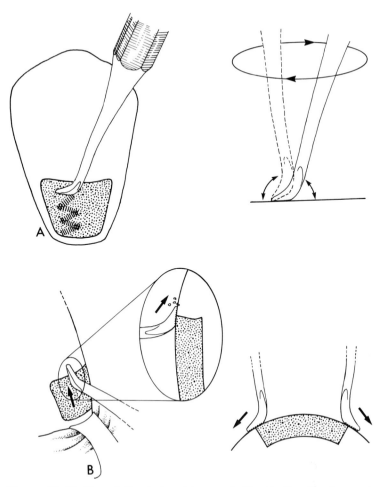

Figure 14–44. Use of the foot condenser. *A,* Combination thrusting and rotational movement allows the foot condenser to "walk" across the surface. *B,* Pinch off fragments of gold against the enamel edge.

Once the initial condensation has taken place, this instrument can often complete the bulk of the condensation (Fig. 14–44).

Finishing the Surface. To obtain excellence in surface smoothness the following sequence is recommended in finishing the direct gold restoration:

1. Contour the surface and remove excess gold from the margins (Fig. 14–45).
    a. Use coarse grit green stone for bulk of contouring in HP at slow speed. Use as large a diameter as possible.
    b. Use files along mesial and distal margins.
    c. Pointed burnisher (GF-33) and gold knife (GF-34). Thrusting the tip of the burnisher rootward between the beak of the clamp and the tooth, the gold is pressed tightly against the gingival margin. Excess metal present can be carefully sliced away with the gold knife.
2. Work harden the surface (burnish the surface) (Fig. 14–46). Pulling GF-33 and GF-36 across the surface under *heavy* pressure "irons" the surface and imparts indirect condensation.
    a. Repeat the use of the stone to dress down the bumps caused by "ironing."

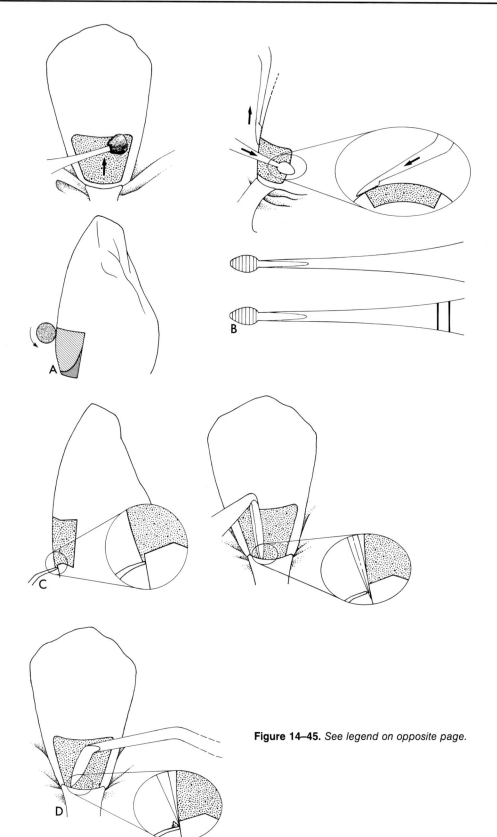

Figure 14–45. *See legend on opposite page.*

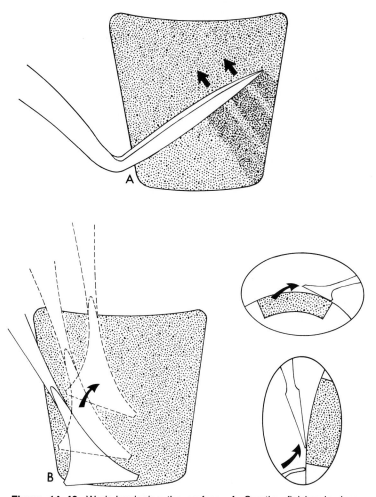

Figure 14–46. Work hardening the surface. *A,* Spratley finisher is drawn diagonally across the surface. Instrument is held with a palm grasp and used with heavy pressure. *B,* "Push" gold knife. A GF-36 is raked across the surface in the opposite direction to create a hard crust free from the microscopic porosities.

   b. Repeat the "ironing" procedure. This time no bumps will remain; the surface will appear smooth and is ready to polish.

3. Polish the surface. Abrade surface with disks, garnet followed by cuttle. Dampened by petroleum jelly, the disk is softer in texture and conforms better to the surface (Figs. 14–47 and 14–48).

   a. Re-inspect margins for excess gold, especially the gingival margin.

   b. Polish surface (Fig. 14–49). Flour pumice may be used wet or dry; Amalgloss and tin oxide are used dry.

Figure 14–45. Contouring of the surface with a coarse grit stone. *A,* It must operate at slow speed with firm pressure. It is never used at the gold/cementum junction lest the soft dentin and cementum become severely abraded (ditched). *B,* Push and pull files; inside cutting, GF-30; outside cutting, GF-31. Files are especially valuable for finishing gold adjacent to cementum. *C,* Finishing margin next to the beak of the clamp. After excess gold has been removed, the tip of the Spratley finisher (GF-33) is thrust rootward between the clamp and the gold/root. The clamp beak springs outward slightly to permit entry of the instrument, which in turn presses the gold against the margin. *D,* Removal of final excess to expose the cavosurface margin. A *sharp* gold knife with its tip can whittle away shavings of gold until the surface of the tooth is exposed. Alternately, between GF-33 and GF-34 the margin can be finished without "ditching" the cementum and dentin.

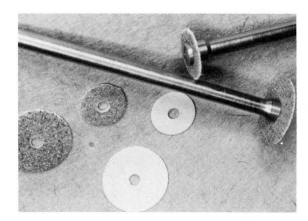

Figure 14–47. Preliminary polishing with garnet disks, followed by cuttle disks (⅜" diameter disks; ¼" for areas of limited access).

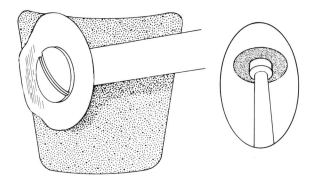

Figure 14–48. Disks in use; the abrasive side faces the handpiece. Vaseline on the disk causes it to soften and conform to the desired contour.

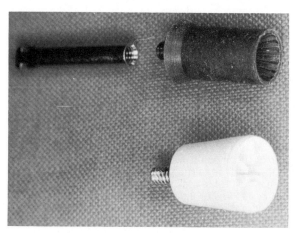

Figure 14–49. Flexible rubber cups of proper texture. The webbed stiff white cup can destroy a nicely contoured surface and is unacceptable. "Gray midget cups" from Youngs' Dental Mfg. Co. are recommended. Caution: Do not use a polishing cup adjacent to the soft cementum and dentin. Abrasive action of the pumice can rapidly erode away the root dentin adjacent to the gold without the operator being aware that it is taking place.

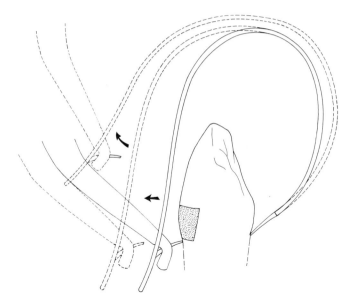

Figure 14–50. Removing the No. 212 type clamp. A blunt instrument, e.g., GF-33, engages the clamp and pulls it outward from the tooth. The compound fractures away as the bows are dislodged.

In all aspects of finishing three things should be avoided: (1) do not overheat the gold; use air coolant, (2) do not ditch the cementum, and (3) avoid rubber impregnated abrasives; stones, disks, and hand instruments are preferred.

To remove the rubber dam, pull the buccal beak outward with a hooked instrument; do not attempt to use the rubber dam forceps. The compound mounting will fracture as the clamp is rotated occlusally (Fig. 14–50).

In the systematic manner described above the placement of a Class V cohesive gold restoration should not be unduly time consuming nor beyond the ability of the average operator.

The greatest joy and sense of satisfaction comes at the conclusion of a successful operation, following the repositioning of the gingiva over the finely finished gold. When one views the permanency of such a restoration in years to come, he realizes the valuable health service that he has been able to provide in this most critical area of the dentition (Fig. 14–51).

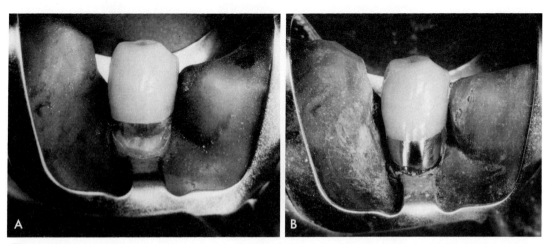

Figure 14–51. Large Class V lesion restored with direct gold. *A,* Preparation stage. *B,* Finish. (Courtesy of Dr. Brian Chiffer)

The Class VI Cavity (Abraded Cusp Tip)

The Class VI cavity (see cavity classification in Chapter 2) is similar in many respects to the Class I. Presenting itself as a worn-off cusp tip, it should be restored in some instances and ignored in others. Those worn-off teeth hollowed out by erosion (see Fig. 2–26) should be restored; those teeth worn but not eroded need not be. When restored, however, direct gold is the material of choice.

The preparation is based on the premise that enamel and gold wear evenly. The preparation therefore does not include any enamel removal, only dentin. A minimal amount of dentin is removed in order to obtain a thickness of approximately 1.5 mm of metal. Retention is minimal and is adequately obtained through parallel walls or possibly a slight undercut where the greatest bulk of dentin is available. Any one of several burs can be used, but a straight fissure bur (e.g., No. 55 or No. 56) is quite effective (Fig. 14–52).

The gold, after condensation, is heavily burnished and finished smooth with the surface. No effort is made to rebuild back the lost contour.

Proximal Cavities

Restoration of proximal lesions involving the replacement of contact points will not be discussed in this chapter; however, a basic difference between the Class V and the proximal lesion is one of access, both for condensation and for finishing (Figs. 14–53 and 14–54). Similar principles for condensation prevail and both Class II and Class III direct gold restorations can be mastered by the average dental student (see pp. 298 to 302 for matrix application).

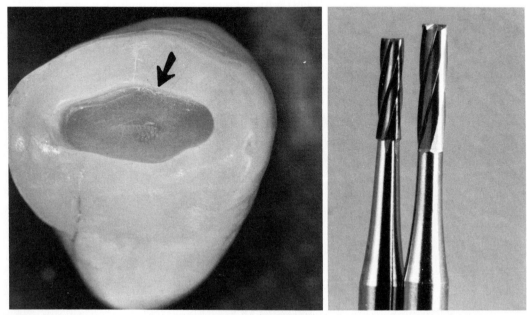

Figure 14–52. Preparation of an abraded canine for restoration with direct gold. The tooth preparation is made with small straight fissure burs (Nos. 55 and 56) and involves only the dentin. The arrow indicates the location of the cavosurface margin.

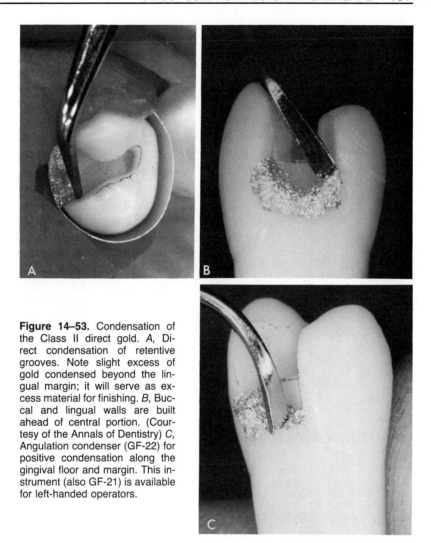

Figure 14–53. Condensation of the Class II direct gold. *A,* Direct condensation of retentive grooves. Note slight excess of gold condensed beyond the lingual margin; it will serve as excess material for finishing. *B,* Buccal and lingual walls are built ahead of central portion. (Courtesy of the Annals of Dentistry) *C,* Angulation condenser (GF-22) for positive condensation along the gingival floor and margin. This instrument (also GF-21) is available for left-handed operators.

As might be anticipated, the finishing of the proximal surface of a gold restoration could be a difficult task. To assist in this regard, the use of a mechanical separator is recommended (see Figs. 12–82 to 12–84). Space provided, even though it is as little as 0.15 mm, permits the passage of an abrasive finishing strip. The Ferrier type separator is more difficult to apply although it is more rigid than the Elliot type.

Like any other sophisticated procedure, direct gold restorations are difficult to place without correct and proper instruments. This is particularly true with the gold knife (Figs. 14–55 and 14–56). Another instance where the correct instrument (small round right angle condenser) must be used is for direct condensation into the incisal angle of the Class III cavity (Fig. 14–57B). Indirect condensation can best be done with a *small* discoid carver (Fig. 14–57C) to "pull" the gold over the crucial labial margin.

Many of the materials used with direct gold procedures are not readily available from local supply houses (e.g., finishing strips, mandrels, instruments) and must be special ordered. These are identified in a list at the end of the chapter along with the source of supply.

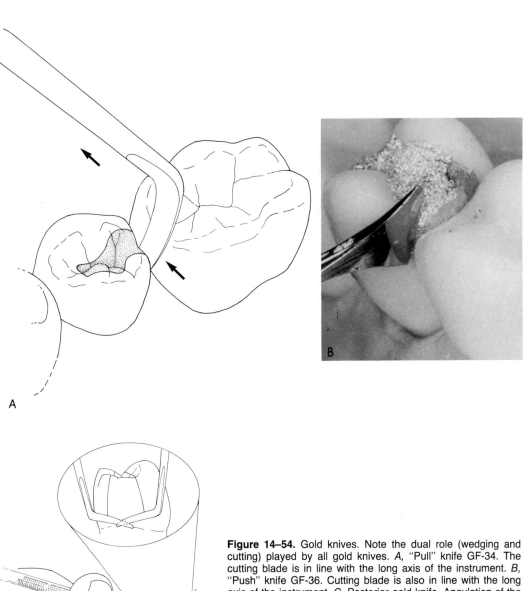

Figure 14–54. Gold knives. Note the dual role (wedging and cutting) played by all gold knives. *A,* "Pull" knife GF-34. The cutting blade is in line with the long axis of the instrument. *B,* "Push" knife GF-36. Cutting blade is also in line with the long axis of the instrument. *C,* Posterior gold knife. Angulation of the blade is *not* in line with the long axis of the instrument. This angulation of the blade to the handle restricts forceful cutting movements.

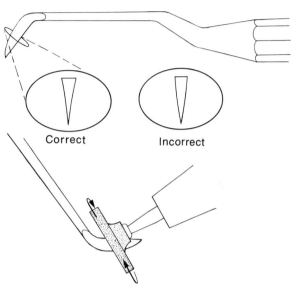

Figure 14–55. Sharpness and contour of the blade is extremely important for wedging contact points and for whittling the gold. Convex sides *(right)* render the instrument virtually useless. A thin blade *(left)*, which is hollow ground with a stone and polished with a rubber wheel, is essential in gold knives. The operator cannot expect the manufacturer to provide the hollow ground surface. He must be prepared to do the grinding himself.

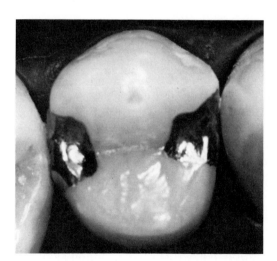

Figure 14–56. Maxillary right first premolar. Mesial and distal lesions have been restored with direct gold.

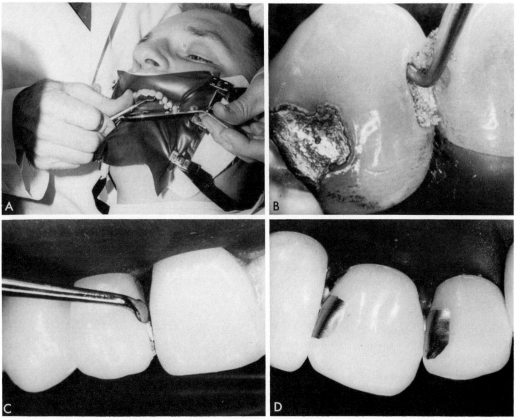

Figure 14–57. Class III direct gold. *A,* Proper position for comfortable condensation. Note the large mirror (see Fig. 6–26). *B,* Condensing gold toward incisal with GF-23. *C,* Forceful adaptation of excess gold along labial margin with discoid carver (GF-32, small end). *D,* Finished restoration. (Courtesy of Drs. Paul P. Hatrel and Richard B. McCoy)

Non-Traditional Uses of Direct Gold

Direct gold is used far too infrequently, particularly for non-traditional purposes. Although direct gold is an excellent restorative for gingival, proximal, and pit and fissure cavities, it lends itself beautifully in other places as well. Figure 14–58, for example, illustrates the restoration of a distal lesion of a lower premolar where access must be obtained from the facial surface.

Far too often a beautiful gold crown is marred by a repair of composite or amalgam. An access opening for endodontic therapy or a faulty margin can very readily be restored with direct gold (Fig. 14–59) instead of amalgam.

It is very common to see a well-contoured and shaded metal-ceramic crown in the mouth, acceptable in all respects except for an open gingivo-labial margin. Sometimes the cement has washed out and the exposed dentin causes patient discomfort. After application of a No. 212 (B-6) clamp to expose the defect, a Class V cavity is prepared partially at the expense of the crown. The preparation may be quite narrow—1.0 to 1.5 mm wide.

After this has been condensed with gold (Fig. 14–60), finished, and polished, the crown is placed in a permanent state of repair. Moreover, the compatibility of gingival tissue to the gold surface and contour will also result in esthetic compatibility as well.

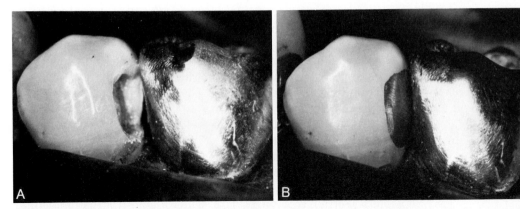

Figure 14–58. Class II restoration of direct gold on distal surface of mandibular left first premolar. Tooth was tilted and rotated, making an occlusal opening impractical.

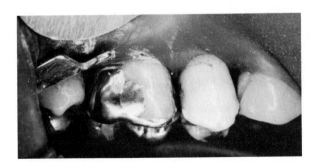

Figure 14–59. Repair of defective enamel adjoining a seven-eighths crown. Repair of defective margins on occlusal as well as axial surfaces is readily accomplished with direct gold.

Figure 14–60. Repair of labial margin of ill-fitting metal-ceramic crown.

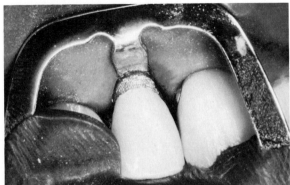

Materials and Supplies

1. Hand instruments: American Dental Mfg. Co., P.O. Box 4546, Missoula, Montana 59801; Thompson Dental Mfg. Co., 1201 S. 6th St., Missoula, Montana 59801.

2. Jeffrey hatchets (for lingual approach Class III preparations). Set of 3, LLGF Nos. 13, 14, and 15, right-handed or left-handed operators.

3. Hand condensers (lingual approach Class III). Set of 2, GF Nos. 21 and 22, right-handed or left-handed.

4. Direct golds (foil, mat, Goldent, Electralloy). Williams Gold Co., 2978 Main St., Buffalo, New York 14214.

5. No. 212 type rubber dam clamp; semi-flexible for customized application. Brinker B-6 designs (wide) and B-5 (narrow), available from Hygienic Dental Mfg. Co., 1245 Home Ave., Akron, Ohio 44310.

6. Separators, Ferrier type, sizes 1, 2, 3. Available from Almore International, P.O. Box 25214, Portland, Oregon 97225.

7. Separators, Elliot type, curved jaw posterior, curved jaw anterior. J. W. Ivory, Inc., 6019 Keystone Street, Philadelphia, Pennsylvania 19135.

8. Mandrels, small, thin-headed; No. 303½ (designed by Dr. Bruce Smith). E. C. Moore Co., 13325 Leonard Street, Dearborn, Michigan 48126.

9. Disks, abrasive, pinhole for above mandrels, E. C. Moore Co. Fine garnet disks and medium cuttle disks, ⅜" and ¼" diameter.

10. Finishing strips, extra long (18 inches). Fine, medium (No. 72830); fine, extra-narrow (No. 72850); extra-fine, extra-narrow (No. 79740). Available from Moyco Industries Inc., 21st & Clearfield Sts., Philadelphia, Pennsylvania 19132.

11. Polishing cups, gray midgets; available with screw-type mandrels (HP and RA) from Young's Dental Mfg. Co., P.O. Box 12806, St. Louis, Missouri 63141.

15

THE CAST GOLD RESTORATION: DESIGN AND PREPARATION

Many of the restorative problems that need solution cannot be resolved by using amalgam or resin. There are definite limitations when using amalgam, resin, or direct gold, for in each instance the completed restoration needs its support from the tooth. When this support is marginal or not available, a cast restoration is usually the restoration of choice (Fig. 15–1).

The process required to make the cast restoration is composed of several individual procedures, each of which must be accomplished within a restricted level of accuracy. The procedure calls for a carefully thought out design and execution of the preparation. The gingival tissue at the margins must be carefully controlled prior to the impression. The impression materials must be manipulated to achieve a result with reliable dimensional qualities. If carefully done, an accurate working model will be made from this impression.

The model will be mounted in an articulating instrument to provide inter-occlusal relationships when forming a wax pattern. The wax pattern must be made accurately to provide the restored tooth with good occlusal contact and anatomic detail. The wax pattern is removed and encased in an investment having accuracy and strength at the temperature required to melt the wax pattern and receive the molten metal into the mold. After recovery, the casting is prepared for placement on the tooth where it is adjusted for proper proximal and occlusal contacts, after which it is cemented and polished.

An alternative method is to form the wax pattern directly in the preparation. This is the method of choice for many of the one- or two-surface preparations. This direct method reduces the total time needed to make a casting as compared with the indirect method involving an impression.

Failure may occur at any of the indicated steps, which results in a casting that does not fit properly as an acceptable restoration. Since the potential for failure is present, it means the dentist and laboratory technician must exercise all possible skill so as to minimize this possibility.

When considering a cast restoration, it is best if the patient has a good understanding of preventive home care as suggested in Chapter 1, for with greater financial involvement the patient will be very interested in long-range success of the restoration. Cast restorations are placed mostly when it can be predicted that they will succeed. This assumes that the patient will follow a careful program of home care.

This restoration will not be routinely placed on young patients through the teen years. During these years the degree of caries activity is unstable and

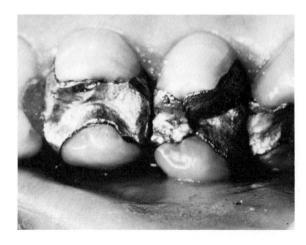

Figure 15–1. Examples of large amalgam restorations with defective margins that would be best replaced by cast restorations.

it is best to wait until this feature is predictable. It is difficult to properly locate and prepare the margins because the tissue level during youth is high and the result produces short clinical crowns.

INDICATIONS FOR CAST GOLD RESTORATION

1. PATIENT PREFERENCE. Many posterior lesions may be restored equally well with either amalgam or cast gold, and the patient may express a preference for the casting, which is a legitimate indication.

2. AMALGAM REPLACEMENT. When large dental amalgam restorations become defective and the cast restoration is the preferred replacement.

3. LARGE CARIOUS LESIONS. If dental amalgam would be poorly supported, a casting is indicated.

4. FIXED AND REMOVABLE DENTURE RETAINERS. To help replace missing teeth.

5. METAL-CERAMIC. A casting is required to support the porcelain used to satisfy esthetics.

6. WORN TEETH. Enamel will wear, exposing dentin, and these teeth must frequently be restored with castings.

A dentist who is successful in the use of castings is very careful with the design of the preparation, for this determines the stability of the casting and the reliability of the margins. The need for stability is obvious, but margins are easily overlooked and may be a source of gingival irritation or recurrent decay. It is possible to have a casting with good occlusal anatomy and good stability that fails because of poor margins. The integrity on the part of the dentist should not allow this to occur.

The process of making cast restorations was introduced to the dental profession around 1906, and Dr. William H. Taggart is given major credit for its introduction. During this time some single-surface cast restorations were made by adapting platinum or gold foil to the prepared cavity, withdrawing the adapted foil, and filling the void with solder. If it was a full crown, a model was made from a modeling compound impression to which 22 carat gold plate was accurately shaped and contoured. A preformed occlusal segment was then soldered to the contoured form to complete the crown. This method required an exacting level of skill to be successful and as a result was not consistently satisfactory.

The various steps in the casting procedure have been under investigation since its introduction, and they have been refined to the point where the process is currently successful.

Inlays and Onlays

Inlays—Class I and II

INDICATIONS

1. Mostly elective on the part of a patient.
2. Used to complement treatment when gold and/or ceramics are the dominant choices for restorations.
3. When form and function are most reliably restored with a casting. For example, it is not advisable to change existing tooth contour by placing an amalgam restoration.
4. Occasional rest seat for a removable partial denture clasp.

The following factors deserve attention when considering Class I and II inlays: (1) the age of the patient, (2) the degree of caries activity, and (3) economics of treatment.

Castings are not routinely placed on patients who are in their early twenties or younger. For Class I and II lesions, amalgam and occasionally direct gold are routinely advised as restorations. Irrespective of age, if a Class I lesion exists, the interproximal area must be carefully analyzed for possible weakness before considering a one-surface inlay. If it appears that the interproximal area is suspect as related to caries activity, an occlusal inlay is not indicated. When a two-surface casting is designated as part of restorative treatment, either as an MO or DO, the remaining proximal surface must be examined carefully and a determination made that caries is not a factor for that surface (Fig. 15–2).

At a time when Class I and II preparations are the most frequent, the cost to the patient is the greatest problem. The budgets of most families have difficulty with a treatment plan emphasizing gold when other options are available.

In spite of the precautions stated, a Class II inlay that is skillfully accomplished, with good margins and anatomy, is a picturesque and a very

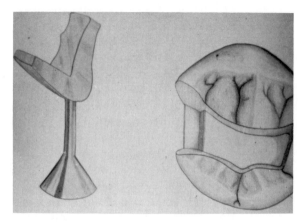

Figure 15–2. A two-surface casting has limited application.

functional restoration. The knowledge and ability to prepare Class II castings is basic to the cast restoration, and its fundamentals should be clearly understood and executed during treatment, as this is one of the classic backgrounds for restorative treatment.

INLAY PREPARATION—CLASS I

Armamentarium
1. Rubber dam supplies
2. Burs: F G Nos. 69, 70, 70L, 170, 171
   Finishing bur
3. Instruments
   Enamel hatchet
   Mon-angle chisel
   Bin-angle chisel
   Marginal trimmer and/or angle former
   Excavator

Procedure
The rubber dam can be used easily with a washed field procedure and its use is advised for the preparation of inlays. As for other operations, the rubber dam is very helpful for the purpose of isolation of the area. It is a great aid to visibility and for partial retraction of the gingival tissue. It is the best way to prevent debris from the preparation from being swallowed or aspirated.

The design requirements for an inlay preparation must allow for the convenience of placing the cast restoration. There must be assurance that when the inlay has been placed the margins will be closed to prevent leakage.

The occlusal walls must be tapered from the pulpal wall to allow the withdrawal of the pattern or casting in an occlusal direction. All occlusal walls are tapered from the pulpal wall toward the occlusal opening.

The enamel is penetrated with a No. 170 or 171 bur at high speed. The penetration is made at the deepest location of the central groove, or if caries has involved the groove, the initial penetration of the bur will occur where this weakness exists. The first objective is to locate the level of the pulpal wall. As a relative guide the pulpal wall will develop on dentin just beyond the dento-enamel junction. When a bur is cutting at high speed, it is recommended that a water spray be directed on the cutting instrument. The spray in turn is removed by using a high-velocity vacuum system.

OUTLINE OF THE PREPARATION. The pulpal wall depth is developed independently of the extent of caries. As far as possible the optimum level for the pulpal wall is initially developed and the removal of carious dentin will follow. The pulpal wall is extended for the length of the central groove, and all grooves are followed to remove existing or potential defects. When developing the buccal and lingual walls, the cutting bur is angulated so as to produce an obtuse angle with the pulpal wall. The outline should reflect conservation of tooth structure. The normal taper of the No. 170 series burs allows for this angulation, but the position of the cutting bur must be carefully controlled to avoid undercutting or over-angulation of the walls. All prepared walls must be aligned to allow for the convenience of inserting the casting but not over-tapered so as to jeopardize the resistance form of the preparation.

All major grooves are followed to clear any existing or potential defect. The outline is a series of coordinated and connecting curves. The buccal to lingual extension will exceed that required for an amalgam to allow for

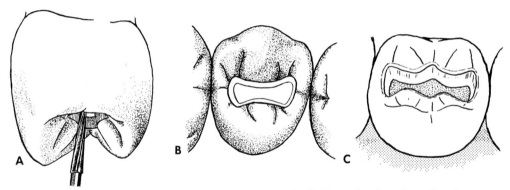

Figure 15–3. *A,* A tapered bur is used to form the occlusal walls. *B,* The outline form for a Class I premolar inlay. *C,* A molar Class I inlay preparation, which includes a cavosurface bevel.

convenience and an adequate line of withdrawal. The pulpal wall is expected to be flat throughout the preparation (Fig. 15–3).

When preparing a Class I preparation, special precautions are observed when approaching the mesial and distal marginal ridges. It is important that these functional ridges be left intact and not in a weakened state. The angulation of the mesial and distal walls is important as a means of preserving the marginal ridges. The mesial and distal margins of the preparation are to terminate on the axial inclines of the marginal ridges.

When occlusal caries invades, undermines, and weakens any of the cusps, the outline of the preparation must be extended to terminate in enamel that has good dentin support. Frequently, the occlusal caries of lower molars extends into the buccal groove, which then should be included in the preparation outline. If this is required, the occlusal groove is terminated on the buccal surface with the same No. 170 bur. Following this the buccal step is extended gingivally as far as required to clear the defect and place the gingival wall in healthy enamel and dentin. The mesial and distal extension of the buccal segment must terminate with dentin-supported enamel. An enamel hatchet or a mon-angle chisel, for example, a 10-4-14, is useful for planing the walls, which are tapered to complement the insertion path of the casting. The axial wall of the buccal extension is positioned on dentin. The gingival cavosurface of the facial wall requires a bevel similar to that used for the gingival wall of the Class II inlay.

When caries penetration extends beyond the normal depth required for the preparation and is a cause of pulpal distress, a base is indicated. Without concern for the penetration of the caries the preparation is positioned at its ideal depth location. Also, enamel that has no support is cut away. At the conclusion of this portion of the preparation the remaining caries is removed and treated as discussed in Chapters 7 and 8. Burs at slow speed and hand instruments are used to produce a smooth surface for the base and the preparation.

INLAY PREPARATION—CLASS II

Procedure

The initial portion of the Class II preparation is the development of the occlusal segment. The occlusal outline and location of the pulpal wall are the same as described for the Class I inlay preparation.

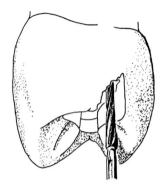

Figure 15–4. The occlusal outline followed by initiation of the proximal box.

PROXIMAL BOX. As the outline and form of the occlusal segment are completed the next step is to enter the proximal portion and begin developing the box form (Fig. 15–4). The occlusal preparation is extended proximally into the marginal ridge, but a thin portion of the marginal ridge is left intact. A No. 69 bur is used to begin the proximal box and it penetrates gingivally with the dentoenamel junction as a guide. The gingival extension is made by cutting both enamel and dentin; if the penetration is done totally at the expense of the dentin, the axial wall might be too close to the pulp.

The proximal box must be positioned gingivally to break contact with the adjacent tooth. It must proceed beyond defective enamel. If the gingival tissue is in a normal position, this will often place the gingival margin within the gingival sulcus. If gingival recession has occurred, there is no attempt to move the gingival wall into the sulcus except as required by the extent of caries.

With most teeth the gingival wall will be positioned at right angles to the long axis of the tooth. The buccal and lingual walls are extended just beyond contact with the adjacent tooth. When this is being done, care must be exercised to avoid any tendency toward placing undercuts in any of the walls. The buccal and lingual extension should not be completed by using burs. This would result in overextension of the walls or possible damage to the adjacent tooth (Fig. 15–5).

Hand instruments are used for final location of proximal walls and margins. The walls and margins must be located to include all defective or weakened tooth structure. The proximal margins must be located so as to conveniently finish the metal-to-enamel interface. This is not a major problem, for even with demanding esthetic criteria most margins may be placed and allow for reasonable finishing convenience (Fig. 15–6).

The angulation of all walls must be arranged to allow for convenience of seating the casting, while providing proper resistance for retention of the

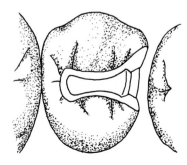

Figure 15–5. The facial-to-lingual extension clears contact with the adjacent tooth.

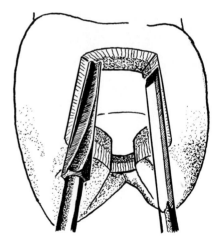

Figure 15–6. Sharp hand instruments are used to extend and complete the preparation.

casting. The axial wall forms a slightly obtuse angle with the gingival wall, which is flat and at right angles to the long axis of the tooth. Proceeding in an occlusal direction, the proximal wall forms a slightly obtuse angle with the gingival wall. As they join the axial wall the proximal walls form an obtuse angle proceeding toward the cavosurface. This helps to minimize the amount of tooth structure sacrificed during the preparation and also helps to produce convenience for placement and finishing.

The final design and internal detail of the preparation are obtained using sharp hand instruments. The usual preference is to use enamel hatchets for lower teeth and bin-angle chisels for the upper teeth. All walls and margins must be smooth and precise following instrumentation. Special emphasis is given to the cavosurface margin to guarantee there will be no loose or irregular enamel remaining. When access permits, it is possible to use cuttle or sandpaper disks to place the final touch on the margins.

Gingival bevels. The gingival wall will have a definite cavosurface bevel. This bevel is required to remove enamel rods that have poor support at this location and also to provide a decrease in the potential opening or discrepancy of fit between the casting and the tooth. This potential discrepancy exists because it is difficult to make a casting that accurately fits the prepared tooth. If poorly supported enamel is left, it may fracture during or following

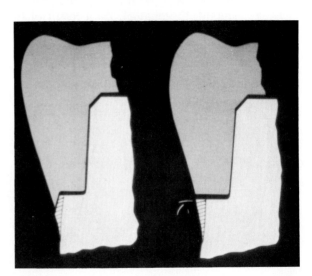

Figure 15–7. Bevels are helpful in minimizing gingival casting discrepancies and provide firm gingival enamel support.

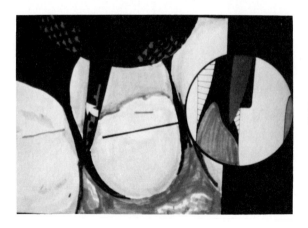

Figure 15–8. The use of a flame-shaped diamond to place a gingival bevel.

placement of the casting, leaving defects in the gingival area that would encourage recurrent caries. If there is no bevel and the casting does not seat completely, the resultant discrepancy extends to the axial wall (Fig. 15–7).

Placing an adequate gingival bevel will reduce the magnitude of this discrepancy. The bevel should be approximately 1.0 mm in width. The bevel must be steep enough to allow the potential opening to be reduced. It is preferred that this bevel blend into the proximal cavosurface margins.

To place the proper bevels one of several instrumentations may be used. A flame-tipped diamond operating at reduced speed will produce a good bevel form. It may tend to overcut if operated at high speed. Carbide finishing burs also with a flame-tipped design will do the same thing and leave a smoother surface than most diamonds (Fig. 15–8). Hand instruments are effective for placing these bevels on interproximal gingival walls. The gingival margin trimmer or angle former is used for this purpose and the former is effective with either upper or lower teeth; the latter because of access is limited to use with maxillary bicuspids. The best control is maintained by choosing the medium or larger size instruments (Fig. 15–9). It is important that when these instruments are sharpened the initial blade angle be maintained.

The finish of the enamel walls is usually accomplished with the same plain fissure bur as used for the preparation. This type of bur is used near its stall-out speed for finishing purposes; otherwise the preparation will be overcut. Enamel finishing burs with 12 or more blades may also be used to smooth the enamel. As a result of the angulation of the occlusal walls, it is not required to provide a cavosurface bevel to the occlusal margins. A soft

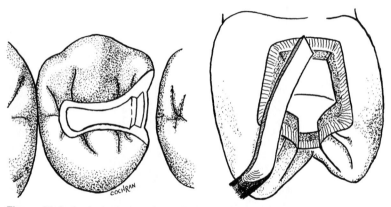

Figure 15–9. Angle formers and marginal trimmers are effective in making gingival bevels.

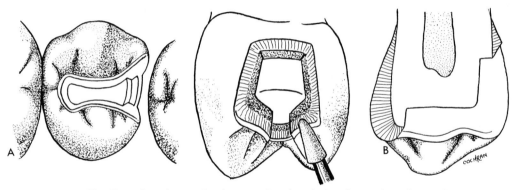

Figure 15–10. The illustration of an occlusal cavosurface bevel when its use is preferred. *B,* The sagittal view of an inlay preparation.

casting gold may be used for small preparations, which simplifies adaptation of the metal margins (Fig. 15–10).

MOD Onlay

When the occlusal morphology has been severely altered by a previous restoration, caries, or physical wear, a two-surface inlay will not be adequate. This leads to a restoration that includes all of the occlusal table. In this capacity an MOD onlay is an effective restoration.

INDICATIONS

1. Replacement of defective amalgam restorations.
2. When the restoration needs to splint the buccal and lingual cusps.
3. Restoration of posterior interproximal caries.
4. Restoration of posterior teeth with heavy occlusal wear.

It is possible for an amalgam or inlay to render the tooth vulnerable to cuspal fracture. A primary asset of a restoration that includes the occlusal surface is one that restores strength to the tooth by splinting the cusps into a single unit.

A popular indication for an onlay is replacing defective amalgam restorations (Fig. 15–11). It is also useful as a restoration to restore carious lesions involving both proximal surfaces. A strong feature of this restoration is that it

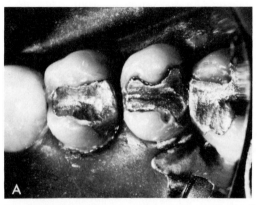
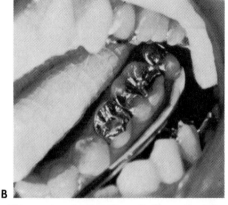

Figure 15–11. *A,* Amalgam restorations, which ideally would be replaced with onlays. *B,* The molar inlay has underextended occlusal margins.

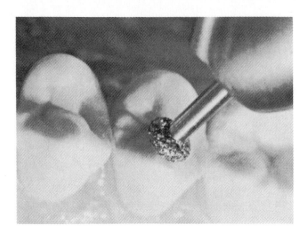

Figure 15–12. Small round diamond wheel (3 mm) used in occlusal reduction of preparation.

preserves most of the tooth tissue associated with the gingiva and this is a helpful periodontal consideration.

MOD ONLAY PREPARATION

Armamentarium
1. Burs: FG Nos. 169, 70, 70L, 170, 171
2. Finishing burs
3. 4 mm diamond wheel
4. Bullet nose diamond
5. Flame-shaped diamond
6. Instruments
   Enamel hatchet
   Bin-angle chisel
   Margin trimmer and/or angle former
   Excavator

Procedure
The basic MOD portion of the preparation is achieved in the same manner as described for the two-surface casting. Both proximal boxes will be prepared and connected to each other with an occlusal isthmus. The method of entry and instrumentation is accomplished in the manner as described for a two-surface inlay.

Frequently the size of the lesion is large enough to allow a No. 70 bur at high speed to penetrate and outline the MOD segment of the preparation. *The operator must be careful not to nick the adjacent tooth during the preparation.* Proximal contact is relieved in all directions and the walls are positioned to provide good structural support.

When the preparation includes defective amalgam the No. 70 bur can be used to provide proximal and occlusal outline. As a rule, all the old amalgam will be removed. A No. 4 bur at slow speed may be used to remove the remote segments of amalgam. If caries is present, either the bur or an excavator is used to remove it and a basing procedure is initiated, as described in Chapter 8.

The buccal and lingual extensions are governed by the extensions of the existing caries or restoration, and they will typically have greater extensions than for a two-surface inlay. If the buccal-lingual extensions for one or both proximals destroy the resistance features that will be needed, it means the preparation will need to be changed and consideration given to using partial or full coverage crowns.

When the proximal outline and box structure have been established, proceed by reducing the remainder of the occlusal surface. This is easily achieved by using a small egg-shaped or round-wheel diamond. Some operators prefer using a straight fluted bur to make this reduction. The amount reduced must allow for a minimum of 1.0 mm of metal in any area that is in function (Fig. 15–12). In non-functioning areas the reduction may be less but must be adequate to allow for a successful casting, which should not be less than 0.5 mm in thickness. The reduction is accomplished to conform to the general morphology of the occlusal anatomy.

An accurate determination of the amount of occlusal reduction is difficult in areas where direct vision is obscure. This is most apparent when a preparation involves lingual surfaces and teeth most remote in the arch. As a direct aid to this problem select a segment of black carding wax or red equalizing wax* that fits the area being reduced and allows adequate excess for handling convenience to the facial. Have the patient close into firm centric occlusion. The thickness of wax that intervenes can easily be observed and measured by a Boley or wax gauge. With a little practice the critical thickness of the intervening wax can be determined by observing the resistance to transmission of light. Usually some of the reduction can be observed by direct vision and, assuming that it is adequate, the remainder can be compared by holding a wax bite to the light and observing if the light transmits at least in equal intensity in the obscure area as compared with that where direct vision gives a clear indication of the amount of tooth reduced.

Following adequate reduction of the occlusal, finish lines or margins are established. The finish lines will appear as bevels on the buccal and lingual surfaces. These bevels provide a convenient location of the final finishing of the cemented restoration. They also provide a means by which the buccal and lingual cusps are splinted together so as to prevent the possibility of future cuspal fracture (Fig. 15–13). These bevels are precisely and smoothly placed with carbide finishing burs with 12 or more cutting blades.

---

*Trubyte Equalizing Wax, Dentsply International Inc., York, Pennsylvania 17405.

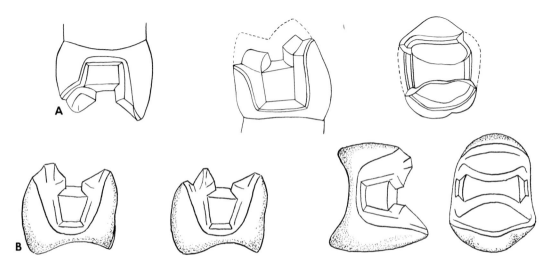

Figure 15–13. *A,* Examples of premolar MOD onlay preparations. *B,* The bevels and finish lines are placed to prevent future fracture.

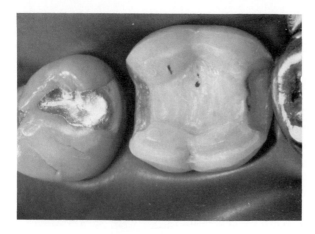

Figure 15–14. A clinical MOD onlay preparation.

Gingival walls will require the placement of bevels, which has been previously described for the two-surface inlay (Fig. 15–14).

Resumé of Inlay and Onlay Preparation
1. With No. 170 bur cut the occlusal outline.
2. Establish pulpal wall depth.
3. The enamel walls require firm dentin support.
4. The preparation may include one or both proximal boxes.
5. A No. 169 or 170 bur is used to cut the proximal box.
6. Contact with the adjacent tooth is severed in all directions.
7. Bin-angle chisels or enamel hatchets are used to complete the extensions and provide smoothness to the walls of the preparation.
8. All proximal and occlusal walls must provide convenience for seating the casting.
9. Gingival bevels are placed on all gingival walls with angle formers, marginal trimmers, or flame-shaped burs.
10. The preparation may require the addition of a base.
11. With a small wheel diamond or a straight bladed bur a minimum of 1.0 mm of the occlusal surface is reduced for clearance.
12. Buccal and lingual bevels are placed with enamel finishing burs.

Partial and Full Crowns

Posterior Three-Quarter Crown

INDICATIONS

1. Replacement of large defective amalgam restorations.
2. Restoration of extensive carious lesions not involving the buccal surface on posterior teeth.
3. Occlusal wear on posterior teeth with short clinical crowns.
4. Fixed partial retainer.
5. Retainer and rest seat for removable partial denture clasp.

CROWN PREPARATION

Armamentarium
1. Burs: FG Nos. 69, 70, 70L
2. Finishing burs
3. 4 mm diamond wheel
4. Bullet nose diamond
5. Flame-shaped diamond
6. Instruments
   Enamel hatchet
   Bin-angle chisel
   Excavator

Procedure

In a sequence of preparation styles one design of a three-quarter preparation is an extension of the MOD onlay. The essential difference is the reduction of the lingual surface, with the placement of a lingual margin or finish line.

The lingual finish line is determined prior to initiation of the preparation. It is influenced by the quality and amount of remaining lingual enamel surface. If the enamel is defective or if the retention for the casting is marginal because the clinical crown is short, the finish line will be located half-way into the free gingival crevice. If the clinical crown is long, the margin may be ideally located above the gingival level approximately 2 to 3 mm above the lingual free gingiva (Fig. 15–15). In either event the margin should not terminate at the same level as the crest of the free marginal gingiva. The amount of reduction should allow for a rigid covering of metal without excessive contour of the restored surface. The reduction is done with a bullet nose diamond.

A preferred style for a posterior three-quarter crown is one that has a groove on the mesial and distal surfaces for the primary source of resistance for the casting. This preparation will retain more tooth structure as compared with a box style and is technically easier to accomplish (Fig. 15–16).

The occlusal reduction is completed first, using the same instruments as used for the onlay preparation. With the teeth closed in contact there should be 1.0 mm clearance as a minimum for adequate metal thickness and this

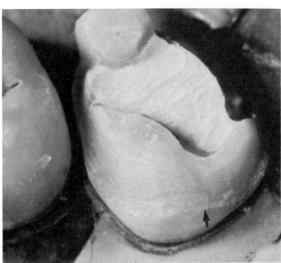

Figure 15–15. When possible, the margin is located above the gingival tissue.

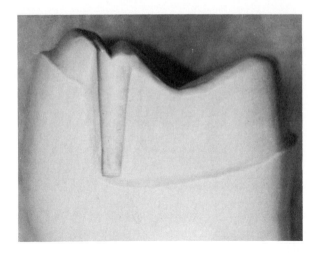

Figure 15–16. Typical three-quarter preparation for mandibular molar. Note the occlusal offset to encompass the facial cusps.

should be verified with a wax bite. During the reduction the general occlusal form is maintained, buccal to lingual and mesial to distal. The lingual finish line is located, according to the preceding criteria, and the same bullet nose diamond is used to prepare the lingual surface until the adjacent tooth in contact presents a problem with access. The lingual reduction should be done so as to have a chamfered finish line. This allows for an adequate thickness of metal for rigidity. The lingual reduction should be styled to enhance the resistance form when related to the proximal grooves or boxes (Fig. 15–17).

The buccal finish line is placed bucally to the contact area, making it convenient to finish the margins of the restoration. To avoid cutting the adjacent tooth or overcutting the proximal of the preparation it is best to use a thin-nosed diamond (Fig. 15–18).

The buccal placement of the margin allows the mesial and distal retention grooves to have as much length as will be needed to stabilize the restoration.

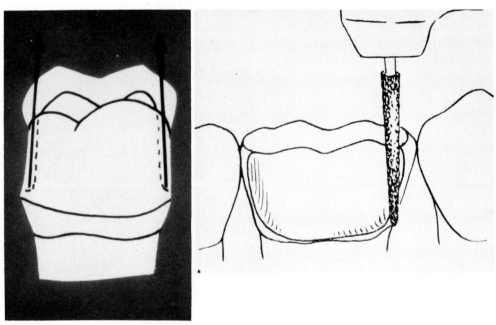

Figure 15–17. Incline the walls to have good resistance form.

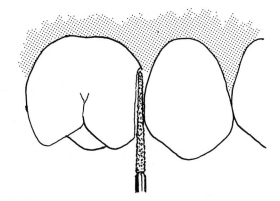

Figure 15–18. A thin diamond is selected for cutting the proximal segment so as to avoid damage to the adjacent tooth.

If the buccal finish lines restrict the groove location, they frequently are too short. If a posterior tooth, as viewed from the proximal side, is divided in thirds, the groove will occur close to the junction of the buccal and middle one-third of the tooth. On some teeth this groove may line up with the tip of the buccal cusp or it may be just lingual to the cusp tip. There is a tendency to place the grooves at the proximal end of the central groove, which leaves them too short to be effective (Fig. 15–19).

Groove placement governs the direction or pathway of insertion of the casting and routinely this coincides with the long axis of the tooth. When the proximal grooves are placed, it is advised to leave them undersized until direction or angulation is verified. Depending on tooth size, the groove is initially placed with a No. 169 or 70 bur. The axial depth of the groove should be placed at 80 per cent of the final depth. The grooves should be carefully analyzed as to location, direction, and depth. If adjustments are needed, they are easily accomplished. Following this, a bur capable of making the proper groove size should be used. For molars it will usually be a No. 701 or 71 bur and for premolars it would be 700 or 70. For many it will be most reliable if the final portions of groove preparation are cut with a slow-speed handpiece. The groove must be cut with adequate precision to guarantee resistance to lingual displacement.

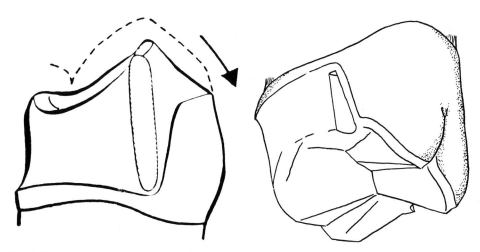

Figure 15–19. The groove should be placed where maximum length can be obtained for the grooves, and the finish line must avoid wear facets.

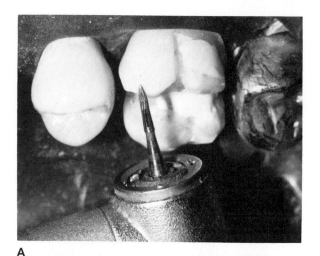

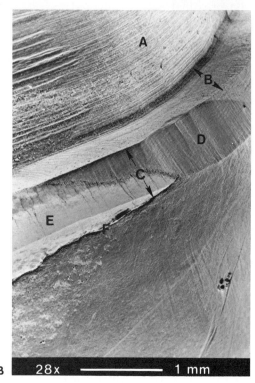

Figure 15–20. *A,* The use of an enamel finishing bur provides a smooth margin. *B,* An SEM view of a margin beveled with a 12-bladed tungsten carbide finishing bur. A, axial well; B, 90° shoulder; C, bevel; D, dentin; E, enamel; F, cemento-enamel junction (28×) (*B* Courtesy of Drs. C. H. Lehner and P. Scharer, University of Zurich, Zurich, Switzerland)

There remains the formation of the bevel at the occlusal margin of the buccal cusp. For upper teeth, the bevel is not expected to have a significant role in the resistance form of the casting. The bevel may be short and precise. The form of the bevel is often influenced by the desire to minimize the display of gold. It is made by proper angulation of a small thin diamond, following which it is smoothed using an enamel finishing bur (Fig. 15–20).

For lower teeth there may be a variation in style because of function. It is normal to have facets of wear on the buccal occlusals of lower posterior teeth. The margin of the casting must not terminate in such a facet and will either be located near the cuspal height to avoid the facet or extend gingivally to fully include the wear facet to avoid compromising the margins (see Fig. 15–19). The remaining enamel is weakened when a margin runs through a

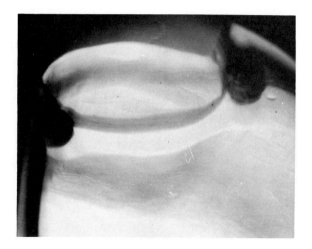

Figure 15–21. A V-shaped connector may be used between the grooves for three-quarter or seven-eighths crowns.

wear facet. When required, placing the buccal margin in a conspicuous facial position on lower teeth usually does not cause great esthetic problems. If the same procedure were to be used on upper posterior teeth, it would produce definite esthetic conflicts.

When more than a conventional bevel is required, a definite buccal wall should be made, which provides aid to the resistance form. This will require a chamfer heavy enough to allow for adequate thickness of metal to accommodate the occlusal morphology. If the chamfer is heavy, it may require a small enamel bevel at the cavosurface.

With some preparations, it is advisable to make a V-shaped connector between the proximal grooves. This is needed to provide adequate rigidity for the casting so that it will not flex at the facial margins when under occlusal stress (Fig. 15–21). The groove can easily be made with a No. 70 or 71 bur at high speed. Usually this connector is made on as direct a line as is possible from one groove to the other. The magnitude of this groove varies according to the needs for stability.

While this discussion for the posterior three-quarter crown has featured grooves as a means of stability, there are many times when the destruction by caries or the design of a previous restoration will lend itself to using a proximal box, or boxes, as the best preparation design. This is easily worked into the design and has been discussed as part of the MOD onlay preparation.

Posterior Seven-Eighths Crown

A restoration that includes more than a three-quarter crown but stops short of full coverage is termed a seven-eighths or four-fifths crown. It is best for the patient to retain as much healthy tooth tissue as possible and yet have proper resistance for the casting. This restoration deserves consideration, as it allows the gingival tissue to have some enamel or cemental contact rather than a lengthy tooth-to-metal interface.

The typical form for this extension is to move the distal margin from the disto-buccal corner to the buccal surface (Fig. 15–22). Many times the distal portion of a tooth is badly destroyed and does not provide the needed tooth structure for adequate resistance within the preparation for a three-quarter crown. To overcome this problem the distal margin is placed onto the buccal surfaces to allow for a reliable margin and stability of the casting. The groove

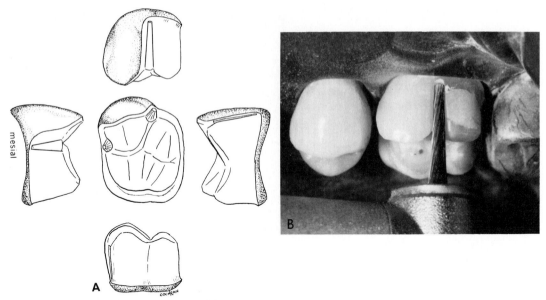

Figure 15–22. *A,* The preparation outline and groove location for a seven-eighths crown on a maxillary molar. *B,* Bur placement for facial groove of a seven-eighths crown.

should be placed directly on the buccal surface to provide adequate resistance for lingual displacement. On molar teeth, if the margin is located distal to the mesio-buccal cusp, esthetics is not a critical problem. For premolars the buccal margin may be esthetically acceptable if placed distal to the buccal ridge (Fig. 15–23).

For the purpose of securing the casting, the groove placed on the buccal surface will have greater length as compared with one placed in the conventional interproximal location. When teeth have short clinical crowns with

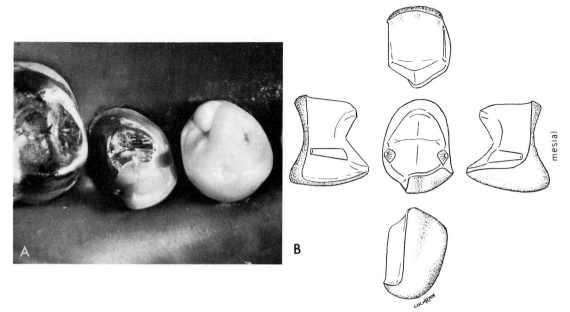

Figure 15–23. *A,* Occlusal view of seven-eighths crown for mandibular premolar. *B,* The location of the finish line for a seven-eighths preparation on an upper premolar.

little potential for interproximal resistance, the seven-eighths crown is a good method of securing a reliable restoration.

The placement of a seven-eighths crown is a workable method for many lower canines as well as for the posterior teeth. There are occasions when the distal portion of a cuspid is destroyed by caries or is unusually short, and at such times it is very helpful to design a needed casting as a seven-eighths crown. This is possible for those patients who are not sensitive about the display of some gold.

Full Crown

INDICATIONS

1. The only option remaining.
2. Usually reserved for molar and lower premolar teeth.
3. Extensive caries or defective restorations.
4. Short clinical crowns.

FULL CROWN PREPARATION

Armamentarium
1. Burs: FG Nos. 69, 70, 70L, 1170
2. Finishing burs
3. 4 mm diamond wheel
4. Bullet nose diamond
5. Flame-shaped diamond
6. Instruments
   Excavator

Procedure

If the problem is such that a partial crown will not function, the only option left is the full crown restoration, and it is the treatment court of last appeal. Full crowns are most frequently placed on molar teeth and occasionally on lower bicuspids.

The situations that require a complete crown include teeth that have extensive but questionable restorations or extensive carious involvement. A significant contributor to this difficulty is a large defective Class V amalgam restoration, and the only way a casting will perform is to make a complete crown. Another situation requiring this type of crown is presented by teeth that are very short and do not provide resistance unless a full crown is utilized.

Many times the locations of the gingival margins are predetermined by the existing restoration or caries and decalcification that must be enclosed. This often dictates that these margins, with emphasis on the interproximal and facial, will be in the gingival sulcus. If adequate resistance for the restoration and effective coverage can be met without placing the margin in the sulcus, that is the recommendation. Many times the lingual surface will be intact and it is easy to terminate the margin above the level of the gingiva, which eases the maintenance problems of the marginal gingiva.

The initial procedure is the occlusal reduction. The reduction may be done using a wheel diamond or a tapered round-end diamond. The same amount of reduction is required as for other posterior teeth, with a minimum of 1 mm wherever function occurs. The occlusal reduction should show correlation with the occlusal morphology of the tooth and not be an arbitrary flattening of the occlusal surface.

Following the occlusal preparation, proceed to the buccal and lingual reduction. A tapered round-end diamond is useful for this purpose. The gingival finish line will have been predetermined by the needs of retention, defective restorations, or caries. The reduction should reflect a chamfer effect at the gingival cavosurface. The buccal and lingual morphology is observed and the reduction is done to produce an even thickness of metal in the completed restoration consistent with the shape of the tooth.

The buccal and lingual walls are structured to provide good resistance to displacement (Fig. 15–24). There is a danger of over-angulating the walls and losing the potential resistance for the casting. This reduction is carried toward the adjacent teeth. To avoid overcutting at the interproximal, a thin flame-shaped diamond is selected.

The finish line must be located gingival to the contact and be on healthy enamel. If an amalgam core or restoration (see Chapter 13) is part of the preparation, it is expected that the finish line for the casting will terminate gingival to the restoration. The proximal walls must relate to each other in the same manner as to the buccal and lingual to provide optimal resistance. They will be slightly inclined toward each other.

This should complete most of the reduction and now with a fine grit finishing diamond or a No. 1170 bur the preparation is made smooth. All sharp corners or angles are slightly rounded. For some of the smoothing it is best that the bur run at a reduced speed to avoid excess cutting.

The occlusal clearance is checked in the same manner as discussed for previous posterior cast preparations.

Consideration must be given to clearance when the patient goes through eccentric movements, and the preparation must have adequate reduction to allow the restoration to have acceptable function in all movements. This information must be placed into a suitable articulator to allow for a reliable wax-up and casting.

The final segment of the preparation is the placement of a groove on the buccal surface and usually this will be in the anatomical buccal groove (Fig. 15–25). This groove is of value, as it helps to provide positive orientation during the placement of the casting. It will tend to limit the potential for slight rotation of the crown during seating, as the groove will guide or key it into the specific placement. At times it will prove of value by providing a degree of supplemental retention, which may be helpful to a restoration with marginal retention. On occasion when the buccal segment of the tooth is badly destroyed this groove may be placed on the lingual portion of the preparation. If the preparation requires a pin-supported amalgam or resin buildup, the groove may be placed in the amalgam or resin.

This groove may be formed by using a thin, tapered round-end diamond, or a No. 171 bur may be used effectively for this purpose. If the bur is used, it is advised to use it at reduced speed to avoid overcutting. This groove extends just short of the gingival finish line (Fig. 15–26).

Resumé of Partial and Full Crown Preparation

1. Gingival finish line when possible should be located occlusal to the gingiva.

2. Grooves with adequate length are preferred over proximal boxes for resistance form.

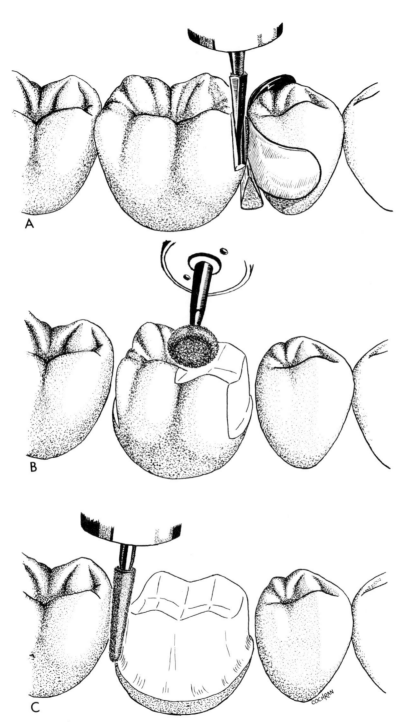

Figure 15–24. A combination of burs and diamonds may be used to make a full crown preparation. Note the design of the finish line and the amount of reduction.

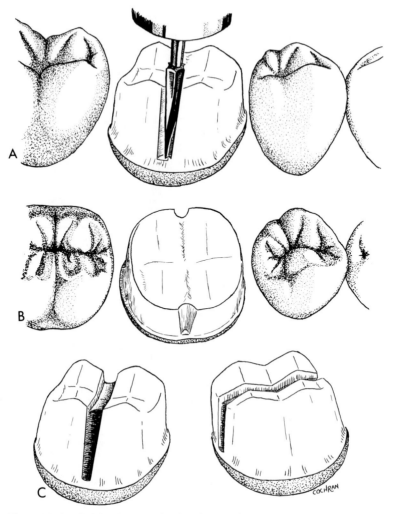

Figure 15–25. *A,* A basic groove is placed most often on the facial surface. *B* and *C,* Variations in groove design are indicated.

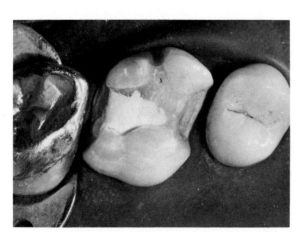

Figure 15–26. The clinical preparation of a partial crown. It is advantageous to use the rubber dam when feasible.

3. Do not terminate a finish line through a wear facet.

4. Occlusal reduction should occur first using wheel or football-shaped diamond. With a wax bite check for a minimum clearance of 1 mm.

5. Lingual reduction with bullet-nose diamond 2D–T.

6. Interproximal reduction with thin or flame-shaped diamond to avoid cutting adjacent tooth.

7. Proximal grooves are located for maximum length and will line up toward the buccal cusp tip.

8. Place buccal bevel toward facial to complement esthetics and function.

9. A V-shaped connector may be used between grooves.

10. With a seven-eighths crown one groove is located on the facial surface.

11. For a full crown preparation the facial reduction is done with the same instrument as for the lingual. A definite chamfer is needed for the buccal finish line.

12. Place a groove on the facial surface of the preparation for positive seating and use of tapered diamond or a No. 171 bur.

Anterior Three-Quarter Crown

INDICATIONS

1. For cuspids when distal lesions are excessive for a Class III metal restoration and not large enough to require full coverage.

2. When proximal loss can be restored with a three-quarter crown casting that has minimum display of gold, leaving the labial surface intact.

3. When the incisal edge, lingual surface, or both are worn, altering function, and the replacement by a casting is not an esthetic problem.

4. Proximal contour requires improvement with a rigid restoration.

5. Fixed partial or splint retainer.

CROWN PREPARATION

Preparation of the anterior three-quarter crown requires the following steps:

1. Proximal reduction.
2. Lingual reduction.
3. Cervical finish line.
4. Incisal bevels and groove.
5. Proximal grooves.

Armamentarium
1. Separating strips and disks
2. Safe side ⅞" diamond disk, slow speed
3. Flame-shaped diamond, 1 DT–L Densco, high speed
4. Tapered diamond, bullet nose, D71 Densco, high speed
5. Football-shaped diamond, 1LC Densco, high speed
6. Small diamond wheel
7. No. 169L bur
8. No. 170L bur
9. Paper disks

Procedure

When an anterior three-quarter crown is possible, it has the potential of being one of the most functional and esthetic restorations. This assumes that the patient will accept some visible display of gold. This restoration has the advantage of leaving intact labial enamel, allowing the periodontal tissue a minimal source of irritation. This restoration is very helpful when trying to restore proper form and function.

This restoration at times is very difficult, as its design features tend to be critical when considering thin teeth. Mandibular incisors and maxillary laterals are frequently poor prospects for three-quarter crowns.

PROXIMAL REDUCTION. When esthetics is a major consideration, the proximal preparation must be executed very carefully. To minimize labial extension a lightening strip is suggested as a means of beginning the proximal reduction by producing clearance at the expense of the contact (Fig. 15–27). It is important that the disk be totally free and not binding in the contact, for if it does bind, the disk may rotate out of control and cause severe soft tissue injury. It may be advisable to first apply a means of slight separation between the teeth with a wedge or mechanical separator to help provide freedom of movement to a lightening strip or disk. This disk is a very slow method of proximal preparation, but it will provide a controlled means of precisely locating the labial extensions and is the most distinct means of limiting any display of gold.

Many times this method is of value for gaining space for a seven-eighths inch safesided diamond disk, which will cut very quickly, simplifying the proximal preparation. As experience is gained, the diamond disk will be used more frequently (Fig. 15–28).

If high speed is chosen, the proximal penetration is done with a narrow or flame-shaped diamond. The reduction begins in the lingual embrasure and is brought toward the labial surface. When esthetics does not pose a problem, as on the distal aspect of cuspids, the labial finish line is located with this diamond. If esthetics is a factor, the thin diamond may stop just short of the labial surface and a disk may be used to locate the labial finish line. In each case a disk is a good instrument for the labial margins, as it leaves the margin straight and very precise.

The inclination of the labial margins is predetermined by the direction required to seat the casting. Usually a line may be drawn through the center of the tooth, and both mesial and distal margins must incline slightly toward the midline.

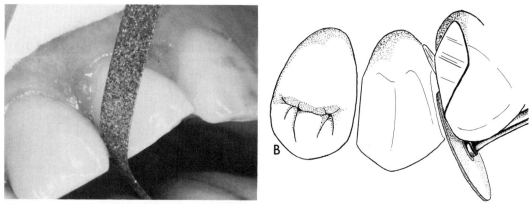

Figure 15–27. A, A metal strip may be used to clear contact. B, The use of a thin disk to clear proximal contact.

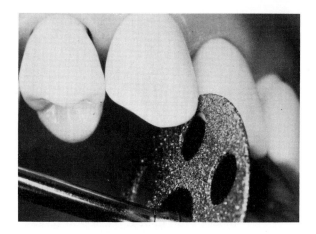

Figure 15–28. The use of diamond disk to prepare the proximal surfaces of upper anterior teeth.

The lingual reduction follows and should be done with a small football- or wheel-shaped diamond. The centric position on the tooth is noted by articulating paper, and in this area it is reduced by 1 mm. The tooth relationship must also be observed in protrusive movement and clearance provided. When the restoration is placed, the force in these movements on the restored tooth should not usually exceed that which occurs in its condition prior to a restoration. An exception to this would be teeth in poor positions that are not really functioning until a restoration is placed.

The reduction should be equal over the lingual surface, and the amount will be determined by visual inspection. The reduction must allow for metal replacement without becoming over-contoured. During lingual reduction try to avoid excessive reduction of the cingulum, for it is best to preserve as much as possible, as it will contribute to the stability of the restoration (Fig. 15–29).

A bullet nose diamond is used to connect the proximal preparations and to enclose the cingulum area. The lingual margin will usually be located slightly below the margin of the gingiva unless there has been tissue recession, and when possible it is best if the margins are above the gingiva. A definite chamfer should be used as the design for the lingual margins (Fig. 15–30).

The incisal reduction may be done with a No. 170 bur or flame-shaped diamond. It is done so as to provide 1 mm of metal, which will be needed for a rigid restoration. The reduction is done at an angle and the reduced surface will reflect toward the lingual. To remove any unsupported enamel a slight contrabevel toward the labial is placed with the No. 170 bur or with a carbide finishing bur. The incisal bevel is placed to avoid any significant display of

Figure 15–29. The use of a small diamond wheel to do the lingual reduction.

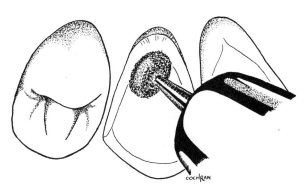

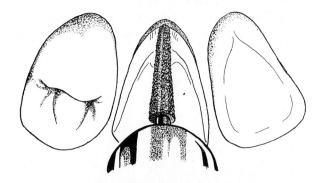

Figure 15–30. The use of a bullet-nosed diamond to produce the lingual chamfer.

metal from the labial surface. The natural curvatures are used to help conceal most of the incisal reduction (Fig. 15–31).

There remains the major component of resistance, which is the formation of the proximal grooves. It may be best to place them before adding the labial bevel to the incisal. These grooves are begun with a No. 169L bur, and their alignment is critical. The grooves usually are expected to be parallel to the slope formed by the incisal two-thirds of the labial surface (Fig. 15–32A and B).

The proximal groove is positioned to provide maximum length. The location must be quite precise to be of value; if too close to the labial surface, the groove will either undermine and weaken the labial enamel or cause an esthetic problem because of needless metal display. If it drifts in a lingual direction, it becomes a retention problem, for the groove will become short very quickly as a result of the lingual slope.

With the No. 169L bur proceed to locate the position the grooves should take and then cut both mesial and distal grooves to near 20 per cent of their expected depth. Examine the initial cut to determine if the grooves are in the proper location as to length and inclination. Then proceed to cut the groove to the desired depth and if some corrections are needed, they are easily made at this time. The grooves must be cut to a depth to allow a positive lock and prevent any tendency toward lingual displacement. If preparations are on lower incisors, the No. 169L bur is used to complete the groove. For most other teeth the groove by this bur would be small, but it is a simple matter to now select the bur to make the right size groove, and it is usually the 170L

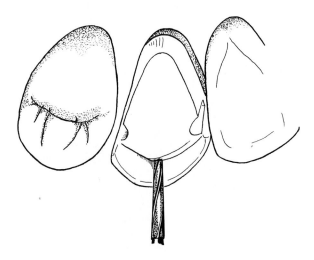

Figure 15–31. The use of a bur to provide the needed incisal clearance and strength.

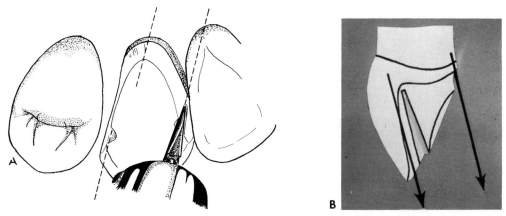

Figure 15–32. *A*, The use of a tapered bur to make the proximal grooves. *B*, The grooves should parallel the incisal two-thirds of the facial surface.

and at times the 171L. It is advisable to use a slow-speed handpiece with the selected bur to ream out the final size because slow speed allows for accurate control. If slight directional corrections are needed, they can be done at this time.

The gingival extension of the groove is located to allow the proximal reduction to provide a finish line gingival to the groove. It is never advised to have the groove extend beyond the limits of the gingival finish line. Frequently the groove extension beyond the finish line will leave a margin that is not closed.

Give the preparation a final inspection to be sure there will be no resistance to placing the restoration; at the same time the preparation design should allow the restorations to be secure. The labial enamel margins may be smoothed with fine paper disks. At the same time look for sharp angles that may interfere with the seating of the casting and round them slightly (Fig. 15–33).

In instances where resistance is marginal, it is advised to place a pin for added support, and the usual place for this is in the cingulum. The direction of this pin must be the same as for the proximal grooves (Fig. 15–34). Pin resistance may be gained by using either a tapered or parallel pin.

Figure 15–33. The enamel is finished with fine grit stone or finishing bur.

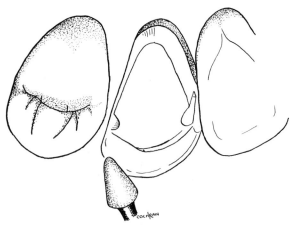

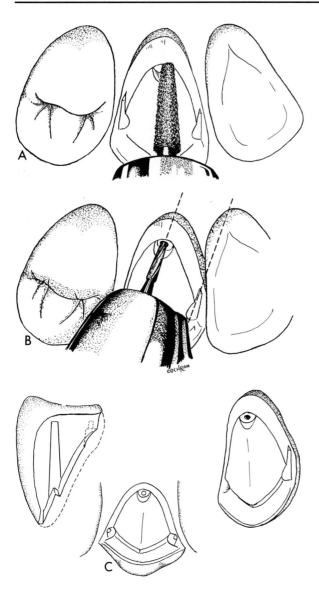

Figure 15–34. *A*, *B*, and *C*, The instrumentation with diamond and bur for the preparation of a lingual pin as an addition to anterior three-quarter crown preparation.

The preparation for a tapered pin is begun by using a No. ½ bur and this bur must be kept on a straight course for good alignment, and the bur should penetrate from 2.0 to 3.0 mm to make it worthwhile. The direction is identical to the proximal grooves. This is followed by a No. 700 slow-speed bur to provide the tapered effect. These burs do not end cut, so a channel must be provided before using them. When pin preparations are employed the operator must be as precise as possible. The size of the preparation should coincide very closely to that of the bur. At the time of the impression a tapered plastic pin* will be placed in the preparation and become part of the impression leading to a wax pattern.

An alternate method for providing pin support will use a parallel pin. The preparation is begun by using a No. ½ bur, which is used to locate the pin and to penetrate any remaining enamel, for the drill that follows will not cut enamel. A 0.024 inch twist drill in a contra-angle is used at slow speed to

*Williams Gold Refining Co., Buffalo, New York 14214.

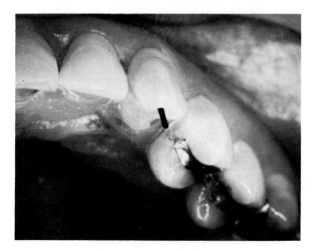

Figure 15–35. The use of a parallel drill and plastic bristle as a supplement to a three-quarter crown preparation.

drill the channel. This channel is drilled to coincide with the proximal grooves to a depth of 2.0 to 3.0 mm. This drill only cuts with the end and when guidance is set; if the drill is sharp it will easily cut the channel. If space allows, it is an advantage to enlarge the channel using a 0.029 inch drill, as this will provide a much more rigid cast pin. For each of these drill sizes there are plastic pins to be used for purposes of the impression and also the eventual wax pattern. It is planned that the size of the cast pin will be 0.004 inch smaller than the channel that was drilled (Fig. 15–35).

CEMENT BASE

There are many cases in which the caries or previous restoration has penetrated deep into the dentin to the extent that the standard form of preparation will not be adequate to allow for the removal of the defect and still remain an adequate preparation design. After the outline and internal features are established the remaining carious dentin is removed and this will indicate the need for pulpal protection and also establish proper pulpal and axial form to the preparation.

The techniques for placing bases are discussed in detail in Chapter 8.

Resumé of Anterior Three-Quarter Crown

1. Patient will need to be tolerant of esthetic problems with display of metal.

2. Provide minimum display of proximal gold by conservative preparations with straight facial margins.

3. Diamond disks or flame-shaped diamonds are used for the proximal preparation.

4. Lingual reduction is achieved with a small wheel- or football-shaped diamond.

5. A bullet nose diamond is used for the gingival chamfer.

6. Incisal reduction is done with a No. 170 bur.

7. Grooves must have maximum length and are begun with a No. 169 bur and finished with a No. 170 bur and are kept within the finish lines.

8. Grooves are parallel to the incisal two-thirds of the tooth.

9. An auxiliary pin may be needed for supplemental resistance.

Restoration Prior to Preparation

Until now cast preparations have been discussed assuming there is adequate remaining tooth tissue in which to design the preparation. Frequently a tooth requiring a partial or full coverage cast restoration will need to be restored before beginning the preparation. For non-vital teeth this consideration occurs in Chapter 19.

For vital teeth the use of a pin-retained amalgam or a resin restoration is a logical means of restoring a tooth prior to making a preparation for a casting. The discussion of retentive pins occurs in Chapter 13. Of the two materials, amalgam is preferred, as it is harder and less resilient than resins and so provides a more reliable base for the casting. Amalgam also offers the advantage of being more effective in discouraging leakage. Acid etching will be of little value in the prevention of leakage with a resin, as there will not be adequate enamel.

Composite resin is attractive as a "build up" mechanism because it hardens quickly, allowing the preparation to proceed at the same appointment. Also, the quick setting high-copper amalgams allow for the same convenience; for more information refer to Chapter 12. A pin-retained composite resin may be used when tooth loss is not a major problem. New developments in gloss ionomer cement show promise as a pin build up.

16

THE CAST GOLD RESTORATION: IMPRESSIONS, OCCLUSAL RECORDS, AND TEMPORARY TREATMENT

Impressions

At the completion of preparations an accurate impression is required of the teeth to be restored. The procedures necessitate careful attention when preparing the tissue area prior to the impression. It may be a time of frustration, for if failure occurs it is often the result of a poor impression, which causes a time loss for both dentist and patient.

Armamentarium
1. Tissue retraction cord
2. Tissue retraction chemical
3. Tissue retraction instruments
4. Impression tray with tray adhesive
5. Impression material
6. Impression syringe
7. Paper mixing pad
8. Mixing spatulas
9. Hydrocolloid conditioner
10. Water-cooled trays
11. Hydrocolloid syringe

Procedure

When finish lines terminate at a level above the gingival tissue, impressions are not a problem, but when portions or entire finish lines are subgingival, a good impression may be very difficult to obtain.

TISSUE RETRACTION

RUBBER DAM. The rubber dam is an aid for impression techniques, as it will tend to mechanically depress tissue, allowing easy access to the margins. Most impressions will require a preliminary mechanical or chemical treatment

443

of the marginal tissue so as to expose the margins and allow accurate duplication. The elastic impression materials commonly used are relatively fluid and will not effectively deflect tissue.

CORD. The most common method of tissue control is with a commercially available chemically saturated string. The chemicals used for this purpose include aluminum chloride, aluminum sulfate, ferric sulfate, and epinephrine.

The texture of the string varies from tightly woven to very loose. The loose string tends to pick up a greater volume of the chemical, but it is more difficult to place as compared with a firm string.

The most prevalent form of retraction cord being marketed currently is braided, which provides a consistently firm retraction cord. The retraction instrument does not penetrate through the cord, which makes for an easier placement of the cord into the gingival sulcus. A recently introduced retraction cord is a knitted cord.* As a result of being slightly elastic it responds very well to the usual techniques of placement. Most retraction cord is predosed with a chemical agent but the knitted cord is free of chemical and the operator makes the chemical selection, excluding epinephrine, and presoaks the cord prior to its placement.

For many years epinephrine has been the most frequently used chemical for tissue retraction and it is proven to be effective. However, undesirable physical side effects have been noted. When using an epinephrine product some patients become very uneasy, with an increase in the heart rate and the pattern of breathing. This drug is readily absorbed through intact mucus membrane and the resulting distress may linger an hour or more after the cord is removed. As a result of these manifestations, it is recommended that this chemical not be used for gingival retraction.

When alum cord is used it is colored yellow for ease of identification. Alum works as a styptic, discouraging local bleeding at the same time it is displacing tissue from the margins. There are no contraindications for using alum, and tissue recovery is very good following its use.

Two other commercial products useful for tissue control are Astringedent* and Hemodent.† Ferric sulfate is the major constituent of the former; aluminum chloride of the latter. They are helpful in the control of bleeding and can be applied to plain cord or cord impregnated with alum or other chemcials— except epinephrine. If the cord is moistened prior to placement it will allow for easier positioning than if dry cord is used. If the rubber dam has been used the gingival crevice will easily accommodate the cord.

A variety of instruments may be employed to insert the retraction cord, including the instruments needed for placing cement bases, interproximal amalgam carvers, explorers, and peridontal probes. There are also serrated instruments designed for the purpose of placing the cord. To simplify placement the cord should be slightly longer than the tooth circumference at the gingival margins. If the cord length is excessive, it is wasteful and difficult to manage (Fig. 16–2).

In situations where bleeding is a problem, ferric solution can be directly deposited at the orifices of the capillaries and cause rapid coagulation. This is done by use of syringe and needle with a tufted cotton tip (Figs. 16–1B and 16–3A), which is rubbed back and forth in the sulcus as the fluid is excreted.

If the bleeding is persistent or if tissue has been severely traumatized,

---

*Ultradent Products Inc., 1345 E. 3900 So., Salt Lake City, Utah 84124.
†Premier Dental Products Co., Philadelphia, Pennsylvania 19107.

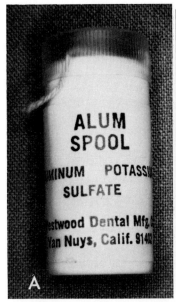
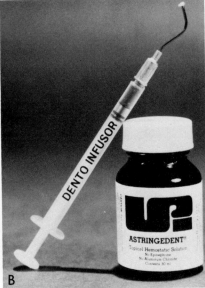
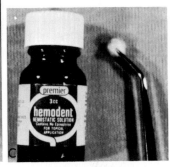

Figure 16–1. Examples of chemicals that are used to manage gingival tissue prior to an elastic impression. *A,* Retraction cord containing aluminum and potassium sulfate. *B,* System employing ferric sulfate. *C,* The major constituent of this chemical is aluminum chloride.

discretion is the better part of valor. The preparation should be temporized for several days to permit epithelialization before re-attempting an impression.

Saliva must be controlled prior to placing the retraction cord and until the impression tray is seated. If saliva makes premature contact with the string, it will neutralize the effects of the chemical in the string. The salivary ducts are blocked by placement of cotton rolls. As with other segments of the procedure, an assistant is very helpful in positioning the cord quickly and in maintaining dryness.

Whenever possible the cord is held tightly around the tooth at the gingival margin with cotton pliers. Then with a suitable instrument it is eased into place by segments (Fig. 16–3). The procedure is to slip the cord between the tooth and the tissue, which provides a lateral pressure on the tissue. It must be positioned in such a way that the finish line is exposed, in order to secure

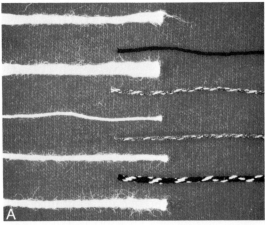
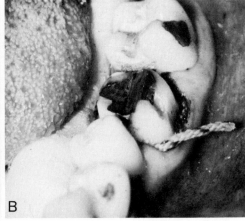

Figure 16–2. *A,* On the left are examples of loose twisted cord and on the right is the more stable braided cord that is currently being used more extensively. *B,* An example of knitted cord in position.

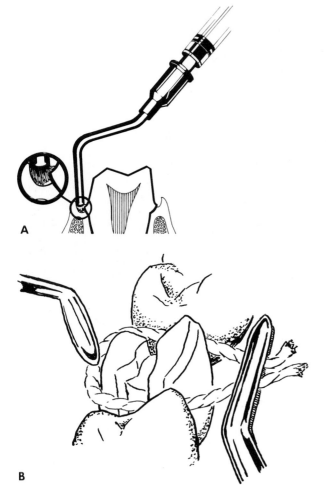

Figure 16–3. *A,* A bleeding area being rubbed with ferric sulfate. *B,* It is helpful to hold the cord firmly around the tooth as it is being placed into the gingival sulcus. (Courtesy of Dr. Dan Fischer and Masson Monographs in Dentistry.)

a satisfactory impression. This often requires a high level of persistence (Fig. 16–4). There are instances that require a second string superimposed on the first.

The string should be in contact with the gingival tissue for a minimum of 8 minutes in order for the tissue to be displaced laterally from the margins. To minimize tissue rebound the string is removed just prior to injection of the impression material. It is best if the string is still slightly moist with the chemical upon removal. If it is dry, it may tend to encourage bleeding as it is removed. As an added precaution the string should not be left in the crevice longer than required to achieve retraction.

In some instances routine chemical control will not suffice, and it will be an advantage to use electrosurgery to properly expose the margins (Fig. 16–5). The instruments for this purpose must be used very carefully, and the technique should be understood before employing it on a patient. For this purpose reference should be made to a text that provides this information.

IMPRESSION TRAYS

The accuracy and reliability of an elastic impression is controlled by the tray in which it is taken. The primary requirements for a tray is that it be rigid and that it conform closely to the area of the impression. The best tray is one

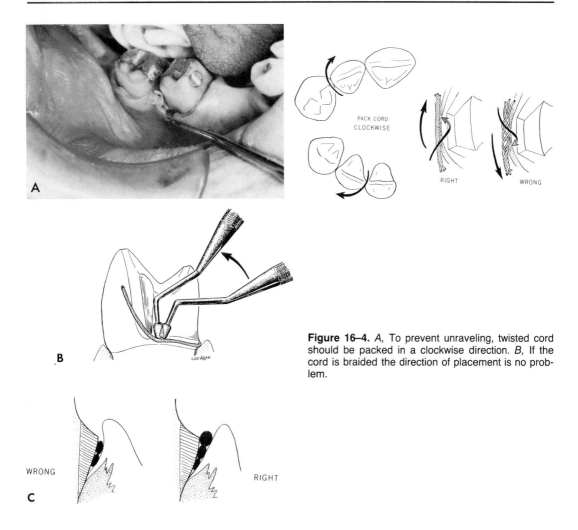

Figure 16–4. *A,* To prevent unraveling, twisted cord should be packed in a clockwise direction. *B,* If the cord is braided the direction of placement is no problem.

Figure 16–5. Electrosurgical techniques are helpful in controlling selected tissue problems.

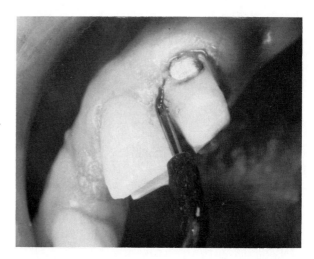

that is custom-made for each patient. In most situations, it is best to take a complete arch impression, which provides maximum reliability.

Tray acrylic, which is provided by several manufacturers, is used to form the tray. A study model provides the basis for forming the tray. To provide space within the completed tray for the impression material the study model is covered with base plate wax. If wax is used, it is advisable to cover it with tin foil to prevent the wax from adhering to the completed tray, thus simplifying the removal of the wax. This material should be adapted so as to permit a thickness of 2 to 3 mm of impression material. This thickness of impression material allows for the development of proper elastic properties and helps to insure accuracy. It also permits the subsequent removal of the model from the impression with a reduced risk of fracturing the stone cast. If the bulk of impression material is greater than approximately 2 to 3 mm, accuracy may be impaired.

To stabilize the tray in the mouth and to secure an impression with uniform thickness, occlusal stops or reference points are created by perforating the wax to the incisal edge of a central, to the occlusal surface of a right and left posterior tooth, and to the palate (Fig. 16–6).

The acrylic powder and liquid (polymer and monomer) as supplied by the manufacturers are combined in a paper cup and mixed together and allowed to become a dough-like mass. The dough is flattened to a sheet approximately 2 mm in thickness. The sheet is placed over the wax and molded to the needed shape. The resin is allowed to cure, after which it is

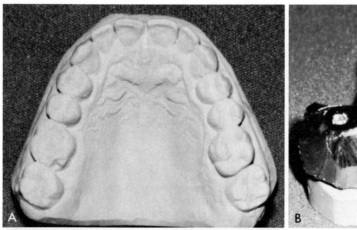

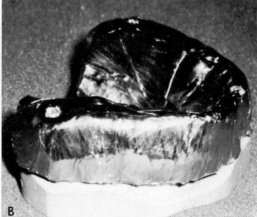

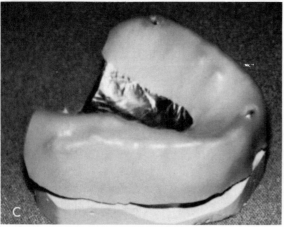

Figure 16–6. *A,* A study model is used for making an impression tray. *B,* The wax spacer is overlaid with tin foil, and strategic perforations are made through the wax to allow for positive occlusal steps. *C,* The model may be covered with tin foil over which a 2 to 3 mm thickness of base plate wax is placed.

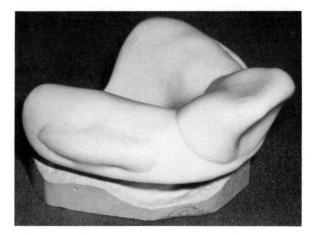

Figure 16–7. In forming the tray, anterior and posterior projections are placed to help with its removal.

removed from the model, and the wax is removed. The periphery of the tray is adjusted to its final shape using acrylic burs or stones on a laboratory lathe.

The tray should extend slightly beyond the margins of the preparation or clinical crowns. This simplifies the removal of the tray and the polymerized impression. These limited extensions provide adequate support for the impression material and minimize restrictions for needed flexibility. The tray is more easily removed if a projection or handle is formed in the incisor region. Also it is convenient to provide a lateral projection from the facial surface at the posterior part of the tray to aid in dislodging it (Fig. 16–7).

Acrylic trays for rubber materials must be coated with tray adhesive to anchor the impression to the tray. If the impression material pulls loose from the tray, distortion will occur. The silicones, polyethers, and polysulfides each have special adhesive liquids that must be used with their respective impression materials, as they are not interchangeable. After being coated the tray must be allowed to dry for a few minutes before being filled with the impression material. It is best if an initial coating of adhesive is applied several hours before needed, followed with a reapplication during the actual appointment (Fig. 16–8).

Preformed perforated plastic trays are available commercially. However, these trays do not allow for a uniform distribution of the impression material and occlusal stops must be added. The perforations are usually adequate for retention of the impression, but it is advisable to use the adhesive cement for added security.

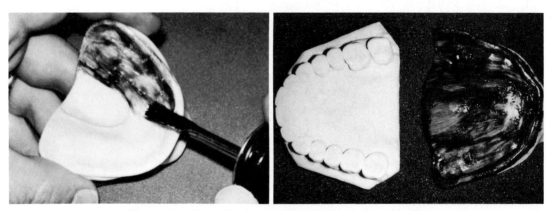

Figure 16–8. Tray adhesive must be placed and allowed to dry.

Selection of Impression Material

The process of changing the elastomeric base, called a liquid polymer, into the final rubberlike material is generally referred to as curing or polymerization. For present purposes, a polymer can be thought of as a chemical compound built up from a number of single elementary units that are linked together during the reaction. As will be seen, there are two basic types of polymerization reactions. One type, called addition polymerization, results in the formation of a polymer without the formation of any other chemical. In the second type, called condensation polymerization, other chemical compounds (called by-products) are produced, which are not part of the polymer.

Chemically, there are four types of elastomeric polymers used for dental impression materials. The respective bases are a polysulfide, a condensation polymerizing silicone, an additional polymerizing silicone, and a polyether. Commercial products that are representative of the four types are seen in Figure 16–9. Since any or all of these are generally referred to as "rubber impression materials," that terminology will be used in the following discussion. The composition, chemistry, and properties of each type will be presented separately, followed by the manipulative techniques to be employed. All four types are comparable in accuracy and faithfully reproduce oral tissues, if handled properly.

In addition to the four chemical types, many commerical products are available in different consistencies or viscosities. The four classes can be identified as (1) very high viscosity, which is actually of putty-like consistency; (2) high viscosity, which is referred to as "heavy body" or tray material; (3) medium viscosity, often called "regular"; and (4) low viscosity, referred to as "light body" or syringe. The reason for the need of these four consistencies will be apparent when we consider the clinical techniques used with rubber impression materials.

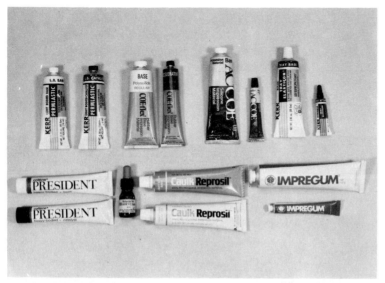

Figure 16–9. The four types of nonaqueous elastomeric impression materials. Two polysulfides are at upper left and two condensation silicones are at upper right. Two additional silicone products are at lower left and center. A polyether is at lower right. (From Phillips, R. W.: Elements of Dental Materials, 4th Ed. W. B. Saunders Co., Philadelphia, 1984, p. 111.)

POLYSULFIDE RUBBER

Polysulfide rubber impression materials are supplied in two tubes (see Fig. 16–9). One of these contains the polysufide rubber base, which is a liquid polymer made into a paste by the addition of certain powdered fillers. Accelerators and retarders may also be added as needed. The basic molecule of the polymer has a sulfhydryl group (SH) attached to a terminal carbon atom.

When this liquid polymer is reacted with an appropriate chemical, usually lead dioxide (PbO_2), the polymer grows or lengthens by polymerization and thereby changes to an elastomeric solid. Sulfur is also employed to facilitate the reaction and to provide better properties. The polymer paste is usually white and is generally labeled as the "base."

The second tube contains the sulfur and lead dioxide. Since both of these substances are powders, a liquid plasticizer is added in order to form a paste. This paste is often labeled by the manufacturer as the "accelerator" or "catalyst." However, the paste should more properly be termed the reactor, since it contains the ingredient (PbO_2) that produces the reaction that forms the soft rubber. This paste is usually brown because of the lead dioxide. However, if an organic peroxide is used as a reactor, it may be another color. Such a mix is more pleasing esthetically and cleaner in handling.

The manipulation of these materials will be discussed in detail later in this chapter. At this time, suffice it to say that the two pastes are proportioned on a mixing pad, usually by squeezing out equal lengths, and then mixed thoroughly with a spatula. The curing reaction begins when the mixing is started and continues in a progressive manner. The mix gains elasticity until a rubbery material is formed that can be withdrawn over the teeth and undercut areas with a minimum amount of permanent deformation.

The properties of the four rubber base materials are summarized in Table 16–1. The polysulfides have a strong odor (due to the SH groups) and will stain clothing. Careful mixing is required to produce a homogeneous mix that is free of streaks. Both the working and setting times are relatively long. The curing reaction is accelerated by increased temperature or in the presence of moisture. Varying the proportions of the base and catalyst should not be done in order to adjust the curing rate.

The use of a chilled mixing slab will increase the working time if the slab is not cooled so much that moisture forms on it. Addition of a drop of water to the mix will decrease the working and setting times. The permanent deformation after removal from undercut areas is relatively high. However, this property continues to improve after the material has reached an initial

Table 16–1. PROPERTIES OF ELASTOMERIC IMPRESSION MATERIALS

Chemical Type	Mixing Time	Working Time (at 20–23° C)	Setting Time (in the mouth)	Permanent Deformation (after removal from undercut areas)	Stiffness	Dimensional Stability (after removal from the mouth)	Tear Resistance
Polysulfide	1 min	3–6 min	10–20 min	high	low	moderate	good†
Condensation Silicone	30–60 sec	2–3 min	6–10 min	low	medium	poor	fair
Polyether	30–45 sec	2–3 min	6–7 min	low	very high	excellent*	poor
Addition Silicone	30–45 sec	2–4 min	6–8 min	very low	high	excellent	poor

*Must be kept dry.
†Material does not fracture easily, but severe permanent distortion occurs.

set. Thus premature removal of a polysulfide impression from the mouth should be avoided. The stiffness is relatively low; hence, these materials are reasonably flexible. This facilitates removal of the impression from the mouth and separation of the cast from the impression. Nonetheless the polysulfides are quite stiff in comparison with the hydrocolloids.

The "tear resistance" of an impression material is important. If it is high, then it will not easily fracture and leave impression material trapped in the interproximal or subgingival areas. The polysulfide rubbers are good in this respect. However, considerable permanent deformation may occur during removal from the mouth if the impression material is caught in these spaces.

The curing reaction for the polysulfides is a condensation reaction (water is the by-product). This leads to a moderate amount of curing shrinkage, which continues after the impression is removed from the mouth. Hence, the polysulfides are not sufficiently dimensionally stable to permit storage of the impression before pouring the cast. Unset gypsum products tend to form a high contact angle on the surface of a polysulfide impression material. Thus, care must be used when pouring the impression to avoid trapping air bubbles.

CONDENSATION SILICONE RUBBER

The silicone rubber base material is usually supplied as a paste in a metal tube (see Fig. 16–9). The reactor is generally in the form of a liquid and may be packaged in a bottle or in a small metal tube. A material of putty-like consistency is often available with the condensation silicone rubber materials and is usually supplied in a jar with a bottle containing the appropriate reactor liquid.

The base material is a silicone-based polymer called a polysiloxane. This liquid polymer is mixed with a powdered silica (SiO_2) to form a paste. Polymerization occurs by a condensation reaction between the silicone base and a second compound, an alkyl silicate. This is done in the presence of a catalyst, tin octoate. The alkyl silicate and tin octoate are combined to form the liquid component, which may be labeled "accelerator" or "catalyst." The by-product of the reaction is ethyl alcohol, which is rapidly lost by evaporation. This leads to a relatively high curing shrinkage and poor dimensional stability after polymerization.

The condensation silicone rubber impression materials are odor free, clean to handle, and relatively easy to mix. Proportioning is done by squeezing out a measured length of base material and adding the specified number of drops of liquid reactor. Varying the amount of reactor is the recommended way of adjusting the working and setting times, although increased temperature will also accelerate curing. Working times do tend to be rather short.

The permanent deformation of the condensation silicones is superior to that of the polysulfides (see Table 16–1). However, the dimensional stability is inferior, and a condensation silicone impression should be poured as soon as possible after removal from the mouth. The contact angle of unset gypsum on a condensation silicone is even higher than on a polysulfide; thus care must again be taken in pouring the impression to avoid trapped air.

ADDITION POLYMERIZING SILICONE RUBBER

The addition polymerizing silicone impression materials represent the most recent development in the rubber elastomer category. Although they are based on silicone polymers, their chemistry and properties are quite different from those of the condensation silicones. They are packaged as a two-paste system in metal tubes (see Fig. 16–9) or in plastic jars in the case of the putty material. They are commonly available in all four viscosity classes for a given product.

Curing occurs by the addition reaction of two different liquid silicone polymers, in the presence of a platinum salt catalyst, to form an elastic solid. No by-product is formed. Hence the curing shrinkage is small and the dimensional stability is excellent. One of the two liquid silicone polymers is a polysiloxane terminated by a vinyl group, which is essential to an addition reaction. Thus manufacturers frequently refer to the addition silicones as poly(vinyl siloxane) impression materials. As usual, powdered solids (silica) are added to the liquid polymers to form the two pastes or putties.

The addition silicones are odor free, clean to handle, and very easy to mix. The working and setting times are quite short. The curing reaction can be retarded by lowering the temperature of the materials and the mixing pad. Alternatively, a liquid retarder (supplied by some manufacturers) can be added to the mix. Base:catalyst ratios should not be altered from those recommended.

Permanent deformation and curing shrinkage are very low. The dimensional stability is excellent, and most manufacturers claim that pouring can be delayed for up to 7 days. The set material is quite stiff and difficulty may be encountered in removing a full arch impression from the mouth. Also care should be exercised when separating the cast from the impression in order to avoid fracturing the gypsum. The tear resistance (of the addition silicones) is poor, but the material does not suffer appreciable plastic deformation before fracture. The wetting of the impression material by the mix of gypsum is similar to that discussed for the condensation silicone. They are the most costly of the available rubber impression materials.

POLYETHER RUBBER

The base is a polyether, which contains end aziridine rings. Activation occurs by a reactor consisting of an aromatic sulfonate ester. Both the base and reactor are supplied as a paste in collapsible tubes. As the set material is quite stiff, a third component, called a body modifier or thinner, is also available to reduce the stiffness. The body modifier will also reduce the viscosity of the unset material. This may be advantageous, since the polyethers are presently marketed only in a regular viscosity consistency (see Fig. 16–9).

The polyethers are clean to handle, odor free, and easy to mix. They have very short working times, which can be extended by the addition of the body modifier or by reducing the amount of reactor used in making a mix.

As can be seen in Table 16–1, the permanent deformation is comparable to that of the addition silicones. Since the polyether curing reaction produces no by-product, the curing shrinkage and dimensional stability are also quite good. In this respect it reflects a marked improvement when compared with polysulfide rubber or condensation silicones. However, the polyethers will absorb water and swell. Thus the impression must be stored in a dry environment until the cast is poured. The set polyether material does have a very high relative stiffness, which may pose clinical difficulties, although, as previously noted, the use of the body modifier will reduce the stiffness. Since the polyethers are somewhat hydrophilic, they form a low contact angle with gypsum and hence are easy to pour.

One additional caution should be noted. The polyether chemistry has been reported to create hypersensitivity in both patients and dental staff who are allergic to the material. If a known allergy exists, this material should be avoided.

Contraction due to polymerization and loss of volatile condensation reaction products is comparable for most silicones and polysulfide polymers. This contraction, which continues for many days after the impression has set, is very much lower for the polyether and the additional polymerizing silicone. Permanent deformation following the strain that occurs during removal of an impression from undercuts is most pronounced for the polysulfide polymers.

Although any of these elastomeric impression materials can be electroplated, the most widely accepted procedure for producing electroformed dies appears to be silver plating, in a basic cyanide bath, of a lead-peroxide–cured type of polysulfide polymer impression.

The stone die should be constructed within the first hour after removal of the impression from the mouth, particularly if a condensation polymerizing silicone or a polysulfide polymer rubber is employed. The vivid effects of distortion upon storage of the impression may be seen in Figure 16–10. As can be noted, a slight discrepancy in fit occurred, even when the stone die was poured within 2 hours. The fit at later times is obviously unsatisfactory.

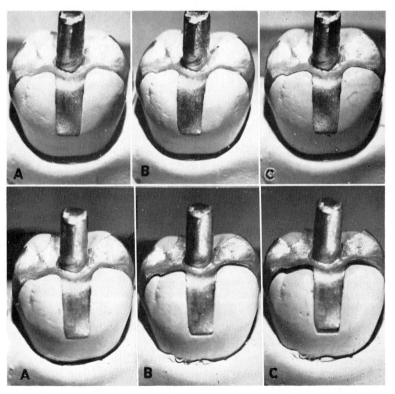

Figure 16–10. Fit of a master casting for a cavity preparation indicative of a practical case. *Upper row,* from a polysulfide rubber impression; *lower row,* from a condensation silicone rubber impression. Stone poured at *A,* 10 minutes; *B,* 6 hours, and *C,* 24 hours.

MULTIPLE MIX TECHNIQUE

To obtain reliable impressions of the preparations a syringe is used to inject the impression material into the details of the preparation. If this is not done, there will be deficiencies in the completed impression, irrespective of the elastic material selected.

In most instances, the manufacturers of elastomeric materials provide two consistencies, one that is used for the tray and a thinner one to be used in a syringe. The syringe type has longer working and setting times as compared with the tray material.

The method of employing both the syringe and tray types of rubber materials is often referred to as the "multiple mix" technique because two separate mixtures are required with two separate mixing pads and spatulas. The required amounts of tray and syringe material are expressed on separate plastic-lined paper pads or glass slabs (Fig. 16–11). Whether the tray or syringe material is mixed first will depend upon the relative working and setting times of the two materials. Simultaneous mixing of the two may be most advantageous. It is important that each base and accelerator combination be mixed very thoroughly and quickly. The final mixture must be homogeneous and not have any visible color streaks, which indicate an incomplete mixture (Fig. 16–12). The curing reaction starts at the beginning of mixing and reaches its maximum rate soon after the spatulation is completed, at which stage a resilient network has started to form. During the final set a material of adequate elasticity and strength is formed and it can be removed over undercuts quite readily.

Prior to making the impression it is important to check all segments of

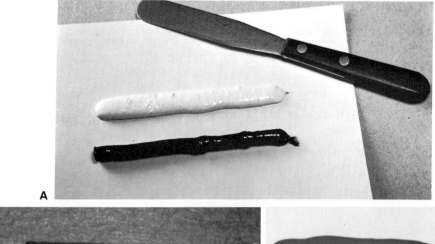

A

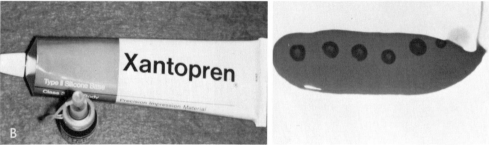

Figure 16–11. *A*, Items needed to prepare a mix of polysulfide impression material. The dark material is the reaction paste, and the white material is the base paste. *B*, A silicone material wherein the catalyst is placed directly on the base.

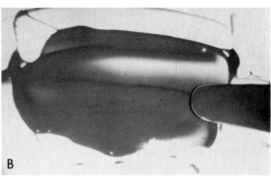

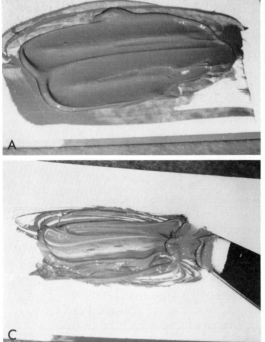

Figure 16–12. Any rubber material must be mixed to be smooth and homogeneous in color whether it is a polysulfide *(A)* or silicone *(B)* material. Streaks must not be left as in *C*.

the arch that will be included in the impression to determine if there will be open interdental spaces as a result of the gingival tissue retraction. This will allow the impression material to fill this space, and the interproximal contacts will be fully encased.

When the impression material sets, it becomes very difficult to remove the impression. Under these conditions release is obtained only by physically tearing the impression material at the contact area. To prevent this it is advisable to place some soft utility wax into these spaces, thus preventing a facial-to-lingual unification of the impression material (Fig. 16–13). However, the wax must be placed so as to avoid interference with any critical portion of the impression. After the impression is completed the wax is quickly removed.

The tray is properly loaded with an equal distribution of material and then the syringe material is mixed if this has not already been done. During

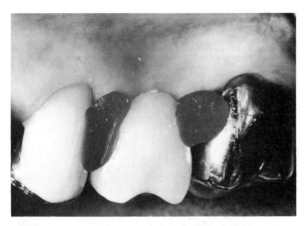

Figure 16–13. Utility wax is placed in the facial and lingual embrasure gingival to the contact to prevent the locking of impression material under the contact.

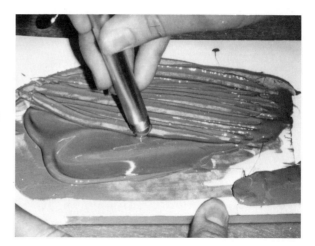

Figure 16–14. A method of filling the syringe from the mixing pad.

this time the tray material becomes more viscous, which is an aid in producing the needed details of the impression. When the syringe material is ready, the syringe, minus the injecting tip, is loaded by scraping it across the surface of the pad, forcing the material into the open end of the syringe. This is the most rapid way of loading the syringe. The barrel end is wiped clean and the plastic tip placed in position (Fig. 16–14). Other syringes are designed so that they can be loaded in a similar fashion but from the top end, leaving the tip in position on the syringe during the polymer pick-up.

The procedure should be timed so that neither the tray nor the syringe material cure to a point that prevents their total unification. If the materials have noticeably cured, an incomplete or distorted impression will result.

At this moment the area of the impression, particularly the preparations, must be free of any form of moisture. The gingival crevice is injected. If the preparation is a partial crown, it is usually best to start at the distal or most remote part of the preparation (Fig. 16–15). Once injection begins for a preparation it should be continuous until completed to avoid entrapment of air bubbles. The syringe tip should first carefully follow the cavosurface margins and then systematically cover the preparation. Special care should be taken regarding fine or unusual details in the preparation and when injection is completed there should be a generous amount of material covering the preparation.

The tray is carefully positioned to its predetermined location, allowing the impression material to flow as it is placed. When excess material extrudes in the palatal region, it should be removed to avoid the possibility of gagging.

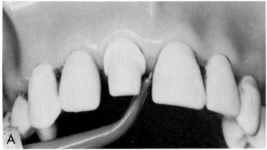
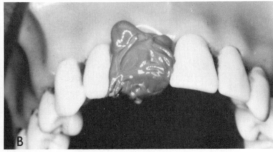

Figure 16–15. The injection of rubber material begins at the most remote or difficult margin *(A)* and continues until the preparations are fully covered *(B)*.

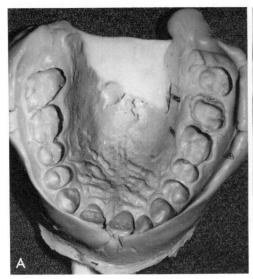

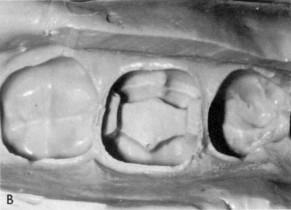

Figure 16–16. Examples of impressions that provide the necessary detail required to make reliable models or dies.

To minimize distortion the impression should not be removed until curing has progressed to a stage that provides adequate elasticity. One method for determining the time of removal is to inject some of the impression material into an interproximal area away from the impression itself. The surface of this material is probed with a blunt instrument and when the elastomer has adequately cured it will return quickly to its original contour, indicating that the impression is ready to be removed. When a multiple mix technique is used it is advisable to test both the syringe and tray materials in this manner, as the curing time may vary for the two consistencies.

A rubber material should be ready for removal within 10 minutes after mixing begins. A range of 6 to 8 minutes in the mouth should be an adequate allowance, except for some polysulfide polymers that undergo considerable strain during removal of the impression.

As with any elastic impression, the method of removal from the mouth is important. The rubber impression should be removed suddenly. The material is subject to less risk of distortion when subjected to sharp stress rather than a slow constant one, as by teasing the impression out of the mouth. This also explains the logic of having an adequate handle on the tray as an aid for tray removal because of the resistance by the impression material (Fig. 16–16).

PUTTY SILICONE

A variation in technique is employed when using the putty silicone impression materals. The stiff putty is dispersed with a scoop, and the recommended number of drops of the liquid catalyst is manipulated into it by use of a stiff spatula until no streaks are present. Mixing may then be completed by molding the material with moist hands, much as if it were softened impression compound. The tray is filled, seated, and then moved in all directions in order to enlarge the space occupied by the teeth. This completed preliminary impression is really a custom-made tray. After the cavity preparations have been made, the matching syringe material is injected around the prepared teeth, and the previously prepared tray is seated. It is held in place until the syringe material has cured.

REVERSIBLE HYDROCOLLOID

One of the popular types of elastic impression material is essentially a colloid. Colloids are suspensions of molecules, or groups of molecules, in some type of dispersing medium. Colloidal systems involve particles of a molecular size somewhere between the small particles of a true solution and the large ones present in a suspension.

The basic constituent of reversible hydrocolloid impression materials is agar-agar in a concentration of 8 to 15 per cent. Extracted from a certain type of seaweed, agar-agar provides a suitable colloid as a base for dental impression materials. When suspended in water, the agar-agar forms a liquid solution at temperatures that can be safely used in the oral cavity and also converts to a gel at a temperature slightly above that of the mouth. The principal ingredient by weight (approximately 80 to 85 per cent) is water.

The hydrocolloid impression material is placed into the cavity preparation as a solution (Fig. 16–17), and by means of water-cooled impression trays the solution is converted into a gel that is firm yet elastic (Fig. 16–18).

The initial investment for such a system requires a financial expenditure to secure a conditioning unit and adequate supply of water-cooled trays. Aside from the initial cost, reversible hydrocolloid is noticeably more economical as compared with the various rubber impression materials. The reliability and accuracy of this material has been well accepted for many years.

In contrast to rubber materials, this material responds in a favorable manner to residual moisture in preparations. Some techniques advocate moistening the preparations prior to making the impression, since one of the basic ingredients of an agar-agar impression material is water. Currently available agar-based materials have a consistency or body style that compares favorably with rubber materials.

The technical instructions given by the manufacturers of materials and equipment to use with this method should be closely followed. The framework of time and temperature needed for good impressions must be carefully observed.

The structure of the gel is such that it will resist a sudden application of force without distortion or fracture more successfully than a force that is

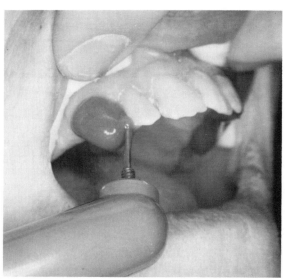

Figure 16–17. The injection of reversible hydrocolloid.

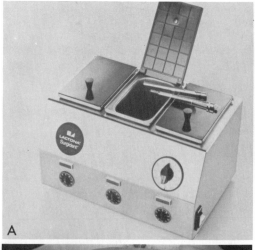

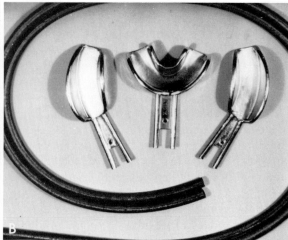

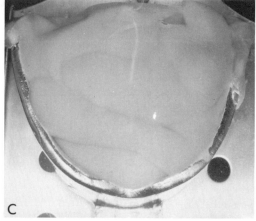

Figure 16–18. *A* and *B,* The equipment and materials that are needed for reversible hydrocolloid impressions. *C,* A full arch hydrocolloid impression in a tempering bath.

applied slowly. Thus, the dentist removes the impression with a sudden snapping movement rather than slowly teasing it out.

Impression Resumé

1. Secure tissue retraction when needed by use of solutions of chemicals described previously.

2. Chemically treated cord is carefully placed for a minimum of 3 minutes and removed when retraction has been achieved. All margins must be exposed.

3. Preferably a preformed acrylic tray is used and coated with tray adhesive.

4. A selection of polylsulfide, silicone, or polyether impression material is mixed according to manufacturer's instructions.

5. The syringe is loaded; the syringe material is carefully injected into and onto the preparation; then the loaded tray is seated.

6. The impression is removed quickly after it has properly polymerized.

7. If reversible hydrocolloid is used, a water-cooled metal tray is selected and the material used according to the manufacturer's instructions.

Occlusal Records

Armamentarium

1. Choice of nonadjustable or semiadjustable articulator

2. Face bow
3. Wax bite wafers
4. Plaster bowl and dental stone spatula

Procedure

Prior to mounting the models into a functional position in an articulator it would be best if a basic knowledge of mandibular movement was understood. For that purpose the reader is advised to refer to texts that discuss that subject in detail.

This section will discuss only at a minimum level the procedure needed to articulate the patient's casts prior to forming the wax pattern. Our techniques are predictably reliable as related to margins and degree of fit, but the occlusal accuracy is frequently secured in the mouth after the casting is made. A minor amount of oral adjustment is desirable to secure accurate occlusal results, but if excessive time and effort are required, it indicates that the basic information was inadequate. Instruments are available that are capable of closely copying mandibular motion, and it would be ideal to construct all castings on such instruments. However, the knowledge and time required to accurately utilize a fully adjustable articulator is not justified for single or routine multiple castings.

For the purpose of providing an easy means of relating upper and lower casts, a visual method of relating the maximum interdigitation of the teeth plus facets of wear as guides for occlulsal position or the use of a semiadjustable articulator will be used.

ARTICULATION OF CASTS USING WEAR FACETS

To minimize the errors possible with this method, full arch models that are free of bubbles on the occlusal surface are required. If wear facets are evident, the upper and lower models can be matched together using the facets as guides and secured with segments of wood and compound (Fig. 16–19).

For single castings it is common practice to use a nonadjustable articulator. However, it must be understood that such a straight line hinge articulator does not reproduce any mandibular movement and merely functions as a

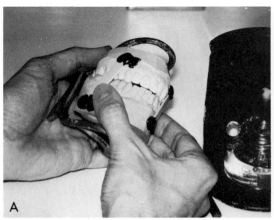
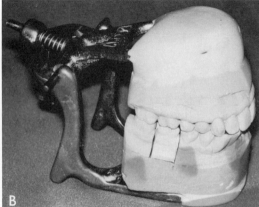

Figure 16–19. *A,* Full-arch models are matched to facets of wear and secured with compound. *B,* The models may be mounted into a hinge articulator.

holder to open and close the casts. It is best if the casts are mounted to such a device without using a wax bite record.

A mix of stone is placed on the lower member of the articulator, and the lower cast is arbitrarily positioned. After this has set the upper cast is placed on the lower, with the upper and lower wear facets matched to each other. A mix of stone is placed on the upper cast, and the upper articulator member is lowered into a position to be attached in the stone. The models should be moistened with water so the new stone will bond the models effectively.

An alternate method is to use preshaped wax wafers for an interocclusal record. The patient closes into this wafer until the teeth are in full contact. The casts are placed in the wax indentations and are attached to the articulator as previously described. This introduces a variable in that it is difficult to be sure that the posterior teeth are in full occlusal contact, since there is a tendency for the posterior teeth to separate slightly. Thus the casting will be fabricated to a slightly open position, which results in the time-consuming effort required for making occlusal adjustments in the mouth.

In the event partial arch models are used, wax occlusal records or zinc oxide–eugenol bite registrations are appropriate to provide an occlusal relationship.

A SEMIADJUSTABLE ARTICULATOR

When forming multiple castings or a single casting for a mouth that has poor landmarks, such as missing or malpositioned teeth, it is recommended that a semiadjustable articulator be used rather than the nonadjustable articulator previously discussed. This will allow the models to be positioned in an instrument that will simulate a condylar hinge axis rotation and mandibular movements. The effectiveness of this instrument is closely related to the accuracy of the information collected from the patient. The action of this instrument will not fully reproduce mandibular movement, but for most cases the instrument provides adequate action to minimize the oral adjustment of the castings.

A face bow is needed to relate the upper cast to the rotational axis of the mandible as the casts are positioned in the articulator. A popular face bow is a caliper-style ear bow.* The reason this is widely used is that it is simple to handle and has a workable accuracy level. It has been validated that by careful positioning of the self-centering ear piece, 75 per cent of the axes obtained will be within 6 mm of the true axis, as determined by a more accurate measurement.

TECHNIQUE OF RECORDING

Place a wafer of bite wax on the bite fork and lute it into position by heating the edge with a wax spatula so it will be immobilized.† Locate it on the upper teeth and impress the wafer forcibly on the teeth to secure a firm indentation of all the teeth and for stabilization so as to avoid any movement or rocking action. It is held in this position or the patient may bite against a bolus of wax on either side to keep it stable (Fig. 16–20).

The caliper face bow is positioned to the bite fork and into the ears for axis relation. The nose piece is placed on the nasion and secured (Fig. 16–21).

*Quick Mount Face-Bow, Whip-Mix Corp., 381 Farmington Ave., Louisville, Kentucky 40217.
†Lactona Corp., 201 Taber Rd., Morris Plains, New Jersey 07950.

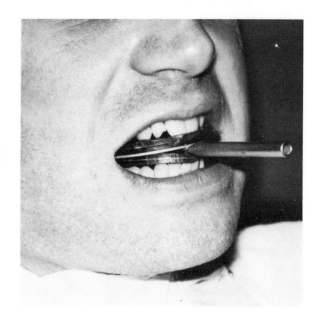

Figure 16–20. A wafer of bite wax on a bite fork is imprinted and held securely against the upper teeth.

This provides a standard height and angulation when the cast is attached to the upper member of the articulator. After all parts are related and secure the nose piece is removed and the assembly is carefully released from the ears and mouth and positioned on the designated axis pins on the articulator (Fig. 16–22).

The upper cast is placed in the wax indentations on the bite fork. The wax may require slight trimming to be sure the model fits accurately into the imprint (Fig. 16–23). Again, with the exception of the teeth the cast should be moistened and some curved undercuts may be needed on the cast to help unite the stone used for mounting to the articulator. The mix of stone should be controlled so as to provide a thickness that allows it to be stacked on the model yet permits it to flow easily to simplify mounting.

The most critical part of the mounting procedure is to accurately relate the lower model to the upper. The optimum accuracy is obtained by having the condyles of the mandible in the rearmost, uppermost, and midmost position in the glenoid fossae at the time when this record is made. It is not assumed that patients automatically have mandibular action from this point of reference because the teeth may contribute to discrepancies in a minor or major way. If told to bite into a wax wafer, most patients will close in an

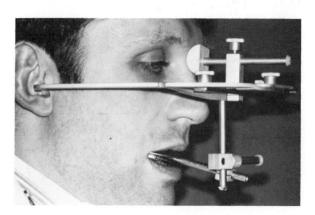

Figure 16–21. The face bow is assembled in position and secured on the bite fork.

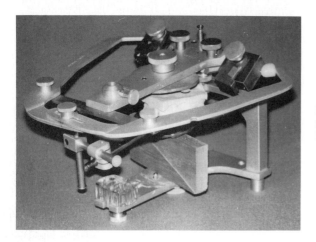

Figure 16–22. The face bow assembly is removed from the mouth and placed on the articulator axis pins.

anterior location so the mandible will need some guidance to achieve best results. Before making a wax record spend a little time having the patient practice closing into the desired position. The operator assists in this by applying manual pressure on the mental protuberance in a distal direction to help locate the condyles. The natural inclination is for the patient to resist this position so it may require some patience until the patient is able to produce a limited arcing movement in the correct position.

A wax wafer is firmly positioned on the upper teeth so as to prevent any movement. The mandible is guided toward centric closure from within as short an arc length as possible (Fig. 16–24). The lower teeth close into the wax, and the closing action should stop just as the teeth are about to make contact, as estimated by the operator. The moment the teeth begin to engage deflection is possible, and it is best if the record avoids this for mounting purposes.

This record is transferred to the upper mounted cast, the articulator is inverted, and the lower model is positioned in the wax record and then attached by stone to the lower member of the articulator (Fig. 16–25). When the stone is set the wax is removed, which will leave a small space between the upper and lower models; but if the models are related to an arc of closure, the possible error will be very small (Fig. 16–26).

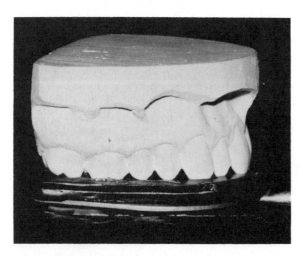

Figure 16–23. The upper cast is accurately fitted into the wax indentations on the bite fork.

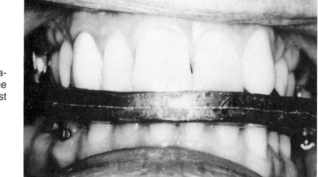

Figure 16–24. A wax recording of centric relation. The teeth are not in contact and the condyles of the mandible are in their most posterior position.

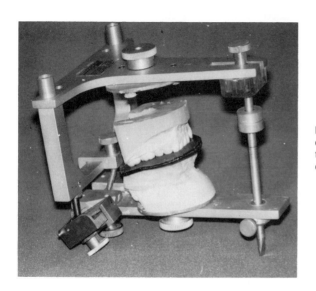

Figure 16–25. With the articulator inverted and the centric wax recording in place on the upper cast, the lower cast is positioned into the indented record.

Figure 16–26. A completed mounting into the articulator.

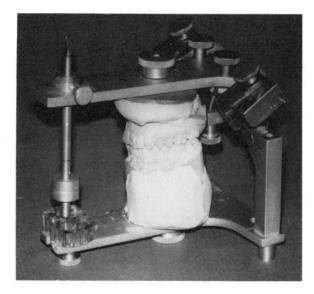

Upon closure of the models some teeth may make premature contact, and it is important to note this either as a basis for correction or to note that it is of little consequence. This is the record from which a casting can be made with minimal oral adjustment.

Additional records are also of value to determine the condyle setting on the articulator. The procedure is similar to that of centric closure but involves the right and left or lateral movements of the mandible. For a right lateral record the patient will be guided toward closure with the right cuspids and the facial cusps of the posterior teeth in an end-to-end position just short of contact. This is repeated on the left side (Fig. 16–27). Each of these records is placed between the models, and for the right lateral record the left condyle is free to move so that the side shift guide is brought into contact with the condyle (Fig. 16–28). This process is then concluded for the opposite side, which now provides the limits of the sideways movement for the mandible. Most wax patterns are developed from this basic information.

One additional step is a record of protrusive movement, which is taken with the anterior teeth closing in an end-to-end position (Fig. 16–29). When this record is used it provides the vertical angulation of the glenoid fossa or the slope over which the condyle glides.

This completes the setting of the articulator and allows waxing of the pattern to proceed within movements demonstrated by the patient. The information assembled represents the external limits of mandibular action, usually called border movements. It is not expected to reveal the details of movement within those limitations.

Resumé for Occlusal Records

1. Simple option—match models to wear facets or their maximum interdigitation and attach them to a non-adjustable articulator.

2. Option with greater accuracy—use a semiadjustable articulator.

3. Obtain a face bow mounting for the upper cast and attach it to the articulator.

4. Secure centric, lateral, and protrusive records.

5. With centric record mount lower cast to the articulator.

6. Use lateral and protrusive records to set the condylar action of the articulator.

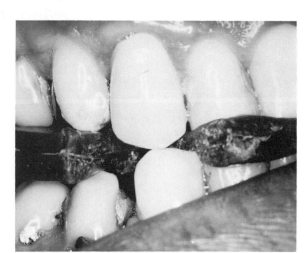

Figure 16–27. A right lateral wax recording wherein the cuspids close near an edge-to-edge relationship, although they should not actually be in contact.

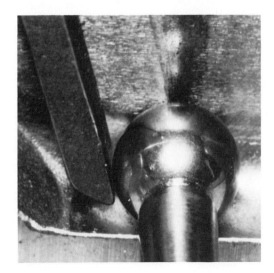

Figure 16–28. With the lateral bite record in position, the side shift guide is placed in contact with the condyle.

Temporary or Interim Treatment of Preparations

Armamentarium
1. Preformed aluminum crowns
2. Autopolymerizing acrylic for temporaries
3. Impression material to form the temporary crown
4. Contouring pliers
5. Crown scissors
6. Zinc oxide–eugenol cement plus cocoa butter
7. Proprietary temporary cement
8. Paper mixing pad
9. Mixing spatula
10. Plastic instrument

Procedure for Fabricating a Temporary (Protective Crown)

When the impression has been completed the preparation will require a temporary restoration. Until the time the casting is ready to be cemented the patient must be comfortable. This includes being free of thermal insult,

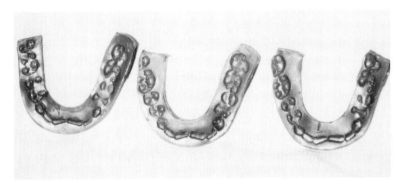

Figure 16–29. A series of bite records with a lateral record on each side and protrusive record in the middle.

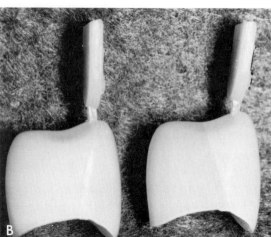

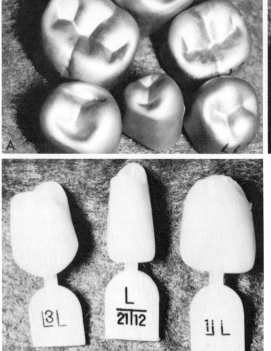

Figure 16–30. Aluminum *(A)* and carboxylate *(B and C)* temporary crowns.

primarily from cold, and the ability to continue with customary mastication of food.

If the preparation is not complicated and does not involve a great portion of the occlusal table, the preparation may be filled with ZOE cement. The restoration will last for several days and the patient will be comfortable. The initial strong taste of eugenol will subside in a short period of time. The essential difficulty with this method is that when the ZOE is to be removed it is tenacious and clings to the wall of the preparation. This may be overcome by placing a few fibers of cotton in the mixture of ZOE prior to placing it in the preparation. The cotton functions as a web and aids in removal of the temporary restoration.

Most of the situations needing temporary treatment will not be so simple, as the entire occlusal surface will frequently be involved. Then the temporary dressing will need to be more sophisticated.

PREFABRICATED TEMPORARIES. One of the solutions will be to use temporary crowns, which are supplied by commercial firms (Fig. 16–30). These temporary crowns will be aluminum* or resin† and they are available in assorted sizes to accommodate both anterior and posterior teeth. They are most easily utilized for posterior teeth. An aluminum crown is easier to adapt to the margins and occlusion as compared with a resin temporary, although the resin has obvious esthetic advantages.

*Unitek Corp., 2724 S. Peck Rd., Monrovia, California 91016.
†Harry Bosworth Co., 7227 N. Hamlin Rd., Skokie, Illinois 60076.

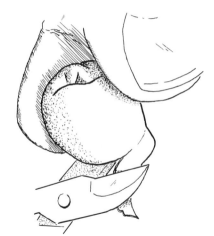

Figure 16–31. A crown scissors is used to partially trim the crown margins.

From among the assorted sizes of prefabricated temporary crowns select the one that comes closest to matching the size of the tooth prepared. If it is too small, it will resist placement; if the size is too large, it will impinge on the gingival tissues and be uncomfortable to the tongue and cheeks. After selection, the gingival portion is trimmed to allow proper placement. The gingival contour is arranged so as to relate to the buccal and lingual contours.

When using an aluminum temporary the gross trimming is done with a crown scissors (Fig. 16–31). When fully seated the temporary should not extend beyond the margins and could terminate 1.0 mm above the margin. To determine if it is properly seated the patient should close his teeth into contact and not have interference from the temporary. Frequently the patient will aid in occlusal contouring by depressing occlusal high spots as he forces his teeth into contact. While the closure is taking place the operator must carefully observe the gingival edge of the temporary and avoid any impingement of gingival tissue and continue adjusting gingival length so as to avoid tissue contact. The final adjustment of the temporary is made by a stone in a straight handpiece, to make sure that there are no rough edges and that the temporary is reasonably smooth. During this time it may be helpful to mold the perimeter of the temporary with a pair of contouring pliers to help locate the margins of the metal adjacent to the margins of the preparation (Fig. 16–32).

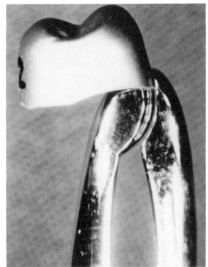

Figure 16–32. The gingival margin is smoothed and, when needed, given a contour with contouring pliers.

If the temporary is of resin, most of the adjusting will be done using a bur in a straight handpiece though some may be partially adjusted using a scissors. A major difficulty with commercial resin temporaries for posterior teeth is the difficulty of occlusal adjustment, which must be done entirely by use of a bur.

The interproximal contacts do not require a great deal of attention other than to allow the temporary to seat properly. This usually occurs during selection when the proper size temporary is chosen. The main function of a temporary is to maintain patient comfort for a short period of time. The proximal contacts usually are closed but if left open it should only be for a few days, for otherwise it will lead to gingival problems as a result of hygiene difficulties.

After a temporary crown form is adjusted so as to provide acceptable contour and margins the acrylic powder and liquid for temporary restorations are combined in a dappen dish.* The cream-like textured acrylic is placed into the crown form. When the acrylic begins to lose its glossy appearance it is placed over the preparation, which has been mildly lubricated with water or a thin film of vaseline (Fig. 16–33). The obvious excess acrylic is quickly removed from the area of the margins or natural undercuts.

Prior to becoming hard it is loosened from the preparation to be sure it can be removed. If this is overlooked, there are times when it is very difficult to separate the developing temporary from its preparation. Normally it is then repositioned and allowed to harden, following which it is removed, trimmed, and smoothed to allow for cementation. The occlusion must be observed and adjusted to prevent premature contacts.

CUSTOM-MADE TEMPORARIES. Another method that is used extensively is to make the temporary with a self-curing resin. This type of temporary has the advantage of producing a reasonable esthetic result. It can also be fabricated to conform closely to individual oral anatomy.

The initial procedure is to secure an elastic impression of the area that requires the temporary. This impression is made prior to beginning the preparation. If the temporary involves a single tooth, a sectional impression will be adequate. If additional preparations are involved, the impression will need to include more of the total arch for purpose of stability when it is reinserted. The usual material used for this procedure is alginate, although some prefer a rubber impression material (Fig. 16–34).

The impression is taken and set aside. If it is alginate, it is wrapped in a moist paper towel. The preparation and a die impression are completed, following which a temporary is made.

The impression that was set aside is re-examined, and all gross extensions are trimmed away. This includes any interseptal projections. It is mandatory that the impression be allowed to seat easily upon its return to the mouth.

When the impression is satisfactory, an acrylic resin, such as already mentioned, is selected. Most are supplied as a powder and liquid. The components are combined in a dappen dish to form a cream-textured material. Some are mixed on paper pads as they are supplied, as a paste to which the catalyst is added. It is then transferred to the section of the tray that contains the preparations. An attempt is made to estimate the volume required and yet provide some excess. The impression must at this time be seated accurately back to its normal position (Fig. 16–35). The teeth that have been prepared should have some lubricant, at least in the form of moisture, so as to ease the

---

*Harry Bosworth Co., 7227 N. Hamlin Rd., Skokie, Illinois 60076.

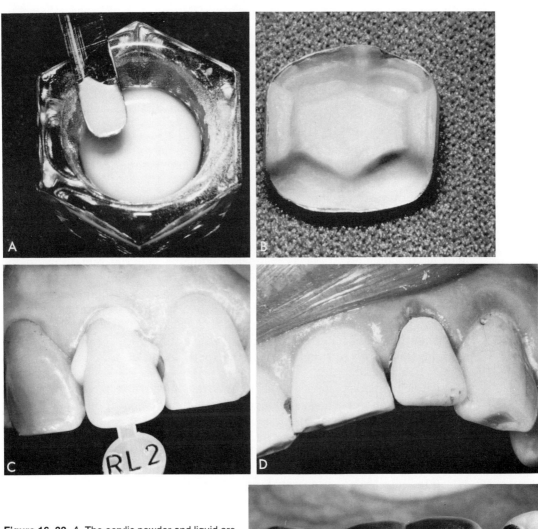

Figure 16–33. *A,* The acrylic powder and liquid are combined in a dappen dish and then placed in a crown form. *B,* In combination with an anodized aluminum crown form the acrylic provides excellent internal detail. *C,* A crown form filled with acrylic and put into position. The gross excess should be quickly removed. *D* and *E,* A lateral and molar crown form in position and ready for temporary cementation.

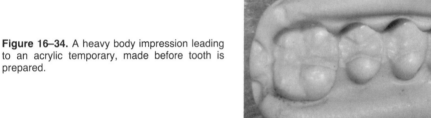

Figure 16–34. A heavy body impression leading to an acrylic temporary, made before tooth is prepared.

removal of the temporary as it polymerizes. Some products include these lubricants, resembling thin ointments, which may be applied to the preparation.

The impression is immobilized until partial polymerization has occurred. This is checked by observing the condition of the material remaining in the dappen dish or by holding some of the resin between the fingers while it polymerizes. If an alginate impression is used, the cooler impression material will delay polymerization, as compared with the material remaining in the hand or the dappen dish. The secret to success is to remove the impression while the temporary is still in a firm, rubbery stage. The temporary may be dislodged with the impression, which is then carefully separated from the impression with an instrument and then replaced on the tooth. With some materials the gross excess can be trimmed with a cuticle scissors. It is important that the temporary be replaced on the tooth to make sure that it can be removed easily.

If the temporary stays in position as the impression is removed, steps should be taken to partially dislodge the temporary before it becomes hard. A stiff explorer or a plastic instrument may be used for this purpose. Again, it is important that the temporary be freely mobile before it fully polymerizes. In all of this the operator will develop experience as to the proper timing for removal of the impression so as to minimize difficulty.

If the impression is separated too quickly, the resin will not be an accurate reproduction of tooth form and it will have to be redone. A more frustrating

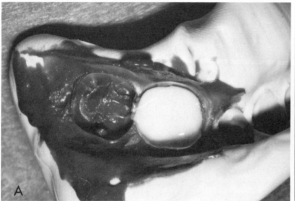

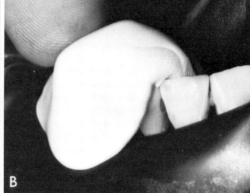

Figure 16–35. *A,* The acrylic is added to the crown space in the impression and *(B)* returned to its position in the mouth.

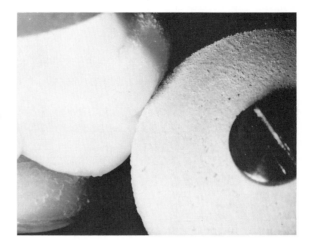

Figure 16–36. A white rubber wheel is used to finish the surface of the acrylic.

problem is when it is left in the mouth too long. The temporary becomes hard and there may be preparation and interproximal interferences that will prevent dislodging of the temporary without a struggle. If the temporary is usable, reliable, and easily removed, it may be placed in hot water to hasten its final curing or hardening. If defects in the form of voids that need correction are evident, this may be done by adding some resin with a camel's hair brush using the bead procedure.

After the temporary is hardened the needed corrections are accomplished using burs and disks in a slow-speed handpiece (Fig. 16–36). If high speed is used, the burs create excess heat in the resin, which softens and then clogs the bur. The occlusion is checked with articulating paper to remove the prematurities. The temporary should be smooth upon completion, although in most cases a high polish is not essential. When polishing is needed, flour of pumice in a rubber cup with a slow-speed handpiece will produce a good surface.

A resin temporary that is completed with proper contours and smoothness will last for a limited period of time. In contrast, an aluminum temporary that is in occlusal function may deteriorate rapidly after a couple of weeks, leaving ragged irritating edges unless lined with acrylic.

The resin temporaries are cemented with a material that will permit easy removal, usually a ZOE material. Several products are available for this

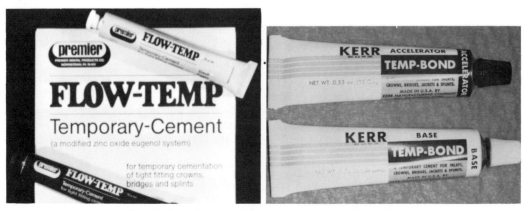

Figure 16–37. Examples of temporary cementing materials.

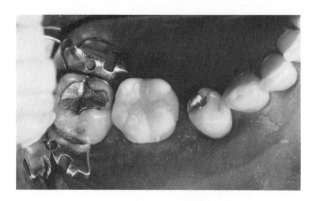

Figure 16–38. An acrylic temporary restoration cemented into place. Some clinicians prefer a non–eugenol temporary cement that does not plasticize the acrylic, which allows repeated cementation. An example is ZONE.*

purpose, for example, Temp-Bond† or Flow-Temp,‡ which are supplied in a two-paste system that is mixed on a paper pad in the required amount. Again the student should learn to be frugal in the amount used and not mix several times the amount needed (Fig. 16–37).

If a commercial temporary cement is not available, there are alternate methods. A conventional ZOE cement may be mixed to a paste-like consistency. To this mixture add a small amount of cocoa butter and again mix it thoroughly. This will make the cement mixture very fluid and allow for ease of cementation. The cocoa butter prevents the ZOE from becoming hard so that the temporary restorations will be easily removed at the proper time. When the temporary has been placed, the excess cement is removed from the marginal areas.

If the temporary is to be used for a short period of time, it is not mandatory to have the margins of the resin precisely meet the margins of the preparation, for the minor deficiencies may be made up in the ZOE cement. Irrespective of the composition, the interface area between temporary and preparation should not be a source of discomfort or tissue irritation (Fig. 16–38). The major problem is that if the cement is exposed to abrasion, it may wear away to expose sensitive dentin.

Resumé of Temporary Treatment
1. Predetermine method of temporization.
2. Select crown form and adapt it to tissue and margins.
3. Or, obtain elastic impression with alginate or rubber as a form for the temporary.
4. Mix self-curing acrylic to a creamy texture and place in the impression.
5. Seat impression and leave until acrylic is at a rubbery or firm state. Check using excess material.
6. Remove impression and partially remove temporary before total polymerization.
7. After temporary hardens, trim the excess to leave smooth margins.
8. Check occlusion of the temporary.
9. Cement temporary with a temporary cement.
10. Check gingival margins to avoid tissue irritation.

---

*CAACO Products Inc., 8890 Regent St., Los Angeles, California 90034.
†Kerr Mfg. Co.—Div. Sybron Corp., Romulus, Michigan 48174.
‡Premier Dental Products Co., 1710 Romano Drive, Norristown, Pennsylvania 19401.

17

THE CAST GOLD RESTORATION: LABORATORY PROCEDURES

Die Formation

The die must be fabricated from the impression within a period of time that is consistent with the physical behavior of the impression material so as to prevent inaccuracies in the model. If the lapsed time is excessive before the impression is poured, an inaccurate casting is likely to result. To prevent distortion all impressions with the exception of those made from addition silicones should be poured within an hour after removal from the mouth.

It is important that the impression material copy some tooth surface gingival from the margins (Fig. 17–1). This simplifies the task of preparing working dies for waxing. There are occasions when this space is limited or non-existent. The space may be limited because the gingival margin is depressed below the gingival level or because the flange of impression material beyond the margin is very thin and short. This makes it difficult to locate the precise margin on the stone die.

Placing a bead of utility wax right at the finish line of the preparation simplifies the problem of locating the margins on the dies. When the model is removed from the impression the wax provides additional marginal space, making it easier to prepare the die (Fig. 17–2). The wax is added using one of the instruments designed for the wax addition technique of forming wax patterns (to be discussed later in the chapter). The wax used for this purpose is utility or boxing wax, which is softer than that used for the wax patterns. With the instrument some wax is picked up and liquefied and a bead is allowed to flow onto the impression material, increasing the thickness of the flange of impression material near the gingival margin.

To form the necessary dies a Class II (Type IV classification in American Dental Association specifications) stone should be used, as it has the physical properties of the best stone possible: strength and minimal setting expansion.

The powder and the water must be accurately proportioned to obtain best results. The water should be measured with an accurate graduated cylinder. The powder can be measured by use of premeasured envelopes supplied by manufacturers or weighed on a balance.

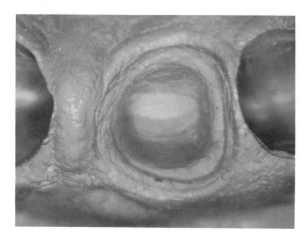

Figure 17-1. Ideal impressions would have a flange of impression beyond the cavosurface margin.

Procedure for Forming a Die

A clean bowl that is free of scratches or abrasions, which would tend to retain previously mixed stone, is used. Water in the amount prescribed by the manufacturer is placed in the bowl. The water should be pure, and in many areas bottled water will be indicated. If there is a high concentration of chemicals in the water, setting time and other properties of the stone may be altered.

The powder is sifted into the water, permitting the particles to be moistened by the water. The bowl is then placed on a vibrator, but the vibration is controlled to avoid a turbulent action on the semi-fluid mass. A stiff spatula is used for mixing and the intention is to minimize the chance for air bubbles to form. This is done by swiping the mix against the sides of the bowl with the spatula and letting the vibrator settle the mass into the bottom of the bowl. This is continued until the mass is homogenous and has a smooth texture. When working by hand, mixing should be concluded within 2 minutes and ready for placement into the impression.

The recommended means of reducing air inclusion is to mix water and stone in a vacuum mixer. The mixing speed should be slow, as high-speed spatulation shortens the working or setting time of the stone, creating diffi-

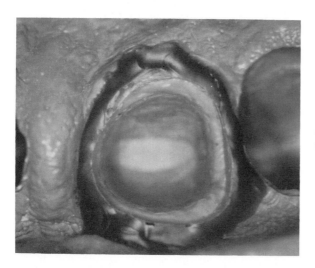

Figure 17-2. Soft wax added to the tissue side of the impression is helpful in preparing the die.

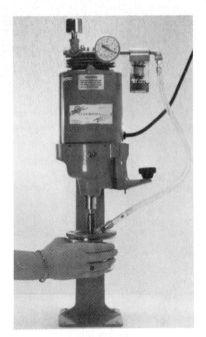

Figure 17–3. Mechanically mixing die stone while under a vacuum.*

culties in pouring stone into the impressions. Commercial mixers are available to facilitate the mixing of gypsum products. Such devices decrease the mixing time and minimize the possibility of porosity (Fig. 17–3).

Placing the stone into the impression is very critical, as it must flow into the details of the impression without trapping air. A vibrator is needed to prevent the formation of bubbles (Fig. 17–4). Frequently when air bubbles become part of the die the die is worthless and an additional impression is required.

When forming the coronal portion of the teeth the stone should flow into

---

*Whip-Mix Corp., 381 Farmington Ave., Louisville, Kentucky 40217.

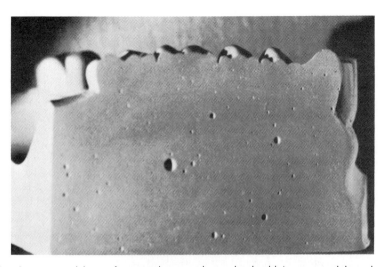

Figure 17–4. Voids occurring either from poor mixing or from carelessness in pouring lead into poor models and dies.

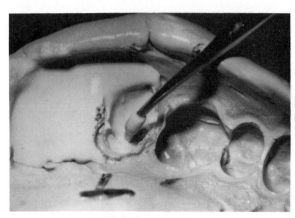

Figure 17–5. A brush or an instrument is useful in placing the stone in the preparation to prevent voids.

the impression in small increments. The stone can be carried to the impression with a spatula or a small sable-hair brush. The vibrator should be adjusted to provide smooth vibratory pattern, as excess agitation promotes bubble formation.

The impression should be held at an angle on the vibrator table, which allows the stone to flow easily and continuously from the same direction. The stone is placed on the ridge area adjacent to the last tooth and from there allowed to flow slowly over the distal aspect into the preparation, slowly filling the individual mold from the bottom. The stone is added slowly and proceeds from the posterior toward the anterior and on to the opposite posterior segment. Sometimes air entrapment is suspected at some specific location, and it is helpful to use a brush or an instrument to physically probe through the area with the intention of breaking up possible air bubbles (Fig. 17–5). While this occurs it is best that the stone be added from the same place continually. When the coronal portion of the impression has been filled the remaining stone may be added quickly. Once beyond the crown details, the potential for air bubbles is reduced.

The flowability of the stone will vary depending on the type of impression material used. An alginate, because of its water content, will allow the stone to flow quite easily, while a rubber material will cause some resistance to flow.

The model must have adequate thickness to its base. This may be achieved by stacking the stone on the impression, which is possible if the stone has developed adequate viscosity. The impression should be left in an upright

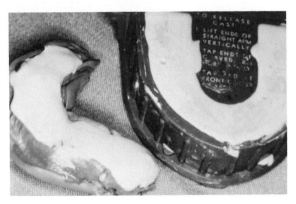

Figure 17–6. While the die stone is fluid the impression should be left upright.

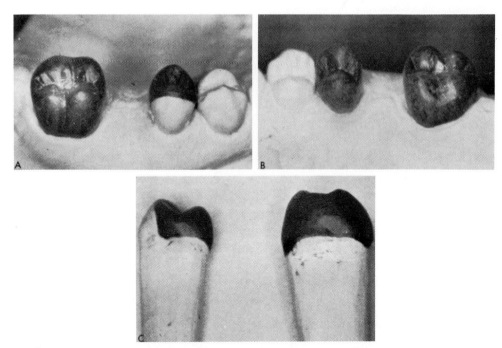

Figure 17–7. The wax pattern is developed on the second pour model and transferred to the first pour dies to refine the margins. (From Johnston, J. F., Phillips, R. W., and Dykema, R. W.: Modern Practice in Crown and Bridge Prosthodontics. Philadelphia, W. B. Saunders Co., 1971)

position until the stone has begun to set. If the impression is inverted prematurely, the stone may drift from the occlusal or incisal portion of the impression (Fig. 17–6). A base is provided to the model by placing the partially set, but filled, impression on a base of thick stone and then molding to shape.

Another means of achieving the same objective is to encase the impression with soft boxing or utility wax and follow the same procedures of forming a model with an adequate base. The space between quadrants in a lower impression may be closed with wax before pouring the model.

Dowel Pin Orientation

When preparations are a part of the impression, in order to form the wax patterns, it is necessary to isolate and remove each die from its environment.

One means used for this purpose is to pour two models from the same impression and separate the dies from the initial model. The wax patterns are formed on these dies, which are the most accurate reproductions. The pattern is transferred to the second model, which will be used to help with alignment, contours, and occlusion. As a final step the pattern is placed on the original die to verify the margins (Fig. 17–7).

A brass dowel pin may be used as a means of orienting dies to the original or master model, which allows the dies to be easily removed and accurately replaced into the model. The pin is tapered and cylindrical but flattened on one side for positive seating. The head is serrated so the pin can be secured into the die portion of the model.

The dowel pin must be suspended over the preparation area prior to

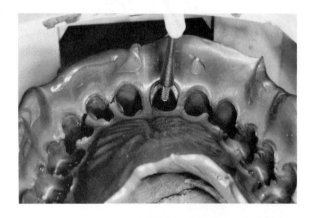

Figure 17–8. A dowel pin in place using a pin positioner.

placing the stone. There are dowl pin holders that may be used to hold the pin in an upright position (Fig. 17–8). The pin must be stationed so as to be parallel to the long axis of the crown so it will be able to move easily in and out of the model.

An alternate method of relating the dowel pin is to place two straight stick pins parallel to each other through the flanges of the impression so as to allow a dowel pin to be held between the pins slightly above the preparation (Fig. 17–9). The dowel pin is stabilized into position between the pins by flowing sticky wax around the junction area.

The die stone is prepared and is vibrated into the impression, as has already been described. There is no attempt to fill all of the impression, rather just the area of and adjacent to the preparations (Fig. 17–10). It is filled to a height at which the head of the dowel pin will be engaged. To help secure the next addition of stone, paper clips may be cut and the curved segments placed into the first pour of stone before it hardens (Fig. 17–11). This mechanically secures the two segments of the model solidly.

After the die stone has hardened it is advantageous to make a depression with a No. 4 bur in the set stone, usually lingual to the pin. This prevents rotation of the die when it is seated into the model (Fig. 17–12).

The area to be included in the die is covered by a separating material. This prevents the die from sticking to the model. The end of the dowel pin is covered with a small ball of utility wax before placing the final portion of stone. This is helpful when locating the end of the dowel pin in the completed model, assuming the dowel pin is covered when adding the final amount of stone.

A new mix of stone is added to form the remainder of the model. This stone may be die stone as used for dies, or if the occlusal segment of the

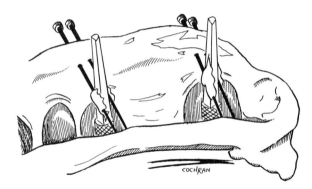

Figure 17–9. A dowel pin waxed into position using stick pins.

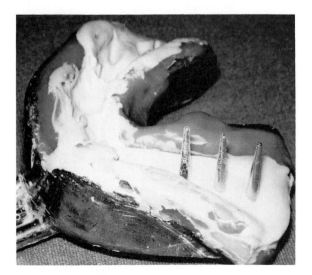

Figure 17–10. Die stone is vibrated into a portion of the impression.

impression is already filled with die stone, conventional stone may be used to form the remaining portion of the model. The occlusal segment should be filled with the same type of stone so as to provide consistent dimensional changes during setting for the cast.

At this time it is ideal to allow the model to set several hours before separating the die from the model. The separation of the die from the model is easily accomplished by using a laboratory saw. The available saw blades will have slight variations in thickness, and selection is based upon the available space between the die preparation and the next tooth. The thinnest blade is .007″ in thickness.

To separate the die, mesial and distal cuts are made to the line of separation between the first and second pouring of stone. At this time the wax over the end of the pin is located and by applying pressure on the end of the dowel pin the die should move free of the model (Fig. 17–13).

The die is trimmed at the margin so as to place the margin in prominent relief to make it easy to wax the margins. It is ideal if the stone is trimmed

Figure 17–11. Segments of paper clips are positioned to secure the second portion of the model.

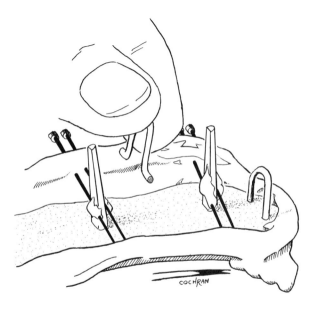

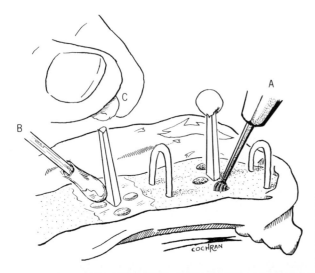

Figure 17–12. *A,* A mechanical depression is made to orient the die in the model. *B,* A lubricant is added so as to allow separation from the model. *C,* Wax is placed on a dowel pin for location after model is poured. *D,* A model being properly oriented.

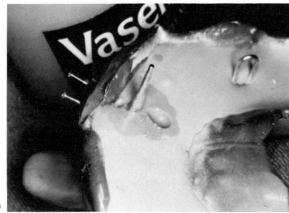

Figure 17–13. Stone is added to complete the model and by using a thin saw blade the die is separated from the model.

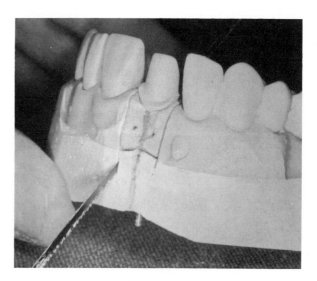

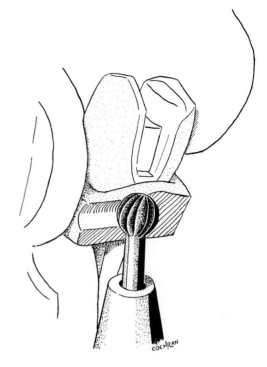

Figure 17–14. A large bur is used to trim most of the stone near the margins.

flush with the margins or if a slight undercut is below the margins (Fig. 17–14).

If there is a large amount of stone to trim, a large part may be cut with a bur or separating disk. Be careful and avoid the margins, for if they are damaged another impression will be needed. The last part of the margin relief should be done with a hand instrument for best control. Among the instruments that may be used are cutting instruments, the cleoid, or small sharp laboratory knives. It is helpful if the die is moistened with water while the final trimming is done (Fig. 17–15).

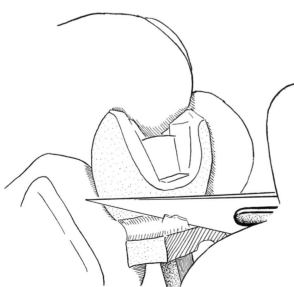

Figure 17–15. The margins are trimmed using a laboratory knife or cutting instrument.

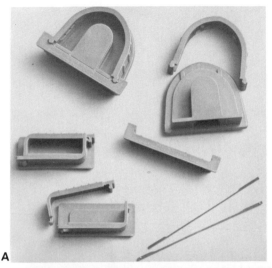

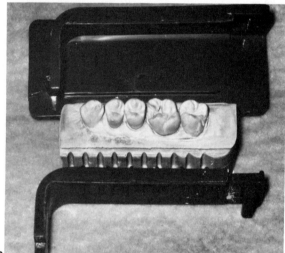

Figure 17–16. *A*, Quarter- and full-arch Di-Lok trays. *B*, A quarter-arch model with its Di-Lok tray.

Die Orientation Using Keyed Trays

Keyed trays provide an alternate method of relating the individual die to the adjacent teeth. An example of such a tray is the Di-Lok Tray.* It is a commercial tray device made of plastic, one arm of which is movable and detaches from the main body to allow easy removal of the individual dies. It is designed to prevent vertical and horizontal movement of the dies when they are secured within the tray (Fig. 17–16).

Its use permits a model to be sectioned and accurately reassembled. The die may be individual or part of the master model. The advantage of its use is that a second impression or a second pour into an impression to provide for a working die is not needed. The second pour into an impression is seldom as accurate as the original.

---

*Lactona Corp., 201 Taber Rd., Morris Plains, New Jersey 07950.

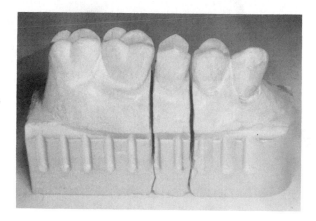

Figure 17–17. The die is separated by using a saw until the die fractures with digital pressure.

The Di-Lok Tray is available in two styles: one is designed to work with a quadrant of teeth and the other with a full arch. The quadrant tray is particularly suited to work with a quadrant-style impression, but it may also be used to orient a portion of a complete arch.

The impression is poured in a conventional manner and allowed to harden. The model is trimmed on a model trimmer and fitted inside the tray. Undercuts are cut into the model base with a separating disk. The assembled tray is partly filled with dental stone of a different color. The model is moistened to assure a good union between the old and new stone and the model is slowly adjusted into the desired position in the tray and allowed to harden until it can be sawed. The model is removed from the tray, and with a thin saw, cuts are made on the mesial and distal sides of the preparation to a depth of three-quarters of the distance through the base. The remainder of the stone is fractured by applying mesial-distal finger pressure on the model (Fig. 17–17).

When the dies are separated the stone is grossly trimmed free of the margins by using a large bur, abrasive wheel, or a separating disk. The small amount of remaining stone is trimmed with an instrument or laboratory scalpel as described with the dowel pin procedure. It is simple to reassemble all the parts back into the tray and have them properly oriented, with no movement as a result of the tray design. The tray must be free of all debris.

The total assembly is attached to the bow of an articulator with a mix of plaster or dental stone and allowed to harden. The occlusal registration of wax or of a zinc oxide–eugenol cement is placed on the attached model and the opposite stone arch is securely placed into the registration and attached to the remaining articulator arm with a new mix of stone.

For occlusal relationships it is most reliable to use full arch models that occlude together. The models may be occluded on the basis of observed wear facets for single restorations. The models are mounted together so as to have the facets of wear coincide with each other. If several teeth are missing or if these facets are not easily detected, it is essential to use an occlusal registration to relate the models to each other to help form the wax pattern. This has been discussed in Chapter 16 in greater detail.

Preparation of Wax Pattern

When a die has been occlusally oriented and trimmed to expose its margins it is ready to be used for making the wax pattern. This requires certain creative ability. The form of the restoration, its ability to function with proximal and opposing teeth, and its esthetics are directly related to the effort necessary to develop a wax pattern. The marginal fit of the casting is dependent on the care taken as the margins are waxed. It is difficult to overemphasize the need for artistic concern for all the details so necessary to making a wax pattern. Unfortunately, many clinical restorations reflect inadequate concern or poor technique.

Before proceeding with a wax pattern it is important to have a mental picture or image of the completed pattern. This requires a good understanding of tooth morphology. Thus it is well to review this subject, using any available source including books and models. Learn to observe the subtle variances of axial and occlusal contours. Then in conjunction with the patient's study models, observe the particular dental anatomy patterns that must be considered as that individual pattern is being made.

Die Relief

Some clinicians may wish to provide a specific amount of relief on the die before making the wax pattern. This is for the purpose of providing a controlled space between the casting and its preparation to accommodate the cement. This is to avoid the need for making relief on the casting before cementation to help extrude excess cement from under the casting.

These materials are painted on the die surface and care is exercised to avoid the margins. Some of these products handle as a conventional lacquer and are easily placed on the die (Fig. 17–18).*

They are applied in multiple layers according to the amount of relief or space desired. Six layers of airplane paint provide 30 ± 4 micrometers of relief. Those who use three or four layers of this material are satisfied with the results obtained. While additional research is needed there is no reported loss of retention for the restoration using this technique of die relief.

Wax Selection

The exact composition of dental waxes is rather guarded by manufacturers. However, the essential ingredients are paraffin wax, gum dammar, and carnauba wax, with some coloring material. All of these substances are of natural origin, derived from either mineral or vegetable sources.

Paraffin is the main ingredient, and it is derived from high boiling point fractions of petroleum. By itself it tends to flake when carved and does not leave a smooth surface. Gum dammar is a natural resin from a specific variety of pine and when added to paraffin it helps resist flaking and allows for a smooth surface. Carnauba wax comes from a tropical palm and is quite hard and tends to decrease the flow of a wax. Carnauba wax is now being largely replaced by synthetic waxes.

Dental wax should be capable of being carved to the thinnest margin without distortion, flaking, or chipping. The color of the wax should be in sharp contrast to that of the die material to aid in visibility during carving. The wax should vaporize as completely as possible without leaving a residue when being eliminated from the mold.

---

*Pactra Industries Inc., Los Angeles, California 90028.

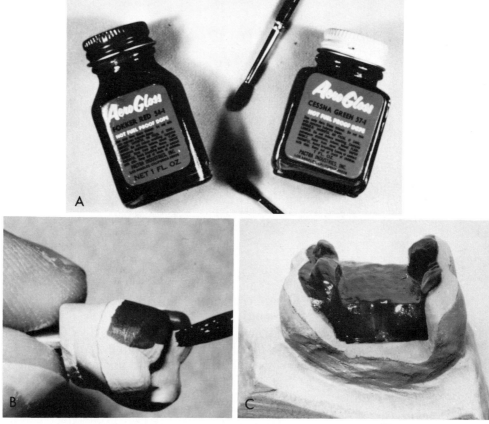

Figure 17–18. *A,* Lacquer-like materials used for die relief. *B* and *C,* Die relief material being placed on the die.

Distortion is probably the most serious problem faced when forming the pattern and removing it from the die. Such distortions arise from thermal changes and from the release of the stress inherent in the pattern. The most practical method of avoiding distortion or damage to a wax pattern is to invest it as quickly as possible after removal from the die.

Technique of Waxing

Armamentarium
1. Die lubricant
2. Cotton pliers
3. Supply of wax
4. No. 7 wax spatula
5. ½–3 Hollenback carver
6. Cleoid-discoid carver
7. Bunsen burner or alcohol lamp
8. P. K. Thomas waxing instruments

PROCEDURE

The first step is to use a sharp black or red pencil and precisely survey all margins. This is valuable when trying to locate them after the wax has been applied (Fig. 17–19).

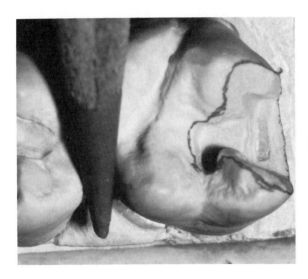

Figure 17–19. The die with the margins surveyed with a pencil.

Next a die lubricant must be applied to the die. This is a light oil-like film.* If not used, it becomes impossible to remove the wax pattern from the die as a single unit. The lubricant must be very thin to avoid a discrepancy between the pattern and the die. It is necessary to apply more than one coat as the first is usually largely absorbed by the stone (Fig. 17–20).

The wax is supplied as small rods or in bulk in a small metal container. Selection is based on personal preference in regard to matters such as carving consistency and color.

The traditional method of forming the pattern is to use a wax spatula and place melted wax on the die in increments. The heat source should be a small well-adjusted flame that will heat the instrument quickly. The heated instrument is used to melt the wax to carry to the die. It may be necessary to reheat the instrument and the wax to properly liquefy the wax so that it will flow easily to the die. It will take some experience in order to learn how to easily control the amount of heat into the instrument to have the wax in the desired consistency. The wax is added by increments to all parts of the die, in an amount that will be in excess of the eventual size (Fig. 17–21).

At this stage it is important to envision the desired form of the pattern and then carve away the excess wax. Among the carving instruments a

---

*Microfilm, a colloidal suspension of wax: Kerr Manufacturing Co., Romulus, Michigan 48174.

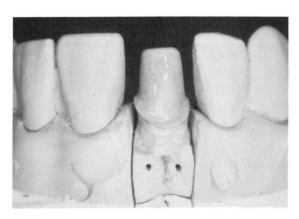

Figure 17–20. A die that has been lubricated before the addition of wax. No die relief has been added.

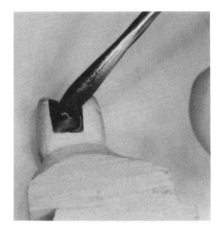

Figure 17–21. A No. 7 wax was spatula being used to place wax on the axial surfaces.

Hollenback ½–3 and a cleoid-discoid are effective instruments for carving the pattern. If there is a large amount of excess wax to remove, it is best to heat the carver to help remove some of the wax, but when detailed carving is needed it should be done with a cool instrument.

Instruments selected for waxing procedures should be reserved for that purpose if they are subject to being heated. The heating removes the temper in the metal and as a result the sharpness is lost. This precludes using an amalgam carver as a wax carver unless overheating is prevented, which is indicated by any color change in the instrument.

First develop the axial contours and then carve the fossa and occlusal pits, blending the cuspal incliners into the occlusal depressions. Then proceed to carve the required anatomy in the wax.

WAX ADDITION PROCEDURE

The initial step in this technique is the same as just described wherein the missing axial contours and their margins are replaced by wax. The axial contours should be related accurately to the adjacent teeth. It is easier to first wax and carve the axial contour to completion and then reduce the occlusal height of the pattern in order to initiate waxing the occlusal anatomy.

In addition to the instruments already listed for carving wax patterns the P. K. Thomas waxing instruments are needed to form the occlusal by incremental additions of wax.

During this technique small segments of the anatomy are developed by adding wax until that part is completed. A planned sequence, based on the anatomical features, is followed as the occlusal is formed and becomes part of a reproducible system of forming wax patterns.

Of the P. K. Thomas instruments, No. 1 or 2 is heated to liquefy the wax and carry it to a specific location. Become familiar with the use of these instruments before attempting detailed wax procedures. Determine how much the instruments should be heated to liquefy the wax to an appropriate consistency. When depositing wax on the pattern, apply the heat just short of the end of the instrument. If heat is applied to the very end, the heat travels up the instrument and carries the wax with it. But when the heat is concentrated just short of the end of the induced heat easily travels to the end and the melted wax is properly positioned for application to the die.

Before beginning the occlusal waxing locate and mark the precise location

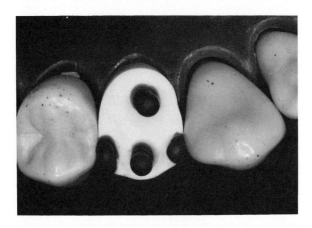

Figure 17–22. The initial waxing step is to locate and place wax cones for the cusp tips followed by cones for the junction of the occlusal and interproximal surfaces.

for the cusp tips on the die. Then proceed to build a cone of wax to its required height. These cones are built in layers and their diameters vary in relation to the cusp size. Usually they should be 2 to 3 mm at the base. The cones should be neither too minute in size nor occupy a large area. These cones are made by learning to pick up the right amount of wax on the No. 2 wax instrument and then reheating it so as to allow it to pool on the surface to form the needed diameter (Fig. 17–22). The height of the cone for the working cusp is determined by the occluding model, which is brought into occlusal contact when the wax is soft. The cusp–fossa relationship controls the height of the working cone. A good occlusal contact of the working cone is expected. The remaining cones are built to an arbitrary height determined by the neighboring mesial or distal cusps, which are on the same alignment.

The exact sequence of the steps beyond this initial step need not be in a specific order, though in general the outside surfaces are completed first, leaving the internal details to the last. Thus the following sequence is one that will work effectively, as it is based on experience.

Locate the junction of the proximal and facial surfaces and at that location place a cone with the No. 2 instrument. The height of this cone is arbitrarily determined by observing the same location of neighboring teeth. From this cone proceed to develop the mesial and distal marginal ridges with the same wax instrument. The marginal ridge height is determined by the occluding contact from the opposite arch or from the height of adjacent marginal ridges (Fig. 17–23).

When cusp cones are developed it is best if the occluding cusp tips fall inside of the marginal ridges, which results in a good cusp–fossa relationship, thereby providing good tooth stability. At times this is not possible and the cusp tip will make contact with the top of the marginal ridge. Placing a cusp tip between the marginal ridges should be avoided. This has the effect of a plunger cusp, which may tend to separate the teeth and allow fibrous food to be impacted below the proximal contact.

Following this the facial and lingual surfaces of the cusp may be added using a No. 1 or No. 2 instrument, depending on the surface area. With the No. 2 instrument begin adding wax to form the ridges for the buccal and lingual cusps. The wax being added is built toward the developmental grooves. Care is exercised to avoid excess addition of wax, which would tend to obliterate the major details of the occlusal surface.

A slight excess of wax in the occlusal development is expected, and to compensate for this the No. 3 instrument is used as a router to locate the pits

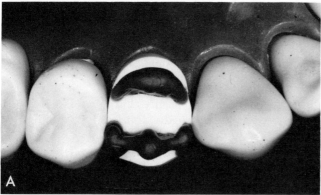

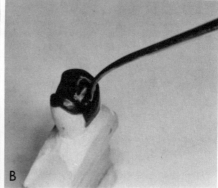

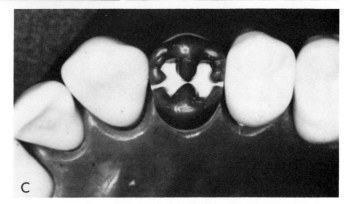

Figure 17–23. *A,* Wax is added to the cusp tip toward the marginal ridge. *B,* A No. 2 instrument places wax for a marginal ridge. *C,* The marginal ridge and external surface are nearing completion.

and grooves (Fig. 17–24). From this reference the grooves and ridges may be carved, using the No. 4 or No. 5 carver. Additional instruments that are useful are the ½ Hollenback No. 3 or the 4–5 cleoid-discoid. It is to be expected that minute additions of wax will be needed. Some of the smaller grooves are made more realistic by heating the smallest end of the No. 2 instrument and fusing the grooves where they have been overcarved.

During this process of occlusal addition close attention must be paid to the occlusal contacts. Determine in advance the number and location of these contacts. Then by articulating the models as wax is added the contact is easily formed while the wax is still warm. When the contact is properly formed guard it very carefully through the remainder of the process. After the casting is seated in the mouth it is anticipated that occlusal contacts will be evident so as to establish the best functioning pattern.

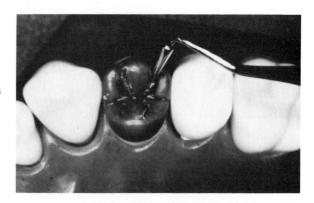

Figure 17–24. Without being heated the No. 3 instrument is used to accentuate the grooves.

At this time using finger pressure very carefully and slowly release the pattern from the die. Just pull on the pattern so that it moves slightly from the margins. Then reposition the pattern, repeat the process, and observe several views of the pattern to be sure the pattern is releasing smoothly and evenly from all parts of the die. Then remove the pattern and examine its internal aspects. Replace the pattern and make corrections if needed. As a final step examine the margins very carefully to assure that they are accurate (Fig. 17–25). It may be necessary to add more die lubricant if significant corrections are to be made.

The final smoothing of the wax pattern is achieved using a large cotton pellet that is moistened with water and warmed. Then using a cotton plier proceed to rub the occlusal surface in order to produce a smooth surface.

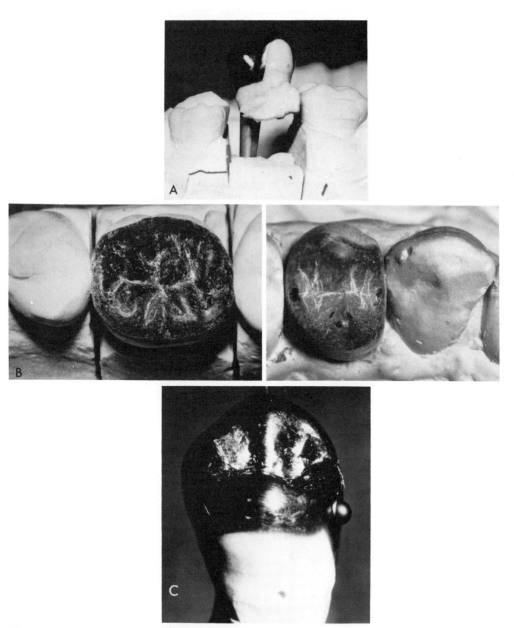

Figure 17–25. *A,* Examine the margins very carefully and use magnification to view the margins. *B,* To check the occlusal contacts stearic acid powder is dusted on the surface. *C,* A projection may be waxed at a convenient place to help remove the casting during the try-in.

Again be cautious to leave the occlusal contacts intact. The axial surfaces are also smoothed in the same manner. As a final step in the sequence a soap solution and a cotton pellet are used to produce a slight polish to the wax surface.

Resumé of Wax Pattern Development

1. Locate and survey the margins of the stone die with a sharp pencil.
2. Place two coats of die lubricant as needed.
3. With a No. 1 instrument add wax for all axial contours.
4. Carve the axial surfaces with a Hollenback ½–3 or similar instrument.
5. Flatten the occlusal segment and locate the cusp centers.
6. With the No. 2 wax instrument build the cusp cones and the proximo-facial corners.
7. With the same instrument add the marginal ridges.
8. With a No. 1 or 2 instrument add the facial and lingual contours.
9. With a No. 2 wax instrument add wax for the occlusal cusp ridges.
10. Use a No. 3 to establish the grooves.
11. Use a No. 4 Hollenback ½–3 and 4–5 cleoid-discoid to finish the grooves.
12. Smooth and polish the wax pattern with moist, warmed cotton followed by a soap solution.

Spruing and Investing the Wax Pattern

Armamentarium
1. Sprue former
2. Sprue pins (wax or hollow metal)
3. Metal ring
4. Liner material
5. Selected investment
6. Mixing spatula
7. Accurate measure for liquid or water
8. Mixing device (mechanical with vacuum preferred)
9. Vibrator (mechanical)

After the wax pattern has been completed the next procedure is to begin the process of its conversion to a metal casting. The compelling but challenging problem, which continues to face the dentist, is to produce a casting that will fit within an acceptable level of clinical tolerance. Variables related to impression and die materials have already been discussed and hopefully minimized by the described techniques.

Assuming the wax pattern is satisfactory, the procedure then centers upon enlarging the mold uniformly and sufficiently to compensate for the casting shrinkage of the gold alloy.

Theoretically, if the shrinkages of the wax and gold are known, the mold can be expanded an amount equal to such a shrinkage and the problem is solved. However, there are variables in the behavior of the materials involved that cannot be fully controlled. The casting procedure is partly empirical and when a routine is firmly established it should be rigidly followed.

Investments

The essential ingredients of the dental investment employed with the conventional gold casting alloys are a hemihydrate of gypsum, some form of silica, reducing agents such as carbon or powdered copper, and other agents used to regulate setting expansion and time. The gypsum is used as a binder because of its strength and it holds the other ingredients together and thus provides the needed rigidity. The investment may contain 25 to 45 percent gypsum.

The silica, SiO_2, is used to provide a heat-resistant material, or refractory, during the heating of the investment and to regulate the thermal expansion. During the heating the investment expands thermally to compensate partially or totally for the casting shrinkage of the gold alloy.

SETTING AND HYGROSCOPIC EXPANSION. A mixture of silica and gypsum results in a setting expansion greater than that of the gypsum alone. In addition to this is hygroscopic expansion that occurs when the material is allowed to set when in contact with water. Hygroscopic expansion is essentially a prolongation of the normal setting expansion and thereby increases the total expansion.

THERMAL EXPANSION. Two forms of silica are used in dental investments—quartz and cristobalite. Actually investments may be classified accordingly. Both forms tend to induce an "inversion" in their crystalline structure when heated, resulting in an expansion. This thermal expansion is the principal cause for mold expansion. The cristobalite form produces greater expansion than does quartz. Likewise the expansion occurs more rapidly and at a lower temperature in the cristobalite-type investment.

Fine particle size of the investment, as with setting expansion, also increases the thermal expansion. The finer particles also produce smooth cast surfaces and help allow for porosity in the set investment so that the mold air will escape in advance of the molten metal and thereby allow the mold to fill completely.

STORAGE AND SELECTION. The investment should be stored in airtight and moisture-proof containers, and during use the containers should be opened for as short a period of time as possible. This helps to prevent any alteration in the setting time and in the expansion of the investment.

As noted, all investments are composed of a number of ingredients, with each possessing a different specific gravity. Under normal storage conditions they tend to separate and this leads to inconsistency in the properties of the material. For these reasons it is advisable to purchase the investment in quantities sufficient for only 6 months.

The selection of an investment by the dentist or technician is largely a matter of personal preference. It will depend upon the choice of technique to be used for shrinkage compensation and for the particular restoration.

The powder should be weighed accurately and the water should be measured with a graduated cylinder. Only in this manner can one control the setting or thermal expansion in relation to the compensation needed for the casting shrinkage. The investment is routinely supplied in pre-weighed packages so that the dentist need only measure the gauging water.

Technique of Spruing

After the wax pattern is completed a sprue pin (sprue former) is attached to the pattern and then is surrounded by the investment. After the investment hardens, the pin is removed, following which the wax is burned out and the molten metal is forced through the sprue or ingate formed by the sprue former into the mold left by the wax.

Spruing may contribute to casting imperfection in the following ways:

1. There may be voids indicating that the mold did not fill completely.

2. There may be voids that are related to the pattern of solidification at the junction of the sprue to the pattern.

3. Debris may enter through the sprue and become lodged in the casting.

4. The sprue may, in part, cause distortion of the wax pattern as it is removed from the die.

The sprue is usually a hollow metal tube, although it may be supplied as circular rods of resin or wax; a choice is made based on personal preference. There may be a temptation to use a carbon steel or iron sprue pin of a proper size and design, but it is likely to rust when in contact with the wet investment. This rust may find its way into the mold during entry of the metal and contaminate the alloy.

The diameter of sprue pins varies in relation to the size of the pattern. Pins are supplied commercially in gauges from No. 10 (2.5 mm) to No. 16 (1.3 mm). The sizes most frequently used are gauges Nos. 12 and 14, which are 2.1 and 1.7 mm in diameter respectively.

If the gold is to be melted directly above the sprue opening, as with an air pressure casting machine, the use of large sprues has to be avoided in order to prevent the molten gold from falling into the ingate under its own weight before the pressure is applied. If the gold is to be melted in a separate crucible, as in a centrifugal casting machine, the diameter of the sprue is not critical except for consistency with the pattern size. When the diameter becomes less than 15 gauge there is a risk that the gold will freeze in the sprue area before the mold is filled. This leads to "shrinkage porosity" in the casting at a point adjacent to the sprue.

The diameter of sprue selected is guided by the greatest cross-section of wax in the pattern, and it is best if the sprue diameter is slightly in excess of this diameter. At this time the wax pattern should be freely removable from the die and the sprue attached to the pattern while it is still on the die.

The sprue pin is selected and if it is a hollow metal sprue, it is filled with red utility wax, which melts at a temperature lower than that of the wax pattern. This provides additional time for attaching the sprue at the proper angle. The hollow sprue tube can be heated adequately while held by the fingers whereas this is more difficult with solid metal sprues. Thus the hollow metal sprues can be located easily, at the proper location, and provide good attachment to the pattern.

The bulkiest part of the pattern is the best location for attaching the sprue. This will usually be on the mesial or distal part of the pattern. The sprue tube is heated to liquefy the wax in the tube and also to allow slight penetration of the metal sprue into the surface of the wax pattern. The direction of the sprue is angled to allow easy flow of molten metal to all parts of the mold.

When the pattern has more than one surface the sprue will be angled at near 45° to a horizontal plane to facilitate metal flow. The wax is allowed to cool, freezing the sprue pin into position. Then additional wax is added at the junction of the sprue to the wax pattern, allowing a flaring of the opening to the mold. To allow easy removal of the pin a thin film of wax should be placed over the pin as this will minimize fracture of investment during its removal. This also increases slightly the diameter of the sprue.

If wax or resin sprues are used, they are waxed into position with the same concern for angulation and flare at the site of attachment.

The sprued wax pattern is carefully removed with every precaution to avoid distortion or physical damage to the pattern. If a metal or resin sprue is

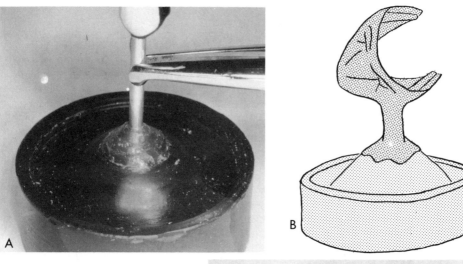

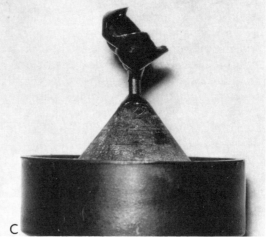

Figure 17–26. *A,* A pair of pliers is used to position a sprued pattern. *B,* Note the angle of the pattern to the sprue. *C,* The pattern is usually sprued into its greatest mass.

used, it is grasped firmly by a pair of pliers and placed into a crucible former (Fig. 17–26). The crucible former is of rubber or metal with a hollow central cone that is filled with utility wax, which permits the pin to be attached by penetration into the wax. This wax addition is domed to help direct the gold flow. The wax pattern is positioned at a distance of 6 to 9 mm from the top of the crucible former. With this short distance a reservoir is not required between the pattern and the former.

Investing

RING AND LINER

For a single-unit wax pattern a metal casting ring 35 mm (1⅜ inch) long, with an outside diameter of 31 mm (1¼ inch), is very convenient. The crucible former must match the dimension of the ring. Rings of varying lengths and dimensions are available for larger and complex types of casting.

The ring is lined with a single layer of asbestos or a substitute (Fig. 17–27). This liner is required for most investing techniques to allow the

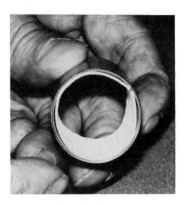

Figure 17–27. A full length of liner is placed inside the ring.

required expansion to take place. Otherwise the metal will restrict and distort the investment expansion. With asbestos it is recommended that the liner extend the full length of the ring. If the investment comes in contact with the metal ring, then the expansion is restricted. It would be ideal if the liner met accurately end to end within the ring. However, this is difficult to obtain so the liner may overlap slightly. To position the liner closely to the metal it is best to dampen the material slightly as it is being adapted. However, it is expected that a uniform thickness will prevail throughout the liner.

In recent years there has been concern that asbestos might be a health hazard, in light of its carcinogenic potential if inhaled in the form of micrometer size particles. However, the type used for lining rings, as described, has a good binder. There is no evidence that it poses any danger with careful use.

Nonetheless, it is possible that asbestos could become unavailable in the foreseeable future. Therefore, manufacturers have been providing substitutes. These are of two general types. One consists of an organic cellulose material that has the same water sorption as asbestos and provides a comparable setting expansion of the investment. However, it does burn away during burnout. This could permit the investment mold to slide out of the ring when lifted out of the furnace. Thus it is essential that such liners be approximately 3 mm (1/8 inch) short of both ends of the ring.

The other substitute consists of a silica–alumina fiber paper. The water sorption of this type of liner is very low but it does have a marked "cushioning" effect and permits some setting expansion and complete thermal expansion of the investment. It also must be kept short of the ends of the ring.

Investing Procedure

The wax pattern should be cleansed of any surface dirt and residue from the die lubricants. A number of commercial products are available for this purpose, or a mild solution of green soap may be used. The pattern is rinsed with room temperature water and then gently air-dried.

For most consistent results in mixing and investing it is best to use a mechanical mixer with a self-contained vacuum system.* This tends to minimize the operator variables and will reduce or eliminate the presence of surface nodules (Fig. 17–28).

---

*Whip-Mix Corp., 381 Farmington Ave., Louisville, Kentucky 40217.

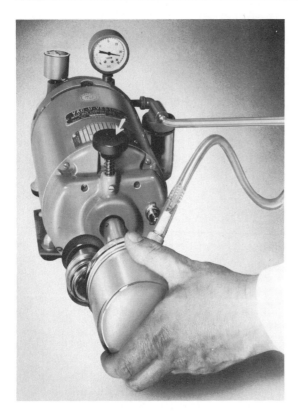

Figure 17–28. A vacuum investing unit. After vacuum mixing, as shown, the mix is held on the vibrator (see white arrow). (Courtesy of R. Neiman)

The investment is selected and the instructions for its use are carefully followed (Fig. 17–29). The crucible and ring assembly are eased into the well in the bowl cover. The rubber "O" ring should be lubricated with the lubricant provided; otherwise the wax pattern may be accidentally jarred loose from the sprue (Fig. 17–30).

For reasons previously mentioned the water and powder, if not preweighed, must be accurately measured. The water is placed into the dry bowl, the powder is added, and with a hand spatula the powder is mixed into the

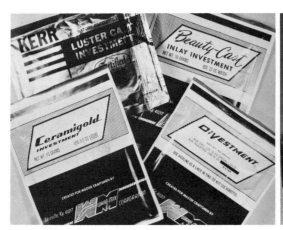
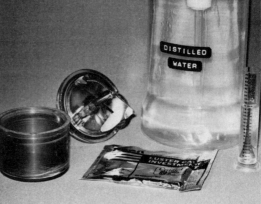

Figure 17–29. Materials used for investing wax patterns.

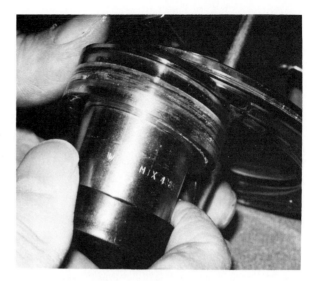

Figure 17–30. The pattern and ring are carefully inserted into position.

water. For consistent results it is recommended that distilled water be used. The cover is placed on the bowl and the vacuum is allowed to become fully effective, following which it is mechanically spatulated for the specific number of seconds required. While the spatulation takes place the vacuum tube is oriented to an up position to minimize the chance for investment to enter the tube. The bowl is placed upright on the vibrator to concentrate the mixture at the bottom of the bowl. The bowl is then tipped on its side with the ring in a down position to vibrate the mixture into the casting ring. The device is designed so that one can see the investment mix gradually fill the ring. It may be necessary to shift the blades to allow the investment to enter the ring unimpeded (Fig. 17–31). The vibrating should be done on the bowl to aid in flowing the mix into the ring. Should the vibration be done on the crucible former it may dislodge the pattern.

The bowl is held in an inverted position and the ring is gently rotated out of the well. If needed, some investment is added to fill the ring flush with the top. It should then set for approximately 1 hour before being placed in a burn-out oven. If the investing unit is near a sink, care should be exercised to prevent the vacuum tube from falling into water, as it would seriously damage the vacuum system. The bowl and paddles must be cleaned meticulously and if to be reused soon, fully dried, for the additional moisture in the bowl would alter the fixed water-powder ratio.

If a vacuum investing unit is not available the investing is done by hand. The water and powder are combined in a small mechanical hand mixer. The mixing should occur on a vibrator, as this will help decrease entrapment of air. The pattern is carefully painted with the investment by using a small soft brush, after which the ring is placed in position and the investment is slowly allowed to flow down one side of the ring until it is filled. The wax surface tends to resist wetting of the investment and care must therefore be exercised during the painting of the pattern.

If the hygroscopic technique is used the freshly filled casting ring is immediately immersed in a water bath at a temperature of 37 to 38°C (98.6 to 100°F). For other techniques the investment is allowed to harden as it sets on the bench.

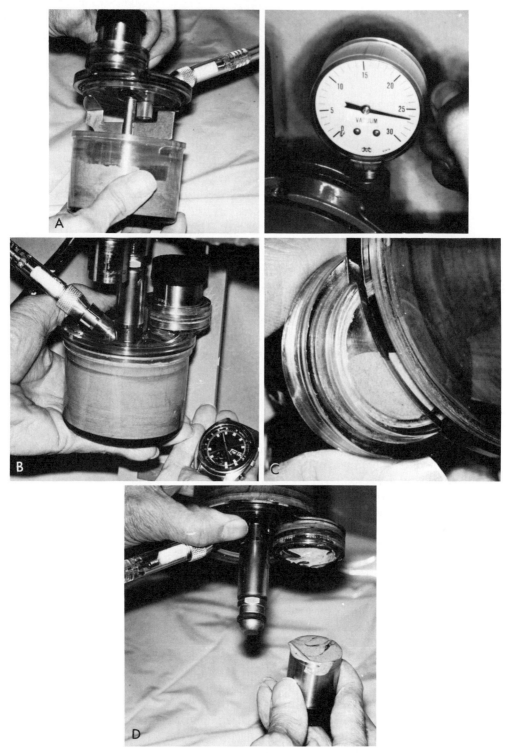

Figure 17–31. *A,* The powder and liquid are fully combined before adding the spatulator and it is determined that an adequate vacuum is available. *B,* Spatulation time is carefully monitored and varies with products used. *C,* The ring is allowed to fill from the lower edge to the top. *D,* Very carefully the ring is rotated out of its compartment.

Wax Elimination and Heating

Armamentarium
1. Burn-out oven
2. Casting machine
3. Gas and air torch or electric crucible
4. Pickling solution with container

After the investment has hardened for 1 hour, one may begin the wax elimination and heating of the investment to the temperature required for casting. The crucible former is carefully removed, but the sprue former or pin remains in the investment. If the sprue is metal, the exposed end is heated over a flame to soften or melt the wax attachment. Then, holding the investment ring so that the sprue pin is facing down, the pin is grasped with a pair of pliers and carefully rotated out (Fig. 17–32). The ring is held in this position to prevent any loose investment particles from falling into the ingate. Any loose particles in the crucible area should be carefully removed.

For most techniques a burn-out oven is used to eliminate the wax and to establish the proper temperature of the investment, and it should have an accurate pyrometer. There are pellets supplied by dental manufacturers that melt at a specific temperature and may be used to check the accuracy of the pyrometer.

The burn-out should be started when the mold is still moist. The water in the pores of the investment reduces the absorption of the wax into the investment, for as the water boils it will tend to flush out the wax, leaving a clean mold. When the mold must be stored for several hours, such as overnight or longer, it should be kept in a humidor. If it has become totally dry, it is recommended that the investment be placed in water for a short time before being placed in the burn-out oven.

The investment ring should be placed in the burn-out oven with the sprue hole down to allow gravity flow of the melting wax (Fig. 17–33). Some furnace muffles may be so airtight that burn-out takes place in a reducing rather than oxidizing atmosphere. If the wax pattern is bulky or if several rings are being burned out, it is advisable to prop open the door of the furnace slightly with some asbestos to provide additional oxygen supply for maximum burn-out efficiency.

When the thermal expansion technique is used, ideally the ring should be placed in a furnace at room temperature and the temperature advanced to 650°C (1200°F) over a 30 to 40 minute period and then held at that temperature

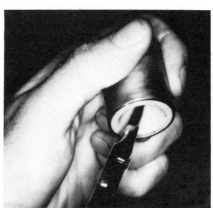

Figure 17–32. The sprue pin is heated and removed by pliers with the orifice in a down position.

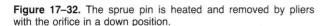

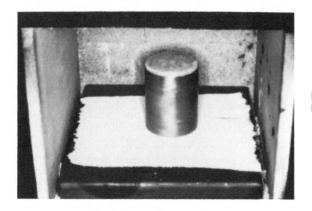

Figure 17–33. Burn-out is begun with the sprue hole in a down position.

for 20 to 30 minutes. Thus the total burn-out and heating time should be a one (1) hour minimum for the average size wax pattern. It will not always be possible to do this in an ideal fashion. A compromise may be required, as at times it will be impractical to wait for the oven to return to room temperature. As an alternate method the ring is placed in the oven at approximately 325°C (600°F). Again it is advanced to final temperature and the total burn-out and heating time should balance out at one (1) hour.

With a hygroscopic or "low heat" technique the ring can be placed in an oven preheated to 482°C (900°F) without fear of the investment cracking during wax elimination. Again one (1) hour is the recommended time for most patterns.

Toward the end of the one (1) hour period, the ring should be inverted in order to have the sprue hole up. This allows oxygen to enter the mold, which helps to provide total elimination of the wax.

If the investment has not been allowed adequate time to harden or if with some investments the heating is too rapid at the start, the generated steam may damage the walls of the mold. In extreme cases the steam pressure will build up to the extent that it will cause an explosion and fracture of the mold. A less dramatic effect from the same cause is the development of a crack in the investment as the outer layers of investment expand more rapidly than the center portions of the investment. This could result in fins or spines in the casting.

Casting

Equipment

The burn-out oven and the casting machine must be convenient to each other to avoid any time loss during the actual casting process. To prevent any noticeable contraction in the investment as the temperature drops, the casting should be made within one (1) minute upon removal from the furnace. This should not pose an unusual difficulty. A cool or cold mold is not indicated for any casting technique. Although the mold temperature in the low-heat casting technique is comparatively low, an accurate casting will result when the mold temperature is maintained, and metal solidification will not be premature.

It can happen that burn-out is completed and for some reason the casting is not made and the mold returns to room temperature. Reheating will result in a reduction of the total expansion and strength of the investment.

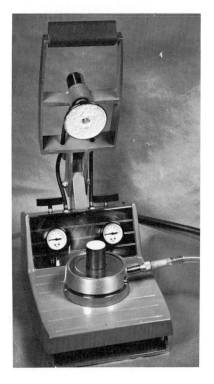

Figure 17–34. An air pressure casting machine with the ring in position. The gold alloy is melted directly in the crucible formed in the investment. Above the ring can be seen the piston through which the air pressure is applied, forcing the molten alloy into the mold.

Currently there are primarily two types of casting machines used. One makes use of air pressure, while the other is a centrifugal casting machine (Fig. 17–34). With an air pressure machine the gold is melted in the investment crucible, and the molten gold is forced into the mold under air pressure. In the more popular broken-arm centrifugal machine, the gold is fused in a crucible separate from the ring (Fig. 17–35). The arm of this machine is spring

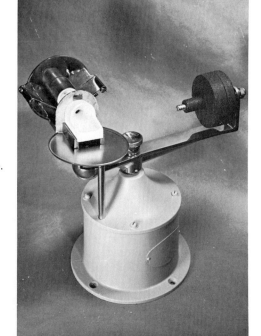

Figure 17–35. A centrifugal casting machine.

loaded and after the metal is fused the spring is released. The initial action is for the broken arm to whip into line, throwing the gold into the mold with centrifugal force. This also permits continuous force on the metal until it has been solidified. To provide adequate force three or four counterturns to lead the spring are sufficient for dental castings. As a precaution it is advised to check the casting ring in the casting cradle to be sure the crucible platform fully secures the ring against the headplate of the casting machine. If it is not secure, the ring will roll out of position upon release of the arm and the gold will not hit the sprue opening. This can be prevented by placing a layer or two of asbestos between the ring and the headplate.

If the gold alloy is to be melted in the crucible formed by the investment, the alloy is premelted on a charcoal block before the ring is removed from the furnace. While the ring is placed into position, the melted gold will have solidified to allow transfer to the crucible where it can be quickly remelted and the casting completed.

There is no practical difference in the physical properties or in the accuracy of the results obtained with either type of machine.

Selection of the Alloy

For the most reliable results the dentist should select only those casting gold alloys that are certified to meet the American Dental Association Specification No. 5. The alloys available are grouped into Types I to IV, with Type IV the hardest.

Type I alloys have Vickers hardness values between 50 and 90 (BHN 40 to 75). They are ductile, have a low proportional limit, and are easily burnished. They are not capable of being hardened by heat treatment. The gold content is high (80 to 96 per cent), and as a result the fusion range is high (950° to 1050°C—1740 to 1920°F). This alloy may be used for restorations where stress is minimal, such as in gingival cavities and small interproximal premolar restorations.

Type II alloys have Vickers values ranging from 90 to 120 (BHN 70 to 100). The copper content is higher as compared with Type I and the fusion temperature is decreased, with a range of 927 to 971°C (1700 to 1780°F). Restorations are of greater durability than with Type I alloys, but the contrast is not readily observed. Thus the indications for its use are somewhat greater in latitude but similar to those of Type I alloys. Both of these groups are readily burnishable because of their high durability.

Type III alloys have Vickers numbers of 120 to 150 (BHN 90 to 140) in a softened condition. A real contrast begins with this group, as they contain some palladium and platinum, which imparts higher strength. These alloys are responsive to age-hardening treatments. Their ductility and elongation decrease. Because of wear resistance and stability most cast dental restorations are made from this type of alloy.

During recent times we have been dramatically reminded that our ability to provide some of our preferred treatment options is influenced by the gyrations in the market place of the metals commodities. The escalation of the gold market has caused restorative dentists to ask about or to use less expensive alloys. Most of the alloy manufacturers have provided alloys that contain less gold than the traditional alloys. These alloys have similar properties and handling characteristics as compared with other alloys in the same classification, and this is most apparent with the type 3 and 4 alloys.

These alloys require nearly 46 per cent gold to maintain the gold color. Tarnish resistance becomes a problem when the noble metal content of the alloy goes below 46 per cent. With careful selection, there are gold alloys that will perform well and offer a financial saving over the long-standing high quality alloys.

Dental manufacturers usually supply a number of alloys within each classification. They differ modestly in matters such as properties, color, and handling characteristics.

Melting the Alloy and Making the Casting

Up to this point in the description of the technique for fabricating cast restorations, a reasonable degree of success may be predicted because definite and fundamental rules are being observed. The actual process of melting the alloy and making the casting is more difficult to control in a precise manner and more difficult to describe by specific instructions. A certain amount of personal judgment now enters the picture. Certain rules will be cited and it is hoped that these plus judgment and discriminating powers of observation will assure the making of a successful casting.

In addition to the burn-out furnace and a casting machine, a gas-air blowpipe, a charcoal block, flux, and alloy are needed.

The major objective in the melting procedure is to develop the most efficient gas-air flame that will quickly yet cleanly melt the metal. The temperature of the flame is easily influenced by the relative proportions of the gas and air. The gas is turned on and ignited and roughly adjusted to develop the size flame that will work the best. Then the air is turned on to again roughly establish the melting flame. The final adjustments are usually made with the air control on the torch.

The parts of the flame can be identified by the conical areas. The first long, blank-appearing cone directly emanating from the nozzle is the zone where the air and gas combine prior to combustion. The next cone is slightly greenish and immediately surrounds the first or inner cone. This is the combustion zone where the gas and air are in partial combustion. This zone is an oxidizing area and it should be kept away from the metal during fusion. The next zone has a bluish cast and is the reducing zone, and this is the hottest part of the flame. The area near the tip of this cone is the part of the flame that must stay on the metal during fusion (Fig. 17–36). Beyond this is the outer or oxidizing zone where conbustion occurs with the oxygen of the air. This part of the flame should never be used to melt the alloy, as its temperature is too low and it will cause oxidation of the metal.

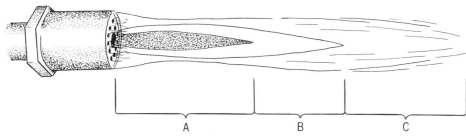

Figure 17–36. *A,* Air and gas combine in this zone. The junction of A and B is the combustion zone. *B,* This area represents the reducing zone and is most effective as it moves toward junction with *C. C,*Oxidizing zone.

Beginners tend to allow an excessive air supply into the flame adjustment, producing a roaring sound that tends to make it "sound hot" when in fact it is a cool flame. It will take some practice to keep the hottest part of the flame in the right place.

When new metal is being used lay it on the side of the crucible, for in this position the operator is able to observe the progress of the melting. An ample amount of metal must be supplied and as a general rule there should be as much metal in the sprue and button as is contained in the casting; frequently this amounts to 2 pennyweight (3 grams) or more of metal. The alloy first appears spongy and then small globules of fused metal appear, following which the bulk of the alloy assumes a spheroidal shape and begins to slide down to the bottom of the crucible. If this is to be a cast by a centrifugal machine, bring the casting ring out of the burn-out oven and place it securely in the casting cradle as the metal begins to liquefy.

As the metal becomes fluid it is always desirable to sprinkle a small amount of borax flux onto the metal. This helps to minimize porosity and to increase the fluidity of the metal, and the film of flux formed on the metal surface helps to prevent oxidation. Reducing fluxes that contain some powdered charcoal are also used for this purpose.

The metal now becomes very fluid and light orange in color and tends to spin as it responds to slight movement of the flame. Ideally at this point the metal should be about 38° to 66°C (100 to 150°F) above its liquidus temperature. When this occurs the casting is made immediately. The flame is kept in constant contact until the casting begins. If air pressure casting is used, the flame stays on the metal in the crucible until the piston closes on the ring. If a centrifugal casting machine is used, the flame does not move until the spring is released and the arm is in motion. It is possible to overheat the alloy, which must be avoided, but this is not likely to occur with a conventional gas and air torch. The duration of time from the point at which the ring is in position in the casting machine until the casting is made should be on the order of 15 to 20 seconds. With experience, the proper zone in contact with the metal can be readily detected by observing the metal surface. When the reducing zone is in contact, the surface of the alloy is bright and mirror-like (Fig. 17–37). Furthermore, the surrounding environment radiates the maximal intensity of color possible. This is quite in contrast to the duller halo with the cloudy, non-reflecting surface in the molten metal when the flame is applied improperly.

When the centrifugal machine is used, the crucible should be lined with a layer of asbestos; otherwise the melt may be contaminated with oxides and fluxes that may be present in the crucible or the natural roughness of the crucible may retain portions of the molten metal as it is being cast (Fig. 17–38).

If asbestos is not available to line the crucible an alternate consideration is to fuse borax flux to all pertinent aspects of the crucible, which provides a smooth and durable surface. It is also advised that if differing alloy systems are being cast, crucibles should be available that are compatible with the various alloys. This prevents contamination of the castings.

It is proper to combine buttons with new gold as long as the alloys are identical and from the same manufacturers. If the buttons are clean, the alloy may be handled as previously described. It is desirable to add some new gold to the used gold in order to maintain a balanced composition. When there is a question about the condition of the old gold, place it on a charcoal block, which is embedded in gypsum so as to last longer. Then the gold is melted as

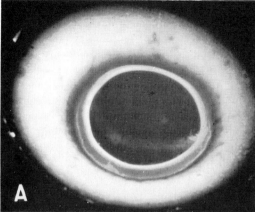

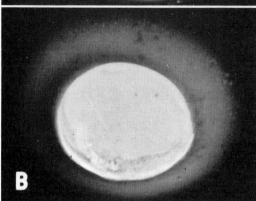

Figure 17–37. *A,* Mirror-like surface of the metal indicates proper fusion. *B,* Cloudy surface indicates surface oxidation by blowpipe flame.

has been described and fluxed with a charcoal-containing flux. After it has been melted, the air is turned off from the torch but the continuing flame kept on the metal as it solidifies. This prevents oxidation of the metal as it cools. Now it may be used in the same manner as described for new metal (Fig. 17–39).

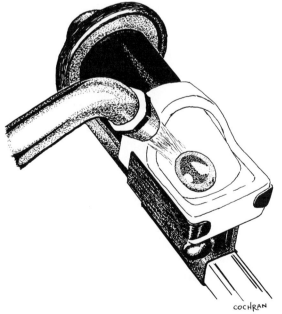

Figure 17–38. The torch is properly positioned to melt the alloy easily.

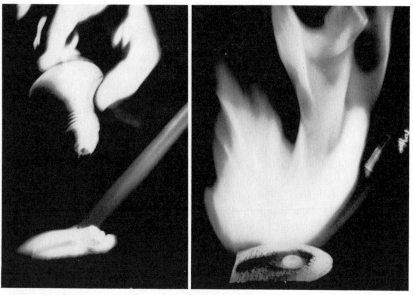

Figure 17–39. *A,* Melting "scrap gold" on a charcoal block. An adequate amount of reducing flux is used. *B,* After the "scrap gold" has been fused, it should be cooled in a luminous gas flame to prevent oxidation and gas occlusion.

There are several devices available for melting the alloy electrically. When the metal reaches a predetermined temperature, it is cast by centrifugal force. The merit of such an induction melting device is that it eliminates certain of the human variables involved in the melting of the alloy. Also the carbon will assume a reducing atmosphere.

When molten alloy is cast using a centrifugal machine there naturally occurs a leading and trailing edge of metal. Because of the direction and forces of acceleration and centrifugal force the alloy is first delivered to the trailing and outermost portion of the mold irrespective of the location of the sprue opening. It appears more effective if the sprue opens from the leading edge.

For most centrifuged castings the position of the ring in the casting cradle is of no concern. For patterns that are complex or that have intricate detail it is an advantage to score the casting ring and relate the pattern to the mark so as to allow the least restriction for the flow of metal.

For most operative castings the use of a mold gas vent is of no value, as adequate venting will occur into the porosities of the investment. When a pattern is bulky, as may occasionally happen with a full crown, a small rod of wax may be attached to the pattern to help relieve mold gas as the casting is made. This vent should be placed near the sprue opening, as this is the last portion of the mold to fill; if attached away from the sprue opening it will fill prematurely with metal and not be able to function as a vent.

As stated, most patterns do not require a special consideration, but again a pattern may have distinct variations as related to its thickness or design, and it is best to influence the pattern of metal solidification to have a solid casting. The metal should begin solidification first in the region where the metal is initially delivered. Small wax projections may be added to this part of the pattern and this will help initiate solidification, as these additions will be the first to cool and will help set an orderly pattern of solidification for the total casting. These function as chill sets and are usually located near the trailing portion of the mold (Fig. 17–40).

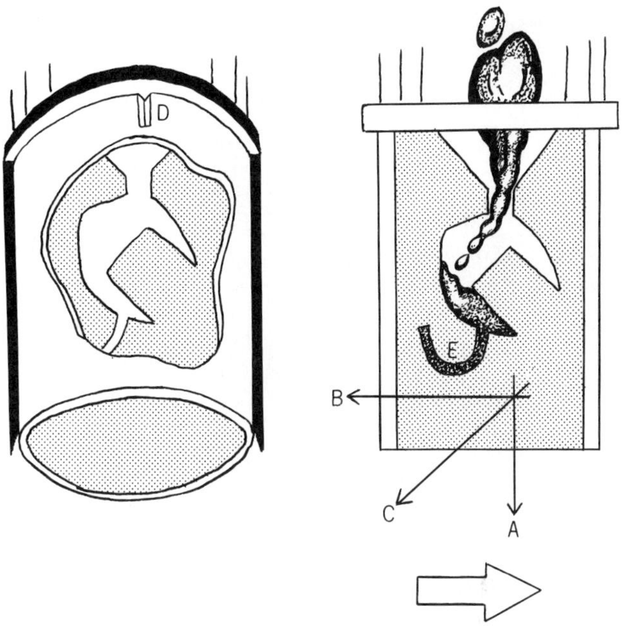

Figure 17–40. The sprue and pattern should be oriented so as to deliver the gold from the leading edge. *A,* Direction of centrifugal force. *B,* Direction of rotational force. *C,* Resultant force. *D,* Ring is marked so as to orient pattern for gold flow. *E,* When needed a projection is added to function as a chill set.

Cleansing the Casting

When the casting has been completed, allow complete solidification of metal to occur before trying to recover the ring from the machine. If it is a centrifugal casting, allow the machine to coast to a stop on its own without applying a braking force to bring it to a quick halt. If it is an air pressure machine, let the ring stand for 2 to 3 minutes.

At this time the button should essentially have lost its reddish color, and it is quenched in water. When the water contacts the hot investment, a violent reaction occurs. Most investments become soft and granular, which simplifies recovery of the casting. It will at least weaken all investments, which is a help in freeing the casting.

If the alloy is a Type III alloy and it is allowed to cool to approximately 260°C (500°F) and then quenched, it will retain its inherent hardness. If quenched while still red hot, it will be in a softened condition and thus will not possess the desired properties to resist dysfunction or attrition. If this age-hardening process is of concern, it should be done under very controlled conditions.

After the casting has been quenched the remaining investment may be brushed free with a small brush under running water. It may be necessary to use a metallic instrument for the removal of some investment. Be sure that the sink drain is stopped to prevent the loss of time, expense, and temper when recovering castings from somewhere within the plumbing system.

Frequently the surface of the casting is dark because of an oxide or tarnish coating. Such a surface film is removed by a process known as "pickling," which consists of careful heating of the casting in an acid. The most effective pickling solution is a 50 per cent hydrochloric acid solution, but its fumes are very corrosive and will damage many metal objects in the office area. Because of this problem it is advised that commercial pickling agents, which are solutions of acid salts, be used. They will act more slowly than hydrochloric acid but will produce acceptable results.

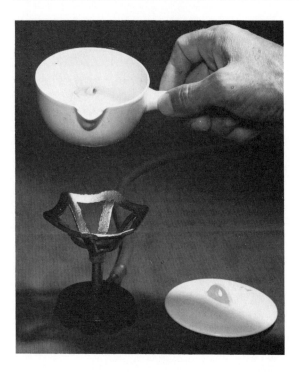

Figure 17–41. The pickling solution placed in a ceramic dish and gently warmed to remove oxides. (From Hollenback, G. M.: Science and Technic of the Cast Restoration. C. V. Mosby, 1964)

It is convenient to store the pickling solution in a covered ceramic pickling dish and place the casting in the solution and then gently heat the solution, which accelerates its action, producing the clean gold-colored casting (Fig. 17–41). It will be necessary to make additional fresh solution or to change it depending on frequency of use. Otherwise it will lose its reactivity.

Steel tongs should not be used when removing the casting from the solution, as the alloy may be partially contaminated by the deposit of copper on the casting. This leads to discoloration and corrosion. There are plastic-tipped tongs available that are effective for this purpose.

An alternate common practice is to heat the casting until it barely emits a perceptible dull glow and then drop it in the pickling solution. This is an effective technique, but there is a risk of distorting delicate margins unless it is done carefully.

After pickling, the casting should be scrubbed under running water. As an added precaution it may be immersed in a solution of sodium bicarbonate,

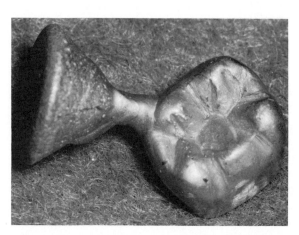

Figure 17–42. Example of a casting ready for finishing.

which will insure that the acid is removed or neutralized before being seated in the mouth (Fig. 17–42).

Resumé of Investing and Casting Procedures

1. Select the investment to be used, which is largely determined by whether a thermal or hygroscopic technique will be used.
2. Select and attach the sprue to the bulkiest part of the pattern.
   a. Flare the junction of the sprue to the pattern with wax.
3. Remove the pattern, without distortion from the die, and attach it to the crucible former.
   a. Cleanse pattern of oil residue and debris.
   b. A distance of 6 to 9 mm should be acceptable between crucible former and pattern.
   c. Line the casting ring with one layer of full-length asbestos or substitute liner material.
4. Place the ring into crucible former.
   a. If a centrifugal casting machine is used, orient the pattern so that the gold will be delivered from the leading into the trailing part of the mold.
5. Accurately measure powder and liquid into mixing bowl.
   a. Mechanical mixing with a vacuum is preferred.
6. Spatulate the investment and fill the casting ring.
   a. Allow the investment to harden for 1 hour.
7. Select burn-out temperature and allow a 1-hour minimum for wax elimination and heating of the mold.
8. Place alloy in casting crucible.
9. If using a gas-air torch, produce the reducing flame, which is the hottest portion of the flame.
10. Apply a borax flux as melting of the alloy begins.
11. When metal is fluid, shiny, and spinning, the casting is made.
12. Cool until color is mostly lost from button and quench in water.
13. Clean the casting.
14. Pickle the casting in a commercial pickling solution, following which remove the acid from the casting with water and/or a sodium bicarbonate solution.

Divestment Technique

An optional modality to casting fabrication is the Divestment* technique (Fig. 17–43). Many practitioners and teachers prefer this to the "pulled pattern" technique previously described. In many respects this is a simplified process; in other respects it is more cumbersome. Briefly it involves investing of the die and pattern together. The die therefore becomes an actual part of the mold cavity. The basic nature of Divestment material is not unlike that of conventional silica and gypsum products, except in the liquid, which is a colloidal silica. It also differs from conventional investments in setting and thermal expansion; Divestment has a large setting expansion with a small thermal expansion.

Briefly the technique is as follows.

---

*Divestment, Whip-Mix Corp., 381 Farmington Ave., Louisville, Kentucky 40217.

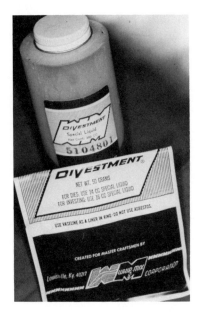

Figure 17–43. Divestment powder and liquid is a gypsum-bound investment.

Pouring the Die

1. Liquid:powder ratios may vary between 13 and 16 ml per 50 gm of powder.

2. The mixed material is somewhat "syrupy" and tends to "run" or "creep" while setting.

3. The material is not as strong as stone die materials, and thin fragile dies may break when removing the model from the impression.

4. Divestment has an affinity for polysulfide rubbers, tending to adhere to the impression after the model has dried (die and model should be separated within 3 hours; setting time is comparable to dental stone). The impression may be sprayed with an aerosol of silicone to offset this difficulty. Silicone rubber does not present this problem.

5. Freshly mixed Divestment will adhere to hardened Divestment, making it possible to block out undercuts on the die.

Wax Pattern

1. As a die relief agent, 1 to 3 coats of aluminum lacquer (Separator No. 2) are painted on the die. It adheres to the die and dries rapidly so the wax can be added. During burn out and casting this coating remains attached to the die. As well as serving as a "relief" it also aids in removal of the die from inside the casting.

2. The margins of the wax pattern terminate exactly at the finish line. If an error occurs in waxing, the edge of the wax should terminate *inside* rather than beyond the finish line. This is an important factor and is opposite to that required of a pulled pattern technique.

Investing and Casting

1. An asbestos liner is replaced by a coat of vaseline inside the casting ring.

2. Investing material is 9 ml H_2O, 9 ml liquid, and 50 gm powder.

3. Burn-out time is 1 hour at 600° to 675°C (1100° to 1250°F).

4. The ring is bench-cooled rather than quenched in water.

5. After cooling, the cylinder of Divestment is pushed out of the ring and the Divestment broken away. After being heated Divestment does not lose its integrity and does not disintegrate as the conventional investments do.

6. After deflasking, the die remains intact within the casting.

7. The casting is contoured and polished before the die material is removed from the inside of the casting.

8. Margins are inspected and relieved of "flash" (minute fin-like projections of gold that may extend beyond the margins). Marginal areas are polished with garnet and cuttle disks.

9. The internal surface of the casting is inspected for minute gold nodules, which are subsequently removed.

Gold that is cast directly against the die inside the mold cavity reproduces an internal surface with extremely fine, detailed reproductions of the impression. This roughened and highly irregular surface, which is not picked up in the pulled pattern, impedes fitting of the casting on the tooth. Relief of these irregularities is necessary if the casting is to seat to place.

Castings made by the Divestment technique are not fitted on a stone die for finishing. As a marked departure from the pulled pattern, the margins of the finished casting are finished in the hand and fitted directly to the tooth.

Because of a tendency for the outer investment to expand away from the die and create a tiny thin peripheral crevice for gold to flow into, the operator must know exactly where the margins end and disk away this flash, if and when it occurs. The use of vaseline instead of an asbestos liner for the ring prevents the investment from expanding away from the die and creating this crevice. If on occasion a flash does develop, it must be removed completely before fitting the casting to the tooth.

As might be expected, when made properly, Divestment castings produce exceptionally accurate and reliable fits. This is to be expected because of the elimination of error that attends removal and investment of the pattern. Until the operator develops some experience with its use, however, it is suggested that he restrict this technique to the fabrication of full crown castings.

For making full crowns and other gold castings, the following method is recommended:

1. Tooth preparation and impression techniques follow the traditional procedure described in previous chapters.

2. Divestment powder and liquid are mixed, the tooth section of the impression is poured, and a dowel pin is inserted (Fig. 17–44).

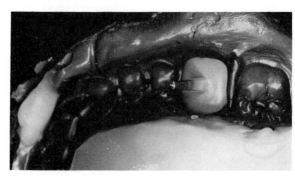

Figure 17–44. Divestment die with dowel pin.

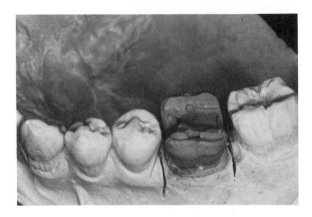

Figure 17–45. Model poured in yellow stone.

3. The dowel pin and Divestment are lubricated lightly with vaseline and the model poured in conventional stone (Fig. 17–45).

4. After separation from the impression the die is freed from the model, the margins carefully identified, and a groove placed below the finish line. (When the finish line is obvious and definite it is not necessary to place a groove.) As with stone dies, margins and sharp edges should be protected against abrasion from the fingers and unnecessary washing with water.

5. Separating medium No. 2 is applied to the die. Axial surfaces are given two or more coats, especially for long parallel surfaces. It is not critical to keep the separator off the margins. Because the separator dries rapidly it should be allowed to flow freely over the surface to give a smooth, even coat and to prevent clumping of the material on the surface (Fig. 17–46).

6. An inlay wax of choice is added to form the contours and occlusion. Care should be taken that the wax extend only to the finish lines. Wax can be added beyond a margin and carved back to terminate exactly at the edge; however, the wax film residue can encourage subsequent gold flash formation during the casting process.

7. The wax is polished in a traditional manner and the sprue attached (Fig. 17–47). It will be noted that the additional bulk to be included in the ring may require the use of a longer casting ring.*

---

*Whip-Mix casting ring, 1¼″ diameter × 1⅞″ long.

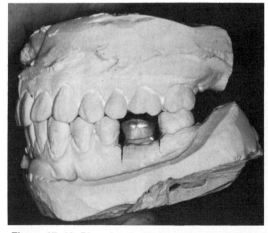

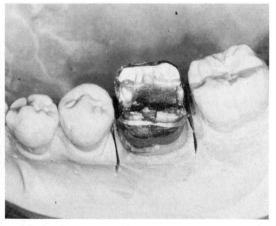

Figure 17–46. Die painted with Separator No. 2. Paint is so thin that it may extend beyond the margin.

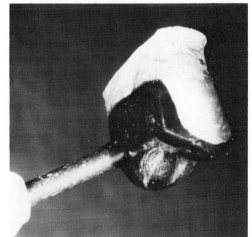

Figure 17–47. Die and pattern ready for investing using a hollow meal sprue. Excess Divestment has been removed.

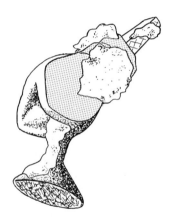

Figure 17–48. Casting removed from ring with an intact die and dowel pin.

Figure 17–49. Sprue has been removed from casting and external surface sandblasted. After dowel pin has been cleansed, it is seated in the model and checked for proximal contact and occlusion.

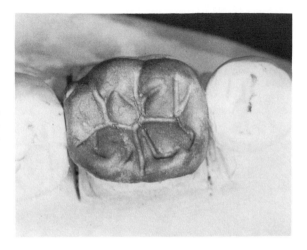

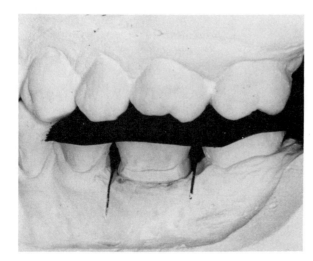

Figure 17–50. Occlusion being checked with carbon paper.

Figure 17–51. Final polish with a rag wheel. Die and dowel pin serve as a handle.

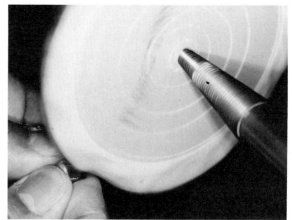

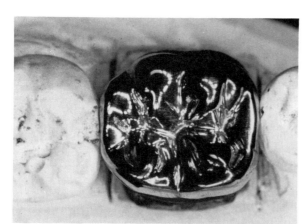

Figure 17–52. Casting with outer surface polished.

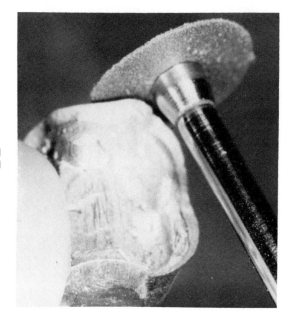

Figure 17–53. The die has been removed, the internal surface sandblasted as necessary, and the marginal area is being polished with a ⅜″ disk (see Fig. 14–47).

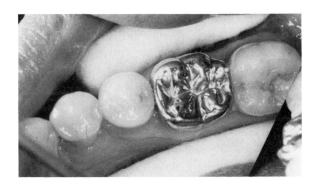

Figure 17–54. Finished casting in the mouth.

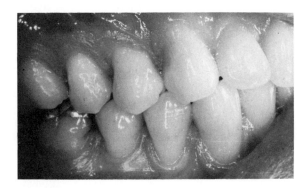

Figure 17–55. Buccal aspect showing the occlusion.

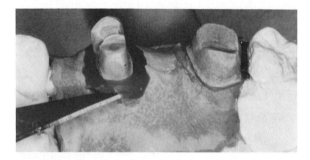

Figure 17–56. Same basic technique for casting a bridge in one piece against Divestment. Note the wax used to help define the die margins.

8. Utility wax is applied to the undersurface of the Divestment die and over the pin. This provides a baffle space so that the dowel pin, the unbroken die, and casting can be recovered in one piece from the ring.

9. The casting ring, having been fitted over the sprue former, is lubricated with vaseline. Divestment is mixed under vacuum for investing (50 gm powder to 9 ml liquid and 9 ml H_2O). Spatulation of as long as 45 seconds seems to produce a smoother surface on the casting.

10. The pattern assembly is not invested under vacuum. Because of its weight and the possibility of its falling off the sprue former, Divestment is poured into the ring. It is optional whether the Divestment die is wet or dry before painting the pattern. Naturally one should be careful of incorporating bubbles against the wax surface or entrapping them within the ring during the investment process.

11. After a minimum of 45 minutes setting time the ring is placed into the oven for the standard burn-out time of approximately 1 hour at a temperature of 600° to 675°C (1100° to 1250°F). It is wise to invert the casting ring so that the sprue hole is turned up the last 10 to 15 minutes of heating.

12. Casting is done in a traditional manner. Vacuum casting is not recommended because Divestment is a relatively dense, non-porous material. *Do not* quench the casting ring in water. It should remain dry and cool in the air.

13. Upon cooling, the investment will shrink and can be readily slipped out of the ring (Fig. 17–48) where it is broken apart. With reasonable care the casting with its gold sprue and button, along with the Divestment and dowel pin, can be salvaged.

14. The sprue is cut off, the oxides and debris scraped away from the surface of the dowel pin, and the die placed back into the model where it is fitted for occlusion and contact (Figs. 17–49 and 17–50).

15. After finishing and polishing all non-marginal areas (Fig. 17–51), the

Figure 17–57. Eight-unit splint cast in one piece against a Divestment model.

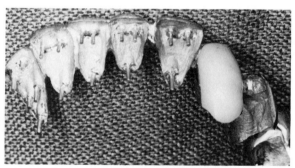

die is cleaned out from inside the casting with round burs or sharp excavators. It is then pickled and inspected for flash and tiny internal nodules or gold bubbles. This is best done with magnification but is a most important step with the Divestment technique. Inasmuch as "flash" and nodules are never present in a "pulled-pattern" it is particularly stressed with Divestment, lest it be overlooked.

16. Using medium or fine garnet disks followed by cuttle disks, the marginal surfaces are smoothed and polished. The casting is then ready to be carried to the mouth where it is fitted to the tooth (Figs. 17–52 through 17–55).

With a variety of modifications, Divestment can also be utilized in bridge fabrication (Fig. 17–56). Divestment is particularly advantageous in gold castings with pins. Pinholes that are reproduced in the impression with nylon bristles are rapidly transported to a Divestment die and subsequently to a gold casting (Fig. 17–57).

18

THE CAST GOLD RESTORATION: FINISH AND CEMENTATION

Finishing

Armamentarium
1. Burs, Nos. ¼, ½, and 2
2. Separating disks and rubber wheels
3. Wire wheel brush (steel or brass)
4. Paper disks: garnet, sand, and cuttle
5. Ribbon articulating paper
6. Armamentarium for local anesthesia
7. Explorers, Nos. 6 and 23
8. Straight and RA stones
9. Gold finishing burs
10. Polishing agents

Inspection of the Casting

After the casting has been pickled and thoroughly washed, it must be carefully examined to determine if any imperfections are present. These include incomplete margins or small nodules on the casting. The nodules are removed by using a ½, round or 33½, inverted cone bur. It is best if this inspection is done with good light and magnification. Be specific when using a bur for removal of small defects and keep the cutting action confined to the defect. The remaining internal surface should remain untouched until after the casting has been initially seated on the die.

If the casting is satisfactory, it is separated from the sprue and button. In order to conserve metal the separation should be made as near to the casting as possible yet without risking damage (Fig. 18–1). The usual means of separation is to use a carborundum disk in a straight handpiece and to cut it free with slow speed. An alternate method is to use a sharp side-cutting pliers, but with caution to prevent the cutter from impinging on the casting, which causes the metal to be distorted. It is acceptable to cut partially with the disk and then use the side cutters to complete the cutting. This helps to minimize the loss of metal. By using the disk the area of the sprue attachment is adjusted to the curvature present at that portion of the casting.

The casting is placed on the die to evaluate the fit and the marginal

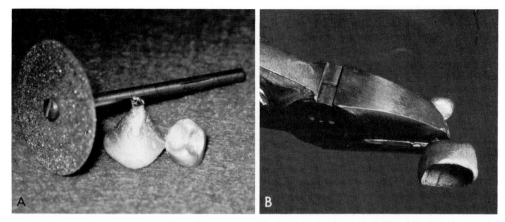

Figure 18–1. The restoration is separated from the sprue and button by a carborundum disc *(A)* or by the careful use of a side cutter *(B)*. (From Hollenback, G. M.: Science and Technic of the Cast Restoration. C. V. Mosby, 1964)

relationship. If proper technology has been used, the margins should relate as accurately as they did in the wax, and the die must not be damaged as this is done (Fig. 18–2). If the casting is made by a process that does not include a die or if it has been destroyed (as in using Divestment), the fit and margins are evaluated on the tooth itself. The internal surface of the casting may need relief (to be discussed later).

If the casting passes inspection, it is polished prior to placing it in the mouth. The smooth surfaces are polished by using paper disks or rubber wheels. This is easy if the wax pattern was left with a smooth surface. The disks are garnet, sandpaper, and cuttle types of paper disks. Disks vary from coarse to fine grit, and garnet is the most coarse. The object is to use as coarse

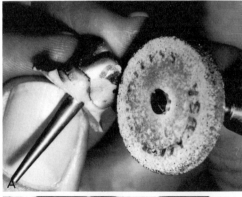

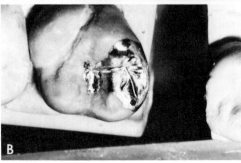

Figure 18–2. *A,* The sprue and contact areas are adjusted so as to return the restoration to the model. *B,* The restoration is repositioned on its die so external finishing can proceed.

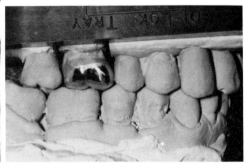

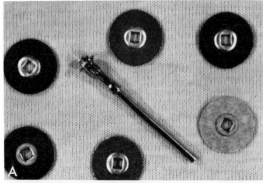

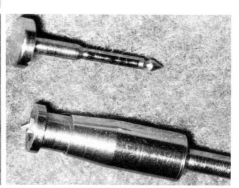

Figure 18–3. A variety of disks and mandrels capable of turning in either a clockwise or a counterclockwise direction. *A*, Moore's snap-on mandrels.* *B*, Spring loaded EZ mandrel.†

*E. C. Moore Co., 13325 Leonard, Dearborn, Michigan 48126.

†Union Broach, 36–40 37th Street, Long Island City, New York 11101.

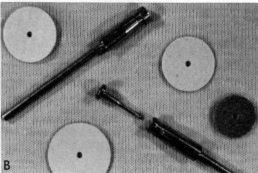

a paper as needed and then graduate to finer paper disks in order to produce a polished surface. A straight handpiece mandrel is recommended for use with these disks (Fig. 18–3).

Rubber wheels are impregnated with carborundum or pumice. While they will not cut metal in any significant amount, they will cut sufficiently to leave a semi-polished surface. When either paper or rubber wheels are used, the margins must be protected to avoid a change in marginal contour or fit. The finishing should be done under good lighting. The occlusal surface may be partly polished with a wire brush in a straight handpiece or a laboratory lathe (Fig. 18–4).

If the casting is on the die, it should be placed back onto the articulated model. First it is important to make an accurate adjustment of the proximal contacts. If a large amount is to be removed, use a carborundum disk or a stone to bring the contact close. Then paper disks or rubber wheels are used to place mesial and distal contact as accurately as possible. If both proximal contacts are involved, avoid overcutting one or both contacts, as they must be in positive contact with the adjacent teeth, assuming the mesial and distal relationships are normal. After contact is established examine the buccal, lingual, and occlusal embrasures, which require good anatomical form. Avoid overcontouring. These adjustments are made using paper disks or rubber wheels to be sure the embrasures are opened without losing the contact.

Observe the relationship of the models with the casting removed. It is to be expected that the same relationship will occur with the casting in position. With articulating paper, check the occlusal contacts and use paper that marks easily but without smearing.* If the markings are exclusively on the casting, they should be reduced by using small finishing burs or stones. This should

*Accufilm, Parkell, Farmingdale, New York 11735; Mark-rite, Charles Holg, Grayslake, Illinois 60030.

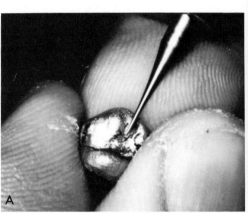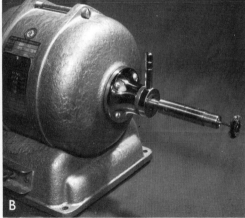

Figure 18–4. *A,* The anatomic detail of the occlusal surface is accentuated using finishing burs. *B,* The occlusal surface can be smoothed by using a wire brush. (From Hollenback, G. M.: Science and Technic of the Cast Restoration. C. V. Mosby, 1964)

be done until the intensity of the occlusal marking with paper is the same on both the casting and the stone model. Proceed over the occlusal surface with slow-speed finishing burs to produce a uniform surface. A small rubber wheel may be used to smooth the highlights. This is followed with a slow-speed wire wheel that leaves a satin finish. The wire wheel is advised because it works very well in both the grooves and the cuspal inclines. Do not place a high shine on the occlusal surface for it is difficult to detect occlusal contacts that may require adjusting if the surface is too shiny.

Intraoral Adjustment

During the procedure leading to cementation the patient should be comfortable and as a rule this includes the administration of a local anesthetic. The friction of trying the casting and exposing the dentin to air is painful to many, and it is exaggerated during the actual cementation. If the try-in is painful, the patient secretes an abnormal amount of saliva and is not relaxed, both of which interfere with accurate adjustment.

REMOVAL OF TEMPORARY

If the temporary is acrylic and cemented with a weak ZOE cement, it may be removed by engaging a margin with a rigid instrument, such as a hand excavator, and then pushed free. Should this method not prove successful, a straight chisel may be placed on the plastic and aligned in a direction closely related to the line of withdrawal of the temporary. It is then lightly tapped with a mallet to dislodge the temporary. Frequently the mouth must be almost closed in order to permit removal of the restoration. When temporaries are of preformed aluminum and have been individually tailored, they are easily removed by using a pair of serrated pliers and lifting the temporary free of the tooth (Fig. 18–5). The preparations must then be thoroughly cleansed of all temporary material by means of water and air and at times a pumice wash.

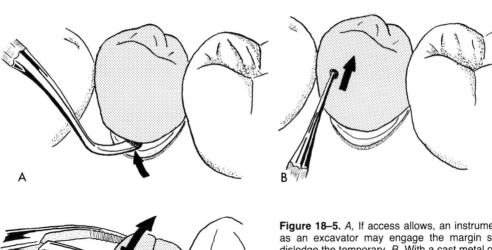

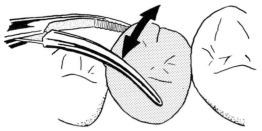

Figure 18–5. *A,* If access allows, an instrument such as an excavator may engage the margin so as to dislodge the temporary. *B,* With a cast metal or acrylic temporary a notch may be placed on mesial facial and a straight chisel used to tap it free. *C,* When the temporary is of preformed metal, a serrated pliers or hemostat is used to remove it.

PROXIMAL CONTACT

The casting is placed on the preparation. If there is resistance to complete seating the first location to check is at the proximal contacts. The restoration must permit the tooth to return to the best possible proximal contacting relationship. Since the casting has been adjusted on a model the contact should be within a very close tolerance but on the plus side. The adjustment can be easily made using paper disks or rubber wheels on the contact area.

If both mesial and distal surfaces are involved, it is a greater problem to adjust for contact. It is not always simple to be sure which contact requires the greatest adjustment, so analyze carefully which area needs the adjusting. Usually it is best to seat the casting as far as possible and, while pressure is maintained, to use dental floss to check the intensity of the contact (Fig. 18–6).

When checking the contact of a restoration that has not been cemented, the dental floss should pass through the restored contact with the same

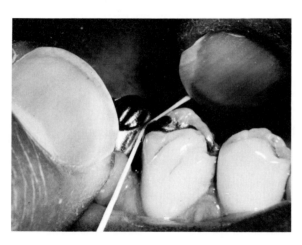

Figure 18–6. The contact area must be adjusted until it provides proper resistance to the dental floss going between contacts.

resistance as between the other teeth in the arch. After the floss has passed by the contact, it is safer to remove it by pulling it facially from under the contact. If it is carelessly pulled back through the contact, it may engage the loose casting and flip it from the preparation. It may fall to the floor, damaging the casting; or worse, the loose casting may be swallowed or inhaled. This *does* happen and obviously is upsetting to all involved. Having the rubber dam in place for as much of the procedure as possible prevents some of these bizarre possibilities.

To seat the casting fully it may be necessary to use direct force on the restoration. This may be applied digitally by the operator, or the patient may apply pressure by biting on an orangewood stick or cotton roll. Light malleting action may be used on an orangewood stick.

When the casting is fully seated the margins of the casting are expected to rest directly against the cavosurface margins of the preparation so as to appear continuous from tooth to restoration. Even with a smooth fit, it is expected that the margins of the casting will need adjusting with stones or disks or both to perfect the closeness of this relationship.

The selection of a stone or disk is made on the basis of the location and amount of adjusting required. If a stone is selected, its design is suggested by convenience. Tapered and inverted cone stones are two popular designs and they may be quite abrasive or fine in their cutting ability (Fig. 18–7). It is normal to use paper disks following the stones to complete the shaping and finishing of the margins. The actual final finishing of the margins occurs

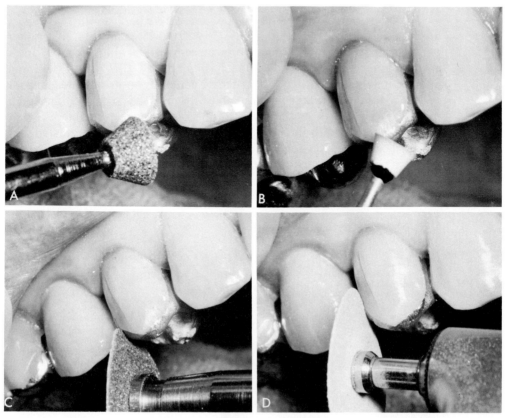

Figure 18–7. *A,* A stone that is very abrasive is used on the metal followed by a stone *(B)* that is not very abrasive. Coarse *(C)* and fine *(D)* disks are used to finish the margins.

during the time the casting is cemented. The abrasive grit used at that time is usually garnet or sand, and the size of disk and mandrel is related to the convenience of reaching the margins (see Figure 18–3). An important rule to observe when employing any of these revolving devices is the requirement that they revolve in the direction going from metal to enamel. Screw-head mandrels pose a problem in this regard in that a counterclockwise direction unscrews the mandrel.

Following the use of stones and disks, the margins are examined to determine the relationship of the casting to the tooth. There must be no detectable space at the tooth-casting interface. The metallic duplication of tooth structure must be as accurate as possible. The examination of the margins is done visually and with tactile sense, using a sharp explorer (Fig. 18–8).

Examination of the margins poses a clinical problem, for even a sharp explorer is large when compared with a human hair, which may measure 40 micrometers. If the tip of the explorer feels any excess of metal, as related to the margins, it is dressed off with a sand or cuttle disk. If a void or deficiency is felt, it must be determined if it is clinically acceptable. This decision will vary depending upon the standards of individual operators and leads to cementation of some restorations that are not reliable. Perfection is the ultimate goal, but this is not always, if ever, achieved and each dentist must determine for himself how much less than total perfection is acceptable. If all explorers were new or sharp, the examination of the margins could be conducted with an acceptable level of confidence. If a dentist uses a dull explorer as a means of checking for discrepancies, it indicates that his criteria for acceptability are of a low order, which is unfortunate.

If any explorer tip, even though sharp, enters between the casting and the tooth when fully seated, the discrepancy is too large and the casting must be considered a failure. The possibility of cement washing out from under the casting must be prevented. If a sharp explorer tip, which will measure approximately 80 micrometers, makes a penetration, it indicates an excessive opening. Naturally when margins are fully exposed to visual inspection, the most accurate assessment of the fit of the casting can be made.

If the casting will not seat after the contacts have been adjusted, examine the internal surface of the casting for possible burnish marks, which may be adjusted with a bur. If the internal surface is shiny, the burnish marks will

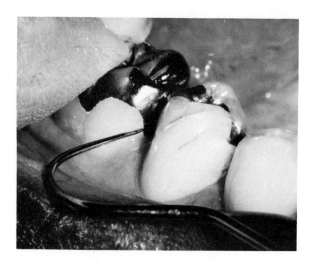

Figure 18–8. A sharp explorer is used to verify all of the margins.

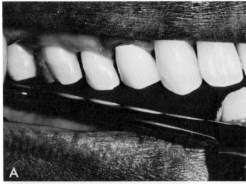

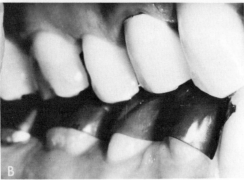

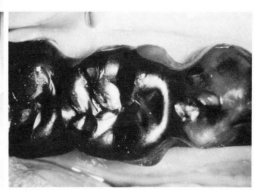

Figure 18–9. *A,* Articular ribbon is held in position to record the occlusal markings. *B,* Ribbons of thin wax may be placed over the teeth and as the teeth occlude it will reveal the specific contacts as the wax is penetrated.

not be displayed. A laboratory sand blasting device, if available, may be used to dull the shiny surface, again allowing burnish marks to be observed when the casting is seated with pressure.

If a casting continually resists being seated, the time involved may become a problem. The experienced operator will limit the amount of time used to fit a casting. In spite of the present levels of technical performance there will be casting failures, and it is best to accept that fact but to strive always to reduce the incidence of failure.

ADJUSTING THE OCCLUSION

Prior to placing the casting have patient close into centric occlusion and observe carefully the occlusal relationships of several teeth. This is done adjacent to the preparation and also on the opposite side of the mouth. As these teeth make occlusal contact it helps to verify the occlusal adjustment of the casting, as these teeth contact in an identical manner both before and after the casting is placed.

To determine occlusal contact, the occlusal surface must be dry, so cotton rolls are used to block saliva.

After the casting is in place use thin articulating paper, which will mark easily but not smear. The patient is asked to close in centric occlusion, thus indicating the marking pattern (Fig. 18–9). It is expected that the initial marking will be the most intense on the casting. These markings are adjusted until they appear equal in intensity and area on the casting as well as on the adjacent teeth. When teeth are noticeably worn the area of the occlusal marking should be less on the casting than on the natural tooth. If the adjustment required is minimal, it is easily done with the casting in position. It may be accomplished with one of several high-speed cutting instruments. Among those recommended are small round finishing burs or a No. 2 or No. 4 cutting bur. Use a light touch to avoid overcutting or needlessly altering the occlusal anatomy. If the marking occurs in a groove or in a fossa, the groove should be deepened to allow the working cusp room to fully seat with the marking or contact occurring on the buccal and lingual sides of the cusp tip. Again observe the opposite segment of the mouth and note if the teeth are in full contact.

When centric occlusal contact is established the lateral movements must be checked. With articulating paper in place the teeth are closed into centric occlusion and from this position the patient is asked to move the mandible both in right and left directions. If the teeth are in their usual alignment the posterior teeth will quickly separate since the lingual inclines of the anterior teeth, especially the cuspids, naturally cause the posterior to separate during lateral movements of the mandible. If markings occur on the casting during these movements, the casting should again be adjusted so as to eliminate this type of marking. Posterior teeth tolerate pressure in a vertical direction very well, but horizontal pressures are generally traumatic.

The protective function of the anterior teeth in relation to the posterior teeth during lateral movement is the preferred occlusal pattern, but this arrangement does not always occur. The usual alternate pattern is for the posterior teeth to stay in contact during lateral movement and share equally in the occlusal force. In this instance the object is to develop markings from the articulating paper that are of equal intensity and are in contact during the same length of lateral movement.

As an additional reference the operator may place his finger over the facial surfaces of the teeth, including the one in the process of restoration, and again have the patient proceed through the mandibular movements. If the impact on the tooth to be restored is heavy, it can be felt as a slight lateral displacement, which will then require adjustment until the movement is non-existent or equalized through the area.

Patients should be asked to close their teeth together, and frequently they are able to discriminate and identify a casting that is in premature contact. Closure should be equalized throughout the mouth. This is not to suggest that patient reactions can be relied upon with complete safety, but frequently they are able to provide valuable clues.

Finishing Prior to Cementation

When the proximal contours and occlusal contacts are satisfactory there remains the final finishing prior to cementation. After occlusal adjustment in the casting it may be smoothed to final contours using small round finishing burs, small paper disks, small rubber wheels, or again using a wire wheel. While this is being done be very careful to guard the final occluding contact spots, for once the occlusion is adjusted the contacts must not be lost.

Additional polishing may also be done by use of a wheel brush with a polishing compound such as Tripoli, lightly over the metal surfaces (Fig. 18–10). Avoid excessive pressure in areas of occlusal contact and do not polish on the margins as this may cause a deficiency. Also be careful that the polishing material is not lodged in the internal portion of the casting.

After blocking the drain in the sink scrub the casting with soap and water using a tooth brush, and then place the casting in the ultrasonic cleaner, following which it should be ready for cementation. With polycarboxylate or glass ionomer cementation the pickled surface of the casting should be mechanically cleansed, as previously noted.

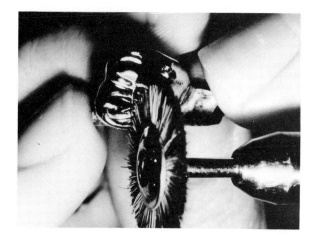

Figure 18–10. A wheel brush and polishing compound are used to polish the surface of the casting.

Correction of Casting Deficiencies

NEGATIVE PROXIMAL CONTACT

On occasion while fabricating a casting a proximal contact will be lost because of inadequate waxing or excessive finishing. This is not acceptable, as this contact must be positive for gingival protection. This at best is an annoying development, but contact may be restored with minimum effort even if it is done at the cementation appointment. Restoration of the proximal contact calls for the addition of solder in the amount needed to restore contact.

The items required to accomplish this restoration include solder, soldering paste flux, antiflux, soldering tweezers, and a Bunsen burner. The requirements for the solder are that it be resistant to corrosion and that it flow at a temperature low enough to avoid damage to the casting. Solder is identified by its fineness, which indicates the gold content of the solder. A recommended solder for restoring contact is 615 or 650 fine, which easily resists tarnish. As a rule, the lower the fineness is, indicating a smaller percentage of gold content, the lower the fusion temperature. If the margins of the casting are delicate, the 615 solder would be a good choice, as its fusion temperature is lower in comparison with a 650 solder, thus decreasing the risk of overheating the casting.

Determine the amount of the deficiency and cut a segment of solder that will provide the contact plus a slight excess. With a soft pencil draw a definite line surrounding the contact area for the purpose of providing definite limits for the solder as it fuses and flows (Fig. 18–11). The molten solder is restricted by the graphite barrier. A thin layer of soldering paste flux is applied over the contact area. The component elements of the paste flux may segregate upon standing, requiring stirring to homogenize. The solder is coated with a film of flux and positioned on the contact and the casting is secured by a self-locking soldering tweezer. The tweezer engages the casting so as to permit the heat to focus on the casting, without first traveling up the tweezer. The casting is held over the hottest segment of the flame of a carefully adjusted Bunsen burner. This flame has the same appearance as was previously discussed for casting the alloy. The casting will heat quickly to a red color and the solder will melt and flow over the contact area. As soon as the solder flows, it is quickly removed from the flame (Fig. 18–12). The casting must again be pickled and finished as previously described.

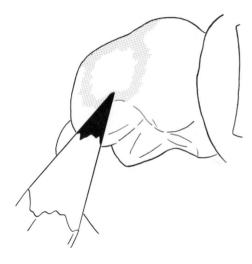

Figure 18–11. The graphite from a soft lead pencil provides a barrier to contain the solder as it melts.

CASTING RELIEF

Castings that fit very snugly may require space between the preparation and the restoration to accommodate the cement and yet allow the casting to fit the margins properly. This may be done on the die, as previously discussed, using a die spacer material. Uniform relief of the metal from the internal part of the casting can be achieved by using an etching solution for non-ferrous alloys. The solution dissolves gold from the exposed parts of the casting, which creates a uniform space. A suggested solution consists of nitric acid (1 part), hydrochloric acid (5 parts), and distilled water (6 parts).

The chemicals should be of reagent quality. When they are mixed the solution remains stable during storage, which should be done in glass reagent

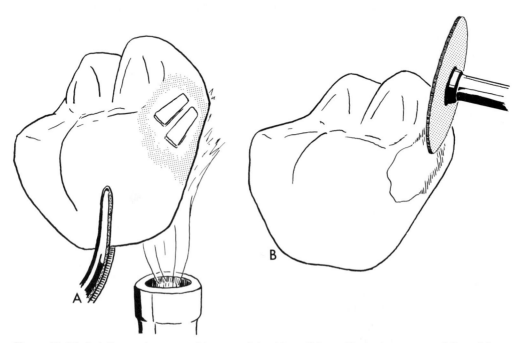

Figure 18–12. *A,* A Bunsen burner provides enough heat to melt the solder and as soon as it flows it is removed from the flame. *B,* After soldering the contact is adjusted with disks or stones and polished.

bottles with ground glass stoppers. The etching itself must be done where there is good air circulation, for the fumes are corrosive to many metals, such as instruments and equipment, that are present in the office or laboratory.

The casting must be prepared by covering the entire external portion with wax and extending the wax approximately 1 mm onto the internal surface of the casting (Fig. 18–13). This permits the solution to dissolve the exposed surface of the casting yet excludes the segment adjacent to the margins. The recommended wax for this purpose should be hard inlay or sticky wax.

The casting is placed in a suitable test tube and covered with the etching solution. The tube is then placed in a water bath at a temperature of 46°C (115°F). A 10-minute etch provides adequate relief for most castings, although the rate of etching varies with the gold content of the alloy. As the gold content decreases, the time required for etching increases. The gold content has been reduced in many alloys as a result of the increased cost of gold, and these alloys cannot be etched as quickly.

Following etching the casting is scrubbed with a tooth brush under cold water and soap. If warm water is used, it may smear the wax into the etched surface, making the wax difficult to remove. The wax is removed and the casting heated to a dull red color to make sure that the wax is melted and burned off. The casting is pickled to remove oxides. Be sure that the solution is clean, as the cast surface must be clean to facilitate successful cementation. Any finishing to the cast surface may be accomplished as previously described.

VENTING AND BURNISHING CASTINGS

The interface between the casting and the cavity preparation is partially influenced by the thickness of the cement that is needed to occupy the space between the casting and the tooth. The film thickness is determined by factors

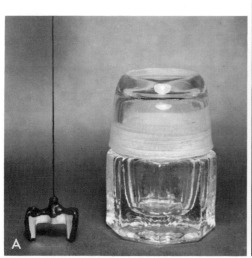
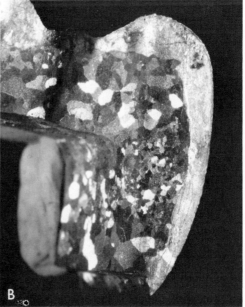

Figure 18–13. A, When etching with aqua regia all margins and external surfaces of the casting are protected by a film of wax, and a string may be attached so as to retrieve it from the aqua regia. B, The action of aqua regia on the casting, which provides space between casting and tooth. Note the display of grain boundaries. (From Hollenback, G. M.: Science and Technic of the Cast Restoration. C. V. Mosby, 1964)

such as the particle size of the cement powder and its thickness or viscosity at the time of cementation. The intention during cementation is to reduce the space to such a minimal degree that no cement line is visible. This is almost impossible to achieve, as the cement must occupy some space. It is not possible to make a perfect restoration, although to the unaided eye castings may appear to be perfectly adapted at the margins. If the marginal area is magnified, a cement line will most often be visible.

The actual cementation is in part a problem of minimizing hydraulic pressure because the casting is trying to squeeze a viscous liquid out of its path of insertion as it is being positioned. This potential for hydraulic interference is increased as the length of the preparation increases and the degree of taper to its wall decreases. It is also highly influenced by the design of the preparation, with the full crown giving the most consistent difficulties as the full impact of hydraulic resistance becomes apparent within such a closed container. This problem is fully recognized by clinicians and researchers but is generally not taken into consideration, except with respect to the force applied to the casting during seating.

For those castings for which hydraulics is a real problem (e.g., a full cast crown with parallel walls), it is advocated that a small hole be cut in the occlusal surface of the casting with a No. 2 or No. 4 bur in a spot that does not interfere with occlusion and is easy to restore (Fig. 18–14). When the casting is placed excess cement will extrude through the hole and allow the casting to be positioned with less difficulty. The placing of a casting vent also allows the casting to seat in its correct position.

The objection to placing a vent in an intact casting is the necessity of restoring the hole with gold in order to preserve the gold surface. This may be done by using a prefabricated gold plug that becomes part of the wax pattern and is removed from the pattern and cemented into position after the casting is seated. The other option is to fill the hole with direct gold.

Burnishing is frequently suggested as a means of improving the marginal adaptation of the casting to the tooth. This means the gold has to be moved or stretched toward the enamel. This is possible if the discrepancy is small and if the Brinell hardness of the alloy does not exceed 100. If the metal is hard and the margins bulky, any attempt at burnishing will frequently cause damage to the enamel, leaving a poor margin.

For burnishing to occur, smooth, thin-beveled margins are required, which result in an equally thin flange of metal that responds slightly to manual bending. This does produce an improvement in the marginal fit but is limited to those parts of the casting that are easily accessible.

Burnishing is accomplished by using a Spratley finisher, an instrument

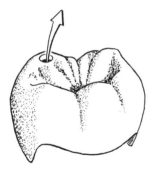

Figure 18–14. A small hole may be placed in a casting to counteract the hydraulics caused by the fluid cement in order to allow seating of the casting; this is commonly known as venting.

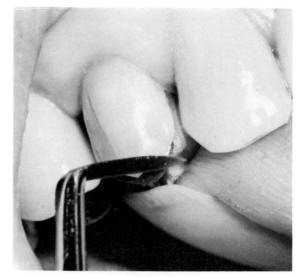

Figure 18–15. A rigid instrument (GF-33) that does not have a sharp cutting edge may be used to burnish accessible margins.

that does not bend while being subjected to burnishing force (Fig. 18–15). Gold files may also be used for this purpose. Worn finishing burs or round burnishers, in a slow-speed handpiece under pressure, can be helpful in producing this effect.

Again, burnishing is very limited as a means of reducing marginal discrepancies. It is not an option for a poor fitting casting. Likewise, if burnishing is excessive, the metal is more subject to corrosion and fracture.

Resumé of Steps Leading to Cementation
1. Inspect casting and remove nodules, etc.
2. Evaluate fit and margins on the die.
3. Polish the external surface with rubber and wire wheels.
4. Administer anesthesia and remove temporary.
5. Adjust interproximal contacts.
6. Occlusal adjustment.
7. Adjust but do not polish accessible margins.
8. Clean the casting.
9. Correct deficiencies if necessary.

Cementation

The final link to a successful cast restoration is dependent upon the care taken during cementation. The process requires that a hard intermediate cementing material be placed between the casting and the tooth for the purpose of immobilizing the restoration.

Some patients have the idea that castings are successful because of the effectiveness of the cement. They need to be informed that the design of the preparation contributes to most of the success achieved by a cast restoration.

The function of the cement is to fill the irregularities on the preparation and those on the casting surface to provide a rigid core mechanically lodged in the surface irregularities, resulting in a secure restoration (Fig. 18–16). It must be emphasized that retention of the restoration is largely due to the mechanics of the cavity preparation itself. However, the cement does enhance the retentive capacity needed to secure the casting.

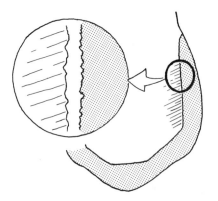

Figure 18–16. An illustration of the mechanical aspect of cementation, with the surface irregularities of both preparation and casting being used to secure the casting.

Cementation of castings is analogous to gluing wood joints, for when two pieces of wood are joined using a suitable wood glue, the liquid glue penetrates into minute openings and crevices. When the glue sets, these extensions provide mechanical retention and unite the two parts as they are placed together. The glue by itself will not be successful if the parts are not well matched, as this places the glue under tension.

Many of the details relating to type of cement, composition, working consistency, strength, acidity, film thickness, and mixing technique have been discussed in Chapter 7.

Zinc Phosphate Cementation

To permit cementation to occur under optimum conditions, moisture must be excluded from the preparation. When feasible, the rubber dam should be used, as this is the best way to maintain a dry field. If the restoration involves the last tooth in the arch or if the margins are positioned gingivally below normal tissue level, the rubber dam may be very difficult to place so that the margins are exposed. Such instances will necessitate the use of cotton rolls as a means of controlling moisture.

The preparation must be safely but fully cleansed of debris before cementation, as a poorly cleansed surface leads to a loss of cement retention. The procedure for cleansing the surface is discussed in Chapter 7 and includes the use of water, 3 per cent hydrogen peroxide, and commercial solutions.

After cleansing and gentle air drying, two thin layers of cavity varnish* are placed over the preparation, the second application being placed after the

*Teledyne Dental Co., Elk Grove Village, Illinois 60007.

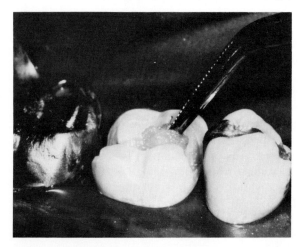

Figure 18–17. Two applications of cavity varnish are placed over the preparation. Note that the rubber dam is in place.

first has been allowed to dry. If the varnish is of a thin viscosity, it does not interfere with retention of the cement. If thick, however, it tends to fill in the tooth surface irregularities and reduces the interlocking effect of the cement (Fig. 18–17).

Armamentarium
1. Plastic instruments
2. Mandrels (include small-head mandrel)
3. Garnet and paper disks
4. Flour pumice and Amalgloss
5. Polishing cups and mandrel
6. Dental floss
7. Explorers, Nos. 6 and 23

PROCEDURE

1. CEMENT COATING. With a plastic instrument coat the preparation side of the casting with a film of cement. Then with the same instrument coat the preparation with a thin layer of cement. If a rubber dam is not used, be sure to apply the cement initially at the gingival portion of the preparation, as this will tend to block any potential gingival moisture (Fig. 18–18).

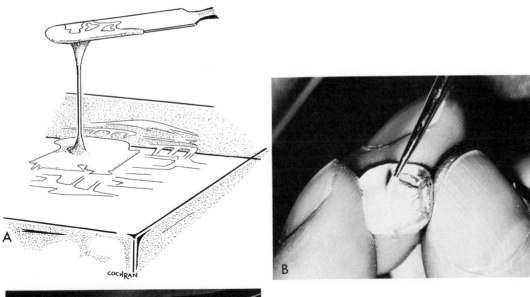

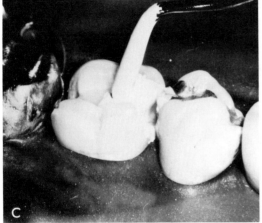

Figure 18–18. *A,* An example of a cement that has been mixed to a proper consistency. *B,* The internal surface of the casting is coated with cement. *C,* The surface of the preparation is coated with cement.

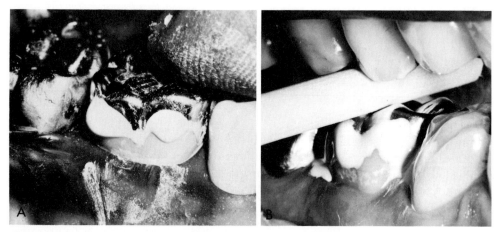

Figure 18–19. *A,* The casting is seated forcefully with heavy digital pressure. *B,* The patient is asked to bite against an orangewood stick with heavy pressure to help seat the casting.

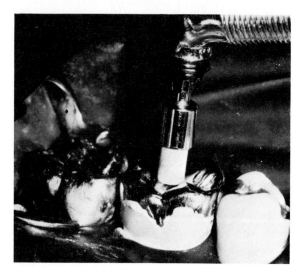

Figure 18–20. A wood insert in a condensing instrument may be used while the cement is still fluid.

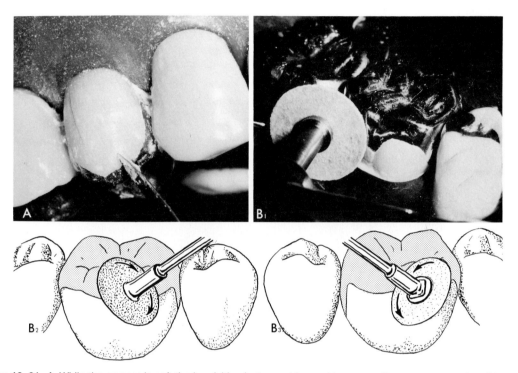

Figure 18–21. *A,* While the cement is soft the burnishing instrument is used to remove the excess cement and to reburnish the margins. *B,* Before the cement hardens go over the margins with sand and/or cuttle paper disks, which must rotate from metal to tooth.

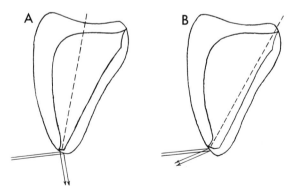

Figure 18–22. The occlusal or incisal margin of gold should be slightly rolled so as to cause light reflection to be less apparent. Casting *A* is not as easily noticed as casting *B.*

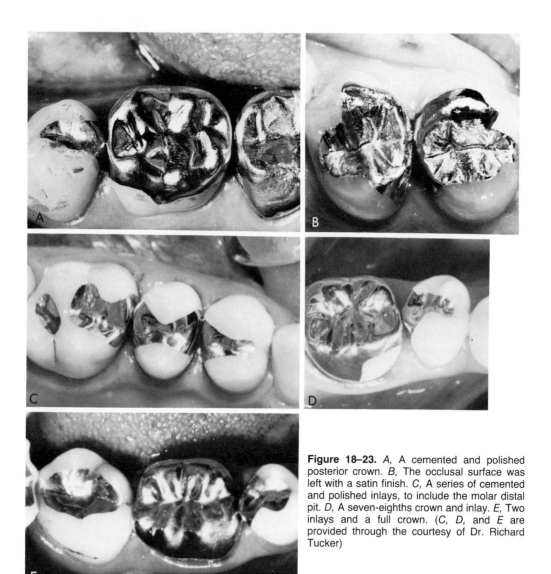

Figure 18–23. *A,* A cemented and polished posterior crown. *B,* The occlusal surface was left with a satin finish. *C,* A series of cemented and polished inlays, to include the molar distal pit. *D,* A seven-eighths crown and inlay. *E,* Two inlays and a full crown. (*C, D,* and *E* are provided through the courtesy of Dr. Richard Tucker)

2. SEATING THE CASTING. The casting is inserted into position, and with finger pressure as much force as possible is placed on the casting to seat it fully. The excess cement is cleared away with a cotton roll, and if at all possible, the margin is exposed to view to see that the casting is fully seated. In addition, an orangewood stick or a cotton roll should be placed on the casting and the patient told to apply pressure with the opposing teeth. Usually with this procedure additional cement will extrude around the margins. This is repeated until cement no longer extrudes from under the casting (Fig. 18–19). The direction in which the opposing teeth engage the casting must be carefully monitored, for if the direction of force is not complementary to the insertion path of the casting, it will cause the casting to be seated askew.

An orangewood stick may also be placed on the occlusal surface of the casting in the direction of the insertion path and with a mallet some tapping blows directed to the casting may be helpful to seating (Fig. 18–20).

An added precaution is to be careful that the casting does not engage the rubber dam or cotton roll at the margin during seating. It is also possible to trap loose tissue while seating a casting, which obviously would be a source of distress.

3. FINAL FINISH OF THE CASTING. As soon as the casting has been seated and the cement is still plastic a sandpaper disk in a straight handpiece mandrel is used to smooth the accessible marginal areas (Fig. 18–21). The operator holds the casting in position and proceeds over the margin with a disk revolving at slow speed and from gold to the enamel. A mandrel that can revolve in either direction is best suited for this purpose. As needed, the use of disks proceeds from coarse to fine in order to achieve a good marginal finish. By this time the cement should be set. As a final step of the finishing procedure a rubber cup is used with flour pumice, followed by Amalgloss, to achieve a high shine.

Polycarboxylate and Glass Ionomer Cementation

The techniques for placing the cemented restoration and for finishing the casting are the same as those discussed for zinc phosphate cementation. There is a strong precaution to be added: carboxylate cement must be removed from the margins either immediately or after it has become hard. If removed while in a rubbery state, it may be pulled out from under the casting or at the margins. Whenever possible, with the use of the glass ionomer cements, the margins should be covered with a cavity varnish after removal of the excess cement.

Final Inspection

As the margins of three-quarter crowns or onlays are being finished, examine the morphology of the margins for esthetics. Occlusal or incisal margins should be slightly rolled, not flat. This allows light to be reflected in a diffuse pattern. Although the gold will be visible, it will be more esthetic (Fig. 18–22).

When the castings have been fully finished, all the debris must carefully be flushed out and removed using intraoral evacuation. Dental floss must be passed through the contact to free any cement that may have lodged around it. Inspect the margins for any possible residual cement and again flush the area with water.

Again inspect the occlusal contacts and movements to verify the desired occlusal harmony. This includes centric closure and lateral movements. The cast restoration should represent a blend of function and art form. The result instills confidence and well-being in the patient and a sense of pride and satisfaction in the dentist (Fig. 18–23).

Resumé of Cementation

1. Isolate the teeth, preferably with a rubber dam, otherwise with cotton rolls.
2. Select the appropriate cement for the restoration.
3. Cleanse the cavity preparation.
4. Apply varnish if required.
5. Proportion and mix the cement.
6. Apply cement first to casting, then to the preparation.
7. Seat the casting.
8. Remove the excess cement.
9. Finish accessible margins while cement is still soft.
10. Complete the finishing procedures.
11. Examine margins and contact for any free cement.
12. Recheck occlusion.

19

REINFORCEMENT OF THE ENDODONTICALLY TREATED TOOTH

Forming a unique problem of its own, the tooth without its pulp usually requires different treatment from the tooth that still retains vitality. In analyzing this restorative problem and the engineering aspects pertaining to it, the following factors distinguish the pulpless tooth.

1. The tooth without its pulp is operable throughout. No pulp horns or vital structure limit the site for cutting dentin or limit the location of pin placement.

2. An endodontically treated tooth is a chronologically old tooth, with a reduction of internal moisture content. Such teeth are in a weakened condition and require that extra precautions be taken to protect against fracture.

3. The tooth is additionally weakened at the cemento-enamel junction from removal of dentin during endodontic therapy.

4. The tooth without its pulp is frequently discolored. In many instances this discoloration is so marked that it requires the removal of sound dentin and enamel and the placement of a crown to create a more acceptable appearance.

Because these endodontically related needs cannot always be met, it is absolutely essential that a favorable restorative potential for a tooth be assured before endodontic therapy is initiated. Frequently a pulpless tooth may be more judiciously treated by removing it and placing a fixed bridge. For example, consider a malaligned maxillary lateral incisor that is in need of endodontic therapy as well as a ceramic-type crown. Examination of the adjacent teeth (central and cuspid) reveals several large broken down and discolored restorations as well as a periodontal pocket between it and the cuspid. One of two treatment plans could be followed: (1) following endodontic and periodontic therapy, all three teeth could be crowned or (2) the lateral could be removed and a three-unit bridge placed from the cuspid to the central. Either plan might be followed, but the latter is likely to be preferred because treatment is more definitive and involves less discomfort and expense to the patient. Moreover, the removal of the lateral would probably eliminate the periodontal pocket on the mesial side of the cuspid.

There is only one basic problem in restoring the endodontically treated tooth—how to strengthen the remaining tooth structure and restore it in such a manner that nothing will fracture. Naturally this is an oversimplification,

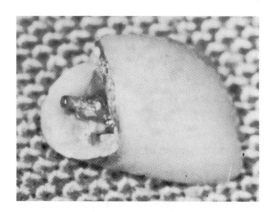

Figure 19–1. Clinical failure resulting from improper post length. (Courtesy of Drs. Earl Collard and Virgil M. S. Lau)

because pulp death is frequently associated with large restorations. Badly broken-down crowns present a challenge under normal conditions. With the added loss of dentin adjoining the pulp chamber, with lesions that often extend sub-gingivally, and with problems in isolation of the working field, restoration of the pulpless tooth is probably the greatest challenge for the operative dentist.

The basic unit of the restorative process is the dowel or its substitute (Figs. 19–1 and 19–2). As a flag pole is rigidly anchored in a concrete base, so the dowel must be anchored in the root. As the flag pole must withstand the windy gale without falling over, so the crown of the tooth must become a member of the masticatory apparatus without the possibility of fracture or dislodgment from its root.

Many pulpless teeth can be restored without a dowel. A clinical crown that is entirely intact except for the endodontic opening (no proximal restorations) needs no reinforcement and can be treated by filling the opening with amalgam, resin, or direct gold. However, most other crowns require dowel reinforcement. The decision to reinforce or not to reinforce is based upon the remaining tooth structure and the stresses that will be applied to this structure. Questions that can be asked are: With what degree of force will the patient execute closure? Is the canal shaped so it will effectively receive a dowel? Will the tooth become an abutment for a bridge? Was the canal, particularly at its orifice, over-instrumented and enlarged during endodontic therapy?

Reinforcement modalities fall into one of two categories: those that can be completed in one appointment and those that require two appointments. The custom-made casting comprises the latter; all other methods, the former.

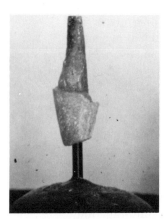

Figure 19–2. Pattern for a post and core. This direct pattern of acrylic resin will be cast in gold and cemented into the root. The plastic post, which extends to the end of the post hole, may be derived from a plastic toothpick or a large broom bristle. (The "post" fits into the root; the "core" supports the crown.)

The Cast Post and Core

The epitome of reinforcement is the cast post and core, which is a two-appointment procedure (Fig. 19–2). It permits an elliptical preparation of the root to match external tooth contours (Fig. 19–3) rather than requiring a circular one, which is characteristic of all pre-fabricated dowels. This is especially desirable, as its irregular shape prevents the restoration from tending to rotate under masticatory usage (Fig. 19–4).

The channel in the root is established with an appropriately sized round bur, followed by a tapered fissure bur for the development of the proper shape and taper. This is quite difficult to prepare without undercuts because the mouth mirror is of little value when the bur is operating. To eliminate undercuts for maxillary anteriors and bicuspid teeth, the use of a straight handpiece is recommended in lieu of a contra-angle.

Having prepared the root to its desired internal form, the operator may make a direct pattern for the post and core or he may take an impression of the prepared root. The former is usually recommended because of the ease of fabrication.

Direct Pattern

Acrylic or wax may be used to make the pattern. Sharp corners of dentin are removed near the orifice of the tapered channel, as they might interfere with making a neat, clean pattern and fitting the casting. If a rubber dam is used, an oily type of separating medium serves to keep the acrylic from adhering to the dentin inside the channel. If the rubber dam is not used, saliva will serve as an acceptable medium.

A plastic rod* approximately 40 mm in length and 1.0 to 1.5 mm in diameter is fitted loosely into the hole. Frequently the plastic rod must be thinned at the end to accommodate the fit. Self-curing resin† is mixed in a

---

*Plastic sprue pins, Williams Gold Ref. Co., 2978 Main St., Buffalo, New York 14214; plastic toothpicks; or plastic bristles from a warehouse broom.

†Duralay, Reliance Dental Mfg. Co., 5805 W. 117th Pl., Worth, Illinois 60482.

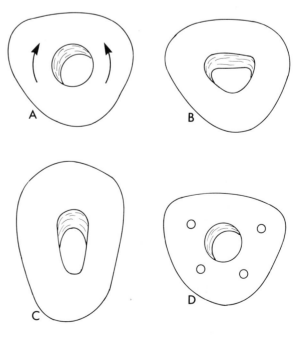

Figure 19–3. Conceptual design for a post that is placed into the root. *A,* Circular design is objectionable. It will not resist rotational forces. *B,* Triangular design for maxillary central is acceptable. *C,* Elliptical shape is acceptable for maxillary canine. *D,* Addition of threaded pins can resist rotational forces around a circular channel.

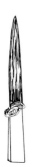

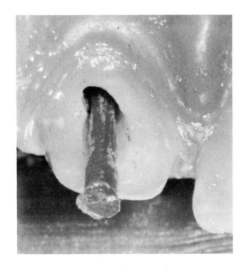

Figure 19–4. Plastic rod or dowel is fitted to the prepared channel. Wax or resin adheres to the rod and reproduces the post hole shape. (Courtesy of Dr. Hugh Cooper Jr.)

dappen dish (see Figs. 12–21, 12–22, and 12–23). After notching the plastic to engage the wet acrylic, a small spindle-shaped mass is added to the bristle, inserted into the hole, and roughly molded to form. Naturally the acrylic must be in a stiff doughy state before this is possible (Figs. 19–4, 19–5, and 19–6). After the resin has reached a stiff rubbery texture, just before its final polymerization, it is removed and inspected for undercuts. The projecting rod serves as a handle for its removal.

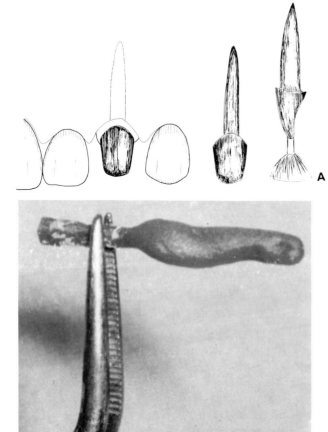

Figure 19–5. Fabrication procedure. *A, Left,* Completed pattern in place. *Center,* Pattern removed ready to be sprued. *Right,* Finished casting. (Courtesy of Dr. Hugh Cooper Jr.) *B,* Resin applied to plastic post ready to be fitted into canal preparation. Canal should be well lubricated.

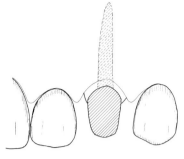

Figure 19–6. Cast post is fitted carefully into the channel. After polishing, post and core are cemented into place. (Courtesy of Dr. Hugh Cooper Jr.)

The resin is not reseated in the tooth until it has completely hardened and small irregularities have been removed with a rotating disk (Fig. 19–7). In refitting the pattern the operator must make certain that it slips freely in and out of its channel without the slightest degree of interference. The acrylic core is contoured as nearly as possible to its desired form, and the extension of the rod beyond the pattern is retained as a sprue for investing the acrylic resin pattern. Inspection of the occlusion may require removal of the natural sprue handle. Any deficiencies in the acrylic pattern may be filled in with inlay wax.

Acrylic patterns must be handled differently from wax patterns. During burn-out, wax softens and melts at approximately 150°F (65°C); not so with acrylic. On heating, it continues to expand even though it does not melt. The expansion of the pattern exerts significant pressures against the investing medium until a temperature in the range of at least 400°F (205°C) is reached. It then softens and burns out of the mold as wax does.

During the initial burn-out period, investment adjacent to the pattern tends to pulverize, especially in thin or fragile sections, unless a hard rigid investment is used.* An ethyl-silicate bonding agent in the liquid instead of plain water (Divestment system) provides the necessary additional strength. A mixture of 14 to 15 ml liquid to one package of Divestment powder provides a suitable investment medium.

After making the casting it is taken to the mouth, fitted, and cemented in place with zinc phosphate cement. To prevent wedging and splitting of the root, it is obvious that the post portion must be fitted with extreme care and never malleted in place. Minor adjustments for contours and for establishment of a good positive finish line on cementum (or enamel) are accomplished after cementation (Fig. 19–8). The tooth is now ready for the impression for making the crown.

---

*Divestment, available from Whip-Mix Corporation.

Figure 19–7. If resin is used, the undercut areas in the pattern are delicately removed with an abrasive disk, so the post encounters no resistance as it is reinserted into the channel. Void spaces in the core are filled with wax before investing.

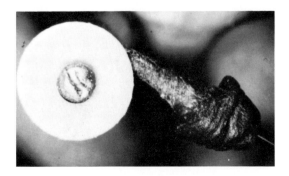

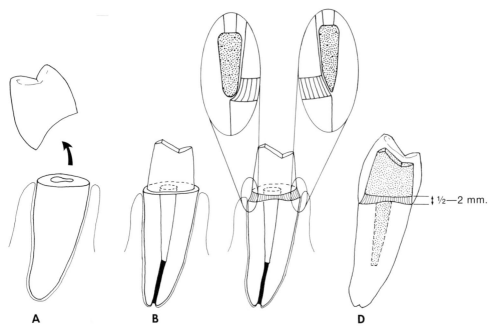

Figure 19–8. *A,* Before preparation. *B,* Post fitted and cemented. *C,* The margins are extended apically so the crown can engage the root with a ferrule of metal. *D,* Finished crown.

Indirect Pattern

If the operator elects to take an impression of the prepared channel rather than make a direct pattern, the tooth is exposed with appropriate gingival retraction, dried, and painted with Microfilm.* Impression material is deposited into the recesses of the channel in one of two ways: (1) a lentulo paste filler can spin soft material into the hole (Fig. 19–9) or (2) a hypodermic needle can be used to bleed the air out of the post hole and permit the elastic material to flow unencumbered to the end of the channel (see Miscellaneous Considerations later in this chapter).

Reinforcement of the impression material can be accomplished by painting

---

*"Microfilm": a colloidal suspension of wax. Available from Kerr Dental Manufacturing Co., Romulus, Michigan 48174.

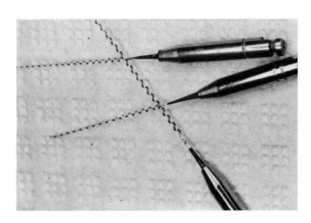

Figure 19–9. Lentulo paste fillers trimmed to about one-half to two-thirds their original length serve as a means for spinning impression material into the post hole (see Fig. 13–42).

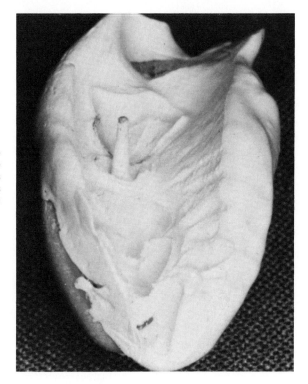

Figure 19–10. Impression of post hole. A large gutta percha point inserted into the filled hole serves as a stiffening agent and reduces chances of distortion of the impression. Tray adhesive is painted on the gutta percha to prevent it from pulling away from the impression material.

a thin coat of tray adhesive over a metal dowel (see Fig. 19–15) and inserting it into the hole after injection with the syringe, but before placement of the impression tray (Fig. 19–10). After removal, a die is poured and a wax pattern made in the conventional manner.

The Prophylactic Dowel

Indications for Usage

The cast post and core restoration involves the replacement of virtually all of the coronal dentin. At the opposite end of the spectrum, the prophylactic dowel eliminates as little coronal dentin as possible. Its function is to prevent a fracture that could separate the root from the crown. It can be placed in a tooth that is completely intact or it can be placed in a tooth prepared for metal–ceramic crown (Figs. 19–11 and 19–12). As stated above its function is prophylactic in nature to prevent a horizontal fracture at the cervical area sometime in the future.

The prophylactic dowel is limited to anterior and premolar teeth. Other indications and contraindications are as follows:

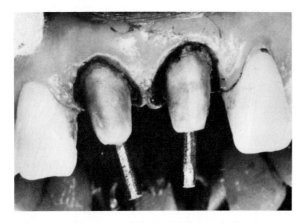

Figure 19–11. Prophylactic dowels in two central incisors. Ordinarily these are fashioned from stainless steel and are cut to length before cementation. Please note that the coronal dentin is entirely intact.

INDICATIONS	CONTRAINDICATIONS
No large restorations present	Large restorations present
Strong-appearing enamel	Mottled, decalcified, or hypoplastic enamel
Thick unworn enamel on the occlusal and facial surfaces	Severe erosion and heavy occlusal facets of wear involving dentin
Adequate bulk of coronal dentin present	Inadequate bulk of coronal dentin present
Reinforcement of a typical crown preparation	Reinforcement of a preparation in which large previous restorations have left voids and undercuts

Unfortunately the prophylactic dowel is used much too seldom. As insurance against breakage it pays big dividends, and its cost is only a few minutes of time and a dowel of stainless steel. Placement of a stiff rod in the center of the tooth should seldom be omitted from the treatment sequence of metal-ceramic crowns for pulpless teeth.

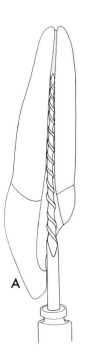
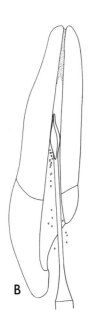
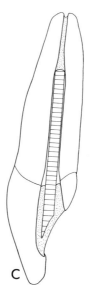

Figure 19–12. Prophylactic dowel inserted into a central incisor. After gutta percha has been removed with a hot instrument: *A*, Enlarge canal with progressively larger file or reamer; *B*, increase channel size with Gates Glidden drill or Muller type pulp bur; *C*, cement selected dowel post into the prepared channel.

Technique for Placement

The pulp bur (Fig. 19–13)* especially makes placement of the prophylactic dowel an easy procedure, augmenting the Peeso reamer and the Gates Glidden drill. The pulp bur cuts on its end. The ultra-thin shank provides excellent chip clearance and prevents the bur from becoming clogged. The thin shank provides excellent flexibility, allowing the bur to follow the channel already established by the endodontic file and the Gates Glidden drill (Figs. 19–13 and 19–14).

For concurrent use with these burs are matching parapost dowels† (Fig. 19–15). Despite root curvatures that might interfere with a hole that has not been reamed straight, the parapost dowel seldom encounters problems in being seated to the complete depth of the prepared channel. Sizes of commonly used drills and parapost dowels are:

DRILL SIZE	PARAPOST SIZE	SPACE FOR CEMENT
No. 18 (1.8 mm diam.)	No. 60	0–0.3 mm
No. 16 (1.6 mm diam.)	No. 50	0–0.35mm
No. 12 (1.2 mm diam.)	No. 40	0–0.2 mm

The difference in diameter between the burs and the dowels provides for cement and for minor deflections in curvature of the root.

Tapered pre-formed dowels, in contrast to cylindrical dowels (parapost), are suitable, but additional problems attend their use. The major problem is the inability of the operator to determine whether the tapered dowel is completely seated. It may wedge against the walls and give the false illusion of being seated (Fig. 19–16). It is quite important that the dowels be completely seated in order to take advantage of the full length of the prepared channel.

---

*Muller pulp burs, available with 1.2 mm, 1.4 mm, 1.6 mm, and 1.8 mm diameters in both SHP and latch types. Available from Brasseler, U.S.A., Inc., 800 King George Blvd., Savannah, Georgia 31419.

†Parapost stainless steel dowels available from Whaledent, Inc., 236 Fifth Ave. New York, New York 10001.

Figure 19–13. Muller type pulp burs. (Available from Brasseler, U.S.A., Inc. in either S. H. P. or R. A.)

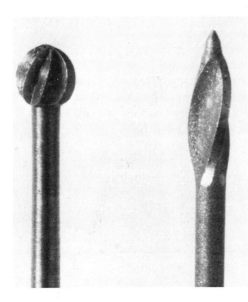

Figure 19–14. Comparison of Gates Glidden drill with pulp bur. Gates drill does not cut on the end (see Fig. 3–7).

In the absence of commercially prepared dowels, a stiff piece of orthodontic wire may be sized to match the channel prepared by the round burs. Dowels may also be cast in hard gold from pre-formed 14 gauge wax rods (Fig. 19–17). Dowels are cemented with zinc phosphate cement.

During the era of silver point endodontics, penetration out the side of the root was a common problem. Perforation can still be a problem whether one uses a bi-bevel drill, a reamer, or a pulp bur, unless the operator is in control of the operation.

Control is impossible without visibility. The operator must be able to see to the end of the channel to verify the presence of the pink gutta percha filler in the center of the hole. Suitable vision is dependent upon reflected light from the mouth mirror. This is true for light that enters the canal, which in turn is reflected back to the operator. The operating light should be positioned

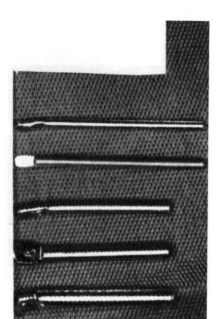

Figure 19–15. Serrated dowels fit into channel prepared by the pulp burs.

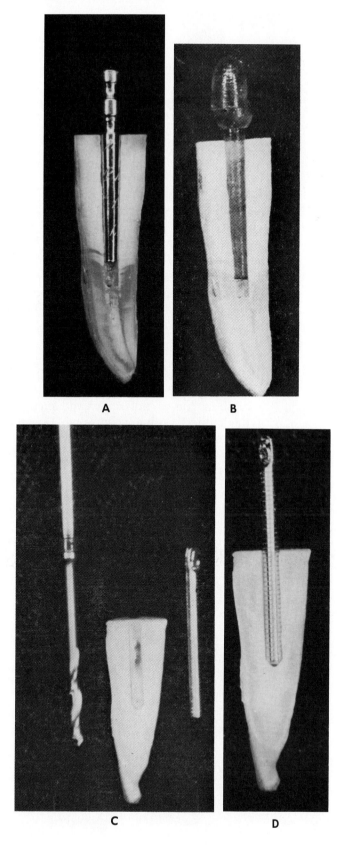

Figure 19–16. Comparison of fit of tapered dowel *(top)* versus cylindrical dowel *(bottom)*. While a snug fit is achieved, a tapered round dowel may or may not be completely seated in its channel. *A,* Tapered prefabricated metal dowel. *B,* Tapered plastic dowel for fabricating a pattern. *C* and *D,* Cylindrical dowel always utilizes the full length of the prepared channel.

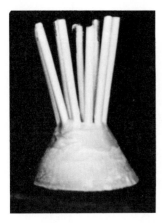

Figure 19–17. Dowel forms cast from hard gold from 14 gauge wax patterns. These match a pulp bur diameter of 1.8 mm.

alongside the head of the operator so the rays to and from the mirror can approach parallelism. Direct vision or direct illumination into the hole is not as effective as reflected light.

The Post and Amalgam (or Resin) Core

Reinforcement with a post and amalgam core is used when a large portion of the clinical crown is missing. Dowels are inserted into the roots, and amalgam (or composite resin) is built over them to re-establish the missing coronal dentin (Figs. 19–18 and 19–19). Where indicated, threaded pins may augment the dowels.

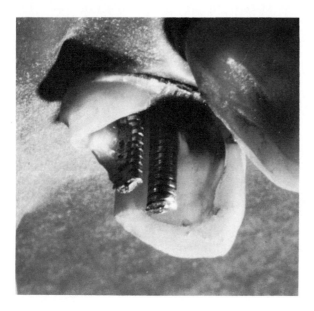

Figure 19–18. Concept of amalgam or composite build-up around dowel posts. With a fair portion of the crown remaining, the dowels inserted into the canals provide anchorage for the amalgam for this premolar.

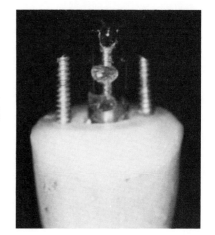

Figure 19–19. Dowel and threaded pins anchor core where no coronal dentin remains. While this type of anchorage may be sufficient for a single tooth restoration, it is inadequate for abutment retainers. A cast gold post and core should be employed instead.

Technique for Placement

Fitting and cementing the dowel is done in the same manner as that described for the prophylactic dowel. Zinc phosphate is the cementing medium of choice. It should be used sparingly lest excess material clog up the serrations of the dowel and fill in the area intended for the amalgam.

All prefabricated posts and dowels rely upon a certain size bur, drill, or reamer for preparation of the hole to receive it. Of necessity, these must all be round or cylindrical. Because they are round, the post has no resistance against rotation. The cast post, on the other hand, because of its irregular shape, does not rotate. The incorporation of threaded pins, which will also engage the amalgam or resin, assists the cylindrical dowel in preventing rotational forces (see Figs. 19–3D and 19–19).

Having prepared the posts (and pins) for reception of the core material, a matrix band (see Figs. 12–31 and 12–38) is selected and the core built to form. Amalgam as a core material is better than composite resin. Amalgam can be condensed against the dentin with probably less potential for microleakage than resin. With a fast setting spherical alloy, amalgam can also be placed and finished in one appointment and provides good rigidity from the standpoint of its modulus of elasticity. Amalgam also provides a smoother surface for taking an impression than does composite resin.

With the acid etch technique resins can be placed with minimal microleakage; however, the absence of enamel inside the tooth makes acid etching irrelevant. In favor of composite resin are ease of placement, rapid setting, and its capacity for being built into thin sections (Fig. 19–20).

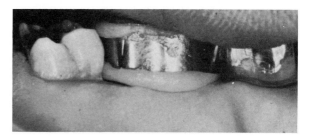

Figure 19–20. Finger held on copper band matrix to maintain positive pressure on the composite resin while it hardens. After hardening, the band will be removed and the composite core will be shaped to its proper form.

Regardless of the "good" or "bad" features of the two materials, the procedure for core fabrication is basically the same for both materials.

With burs and diamond stones the restoration and adjoining tooth structure are blended into the finished preparation. A continuous and smooth finish line produces the most accurate fit for the crown, as well as for the metal collar that encircles the remaining tooth structure.

The impression is taken, the bite registration made, and the restoration fabricated in the conventional manner. One suggestion about the impression is worthy of note. Freshly cut composite resin has an affinity for the polysulfide rubbers, and the use of a mold release agent is suggested when taking an impression of a composite core during the same appointment it is placed. Microfilm or a very thin coat of vaseline on the resin core will prevent the rubber from adhering to it.

The Amalgam Post and Core Without a Dowel

If sufficient space is present, amalgam does have sufficient strength to serve as an anchoring medium in the pulp chambers of molars. The pulp orifices to the canals lie well below the cervical line. When ample tooth structure remains around the pulp chamber and the buccal and lingual plates of the crown, amalgam alone can provide the necessary anchorage.

If sufficient adjoining dentin is not present and radicular anchorage is needed beyond the orifice of the canals, a dowel can be cemented in the distal root of lower molars and in the lingual root of upper molars (Figs. 19–21 and 19–22).

Contrary to what might be expected, little if any preparation is done inside the pulp chamber. Only in the orifices of the canals is the gutta percha removed to provide a clean interface between amalgam and dentin (Fig. 19–23).

With the advent of the high copper amalgam alloys, with their added strength, it is reasonable to expect that many amalgam core buildups can be shaped and carved as finished restorations (Fig. 19–24).

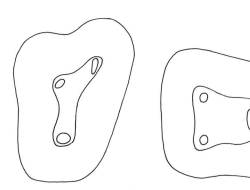

Figure 19–21. Upper (left) and lower (right) molars sectioned through the pulp chambers. Although it is possible to anchor dowels in all the canals, the large openings in the lingual root of the maxillary molar and the distal root of the mandibular make them ideal sites for dowel placement.

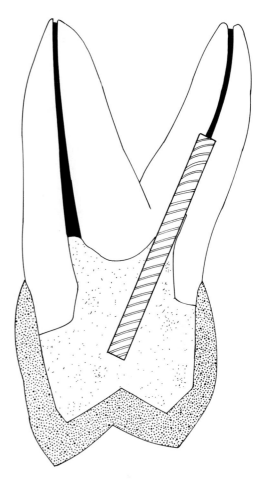

Figure 19–22. Dowel in combination with amalgam core. The same design would prevail for a mandibular molar.

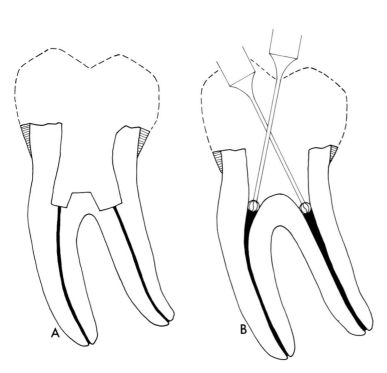

Figure 19–23. Preparation inside the pulp chamber. *A,* Internal retention. Undercuts placed around the pulp chamber may be more harmful than beneficial. *B,* Adequate support can be obtained by countersinking the orifice of the canals. (Courtesy of Dr. Douglass B. Roberts; redrawn from Masson Monographs in Dentistry)

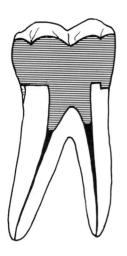
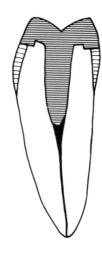

Figure 19–24. Amalgam post supporting the entire restoration (an MOD capping buccal and lingual cusps). In selected cases with sufficient buccal and lingual tooth structure, it is not necessary to place a gold crown. (Courtesy of Dr. Douglass B. Roberts; redrawn from Masson Monographs in Dentistry)

Miscellaneous Considerations

Length and Size of the Post (Dowel)

The distance that the dowel should extend into the root is arbitrarily determined by simultaneously considering many factors, e.g., the root to crown ratio, the force of the occlusion, and the adjoining supportive dentin. Fracture of the root and dislodgment of the crown are the basic considerations involved. Too short a dowel will probably result in dislodgment. Fracture is likely to occur from an accident if the walls of the root are very thin and the post length is too short (Fig. 19–25).

Common sense and judgment should prevail in the placement of all posts. The size of the post should resist tipping forces on the crown, which could cause it to bend or fracture. Although the size (diameter) is important, the length is probably the one single entity that invites most failures.

An excellent method for the preparation of a post hole is to measure the depth against the x-ray, place a rubber dam marker at the occlusal plane level, and use this mark as a guide while drilling the channel (Fig. 19–26).

The diameter of the dowel can be too small or too large. Small dowels are subject to bending; larger ones will weaken and fracture the root (Fig. 19–27).

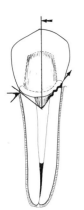
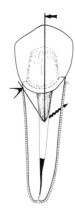
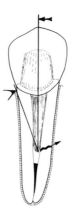
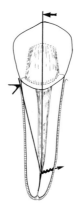

Figure 19–25. Forces applied at the cusp tip of devitalized teeth tend to use the height of periodontal attachment as a pressure fulcrum. Long post length reduces the incidence of resulting fractures. (Courtesy of Dr. Hugh Cooper Jr.)

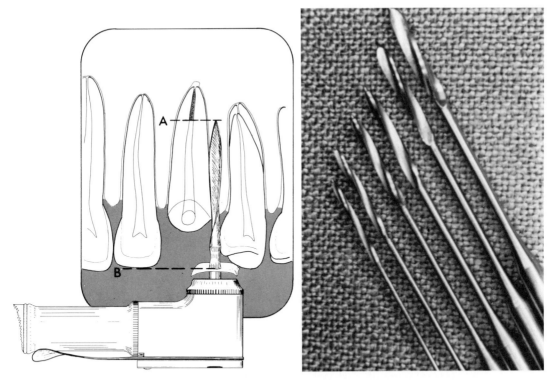

Figure 19–26. *Left,* Accurately determining post depth. A, Measuring the distance on the x-ray film and inserting a piece of rubber dam over the reamer at occlusal plane height. B, Transferring the marker to the drill site in the mouth to measure the depth. (Courtesy of Dr. Hugh Cooper Jr.) The use of a Peeso reamer is excellent for final preparation of a canal for a cast post and core. Undercuts are eliminated and a smooth internal surface is created in the channel. *Right,* Peeso reamers of varied sizes.

UNDERCUTS: HOW TO AVOID

The prefabricated post is simpler and easier to place than the cast post because the former does not require a tapered channel and one without any undercuts. In the latter, however, parallelism is vitally important, both in making a pattern and in cementing the casting. Invariably a dentist at some point in time has been distraught when fitting a cast post to discover than an irregularity in the channel has caused a warped pattern and the preparation must be refined before attempting a remake of the casting.

Figure 19–27. Potential problems with a dowel of the incorrect size. *A,* Small dowel bends or fractures; it is too flimsy. *B,* Large dowel weakens the root and subjects it to subsequent fracture. (Courtesy of Dr. Douglass B. Roberts; redrawn from Masson Monographs in Dentistry)

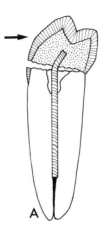
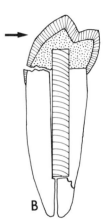

Three cardinal rules should prevail when preparing a channel for a cast post.

1. *Do not* use high-speed cutting inside the canal.

2. *Do not* use a bur with a flat end to prepare the channel (a bur with a squared end, e.g., No. 702, is acceptable for the *last* final step if one chooses to refine the terminal end with a flat seat).

3. *Do not* attempt to instrument the channel with lateral cutting until the *full* desired *depth* has been obtained with a pilot drill first.

Most teeth have relatively straight canals and most undercuts that occur are dentist induced. The procedure is basically to prepare a small hole—eliminating the gutta percha—to the full depth desired. Then select a rotating instrument for a slow-speed handpiece that has a round or pointed end and long blades (e.g., Peeso reamer, see Fig. 19–26) to shape the canal to its elliptical or triangular form (see Fig. 19–3B and C). An excellent instrument—particularly for large channels—is the multi-bladed finishing bur in a *slow-speed* handpiece (see Fig. 6–38).

The best way to eliminate undercuts is to avoid making them. Deliberate cutting with patience and care will result in a beautiful channel that will readily produce an accurate pattern and a well-fitting casting.

Impression Technique Employing a Hypodermic Needle

Impressions of post holes are often a challenge because of the difficulty of *eliminating the air bubbles in the post hole*. Naturally a good impression must reproduce the end of the post hole if it is to be satisfactory. The problem is how to eliminate the air entrapped inside the hole, because once the air is gone the rubber can flow in. The sticky nature of the rubber impression material seems to automatically seal the orifice of the hole, thereby trapping the air inside. A small passageway for the release of this entrapped air is provided by a hypodermic needle.

A 27 gauge needle is cut with a disk to approximately ½ to ¾ inch length. Clipping it off with nippers pinches the orifice and seals the lumen shut. The object is to eliminate the cutting bevel of the needle as well. It should be clearly understood that *no impression material travels through the needle; only the air inside the hole*. As the material is injected into the hole it travels freely to the end because the pressure created thereby forces the air out the lumen of the needle (Fig. 19–28). When the material fills the hole and rubber occludes the lumen of the lumen of the needle, the needle is removed and discarded.

A metal dowel that is to serve as a reinforcing agent prepainted with tray adhesive is now inserted into the hole. As the retraction cord is removed the sulcus is injected with the syringe, and the impression tray is seated in the standard manner described in Chapter 16 (Fig. 19–29).

The impression tray for the cast post and core should be *very* small. A full arch or even a large sectional tray should be avoided because its removal from the mouth should be as unrestricted as possible. In fact best results are obtained by using a simple bur box as the impression tray. With adhesive applied to its surface and with wax stops at either end, the tray can be seated and removed with accuracy and predictability (Fig. 19–30).

Along with using a small tray, a second precaution is the lubrication of the canal so the rubber impression material does not adhere to the dry dentin

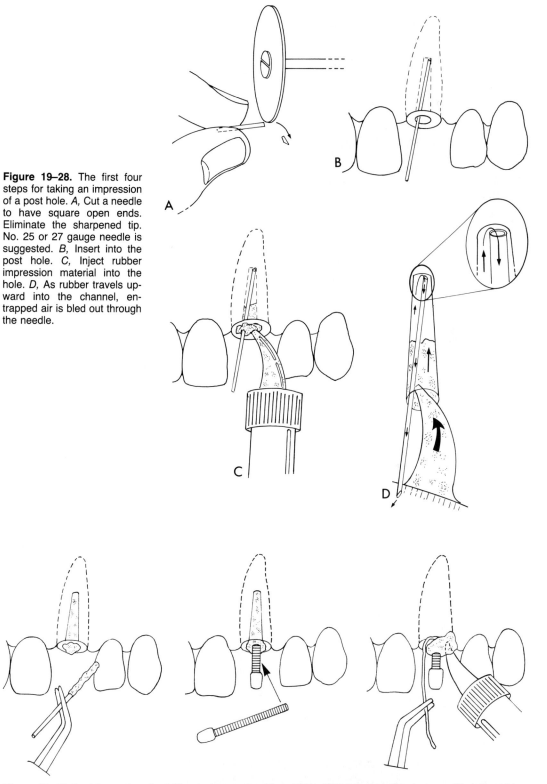

Figure 19–28. The first four steps for taking an impression of a post hole. *A,* Cut a needle to have square open ends. Eliminate the sharpened tip. No. 25 or 27 gauge needle is suggested. *B,* Insert into the post hole. *C,* Inject rubber impression material into the hole. *D,* As rubber travels upward into the channel, entrapped air is bled out through the needle.

Figure 19–29. Last three steps for taking an impression of post hole. When the hole has become filled, the rubber automatically occludes the lumen. The needle is then pulled out and discarded. A metal dowel (e.g., para post) is cut to length, painted with tray adhesive, and inserted in the hole. As the retraction cord is removed, impression material is injected in a standard manner. The impression tray naturally follows injection of the material into the sulcus.

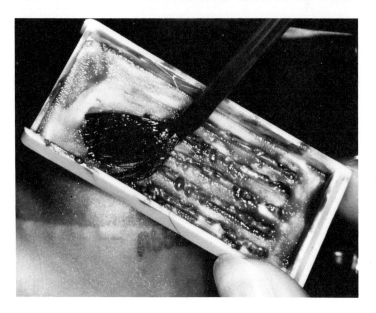

Figure 19–30. Bur box painted with tray adhesive for impression of a prepared root canal. Wax stops are placed on either end to brace the tray against the occlusal surface of the teeth.

inside it. "Microfilm" lubricant (Kerr Mfg. Co.) is a colloidal suspension of wax that is well suited for this purpose. After applying it with a cotton pellet twisted into a spindle, the excess is blown away and the impression material is injected as described above. After setting, the impression is gingerly removed while alternately spraying air and water around the edges while teasing it loose (Fig. 19–31) without stretching the rubber post.

Although the small tray does not always provide ideal orientation to proximal teeth or occlusion of opposing ones, a full arch impression in simple alginate with its model can give the technician a reasonable guestimate as to the shape and form of the wax core, a form that can readily be altered during the try-in stage of the casting.

"DIVESTMENT" FOR CAST POSTS

The Divestment technique for dental castings is described and illustrated in Chapter 17. Although this technique is excellent for casting onlays, crowns, and so on, the cast post and core is the ideal application of it.

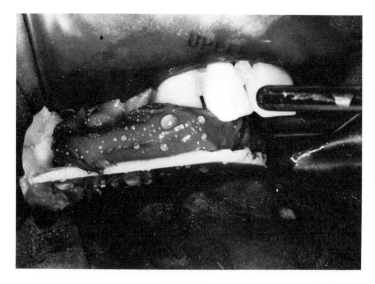

Figure 19–31. Removing the tray from the mouth. A small tray is less likely to distort the impression during removal than a large tray with flanges. Air/water spray helps release the material from the teeth so it can be removed with minimal distortion.

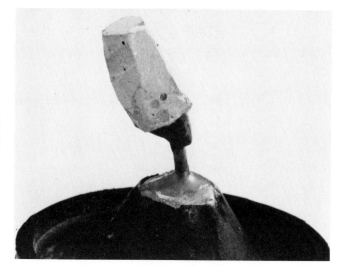

Figure 19–32. Post and core using the Divestment technique. Wax pattern sprued and ready to invest in a casting ring. The die is invested along with the pattern and will become part of the mold cavity for casting the post.

One of the reasons for the popularity of the direct pattern for fabricating a cast post and core is the apparent difficulty in obtaining an impression of the core and also the difficulty of producing a good wax pattern from the die. The Divestment technique, in conjunction with the impression technique described above, go hand in hand to provide the operator with a system that is easy, fast, and extremely accurate.

The laboratory procedure is quite simple. The impression of the post is poured in Divestment (powder and liquid), which is mixed to a rather stiff consistency. After separating the rubber impression, which must be done within the first 2 hours, the die is prepared so it will be suitable for waxing. Separator No. 2 is applied (see Fig. 17–46) and the wax is built to the desired form for the core. Because it would be burned out in the casting process no effort need be made to flow wax all the way into the depth of the hole.

The excess Divestment from the "die" is cut away, a hollow metal sprue is attached to the wax, and the pattern and die are invested together (Fig. 19–32) as described in Chapter 17. The finished casting is sandblasted and relieved in any area that might appear to restrict its seating. After adjusting the core for parallelism, occlusion, and axial alignment it is cemented into place.

The One Piece Casting (Post and Crown)

In an effort to save time and reduce the number of steps in the restorative procedure, some operators cast the post and crown in one piece, cementing the finished crown directly into the prepared root (Fig. 19–33). This is inadvisable for two reasons: (1) The one-piece assembly cannot be removed for reoperation on the tooth at a future date, whereas the two-piece assembly permits removal of the crown without disturbing the post in the canal. (2) Except in the hands of the most careful operators and technicians, the one-piece procedure is difficult to accomplish with accuracy of fit.

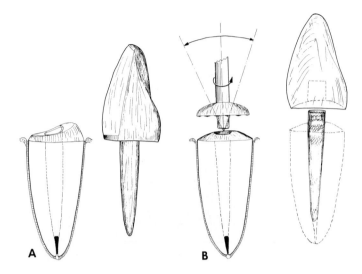

Figure 19–33. Post and clinical crowns prepared as single cemented units. Richmond Crown: *A,* Prefabricated dowel soldered or cast with an esthetic veneer crown. *B,* Prefabricated posts and ceramic crowns cemented to a prepared root stump. (Courtesy of Dr. Hugh Cooper Jr.)

Interlocking Castings

If the canals of the multi-rooted teeth, e.g., the maxillary first premolar, are parallel with each other and provide ease of pattern withdrawal, one-piece castings can be made to provide the post and core. If the roots are divergent, castings must be made that will fit the respective canals yet interlock with each other (Fig. 19–34). There are several methods for designing interlocking castings, none of which enjoy great popularity. This lack of popularity is probably due to the added effort required for fabricating castings, as well as to the technical skill required by the operator for expediting the procedure. Categorically, multi-rooted teeth do not ordinarily lend themselves well to cast posts and cores. Other methods utilizing prefabricated parts are usually preferred.

Crown Fractures

Throughout the chapter our attention has been directed to maintaining integrity by strengthening the inside of the tooth. Problems of splitting pieces off the outside of the tooth as shown in Figure 1–13 must be faced as well. A

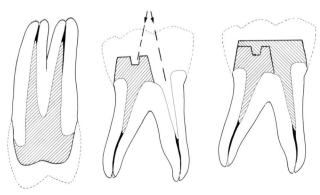

Figure 19–34. Cast post and cores for multi-rooted teeth. *A,* Parallel canals and absence of undercuts permits the use of a one-piece casting. *B,* Divergent canals require a design where two castings can interlock with each other. (Courtesy of Dr. Hugh Cooper Jr.)

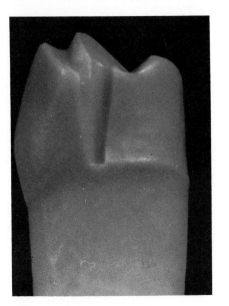

Figure 19–35. Three-quarter crown preparation to protect the lower second bicuspid against fracture. Substantial support is derived from an apron of gold covering the distal part of the buccal surface. Mesial view of preparation. (Courtesy of Dr. Judson Klooster)

complete crown of gold or ceramometal is very often chosen to bind and tie the tooth together; however, this is not necessary much of the time. Figure 19–35 illustrates a ¾ crown that effectively provides necessary support while preserving the facial surface of the enamel. MOD onlays that cover the occlusal surface are also very effective against post-endodontic splitting. The challenge at times is to design a protective casting that shows only a minimal amount of gold, e.g., the ⅞ crown for the molar and a reverse flare on the distofacial side of the premolar (Fig. 19–36).

The operator is restricted in his esthetic pursuits where the mandibular posterior teeth are concerned. Showing gold is usually acceptable to most patients where the molar teeth are concerned, but mandibular premolars, especially mandibular first premolars, are quite obvious during conversation or when one smiles. Moreover, the buccal cusp with its prominent facial slope appears as part of the occlusal surface of the lower posterior teeth.

The mandibular first premolar with its *very* prominent facial slope and its rudimentary lingual cusp is quite unique and stands apart anatomically from the other posterior teeth (Fig. 19–37). This characteristic of the first premolar where the tip of the buccal cusp lies almost in line with the long axis of the tooth affects tooth preparation in vital teeth (see Fig. 11–63) but especially in endodontically treated teeth as well. In a sense the facial cusp of this tooth serves as a pestle in the masticatory apparatus and is very seldom split away from the lingual cusp as is so often the case with the maxillary

Figure 19–36. Buccal portion of the maxillary tooth tied in with a generous distal reverse bevel (bicuspid) and a seven-eighths crown (molar).

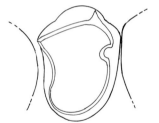
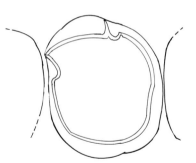

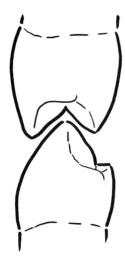

Figure 19–37. Anatomic differences between bicuspids. The maxillary tooth is much more subject to splitting than is the mandibular.

premolars. Another observation in practice is that the very tip of this cusp is seldom undermined by a deep carious lesion. Consequently the post-endodontic treatment for a mandibular first premolar as often as not does not require a crown or other type of casting reinforcement (Fig. 19–38). A simple amalgam restoration can serve the need unless of course the attrition and abrasion has substantially reduced the enamel on the cusp tip. In these cases where heavy occlusion is involved one will probably resort to placing a metal-ceramic crown instead.

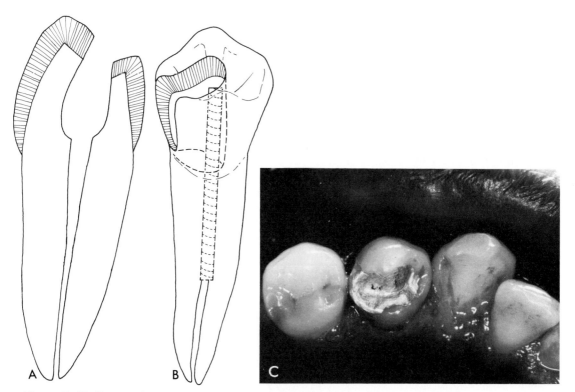

Figure 19–38. Conservative restorative treatment of a mandibular first premolar that has undergone endodontic therapy. *A,* Sectional view shows cusp tip nearly in direct line with long axis of the tooth. Caries had not involved the cusp tip. *B,* Dowel cemented in position and ready for amalgam condensation. *C,* Amalgam inserted.

Other Prefabricated Dowels and Reinforcement Units

Despite the popularity of the prefabricated units and their effort and time saving advantages, the cast post and core still remains as the standard reinforcement system by which all others are judged. In many instances either method can be used but in other cases the cast system is clearly indicated.

One such instance pertains to the realignment of a crown. Orthodontic treatment is the traditional method for repositioning teeth; however, crowning may also be employed (see Fig. 5–2). Occasionally the desired correction is so severe the pulp is exposed and its devitalization is required. The insertion of a cast post and core in its new position, a feat that would be impossible to achieve with the prefabricated system, permits gross recontouring of the crown (Fig. 19–39).

With the acquired popularity of retentive pins and composite resin, many designs of dowels and posts have emerged (Figs. 19–40, 19–41, and 19–42). Following the principles described earlier in the chapter, these can be utilized to the benefit of both patient and dentist. Experimentation in the laboratory on an extracted tooth should precede the use in the mouth of a new and unfamiliar product.

Repair of a Broken Crown

A sad commentary on the dental profession is the metal-ceramic crown that breaks off the tooth because no reinforcement was used. Although this does happen, a repair is often possible if the fracture is clean and follows within the peripheral finish line of the crown and if the fracture leaves a cleanly sheared root stump. After removal of the dentin and cement from

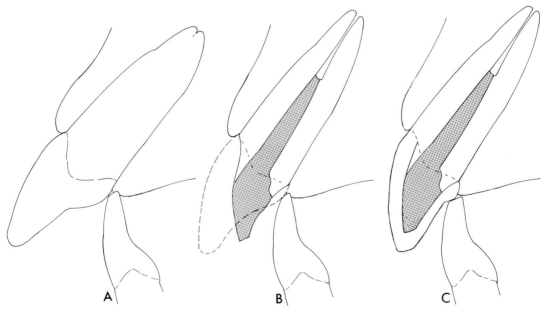

Figure 19–39. Modification of anterior crown alignment. *A,* Maxillary central incisor tipped labialward. Mandibular incisor elongated and occlusing in the lingual sulcus. *B,* Cementation of cast post and core with incisal edge angled to the lingual. *C,* Clinical crown replaced at its corrected angle. Mandibular incisors have been shortened to provide positive centric "stop." (Courtesy of Dr. Virgil M. S. Lau)

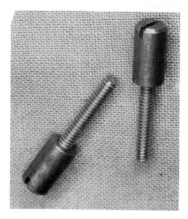

Figure 19–40. Kurer anchor post (see Fig. 2–8). A brass core is attached to a stainless steel threaded dowel. After being firmly seated and cemented into the root the brass core is shaped to provide the desired preparation for taking the impression for the crown.

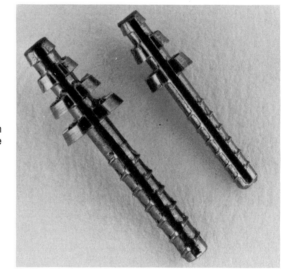

Figure 19–41. Prefabricated post to be cemented in a prepared hole in the root. The lateral fins stabilize the core material.

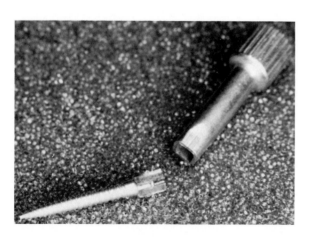

Figure 19–42. The Dentatus screw post: The screw post is fabricated from a softer metal than the parapost dowels. The wrench screwdriver method for placement is a distinct advantage.

inside the crown, it can be repositioned on its stump and can enjoy the same marginal fit that it did before the fracture.

Using several self-threading pins (3 to 5), with patience and care the crown can probably be put back into service. Dentin inside the crown is removed to make space for the pins, which are inserted into the root. By drilling and fitting only one pin at a time, each can be inserted and bent so its end projects upward into the crown without interference. Pin insertion should be delicate, without stressing the dentin lest it become weakened and fracture again later (Fig. 19–43).

Composite resin is mixed, placed into the crown, injected around the pins, and the crown seated to place. Extreme care must be exerted to be sure the crown is completely seated.

Fractured Roots

Vertical fractures are particularly devastating to a patient because they usually involve abutment teeth. In Figure 19–44 the cause for the fractured cuspid is uncertain; however, one can readily see the glass-like texture of the root dentin. It can also be observed that there is not a snug fit of the post into the prepared channel. Whether relevant or not fractured roots do occur more frequently in teeth that have had endodontic treatment than in teeth that have not.

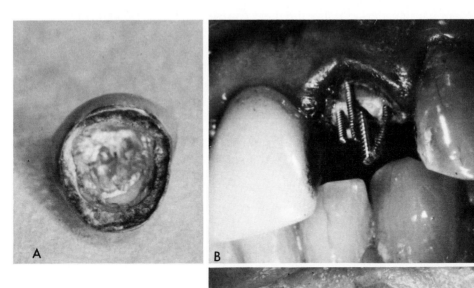

Figure 19–43. Replacement of metal-ceramic crown that was fractured from the root. Shearing of the dentin occurred at or inside the finish line of the preparation. *A,* Cement and dentin removed; crown margins are still intact. *B,* TMS pins have been inserted in the root face and bent inward. A parapost has also been inserted into the channel. *C,* Recemented with composite resin. Complete seating is essential.

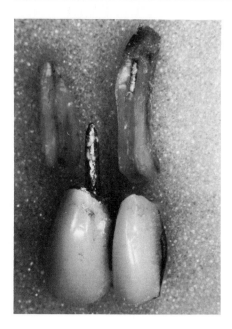

Figure 19–44. Root with a vertical fracture. (Courtesy of Dr. Michael Sponzo)

Modified Preparation: Anterior Teeth

An alternate structural component can be built into the post and core by preparing a root cleat on the lingual surface. Subsequent to the crown preparation, a tapered fissure bur is used to cut a slot approximately 2 mm deep, 2 mm long, and 1.0 mm wide (Fig. 19–45). This is reproduced in the impression and subsequently incorporated into the final casting (Figs. 19–46 and 19–47). This gold-dentin interface provides direct contact between crown and root, which is very effective against rotational and tipping forces.

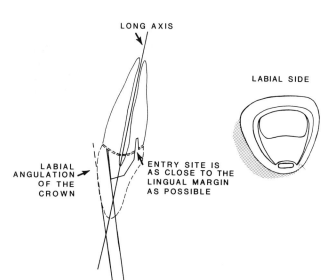

LONG AXIS

LABIAL SIDE

LABIAL ANGULATION OF THE CROWN

ENTRY SITE IS AS CLOSE TO THE LINGUAL MARGIN AS POSSIBLE

Figure 19–45. Diagram of a cingulum (lingual) cleat preparation, which permits the crown to directly engage the dentin of the root. (Courtesy of the Journal of the Conn. State Dental Assn.)

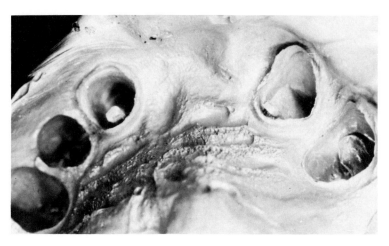

Figure 19–46. Impression of the cingulum cleats. The method described in Figures 19–28 and 19–29 may be helpful in obtaining an impression. (Courtesy of the Journal of the Conn. State Dental Assn.)

Diagnosis and Treatment Planning

The operative dentist is concerned that as many teeth as possible be saved by endodontic therapy. He should likewise be sensitive to overly heroic treatment directed toward saving teeth that should actually be removed. It is possible in many instances to save a tooth endodontically only to discover that it is not restorable.

One should have reservations about restoring maxillary first premolars, maxillary lateral incisors, and all mandibular incisors. The first premolar with its kidney-shaped root, the lateral with its small round root, as well as the mandibular incisors with their delicate ribbon-like root forms, present operational hazards that can make post and core placement most difficult. These teeth should be examined carefully, both orally and radiographically, to be sure sufficient root substance remains to permit anchorage of the post and cores. Concern for these above-mentioned teeth is especially important when metal-ceramic crowns are planned as the final restorations.

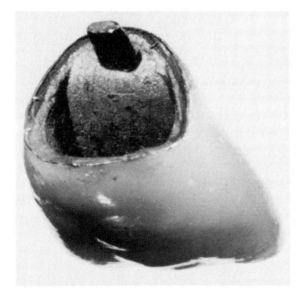

Figure 19–47. Metal-ceramic crown with cingulum cleat.

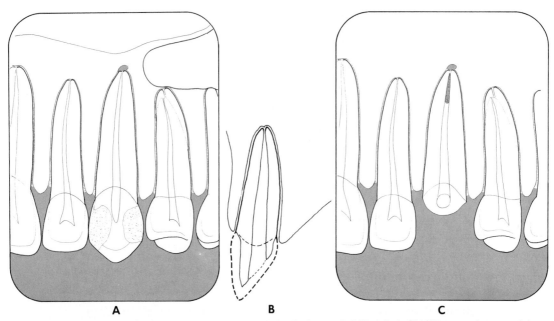

Figure 19–48. Planning operative treatment before endodontic therapy is initiated. *A,* Old fillings weaken remaining crown. *B,* After crown preparation, during which a large amount of facial tooth substance will be removed. Combined with access opening for endodontic therapy, only a few spicules of dentin will remain. Often these should be removed and a complete post and core fabricated. *C,* Completed root canal filling and crown reduction. (Courtesy of Dr. Hugh Cooper Jr.)

Along with biomechanical considerations and cost factors, patient comfort and welfare should also be considered in planning endodontic as well as restorative therapy. Endodontic therapy is expensive and in many instances extremely complicated. Only after these factors have been considered in detail should endodontic therapy begin.

As indicated earlier almost all anterior teeth that are endodontically treated require a dowel or post and core reinforcement before crown placement. To obtain optimal retention and strength, many anteriors require replacement of all coronal dentin (Fig. 19–48). The deciding factor is probably the magnitude of the stress to which the tooth will be subjected. A central or lateral serving as a bridge abutment or under marked occlusal stress should be treated with a well fitting cast post and core. On the other hand the non-splinted tooth

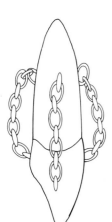

Figure 19–49. Basic concept of reinforcement of the endodontically treated tooth. The challenge is to keep the crown and root intact and attached to each other.

with evidence of only mild occlusion can be adequately handled with only a pre-formed dowel in conjunction with a pin build-up.

It is to the advantage of the patient and operator to preserve ridges and masses of coronal dentin where possible. This is more readily accomplished when using pre-formed rather than cast posts, which often necessitate removal of structural dentin in order to eliminate undercuts that can prevent withdrawal and insertion of a wax pattern and casting.

Resumé of Reinforcement Systems

Single-rooted teeth with only one canal can be best restored with a cast post and core. With both the post and the core customized into one piece, optimal support is provided to the system. When another substance is adapted around a post where it hardens to become a core, the anchorage and fixation is naturally compromised.

Cast posts and cores therefore should be given serious consideration for:

1. single-rooted teeth under stress, e.g., bridge abutments or supports for partial denture clasps.

2. teeth that may require the removal of the crown several years hence. In removing a crown over a resin core the composite would likely be pulverized in the process.

3. teeth for which crowns are to be realigned.

4. interlocking castings for teeth with divergent roots.

Pre-fabricated posts with amalgam cores would be used for:

1. all molars under heavy stress.

2. maxillary first bicuspids with divergent roots. Final restoration will be partial coverage, e.g., three-quarters crown.

3. most other teeth under moderate stress (may or may not be abutment teeth).

Pre-fabricated posts with composite cores would be used for:

1. multi-rooted teeth under moderate stress, especially where walls of dentin still provide substantial support.

2. single-rooted teeth under moderate stress, with at least one strong wall of dentin present.

3. single-rooted teeth under minimal stress, in which no coronal dentin remains; also included would be threaded pins anchored into the root.

Regardless of treatment chosen (dowel, composite, amalgam, or cast post and core), structural integrity is the vital element of concern and should never be sacrificed (Fig. 19–49). The endodontist saves the root; the operative dentist restores the crown. If a restoration failure occurs, perhaps because the endodontist removed too much dentin inside the canal, the blame will fall on the shoulders of the operative dentist.

In summary, it is the clinical judgment of the operative dentist that determines whether endodontic therapy should take place and what type of restoration should be used for the best interests of the patient.

20

THE METAL–CERAMIC RESTORATION

For years, the porcelain jacket crown was the restoration used for anterior esthetic problems. It was made by placing ceramic powder on a platinum matrix, arranging its contours, and then by careful control of time and temperature fusing it in an oven designed for dental ceramics.

The quality of esthetic results was governed by the talents of the dentist and his ceramist. The final appearance of the jacket could also be manipulated by the color of the cement. The problem with this restoration was its weakness when subjected to tensile forces, as it was brittle and would fracture easily when subjected to the stresses of mastication.

Alumina is now being used to replace the quartz portion of the porcelain and is known as aluminous porcelain. This material has higher strength and greater resistance to fracture when compared with a quartz porcelain. With this improved porcelain the jacket crown is a very good restoration in selected cases.

The natural weakness of the porcelain jacket has largely been reduced during recent years by using ceramics as a veneer on a metal casting. This allows both strength and esthetics to be combined in the same restoration (Fig. 20–1).

As an added consideration the porcelain inlay is a good esthetic option for treating some of the cervical lesions of premolar and anterior teeth.

By necessity the following discussion will be limited in scope, and the reader is referred to a crown and bridge text for an in-depth treatment of the subject.

Physical Properties

Metal–Ceramic Bond

The process of combining dental ceramics and metal is similar to the process for applying an enamel or ceramic surface to bathtubs or cooking utensils, which is a very old technique. Such a restoration is referred to as a metal–ceramic or porcelain-fused-to-metal restoration. Both the metal and the ceramic must have coefficients of thermal expansion that are closely matched during and after cooling to inhibit undesirable tensile stresses at the interface. The metal must be rigid to prevent ceramic crazing or fracture. Obviously the tenacity of the metal–ceramic bond is critical to the durability of the restoration.

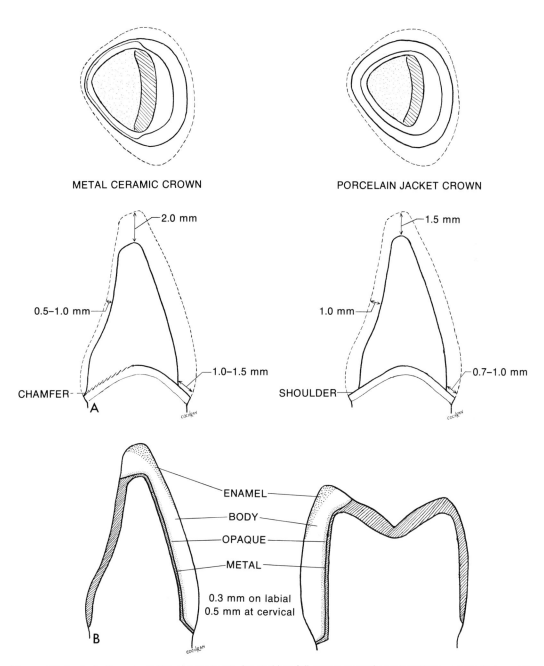

METAL CERAMIC CROWN

PORCELAIN JACKET CROWN

2.0 mm

1.5 mm

0.5–1.0 mm

1.0 mm

1.0–1.5 mm

0.7–1.0 mm

CHAMFER

SHOULDER

A

ENAMEL

BODY

OPAQUE

METAL

0.3 mm on labial
0.5 mm at cervical

B

Figure 20–1. *A,* A diagram of the requirements for making full-crown ceramic preparations, contrasting metal–ceramic with porcelain jacket preparations. *B,* A schematic portrayal of the metal and porcelain combination for a metal-ceramic restoration.

The main constituent of the noble metal alloys used in metal–ceramic techniques is gold. Platinum and palladium are added to raise the melting temperatures, to reduce the coefficient of thermal expansion, and to strengthen the alloys. Small proportions of base metals—e.g., indium, zinc, and tin—are included to produce a surface oxide film needed in the bonding process.

The melting temperature of these alloys is greater than 1093°C (2000°F). The melting (solidus) temperature of such alloys must exceed the maturing temperature of the ceramic enamel or the temperature required to condition the metal prior to the placement of porcelain.

The bond between the noble metal alloys and the dental porcelain can be divided into three main components: mechanical, compressive, and chemical. Mechanical retention is dependent upon good wetting of the metal or metal oxide surface by the porcelain. A form of mechanical interlocking takes place by penetration of the porcelain within the roughness of the casting surface. Compressive stresses are set up during the curing of the porcelain veneers. Metal–ceramic systems are deliberately designed with a very small degree of thermal mismatch in order to leave the porcelain in a state of compression. This plays a part in improving the strength of the metal–ceramic bond. There is strong evidence that there is also a form of chemical bonding involving the migration of indium or tin to the alloy surface to form an oxide that combines with the porcelain during its firing.

Base metal alloys are also available for metal–ceramic restorations. These alloys have been introduced principally to reduce the cost and increase the modulus of elasticity, as compared with the precious metal alloys. Although a number of formulations have been marketed, they are generally chromium–nickel alloys, which may also contain beryllium or molybdenum. At least one such formulation contains palladium.

The physical properties of these silver-colored base metal alloys are comparable or superior to those of the gold alloys used for this purpose. For example, the modulus of elasticity of certain products is twice that of the precious metal alloys. However, they are somewhat inferior in handling characteristics. For example, it is considerably more difficult to secure well-fitting castings from these alloys, i.e., they are more technique sensitive.

At this time the market price of noble metals, especially gold, fluctuates very easily and at a level that is disagreeable to all. The use of noble metal alloys is currently encouraged in spite of the elevated cost. The difficulty in fabricating and handling base metal alloys tends to equalize the cost factors when deciding whether to use base or noble metals. The discussion to follow relates to basic fundamentals regardless of the alloy used. One biological consideration should be made. A small proportion of the population is allergic to nickel. Thus the use of nickel-containing alloys is contraindicated for patients who have a known nickel allergy.

Color

While it is possible to make a functional metal–ceramic restoration, its esthetic value will largely depend on the accuracy of color interpretation. Unfortunately there are indications suggesting that many dentists' greatest concern with color is in interior decorating. They are careful in selecting colors for equipment, waiting room, and wall decor; but the selection of color for restorations is left to chance or to a distant ceramist, with the hope of getting a color match close enough to satisfy the patient. This lack of concern is indicated by prescriptions to the ceramist that give a shade selection and then tell the ceramist to make it a "little lighter" or "darker" than the selection offered. The problem of shade selection is perpetuated because most dentists have little background for dealing accurately with color, as the subject is rarely included in the undergraduate curriculum.

The subject of color can be given exhaustive consideration, as there are many considerations that will improve the quality of the final restoration. However, initially it is important that the dentist have some understanding of the terms hue, saturation, and value, and it would also be of value to understand the color wheel.

HUE. Hue refers to the actual name of a color, and it allows us to distinguish one color from another. Color discrimination occurs because each hue transmits energy in the form of varied but well-defined wavelengths that are received by the observer. In the case of the dentist, these wavelengths must be interpreted and reproduced in an esthetic restoration.

SATURATION. Saturation is the quality that allows us to distinguish weak colors from strong and refers to the intensity of the color. This quality is illustrated by placing drops of food coloring in a glass of water. The first drop mildly colors the water, but as drops are added the saturation of the color increases, although the hue has not changed. In a tooth the saturation of the color may be high at the gingival margin but noticeably reduced toward the incisal edge.

VALUE. The value of a color allows us to distinguish light colors from dark. Value refers to the brightness of a color and is influenced by the amount of white or gray contained within the color. In the mouth this quality determines the vital appearance of the teeth. Hue and saturation may vary from tooth to tooth, but value will not, which makes the teeth appear as a matched set. If the value in a single tooth restoration is higher than in the natural teeth, the restored tooth will not appear realistic; if the value is lower, the restored tooth will appear devitalized. The value of a ceramic restoration may be decreased, or darkened, by making additions; but if the value is too low, it is almost impossible to adjust it (increase the value) so as to make it lighter.

Pretreatment Diagnosis

Before preparations are attempted the patient must be informed of the expected results. If alignment irregularities are to be modified, it may be advisable to use a study model, adding wax or reducing the stone to demonstrate the anticipated result to the patient. Always make sure to retain a study model depicting the situation as first presented. If there are obvious problems of which the patient should be aware, inform the patient at the outset of treatment, rather than try to explain the problem after treatment is under way.

If the patient is a teenage person, the degree of success with a metal–ceramic crown is marginal. The pulpal anatomy may be very large as compared with the tooth, which makes it difficult to properly prepare the tooth and maintain the viability of the pulp. The level of the gingival tissue is not stabilized at that age, and later changes will frequently expose the tooth–restoration junction after the restoration has been placed. This detracts from the esthetics. If possible, it is best to use a long-range temporary until the pulp and tissue levels are predictable. If that treatment plan is not feasible, the patient and parent should know that the tissue level and color pattern may shift within a few years, making a new restoration a strong possibility.

Some teeth, such as lower incisors and upper lateral incisors, are so thin that a proper preparation may be impossible and this leads to an overcontoured restoration or to one with a mismatched color. With the exception of concerns such as these, the metal–ceramic restoration has wide acceptance and versatility.

Armamentarium
1. All available ceramic shade guides
2. Diamonds for high speed—bullet nose, flame, wheel, and football shapes
3. Burs, No. 256 or 1170L
4. 10-4-8 or 8-4-10 hand instrument
5. Large spoon excavator
6. Sandpaper disks
7. Refer to Chapter 16 for impression techniques

Procedure

Shade Selection

The ease and accuracy of shade selection is easily influenced by the conditions and the environment in which the selection is made, and when possible these factors should be controlled so selection will occur in as consistent a manner as possible. The color perceptions of the operator are subject to change if the environment of selection varies a great deal.

The best dental operatory for shade selection is one with natural lighting and neutral colors on the walls. If walls are dark or heavily colored, they may

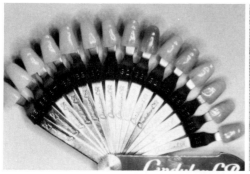
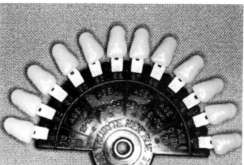
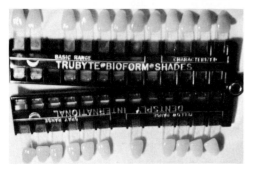

Figure 20–2. For accurate selection of shade it is necessary to have several porcelain guides.

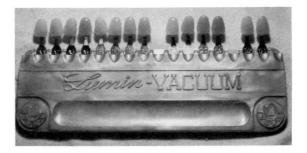

Figure 20–3. The shade tabs are more reliable if the cervical porcelain is removed.

influence color perception when the operator looks away from the subject. It is proper to consider the problems of shade selection when decorating the office; however, this does not mean that the walls should be drab and uninteresting.

Lighting conditions are important to successful shade selection. The best lighting is natural light from a northern exposure; it is the most diffuse and combines all the possible wavelengths in a natural manner. This is not universally practical, as in many situations the office arrangement or the time of day or weather may preclude the use of natural light. The most consistent results are obtained if shade selection is made under a color-corrected light source closely approximating natural light.*

Use a towel to cover bright clothing and provide a neutral background. For the same reason have the patient remove colored lipstick. Do not attempt a selection following isolation of teeth by a rubber dam or cotton rolls, for there is a definite color shift when teeth are dry and the original color does not return immediately after the teeth become wet.

Try to secure all available ceramic shade guides, as a greater assortment gives more versatility to the selection process (Fig. 20–2). None of the available guides accurately reflects the total spectrum of selection. Do not use a resin shade guide for ceramics, as light refracts differently from plastic as compared with porcelain. The preferred guide is one that is balanced to the porcelain system anticipated for use in the restoration. This may require searching for a ceramist who uses the porcelain desired. To do otherwise means that the ceramist must interpolate between systems, and the results are seldom as good as they should be.

It is advisable to cut the necks of the tabs, leaving intact the labial surface, which is the working surface. The highly colored neck is a distraction (Fig. 20–3).

MECHANICS OF SELECTION

The patient should be seated in an upright position, which duplicates the position from which the patient's teeth will be seen most frequently. Actually the selection can be made when the patient is first seen if a ceramic restoration is a strong possibility as the restorative procedure. Selection can then be verified prior to doing the preparation.

Have the patient's teeth and the shade tab moistened frequently during the process of shade selection. Be seated at eye level with the patient and at an arm's length so as to accurately view the shade tab when placed. The shade tabs should not be run by the patient as if they were keys on a piano. Try first

*Verd-A-Ray Corp., 615 Front St., Toledo, Ohio 43605.

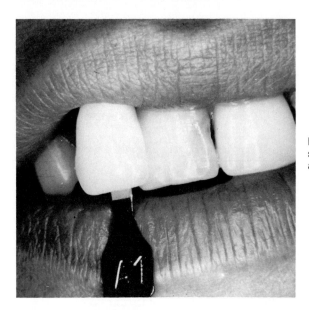

Figure 20–4. For observation and selection, the shade tab is placed adjacent to the tooth used for a model.

to determine the dominant color without looking for a specific tab. Decide if the basic color is yellow, gray, brown, or red in relation to sections of the guide. If this can be determined, then all that remains is to match the saturation and the value from among the related tabs. Otherwise selection becomes a process of elimination until the right tab is found.

To evaluate the tab, glance momentarily at the porcelain and tooth, for the first impressions are the most accurate (Fig. 20–4). Do not stare continuously at the tab, for color fatigue sets in quickly, causing an inaccurate result. In some cases selection will be difficult and the time required for shade selection may be the same as that needed for the preparation. It may be necessary to divide the tooth into sections and match each section to a shade tab (Fig. 20–5). Sometimes the selection is done with just a portion of a shade tab.

When possible the selection should be verified in lighting conditions similar to those of the living or working conditions in which the patient spends most of his time. As an aid to selection it is desirable to have the assistant verify or question a selection from several feet away.

Patients should not participate in the shade selection, as they are not able to objectively discriminate among the subtle differences. For the patient who

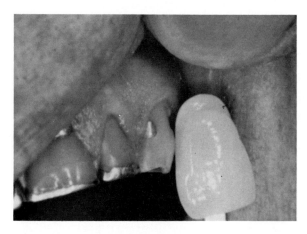

Figure 20–5. Frequently it is an advantage to make shade selections for specific segments of a tooth.

is very curious the process may be casually reviewed with the aid of a hand mirror after it has been completed.

Color blindness of varying degrees is a problem in nearly 10 per cent of the male population. It is advisable for male dentists to learn the accuracy of their vision. Those with incomplete color vision should train the dental assistant to take an active part in shade selection.

A Polaroid picture of the teeth to be matched is a helpful aid for the ceramist. This does not help with actual shade selection, but it provides good clues for the blending of color and for surface characterization and morphology.

Preparation for the Metal–Ceramic Crown

The preparation must permit proper stability and function of the casting and must also permit good esthetics by the ceramist. The preparation requires extensive removal of tooth tissue, and the precautions required during this preparation have been discussed in Chapter 4.

A predetermined plan for making this preparation is of greater importance than with conventional cast preparations, as surface reference guides will be needed to develop proper tooth reduction.

Incisal Reduction. The length of the incisal edge of anterior teeth should be reduced by 2.0 mm, as this provides the ceramist with space to reproduce ceramic incisal that appears natural. If the tooth is longer than usual, and the location of the pulp is no problem, it may be reduced in excess of 2.0 mm, which simplifies making the restoration.

An initial cut is made from labial to lingual with a bullet nose or wheel diamond through the incisal edge at a depth of 2.0 mm (Figs. 20–6 and 20–7). With this as a guide the entire incisal edge is reduced to that level. For an upper anterior tooth this reduction is given an angulation slightly facing the lingual. If the incisal reduction is done without guide cuts, mistakes in reduction may occur, as it is difficult to gauge accurately the amount of reduction as it occurs.

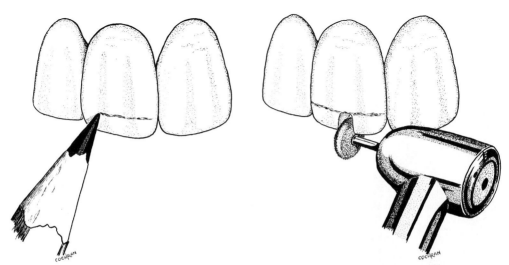

Figure 20–6. The amount of incisal reduction is predetermined by placing a line and a specific cut in the incisal edge.

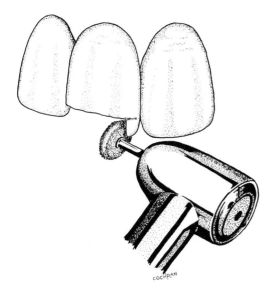

Figure 20–7. After the incisal depth is located, the entire incisal is prepared.

Labial Reduction. It is advisable to use a bullet nose diamond to make a guide cut in the middle of the labial surface to a depth needed for the completed preparation (Fig. 20–8). This cut is initiated by placing the end of the diamond near the gingival border. The depth is determined by knowing the diameter of the diamond. Because of incisal curvature it is best to do this in two stages: first cut the gingival half and then adjust the cutting instrument to accommodate the incisal half, as the labial guide cut must accurately reflect the depth of the preparation from gingival to incisal.

The basic reduction required is 1.5 mm, which will allow a metal base to be covered with opaque porcelain, leaving approximately 1.0 mm for dentin and enamel porcelain, which is required as a minimum for esthetic needs. If the preparation does not provide adequate room, the ceramist will overcontour the restoration, which may lead to esthetic and soft tissue problems.

With the same diamond reduce the labial surface and follow the guide cuts (Fig. 20–9). At this time the gingival reduction should end just where the gingival tissue contacts the tooth. Again be sure the reduction follows the

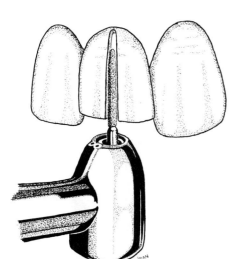

Figure 20–8. To initiate facial reduction, a depth-guide cut is placed in the facial surface.

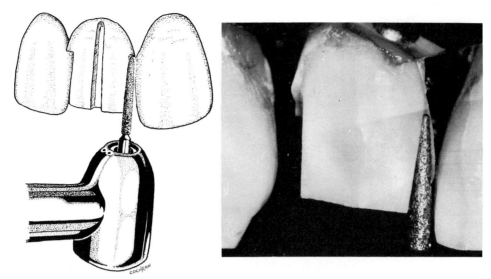

Figure 20–9. The diamond selected must provide good proximal inclination to the preparation and avoid damage to the adjacent tooth. (Photograph courtesy of Dr. Ted Hunley)

general contour of the labial surface, for when the labial incisal does not have the proper reduction the restoration will be overcontoured. This reduction follows the surface into the interproximal area and should extend one-half the distance through the normal contact.

Interproximal Reduction. The diamond is now exchanged for one that is flame-shaped and thinner. This allows the preparation to continue from the labial through contact to the lingual embrasure. The thin diamond helps prevent overcutting the inclination of the interproximal wall and also avoids cutting the adjacent tooth.

The proximal walls will converge slightly toward the incisal to provide a path of insertion for the restoration and also to create good resistance form, as required for all complete crowns (Fig. 20–10). The interproximal reduction will also provide ceramic translucency at the incisal angles. The gingival margin will most frequently end in the gingival crevice.

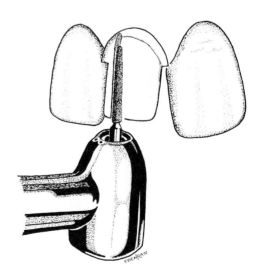

Figure 20–10. The facial surface is reduced to the level of the guide cut, observing the facial contours of the tooth.

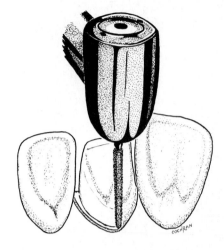

Figure 20–11. The lingual margin is designed as a chamfer.

Lingual Reduction. The same diamond may be used to prepare the entire lingual margin and most frequently it will end in the gingival sulcus under the height of the free gingiva. The magnitude of reduction is the same as for a conventional three-quarter crown that might be placed on the tooth (Fig. 20–11). The requirement is that the metal have enough thickness to prevent flexing under stress.

The actual lingual reduction is done with a wheel- or football-shaped diamond (Fig. 20–12). This reduction is for the purposes of providing proper thickness of metal and preserving part of the lingual shape to support the restoration. Try to maintain the cingulum morphology if at all possible.

The part of the tooth that is in function should have a minimum of 1.0 mm reduction, while in areas where function is not anticipated the reduction may be at a minimum of 0.5 mm. The football-shaped diamond has the advantage that it does not leave a grooved appearance to the preparation, as may occur with a small wheel diamond.

Labial Shoulder and Finish. The major remaining feature of the instrumentation is to place the labial shoulder in its final location and finish the preparation. The principal reason the margin of the restoration must be under the gingival tissue is that of esthetics, for the tooth–restoration junction is

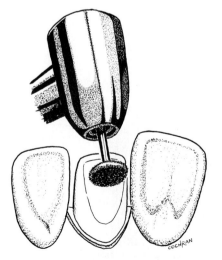

Figure 20–12. The lingual is reduced so as to provide a concavity to the lingual surface.

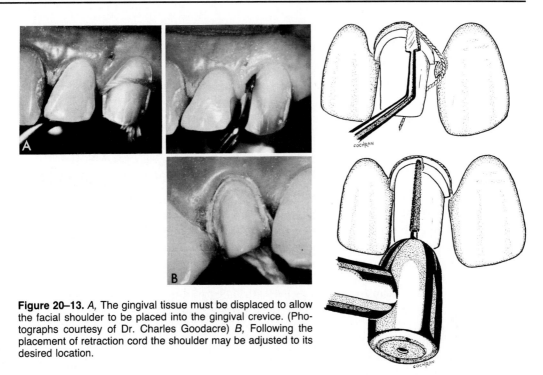

Figure 20–13. *A,* The gingival tissue must be displaced to allow the facial shoulder to be placed into the gingival crevice. (Photographs courtesy of Dr. Charles Goodacre) *B,* Following the placement of retraction cord the shoulder may be adjusted to its desired location.

distracting. Another reason is the occasional need for additional length of preparation to provide needed resistance form.

It is expected that the finished restoration will have a labial margin of 1.0 mm to 1.5 mm within a healthy gingival sulcus. Burs can be effectively used to depress the labial shoulder, and among those burs that may be used are Nos. 56, 256, 170L, and 1171L or diamonds. They have a diameter of approximately 1.0 mm that can be used to provide a gingival width of 1.5 mm. While the shoulder is being prepared the gingival tissue must be fully protected to prevent damage (Fig. 20–13). If the tissue is mechanically lacerated, it creates problems for the impression. In addition it may cause gingival recession upon healing, which exposes the margins and results in poor esthetics.

Figure 20–14. A flat metal instrument may be used to reflect gingival tissue while the shoulder location is being completed.

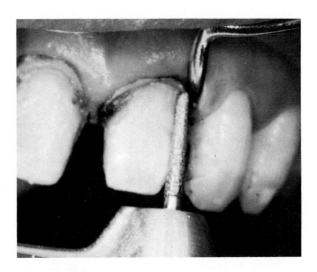

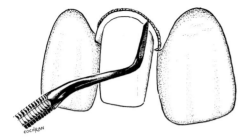

Figure 20–15. Hand instruments are used to provide the final finish to the gingival shoulder.

The gingival tissue may be protected by having an assistant place a flat plastic instrument into the sulcus and locally reflect the gingival tissue from the margin (Fig. 20–14). The bur and the metal blade follow each other around the margin as the shoulder is being positioned. This instrument rapidly becomes badly scarred and is of no value for any other purpose. Another method that helps is to place retraction cord into the sulcus, which moves the tissue away from the tooth while the shoulder is being prepared. The time available to complete the task with this method is very limited after the cord is removed.

The labial shoulder should follow carefully the gingival contour from the labial into the interproximal. A mistake may occur as the shoulder moves from the labial toward the proximal contact in that the shoulder tends to drop gingivally and endanger the attachment of the interproximal tissue. This causes tissue damage and difficulty in securing an accurate impression.

The shoulder is finished with hand instruments in order to leave a smooth surface, and a mon-angle chisel (10-4-8 or 8-4-10) is used for this purpose (Fig. 20–15). The walls of the preparation may be smoothed by using burs such as Midwest No. 7664 or sandpaper disks (Fig. 20–16; see also Fig. 6–31).

Avoid leaving sharp angles on the preparation, for seating of the restoration is simplified when the incisal and interproximal corners are rounded (Fig. 20–17).

Impression

The procedure for making the impression has been described in Chapter 16.

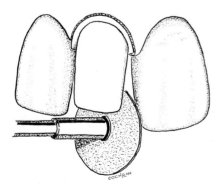

Figure 20–16. Paper disks are useful to make the surface of the preparation smooth.

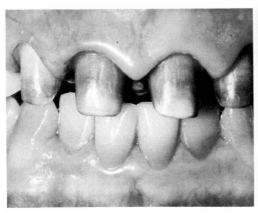
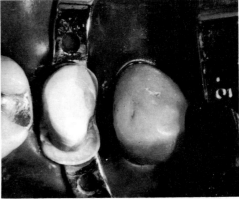

Figure 20–17. Completed preparations for metal-ceramic crowns. (Courtesy of Drs. Charles Goodacre and Michael Hanst)

Temporary Restoration

The temporary restoration is made of acrylic by the method described in Chapter 16. There is one additional precaution: the color of the temporary should not be as good a color match as would be expected of the permanent restoration (Fig. 20–18). It is a little hard to explain to the patient why the temporary was a better match than the final restoration. However, the margins and contour of the temporary must be accurately adapted to provide good gingival protection.

Prescription to the Ceramist

The dentist must approve the models and die that will be used to make the restoration. The stone should be trimmed from the margins so that they are fully exposed. The technicians should not be required to guess at the location of the margins; the dentist should survey them with a pencil (Fig. 20–19).

The study models should be sent to the ceramist, since they are a good source of information. They may be modified by the addition of wax or carved to provide a morphology guide. The dentist should always retain original study models as part of the patient's permanent record (Fig. 20–20).

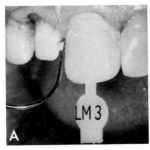
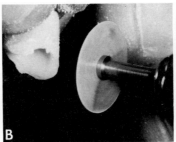
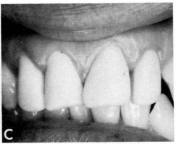

Figure 20–18. *A,* A crown form plus acrylic is placed on the preparation to form the temporary. *B,* Upon removal the temporary is adjusted for margins and contour. *C,* The acrylic temporary crowns must be smooth and with good margins.

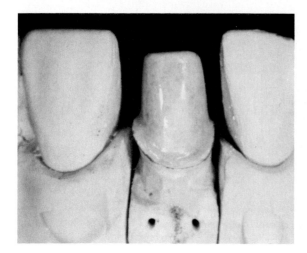

Figure 20–19. The dies should be carefully trimmed and surveyed with a pencil line.

It is the responsibility of the dentist to provide a prescription to the ceramist with as much reliable information as possible. The written prescription should include all the details noted during the shade selection process. Frequently this requires a detailed diagram to picture the variations in the color patterns. This is also required for depicting stain and check lines or the location of areas of decalcification (Fig. 20–21).

Give as much guidance for contour and characterization as possible. In some instances it will be necessary to state that the contact should be left open or closed. It is preferred to have centric closure occur on metal, but there also are times when this is not feasible and the ceramist should be advised.

Allow a reasonable amount of time for completion of the restoration, as the ceramist will provide better and more consistent results if given adequate time.

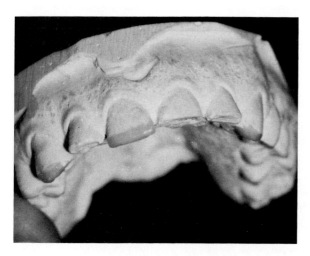

Figure 20–20. A study model that has been altered as a guide for a ceramist.

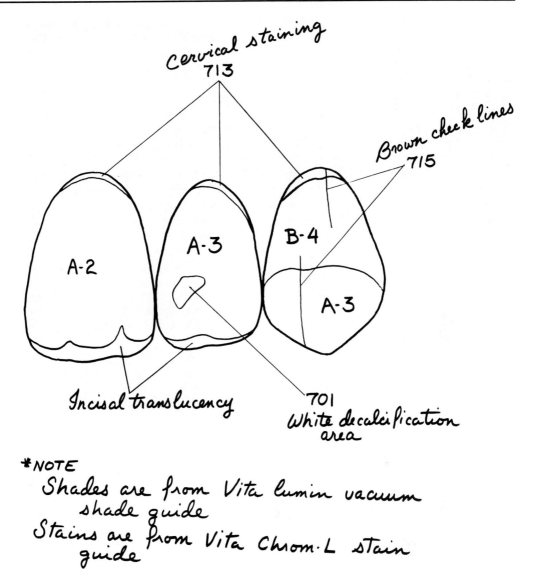

Figure 20–21. An example of a diagram to be sent to the ceramist to help with staining and facial surface variations.

Try-in of Restoration

When the restoration is completed it is seated in the same manner as a casting. The margins as well as proximal and occlusal contacts must bear the same scrutiny for acceptance. Some adjustments may be required in the proximal and lingual porcelain, using fine abrasive wheels. If the area is small, these spots may be polished with porcelain polishing wheels or commercial polishing materials* (see Fig. 3–25). Otherwise they should be reglazed.

During the time of try-in color accuracy is determined. For satisfactory esthetics, the restored tooth must appear as if it belongs with the other teeth. Examine the surface contour carefully. It may be necessary to make some modifications either in its major contour or in some of the surface irregularities.

---

*Dental Ventures of America, P.O. Box 2164, Yorba Linda, California 92686.

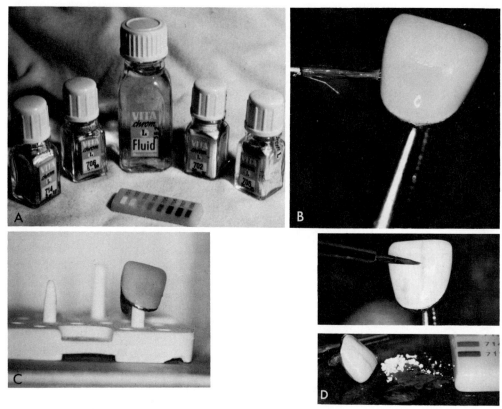

Figure 20–22. *A,* Part of a stain kit used to modify the color of porcelain.* *B,* The staining powder and liquid are mixed to a thick consistency and applied to the ceramic surface with a brush. *C,* Following application of stain it is fired in a porcelain furnace at the prescribed temperature. *D,* In a similar but more precise manner a selected stain is applied to the ceramic surface for the purpose of characterization.

*Unitek Corp., Monrovia, California 91016.

A crown that has correct contouring and that obviously blends with the other teeth can tolerate a small degree of color mismatch and yet appear natural.

If the color is a mismatch and the crown is on the light side, the hue and value can frequently be altered by staining and reglazing. Staining is not difficult but best results occur when staining is accomplished internally during the porcelain build-up. It can be done on a trial and error basis, although those who understand color will achieve results more quickly. For example, adding gray stain to a hue will reduce its value and its degree of saturation. If the distracting hue can be identified, it can be partially neutralized by using its complement; for example, violet may be added to a yellow hue. Some alloys have had an increase in silver content, which tends to provide a greenish cast; this may be neutralized by using pink (Fig. 20–22).

Characterization can easily be done at this time, and the esthetic results justify the additional effort. Those who are particularly interested in this field will have in their office an oven capable of glazing.

If the color is dark, it is likely that a new application of porcelain will be needed. Check the restoration with the shades requested to see if they match, and if they do, it means reselecting the shade.

If there is a problem with the restoration, do not blame the technician in the presence of the patient, for all too often the basis for the difficulty lies

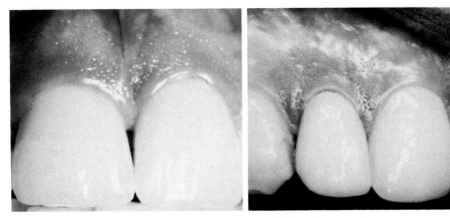

Figure 20–23. Examples of metal-ceramic restorations.

with the dentist. Even if the fault lies with the technician, the patient trusts the judgment of the dentist to choose good technical support.

When this restoration is completed, both patient and dentist should feel satisfied because of the function and the esthetics it provides (Fig. 20–23). Cementation is done in the manner discussed in Chapter 18.

Resumé of Metal–Ceramic Restoration
1. Pretreatment diagnosis
2. Select the shade required
3. Preparation for metal–ceramic crown
   a. Incisal reduction of 2 mm
   b. Labial reduction to provide 1.5 mm for casting and porcelain
   c. Interproximal reduction
   d. Lingual reduction of 1.0 mm where occlusal function occurs
   e. Retain cingulum and prepare lingual margin as for three-quarter crown
   f. Labial shoulder is placed into the gingival sulcus for at least 1.0 mm
   g. Protection of gingival tissue
   h. Do not leave sharp corners or wall junctions
4. Impression and temporary
5. Directions given to the ceramist
6. Try-in of restoration with alteration by staining and contouring if needed
7. Cementation of restoration

INDEX

Note: Page numbers in *italic* indicate figures, page numbers followed by (t) refer to tables.